CONGRATULATIONS

D0549333

You now have **FREE** Internet Access to *Mosby's Drug Consult* for 6 months!

2 2 MAY 2022   WITHDRAWN

Register at:

http://www.mosbysdrugconsult.com

2006

Mosby's Drug Consult™

www.mosbysdrugconsult.com

The trusted drug information found on MDConsult

CD-ROM INCLUDED

HERBAL SECTION INSIDE

MOSBY ELSEVIER

Here's what's included on *Mosby's Drug Consult* electronic products:

An incomparable combination...

- Accurate and unbiased coverage
- *Drug Master Plus* drug interaction tool with more than 5000 interactions
- Customizable, printable patient teaching drug information handouts available in English and Spanish
- Links to Key Suppliers
- New Drug Indications
- New Drug Approvals
- Safety Notices

PLUS — Hard-to-Find Facts and Figures...

- Required Child and Adult Immunizations
- Pregnancy Categories
- FDA Drug Class
- DEA Controlled Substances Schedules
- Comparative Tables
- NDC Numbers
- CDC Dosage Recommendations
- List of Oral Solid Dosage Forms Not To Be Crushed
- FDA Approval Date
- Cost of Therapy
- Top-Selling Drugs

...and much more!

GLAPTQDGADKG

Free *Mosby's Drug Consult* access on the Internet with this passcode!

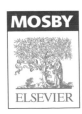

MOSBY

ELSEVIER

evolve

•• *To access you*

http://evolve ... macology

Evolve® Student ... *ogy for Physical Therapists* offers th...

Student Reso...

- **WebLinks**
  An exciting re... tes carefully chosen to sup...

- **Activities**
  Activities and ... dies in each chapter

- **Answers**
  Answers and ...

- **Mosby's Ele...** macology
  Illustrate and ...

- **Sample Exar...**
  More than 50 ... e learned

- **Drug Update Column**
  Provides up-to-date information on the latest drugs

- **New Articles of Interest**
  Will list the most current resources available for drug-related information

...volve.elsevier.com/Gladson/Pharmacology

PHARMACOLOGY
for PHYSICAL THERAPISTS

PHARMACOLOGY
for PHYSICAL THERAPISTS

Barbara Gladson, PhD, PT, OTR

Graduate Program in Physical Therapy

University of Medicine and Dentistry of New Jersey

Newark, New Jersey

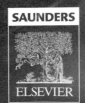

SAUNDERS

ELSEVIER

SAUNDERS
ELSEVIER

11830 Westline Industrial Drive
St. Louis, Missouri 63146

PHARMACOLOGY FOR PHYSICAL THERAPISTS
Copyright © 2006 Elsevier Inc.

ISBN 13: 978-0-7216-0929-4
ISBN 10: 0-7216-0929-5

Notice

Knowledge and best practice in this field are constantly changing. As new research and experience broaden our knowledge, changes in practice, treatment and drug therapy may become necessary or appropriate. Readers are advised to check the most current information provided (i) on procedures featured or (ii) by the manufacturer of each product to be administered, to verify the recommended dose or formula, the method and duration of administration, and contraindications. It is the responsibility of the practitioner, relying on their own experience and knowledge of the patient, to make diagnoses, to determine dosages and the best treatment for each individual patient, and to take all appropriate safety precautions. To the fullest extent of the law, neither the Publisher nor the Author assumes any liability for any injury and/or damage to persons or property arising out or related to any use of the material contained in this book.

The Publisher

ISBN 13: 978-0-7216-0929-4
ISBN 10: 0-7216-0929-5

Acquisitions Editor: Marion Waldman
Publishing Services Manager: Pat Joiner
Designer: Jyotika Shroff

Printed in the United States of America

Last digit is the print number: 9 8 7 6 5 4 3 2 1

In loving memory of my father, Dr. Stuart Holz, who taught me to value not only knowledge, but also kindness, fairness, and perseverance.

For my children, Jennifer, Sam, and Carly in the hope that I have and may continue to pass along these lessons to you.

Contributors

Lee Dibble, PT, PhD, ATC

Clinical Associate Professor
University of Utah
Division of Physical therapy
Salt Lake City, Utah

Mary Jane Myslinski, PT, EdD

Associate Professor
Doctoral Program of Physical Therapy
University of Medicine and Dentistry of New Jersey
Newark, New Jersey

Sue Ann Sisto, PT, MA, PhD

Director, Human Performance and Movement Analysis Laboratory
Kessler Medical Rehabilitation Research and Education Corporation;
Associate Professor, New Jersey Medical School
University of Medicine and Dentistry of New Jersey;
Assistant Clinical Professor of Physical Therapy
School of Health Related Professions
University of Medicine and Dentistry of New Jersey;
Associate Research Professor
New Jersey Institute of Technology
Newark, New Jersey;
Clinical Assistant Professor of Physical Therapy
Columbia University
New York, New York

Preface

Pharmacology for Physical Therapists presents basic pharmacological principles along with the mechanism of action and side effects of major drug categories seen in physical therapy practice. Chapters are organized using the systems approach. Each section begins with the pathophysiology and continues with a discussion of the drug groups used for treatment. Most sections end with a discussion about how drugs affect physical therapy intervention and how physical therapy may affect drug effectiveness. Special emphasis, when known, is placed on what type of exercises or modalities are contraindicated for a patient on a particular drug. In addition, adverse drug events that may occur during therapy are reviewed, and the therapist is then counseled on the intervention necessary. The chapters conclude with discussion activities that help the student learn the material and integrate it into practice without having to resort to rote memory. The last chapter of the book provides an in-depth discussion of the medication and exercise response as it pertains to cardiopulmonary illnesses and diabetes. This chapter explores recent studies on medication and exercise and will assist the therapist in designing exercise programs based on evidence. Finally, the appendices provide useful information on how to navigate through the *Physicians' Desk Reference* and the Internet for online drug information. They also provide generic and trade names for commonly used drugs.

The discussion activities at the end of each chapter are unique to this text, requiring that the student apply chapter information to physical therapy case scenarios. The case studies are followed by challenging questions that require critical thinking. Some of the discussion activities also require a literature search and a critical appraisal of research before answering, and still others require interviewing a patient and taking an adequate drug history. In addition, these activities can be answered by individual students, as well as by groups. The answers to these discussion activities can be found on the book's website which is available for students who purchase this book.

There are many advantages to *Pharmacology for Physical Therapists* compared with other pharmacology textbooks. First, it is uniquely designed for physical therapists and thus discusses drugs within the confines of what might be seen in the clinic or in a home care situation. Second, the level of presentation is consistent with physical therapy education. The book offers a mix of basic and clinical science. Third, the website not only provides the answers to the discussion activities, but it also provides pharmacology updates as they occur and links to supplemental resources. Last, the student who purchases this book will receive a 6-month free subscription to *Mosby's Drug Consult*, a reliable and trustworthy Internet drug reference. Students and therapists will have access to the most current, unbiased, and accurate information available on prescription and over-the-counter agents, including new drug approvals, safety announcements for established drugs, and links to the pharmaceutical companies.

— *Barbara Gladson*

Acknowledgments ✢

No author works in a vacuum, and I especially have had the good fortune to be supported by a dedicated legion of family, friends, and colleagues. In the end, it has been their project as much as mine, and I would be remiss if I did not acknowledge their contributions of time, knowledge, and enthusiasm. I am thankful for the unique perspectives of my contributing authors, Dr. Lee Dibble, Dr. Sue Ann Sisto, and Dr. Mary Jane Myslinski, which truly set this book apart from its peers. And without the unrelenting encouragement of my champions in the School of Health Related Professions at the University of Medicine and Dentistry of New Jersey, this text could never have been completed. To them I am ever grateful. Many thanks as well to Marion Waldman at Elsevier and Teri Zak, who were my guides throughout this journey.

Barbara Gladson

Contents ✤

SECTION 3

TREATMENT FOR PULMONARY AND GASTROINTESTINAL DISORDERS

SECTION 4

PAIN CONTROL

SECTION 10

THE RELATIONSHIP BETWEEN DRUG THERAPY AND EXERCISE

PHARMACOLOGY
for PHYSICAL THERAPISTS

Principles of Pharmacology

INTRODUCTION

WHAT IS PHARMACOLOGY?

Pharmacology is defined as the study of how chemical substances affect living tissue, and it includes the monitoring of how these agents bind to receptors to enhance or inhibit normal function.[1,2] The study of pharmacology may be divided into two main areas, **pharmacotherapeutics** (also known as *medical pharmacology*) and **toxicology**. Pharmacotherapeutics is the use of chemical agents to prevent, diagnose, and cure disease; whereas toxicology is the study of the negative effects of chemicals on living things, including cells, plants, animals, and humans. Pharmacology is separate from pharmacy, which refers to the mixing and dispensing of drugs, as well as to clinical functions, including monitoring drug prescriptions for appropriateness and monitoring patients for adverse drug interactions.[3,4]

Pharmacotherapeutics may be further divided into two domains, **pharmacokinetics** and **pharmacodynamics**. When we think of the word *kinetics*, we think of mathematical formulas and rates. When the word *kinetics* is applied to pharmacology, it is the study of how fast and how much of the drug is absorbed into the body, how it is distributed to the various organs, and how it is ultimately metabolized and excreted by the body. Computing the concentration of drug absorbed or excreted is part of a pharmacokinetic study.

Pharmacodynamics describes what the drug does to the body and its beneficial or adverse effects at the cellular or organ level. Pharmacodynamic studies identify the mechanism of action and compare effects of different drugs for potency and efficacy. Pharmacodynamic principles are often presented in a graphic form called a *dose-response curve*.[2] This curve demonstrates the effect of increasing drug doses on a particular response (see Figures 2-10 and 2-11). The dose-response curve helps explain the nature of the drug-receptor interaction and is useful for comparing drugs in similar categories for strength and effectiveness (see Chapter 2).

Although this schema for describing the basis of pharmacology is simple and easily understood, in actuality, it should be expanded to include not only the traditional areas of pharmacology driven by a systems approach, but also some new specialty areas such as pharmacogenetics, pharmacogenomics, pharmacoepidemiology, and pharmacoeconomics[5,6] (Figure 1-1). Pharmacogenetics and the related field of pharmacogenomics examine how our genetic make-up produces unexpected and peculiar reactions to drugs and help direct therapeutics according to a person's genotype. Pharmacoepidemiology is concerned with the effects of a drug when it is consumed by large populations as opposed to when it is consumed by individuals. This specialty also scrutinizes all factors, including compliance, that are involved in the real-life situation of taking a medication. And last, pharmacoeconomics is the area of pharmacology that quantifies in dollar amounts the cost versus benefits of therapeutics.

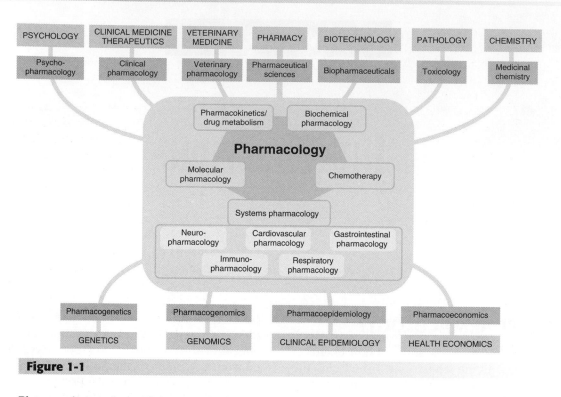

Figure 1-1

Pharmacology today with its various subdivisions. Interface disciplines link pharmacology to other mainstream disciplines. (From Rang HP, Dale MM, Ritter JM, Moore JL. *Pharmacology.* 5th ed. New York: Churchill Livingstone; 2003.)

WHY SHOULD PHYSICAL THERAPISTS STUDY PHARMACOLOGY?

The field of pharmacology is constantly changing. Almost daily, new drugs appear on the market, and new information about older drugs is presented in medical journals. Drug therapy is pervasive among our physical therapy clients, and therefore we must have some understanding of drugs' mechanisms of action and adverse drug reactions. Perhaps even more important is an understanding of how drugs affect physical therapy practice. Some beneficial effects of drugs may be enhanced by our interventions, and in some cases, our interventions may be able to lessen some of the negative effects of medication. However, we must also be aware that physical therapy intervention may exacerbate some of the adverse effects of drugs and necessitate a change in treatment. Excellent examples of interventions producing adverse effects include massage procedures and strengthening exercises performed

in an area recently injected with insulin. Both of these interventions accelerate the absorption of insulin and may lead to hypoglycemia.[7,8]

There are four specific reasons that physical therapists should study pharmacology. First, physical therapists must understand the patient's response to different drugs. Drugs often cause fatigue that interferes with cognitive and motor function. Examples of drugs that cause fatigue are sedatives, opioids, and muscle relaxants; however, many other drugs produce sedation and affect muscle strength.[9-14] A second reason to study medication is for optimum scheduling purposes. A physical therapist may want to see a patient during the time when his or her pain medication has reached its peak effect; however, the therapist would not want to treat a patient at peak sedation. The same is true for a patient taking anitparkinsonian medication: the patient should be experiencing the peak anti-tremor effect during the scheduled physical therapy session. The third reason for studying pharmacology is to learn to recognize drug-therapy interactions. Whirlpool treatments and other heat-related modalities produce peripheral vasodilation, which can exacerbate the orthostatic hypotension produced by certain antihypertensive agents and lead to syncope.[15-17] Lastly, it is estimated that 6.7% of hospital admissions are due to serious adverse drug reactions (ADRs), and at least in 1994, fatal ADRs ranked somewhere between the fourth and sixth leading causes of death in U.S. hospitals.[18] Many of these ADRs are preventable, and therapists must recognize these reactions and report them immediately to the patient's physician.

DRUG DEVELOPMENT AND REGULATION PROCESS

The Food and Drug Administration (FDA) is the administrative arm of the United States government that directs the drug development process and gives approval for marketing a new drug or approves a new use for an older drug. The FDA's power comes from a series of legislation enacted since the passage of The Pure Food and Drug Act of 1906.[19] This act represented the U.S. government's earliest attempts to protect public health and resulted from the discovery of unsanitary practices in the meatpacking industry. Later on, the Food, Drug, and Cosmetic Act of 1938 was passed; it required that drugs be safe and of good quality but did not require evidence of efficacy. It was not until the Kefauver-Harris Amendments to the Food, Drug, and Cosmetic Act were signed in 1962 that drug approval was contingent upon both safety and efficacy. This legislation was a reaction to the evidence that thalidomide, a supposedly nontoxic hypnotic, when taken during pregnancy was responsible for phocomelia, a rare birth defect involving the shortening or absence of limbs.[19] Some other legislation that has been passed includes the Comprehensive Drug Abuse Prevention and Control Act of 1970, which limited access to drugs of abuse, and the Expedited Drug Approval Act of 1992, fueled by the AIDs crisis, which shortened the drug development process for certain life-saving medications. However, it was not until 1997 that legislation requiring pharmaceutical companies to provide information on side effects of drugs to consumers was passed (Agriculture, Rural Development, Food and Drug Administration and Related Agencies Appropriations Act, 1997).[20] In Senator Kennedy's amendment speech to this bill, he is quoted as saying, "Millions of Americans are affected and billions of dollars are spent on medical problems caused by prescription drugs. The nation spends as much to cure the illnesses caused by prescription drugs as we spend on the drugs themselves."[21]

Drug regulation is essential to ensure a safe and effective product. The purposes of regulation include balancing the need of the pharmaceutical companies to show a profit with the need of patients to have easy access to medications, especially nonprofitable drugs or orphan drugs (drugs for rare diseases); to ensure safety and efficacy by detailed review of all research studies, as well as review of the product labeling; to regulate the manufacturing process to ensure stability in the product; and to control public access to drugs that have abuse potential.[22] In the United States, the FDA is charged with this responsibility, but in Europe and the rest of the world, there are both centralized and decentralized procedural methods for drug approval. Europe is united under the European Union (European Medicines Evaluation Agency [EMEA]), which replaces the previously individual country approval process. In order for a pharmaceutical firm to market a drug in a foreign country, the drug must receive approval by the governing regulatory agency. However, in general, the process is less restrictive than in the United States, and these agencies take a more passive role in the approval process. According to T. Reiss, Executive Director of Clinical Pharmacology at Merck & Company, Japan appears to have a stricter policy regarding drug approval, requiring that clinical testing be performed on Japanese people before the distribution of drugs is approved (personal communication, October 2003). The reason for tighter control in Japan is biological; different ethnic groups may respond in different ways to a particular drug.

Although some centralized control over drug regulation is exercised, individual countries have their own rules regarding possession and prescription of drugs, and these rules vary greatly. In some countries patients can obtain drugs without a prescription, whereas in other nations purchase of drugs is tightly controlled. In addition, vitamins, dietary supplements, and herbal remedies are not regulated as drugs in this and many other countries, and therefore manufacturers of these items do not have to abide by the strict regulations for safety, purity, and efficacy governing distribution of prescription drugs.[23]

Drug Development

The first step in the drug development process is for the drug company to target a market. For example, let's say that Drug Company X decides that there is a need for an oral form of insulin. Insulin is commonly delivered by means of a subcutaneous injection, a form of drug delivery that is less desirable by patients. First, the drug company enlists some chemists to perform research and provide support. The chemists recruited will be knowledgeable on the structure of the insulin receptor and will therefore develop chemical compounds to bind to the receptor. These compounds will then be passed along to the pharmacologist for drug screening. A variety of biological assays will be used to test the compounds at the molecular and cellular levels, as well as at the organ and animal levels. The tissues chosen for testing will be ones influenced by insulin, and the animals chosen for testing will be ones that have insulin receptors that are similar to those of humans. An evaluation of cardiovascular and renal function will be performed on healthy animals for safety. Efficacy testing will be conducted on animals bred to become diabetic. Additional testing on the respiratory, gastrointestinal, reproductive, and central nervous systems is also performed. These experiments constitute the **preclinical testing** phase, which lasts 2 to 6 years.[19] At the end of this phase, representatives from Drug Company X will take the data on their lead compound to the FDA and seek approval to begin testing the oral insulin in humans. In addition to data to support that the compound does what it is supposed to do, information on the effects of a single large dose up to a toxic level, the effect of multiple dosing, and the drug's teratogenicity and mutagenicity will be given to the FDA. If the compound is thought to be ready to be studied in humans, a Notice of Claimed Investigational Exemption for a New Drug is filed with the FDA. Human testing begins once the FDA approves the Investigational New Drug (IND) and consists of four phases.

Phase 1 is the safety assessment study.[24] In this study the oral insulin is given to a small number of healthy volunteers (about 25 to 50), and a safety profile is established. These studies are conducted to identify any toxic effects and to begin to establish a safe dosage range. Pharmacokinetic studies are also performed. If the drug is thought to have significant toxic effects, testing will be conducted with volunteer patients who have the disease being targeted instead of with healthy control subjects. This is often the case for AIDS drugs or drugs designed for resistant types of cancers. This phase lasts another 1 to 2 years.

Phase 2 is the drug effectiveness study.[24] In this phase a small number of patients (approximately 200) who have the targeted disease will receive the drug. In our example, phase 2 would be conducted with diabetic patients who require insulin to control their blood sugar levels. The study design is usually single-blind in which the new drug is compared with a placebo (a nonactive compound) and also with an older active drug with known safety and efficacy. The questions that must be answered include: Is this drug safe for diabetic patients and is it effective in lowering blood glucose levels? This phase will also last for another 1 to 2 years but is variable, depending on the specific endpoint being studied. In our example a lowered blood glucose level is the endpoint, but the study might track time to development of disease or retinal damage, which would extend the length of the study.

Phase 3 is a much larger study including many more diabetic subjects than in the previous phase (5000 to 10,000 subjects or more). In addition, the duration of the study is usually extended to 3 to 6 years. Investigators and study sites for these trials are recruited from all over the world. Safety and effectiveness are again studied but on a much larger scale. In phase 3 trials, investigators attempt to determine the contribution of the investigational drug compared with placebo for reducing symptoms of a particular disease. The investigators usually perform double-blind, randomized, controlled studies that are parallel or crossover in design. Parallel designs test at least two therapies at the same time, but each patient group is assigned only one drug. In studies with crossover designs, patients act as their own control subjects by receiving therapies in sequence. Some patients may receive Drug A first then Drug B, and other patients will receive Drug B first then Drug A. Phase 3 studies tend to be performed in larger tertiary care centers by experts in the targeted disease. Again, if we use the example of oral insulin, test sites would be set up around the country and in Europe and Japan, preferably at centers for the study of diabetes. These centers receive funding from the pharmaceutical company to recruit and pay subjects, set up data collection systems, and obtain any other supplies or equipment needed to support the research. Clinical researchers from the drug company will closely monitor all the data to make sure that the oral insulin is effective and safe throughout phase 3.

If phase 3 studies are successful, the drug company will file a **new drug application (NDA)** with the FDA. As part of this application, the company will submit all preclinical and clinical data on the oral insulin. The FDA will then review the materials, and if the drug seems to be effective and without significant adverse effects, the FDA will give permission to the company to market the insulin to the public.

Phase 4 begins when the drug is approved for public use. It is called the *postmarketing surveillance* phase and is a much larger study than any previously performed.[24] This phase constitutes monitoring the drug for safety under real-life conditions in large numbers of patients. During this phase members of the public who have diabetes unknowingly become study subjects. Many adverse drug reactions are discovered during this phase, and if they present significant health risks, the drug may be recalled. Technically, phase 4 has infinite duration because the drug company will continue monitoring for any problems throughout the marketing process. However, even though the drug has been released for public consumption after phase 3, it might be prudent to wait until it has been on the market for at least 2 years before taking it. It is responsible health care to prescribe an older drug with a proven track record first and then to switch to a newer drug after all the ADRs have been identified. This process underscores the attitude among many health care professionals that every drug prescription should be viewed as a therapeutic experiment. We are all subjects in drug studies.

The time it takes to bring a drug to market may be as long as 10 years[22] and cost more than 300 to 800 million dollars (F. J. Grogan, personal communication, October 2003).[25] It is a labor-intensive process that does not always lead to success. For every compound that makes it to our medicine cabinets, about 200 have been abandoned because of safety or effectiveness issues.

Drug companies fight hard to extend their patents by coming up with new uses for their drugs to balance out the lengthy review process and cost of failed compounds.

Patents are issued around the time that phase 1 studies begin and are in effect for only 20 years.

Ownership of the patent means that the pharmaceutical company that developed the drug is the only company that can market it to the public. When the patent expires, any company may produce and sell the drug as a generic without having to pay any fees to the original company, but the licensed trade name given to the drug remains the property of the original drug maker. For a lengthy FDA review process, the patent may be extended for up to 5 years.[19]

Although the FDA approves drugs for specific indications that then become listed in the package insert, it does not limit the use of drugs to these described conditions. Physicians have the final say on how a drug may be used. Prescribing a drug for off-label or unapproved uses is common and legally permitted.[25]

Orphan Drugs and Treatment Investigational New Drugs

Because drug development is an extremely expensive and lengthy process, drugs for rare diseases, so-called orphan drugs, tend not to be researched or marketed by the drug companies. Therefore in 1983 the Orphan Drug Act was passed to provide research grants for the study of diseases affecting fewer than 200,000 patients in the United States.[19] This act provides special financial incentives to companies to help offset their development costs, although lack of profit is not the only reason that these drugs are rarely studied. Orphan drugs present some scientific dilemmas because it is difficult to establish safety and effectiveness in small numbers of patients. In addition, many rare diseases occur in children, but investigators do not want to include children in early clinical trials.[25] However, since the early 1980s, almost 500 drugs have been developed as a result of this act.[26] Some of the disorders that have benefited include cystic fibrosis, AIDs, and leprosy.

The FDA has also provided guidelines to streamline the development of certain drugs for life-threatening conditions such as AIDs and certain cancers. These drugs receive **Treatment IND** status, allowing them special priority throughout the review procedure.[25] This status also allows patients outside the ongoing studies to be treated with investigational drugs. Treatment IND status is issued for a drug designed to treat serious life-threatening illnesses when there is no other acceptable alternative on the market. The drug must already be involved in a clinical trial, and the pharmaceutical company must show that it is proceeding with the normal steps involved in drug approval. If a physician wants to prescribe a drug that is in clinical study but lacks the treatment IND status, the drug may still be obtained for a patient under a "compassionate use" clause.

Barriers to Drug Development

Many barriers to development of new drugs exist, particularly for diseases that progress over time such as multiple sclerosis and Parkinson's disease. First, of course, is the issue of funding. This barrier affects rare diseases much more so than the more common ones, but even for common illnesses, new drug discovery is risky and quite expensive. Drug researchers suggest that charity organizations and government support programs continue to be emphasized as funding sources.[27]

Another barrier to development is the fact that many diseases are considered clinical syndromes that lack specific markers of identification or lack consensus regarding clinical trial endpoints, thus making treatment progress difficult to document. An example is Alzheimer's disease in which an absolute diagnosis can only be made at autopsy when β-amyloid plaques and tangles can be identified in the brain.[27] In addition, Alzheimer's disease is a multifactorial condition demonstrating impairments in language, memory, motor planning, and cognitive domains. Functional testing in all these areas is necessary to prove that a medication is effective. Even when markers have been identified, researchers in the field do not always agree on the level of significance that these markers provide in terms of documenting improvement. For example, manufacturers of arthritis drugs may show a reduction in signs and symptoms (e.g., redness, swollen joints) in rheumatoid arthritis and claim that the drug is effective, but others may insist that effectiveness claims be based on a slowing of disease progression as determined by radiography.[28] Because the lack of a specific drug target or marker is a function of our incomplete understanding of the anatomy, we can hope that in the future further study will lead to more effective drugs.

Another problem with the drug discovery process is the lack of animal models for drug screening.[27] There exist animals that can grow specific tumors, animals that are bred to have diabetes, and even animal models for epilepsy; but animal models are lacking for many illnesses. Again, Alzheimer's disease is a good example because it does not have an existing animal model for the testing of different compounds.

Barriers to the implementation of clinical trials also exist. For drug approval, the FDA and the European Medicines Evaluation Agency require two significant studies demonstrating efficacy, whereas Japanese regulators require only one study; and depending on the country, the duration of study may last between 3 and 12 months.[27] Ideally, the longer the study, the more information about an experimental agent can be obtained. However, long-term trials produce certain ethical dilemmas, particularly for placebo-controlled trials. Researchers working in the area of psychiatric drug discovery have expressed concern over administering placebo and withholding treatment for extended periods. Some researchers are particularly concerned about an increased risk of suicide among the population receiving placebo, although a recent study showed no difference in suicide rates between placebo and treatment groups.[29] Another dilemma is whether it is ethical to withhold treatment for rheumatoid arthritis while irreversible structural damage continues.

Another problem is the reluctance to include women and children in clinical trials, largely because of differences in pharmacokinetics and pharmacodynamics in these populations. One solution to this has been the establishment of the Office of Women's Health within the FDA in 1994.[30] This office has promoted the development and approval of drugs for diseases affecting women. In addition, this office is dedicated to identifying how drugs affect women because traditionally most clinical trials have been conducted on men.

Drug development is a labor-intensive, expensive, risky, and time-consuming process. Although this process is widely accepted and adhered to, there is growing discussion regarding alternative methods to prove drug safety and efficacy.[31,32] Improved postmarketing surveillance, involving a coordinated data collection system from around the world, has been suggested to detect unanticipated events, either positive or negative, that could lead to greater accuracy in identifying treatment options. The use of meta-analyses for analyzing many trials simultaneously has also been suggested as a way of improving therapy. In some cases a meta-analysis of multiple small trials can be used to identify a drug effect not previously recognized by individual trials. Pharmacoeconomics, consisting of studies that determine the cost/benefit ratio of drugs, is likely to become a growing field as research dollars continue to shrink. Pharmacoeconomic studies examine overall outcome in clinical practice and are used to inform changes in practice.[22] These suggestions are not likely to become standard operating procedures in the drug delivery process yet, but the FDA has instituted a number of changes that will ultimately benefit patients. Approvals of drugs via the "fast-track" and greater inclusion of women in clinical trials represent two recent changes in drug processing. In addition, the FDA has begun using outside help, groups of clinical specialists in a variety of fields, in evaluating studies to hasten the review process. Further changes focused on streamlining the process and improving data collection are expected as time goes on.

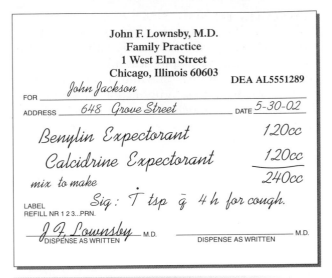

Figure 1-2

Sample prescription. (From Asperheim MK. *Introduction to Pharmacology.* 9th ed. Philadelphia: Saunders; 2002.)

ELEMENTS OF A PRESCRIPTION

The prescription is an order written by a licensed practitioner (e.g., physician, dentist, veterinarian, or podiatrist) to instruct the pharmacist to provide a specific medication needed by a patient.[25] The elements contained in the prescription include the following[33] (Figure 1-2):

1. The prescribing physician's name, address, and telephone number.
2. The date and the patient's name and address.
3. **Rx,** called the *superscription,* which tells how the drug is to be administered to the patient (e.g., orally or by injection). Rx is an abbreviation of the Latin word for "recipe" and "receive thou."
4. **Inscription,** which includes the drug name, dose, and quantity to dispense.
5. **Subscription,** which gives directions to the pharmacist as to the mixing instructions. This may be excluded because many physicians do not have adequate knowledge about compounding.
6. The **Signa** or **Sig,** which gives directions to the patient, including how often to take the drug, how much drug to take, and additional instructions such as "shake well" or "take with food." Signa is Latin for "label." The

patient instructions are usually written with Latin abbreviations.
7. **Refill** information.
8. **Prescriber's signature.**
9. **DEA** number, which is required for controlled substances, as well as for insurance claims processing.

CONTROLLED SUBSTANCES

Controlled substances are drugs classified according to their potential for abuse. They are regulated under the Controlled Substances Act (CSA), which classifies these compounds into schedules (levels) from I to V.[26,34] This law was enacted in 1971 and also provides provisions for research into drug abuse and treatment programs for dependency. This act, along with assistance from the Drug Enforcement Administration (DEA), controls the distribution of drugs of abuse.

Schedule I

Schedule I drugs are available only for research. They have a high abuse potential, leading to dependence without any acceptable medical indication. Some examples include heroin, LSD, mescaline, and marijuana. Special approval is necessary before any of these agents can be used.

Schedule II

Schedule II drugs also have a high abuse potential with the likelihood of physical and psychological dependence, but unlike schedule I drugs, they have accepted medical uses. Drugs classified at this level include stimulants such as amphetamines; opioids including morphine, fentanyl, and oxycodone; and some barbiturates. Automatic refills are not allowed, and the prescriber must write a new prescription each time a refill is needed. In the hospital setting if an order is written on an as-needed basis, it is only valid for 72 hours.

Schedule III

Schedule III drugs have a lower abuse potential than those in schedules I or II; however, they may also be abused, resulting in some physical and psychological dependence. Refills are allowed, but no more than five refills are permitted within a 6-month period. Mild to moderately strong opioids, barbiturates, and steroids are categorized at this level. Opioids that are formulated with aspirin and acetaminophen and anabolic steroids are also included under schedule III.

Schedule IV

Schedule IV drugs have less of an abuse potential than those in schedule III; however, this does not mean that they are not popular among drug abusers. They include opioids such as propoxyphene (Darvon), benzodiazepines such as diazepam (Valium), and some stimulants. No more than five refills within 6 months are allowed under one prescription.

Schedule V

Schedule V drugs have the lowest abuse potential and may even be available without a prescription. Actual availability without a prescription is state regulated, so laws governing their use vary. Various cold and cough medicines containing codeine are listed in this category.

Rules Governing Narcotics

It is against the law for any person to possess a scheduled drug unless it has been obtained with a prescription. It is also illegal to transfer possession of any scheduled drug to another person.[26] In the hospital setting if a narcotic is ordered for a patient and then not used, it must be returned to the hospital pharmacy. In addition, if a narcotic falls on the floor and becomes contaminated, it must also be returned to the pharmacy. Every dose of a schedule II drug ordered for a patient must be accounted for. For this reason, any drug found by a physical therapist on the floor, table, or anywhere else in a patient's room must be turned in to the nursing station so that proper accounting of these drugs can be made.

DRUG NAMING AND CLASSIFICATION SYSTEMS

Drugs have chemical, generic, and trade names. The chemical name is based on the specific structure of the compound. It tends to be long, and this name is often not used by either the public or the health care team. The generic name is considered the official name of the compound and may have some resemblance to the names of other drugs that fall within the same category or have the same purpose. It is the name listed in the official drug compendia, *The United States Pharmacopeia,* and stays with the compound, no matter how many trade names it accumulates.[26] The generic names are also the only names recognized for use in the scientific journals, although these too can vary from one country to another; for example, acetaminophen in the United States is known as *paracetamol* in the United Kingdom. The trade name or brand name is the name given to the drug by the pharmaceutical company and is copyrighted to that company. In recent years there has been a push for trendy names that the public will recognize. An example is the drug Singulair. Singulair, taken from the word *single,* is supposed to remind the public that it has once-a-day dosing and is thus a more desirable drug than one that must be administered several times a day.[35] These names, although they are helpful in steering the public toward a particular drug, actually add more confusion to the system of naming and increase the possibility that someone might make a mistake when writing a prescription. Once a patent expires, other pharmaceutical companies have a right to market the drug and assign their own trade names. Because there may be several trade names given to one generic drug, use of these names should be avoided.[36]

Drug Classification

Drugs are often classified into specific categories. These categories do not represent a universally accepted system, and one drug may be placed into a variety of different classes. The classes do, however, provide a useful framework for studying pharmacology. The pharmacotherapeutic classification describes the overall pharmacological action on a specific disease process.[36] Examples of drugs classified in this manner are antivirals, antibiotics, and antihypertensives. A mistake that is often made when drugs delineated within this category are studied is the assumption that all the drugs classified under the same heading act in the same manner. Not all drugs for hypertension have the same mechanism of action.

Drugs may also be categorized according to their pharmacological action.[36] Examples include arterial vasodilators and anesthetic agents. This is also an imprecise way to classify drugs, which includes the assumption that all drugs within the same category act in the same way. Some drugs act directly on smooth muscle to vasodilate arterioles and lower blood pressure. However, some vasodilators act by blocking receptors on arterioles that would ordinarily produce constriction. The result is the same, but the mechanism of action is different.

A third way in which drugs may be classified is according to their molecular action.[36] The molecular action is described by identifying the molecular target of the drug. These targets consist of receptors for hormones and neurotransmitters, enzymes, ion channels, and cell membrane transporters. Examples include calcium channel blockers used to decrease cardiac contractility to lower blood pressure and sodium channel blockers used to inhibit pain impulses.

The last method for categorizing drugs is a classification based on either chemical make-up or the source for the drug.[36] Plant material provides a good natural source for many compounds. Atropine is named after the *Atropa* species of plant. Penicillin is part of a group of compounds described as β-lactam antibiotics because they contain a β-lactam ring, a four-member nitrogen-containing carbon structure.

This drug classification system adds another layer of confusion to the drug-naming schema. Although this naming system describes drug actions that might be more understandable by the patient, this system is imprecise and implies that all drugs within the same classification group act in a similar manner. Given the potential for mistakes when trade or proprietary names are used and the inaccuracies implied in using functional categories for naming, there is a push to use the official or generic names of drugs when speaking to patients and health professionals or when writing prescriptions.[37] However, pharmaceutical companies continue to market their drugs with trendy trade names.

ACTIVITIES 1

■ 1. Describe the following drugs using the pharmacotherapeutic, pharmacologic, and molecular categories of drug naming.

Propranolol
Prazosin
Captopril
Losartan
Nifedipine
Hydrochlorothiazide

■ 2. You are in the process of conducting an initial evaluation on a patient with knee pain. This patient has a complicated medical history and has experienced a variety of illnesses. While taking the medical history, you realize that this gentleman is taking multiple medications, many of which you are not familiar with. Review the information in this chapter, as well as in Appendixes A and B, and outline some sources of drug information that might be helpful to you while reading this text.

References

1. Katzung BG. Introduction. In: Katzung BG, ed. *Basic & Clinical Pharmacology*. 8th ed. New York: McGraw-Hill; 2001:1-8.
2. Sutter MC, Walker MJ. Introduction. In: Page CP, Curtis MJ, Sutter MC, Walker MJ, Hoffman BB, eds. *Integrated Pharmacology*. 2nd ed. Philadelphia: Mosby; 2002.
3. Definition of pharmacy. Available at: http://www.free-definition.com/pharmacy.html. Accessed September 10, 2004.
4. Carmichael JM, O'Connell MB, Devine B, et al. Collaborative drug therapy management by pharmacists. *Pharmacotherapy*. 1997;17(5):1050-1061.
5. Rang HP, Dale MM, Ritter JM, Moore JL. *Pharmacology*. 5th ed. New York: Churchill Livingstone; 2003.
6. Ingelman-Sundberg M. Pharmacogenetics: an opportunity for a safer and more efficient pharmacotherapy. *J Intern Med*. 2001;250:186-200.
7. Koivisto VA, Felig P. Effects of leg exercise on insulin absorption in diabetic patients. *N Engl J Med*. 1978; 298(2):79-83.
8. Linde B. Dissociation of insulin absorption and blood flow during massage of a subcutaneous injection site. *Diabetes Care*. 1986;9(6):570-574.
9. Allen GJ, Hartl TL, Duffany S, et al. Cognitive and motor function after administration of hydrocodone bitartrate plus ibuprofen, ibuprofen alone, or placebo in healthy subjects with exercise-induced muscle damage: a randomized, repeated-dose, placebo-controlled study. *Psychopharmacology*. 2003;166(3):228-233.
10. Bower EA, Moore JL, Mos M, Selby KA, Austin M, Meeves S. The effects of single-dose fexofenadine, diphenhydramine, and placebo on cognitive performance in flight personnel. *Aviat Space Environ Med*. 2003; 74(2):145-152.
11. Mattila MJ, Vanakoski J, Kalska H, Seppala T. Effects of alcohol, zolpidem, and some other sedatives and hypnotics on human performance and memory. *Pharmacol Biochem Behav*. 1998;59(4):917-923.
12. Gracies JM, Elovic E, McGuire J, Simpson DM. Traditional pharmacological treatments for spasticity. Part I: Local treatments. *Muscle Nerve*. 1997;(suppl 6):S61-S92.
13. Gracies JM, Nance P, Elovic E, McGuire J, Simpson DM. Traditional pharmacological treatments for spasticity. Part II: General and regional treatments. *Muscle Nerve*. 1997;(suppl 6):S92-S120.
14. Giardina WJ, Wismer CT. The rat-pull test procedure: a method for assessing the strength of rats. *Pharmacol Biochem Behav*. 1995;50(4):517-519.
15. Drugs for hypertension. *Treat Guidel Med Lett*. 2003; 1(6):33-40.
16. Nagasawa Y, Komori S, Sato M, et al. Effects of hot bath immersion on autonomic activity and hemodynamics: comparison of the elderly patient and the healthy young. *Jpn Circ J*. 2001;65:587-592.
17. Allison TG, Maresh CM, Armstrong LE. Cardiovascular responses in a whirlpool bath at 40 degrees C versus user-controlled water temperatures. *Mayo Clinic Proc*. 1998;73(3):210-215.
18. Lazarou J, Pomeranz BH, Corey PN. Incidence of adverse drug reactions in hospitalized patients. *JAMA*. 1998; 279(15):1200-1205.
19. Berkowitz BA, Katzung BG. Basic & clinical evaluation of new drugs. In: Katzung BG, ed. *Basic & Clinical Pharmacology*. 8th ed. New York: McGraw-Hill; 2001.
20. Making Appropriations for Agriculture, Rural Development, Food and Drug Administration, and Related Agencies Act, Pub L No. 104-180, 110 Stat 1569.
21. Gray J. Senate backs bill to require data on drugs for consumers. *New York Times*. July 25, 1996;sect. 19.
22. Mamelok RD. Regulation of drug use. In: Page CP, Curtis MJ, Sutter MC, Walker MJ, Hoffman BB, eds. *Integrated Pharmacology*. 2nd ed. Philadelphia: Mosby; 2002.
23. How the Dietary Supplement Health and Education Act of 1994 weakened the FDA. Quackwatch, 2000. Available at: http://www.quackwatch.org. Accessed September 20, 2004.
24. Stein G. Related drug development and usage. In: Brody TM, Larner J, Minneman KP, eds. *Human Pharmacology: Molecular to Clinical*. New York: Mosby; 1998:903-908.
25. Committee on Drugs. Uses of drugs not described in the package insert (off-label uses). *Pediatrics*. 2002;110(1).
26. Salerno E. *Pharmacology for health professionals*. New York: Mosby; 1999.
27. Fillit HM, O'Connell AW, Brown WM, et al. Barriers to drug discovery and development for Alzheimer disease. *Alzheimer Dis Assoc Disord*. 2002;16(suppl 1):S1-S8.
28. Witter J. Drug development in rheumatoid arthritis. *Curr Opin Rheumatol*. 2002;14:276-280.
29. Storosum JG, Van Zwieten BJ, Wohlfarth T, de Haan L, Khan A, van den Brink W. Suicide risk in placebo vs active treatment in placebo-controlled trials for schizophrenia. *Arch Gen Psychiatry*. 2003;60:365-368.
30. Sheppard A. US Food and Drug Office of Women's Health: Update. *J Am Med Womens Assoc*. 1999;54(2):97-98.
31. Hogel J, Gaus W. The procedure of new drug application and the philosophy of critical rationalism or the limits of quality assurance with good clinical practice. *Control Clin Trials*. 1999;20:511-518.
32. Carpenter WT. From clinical trial to prescription. *Arch Gen Psychiatry*. 2002;59:282-285.
33. Blaschke TS. Writing prescriptions. In: Carruthers SG, Hoffman BB, Melmon KL, Nierenberg DW, eds. *Melmon and Morrelli's Clinical Pharmacology*. 4th ed. New York: McGraw Hill; 2000:1267-1288.
34. Kuhn M. *Pharmacotherapeutics: A Nursing Process Approach*. 4th ed. Philadelphia: FA Davis; 1998.
35. Reiss TF. Montelukast, a once daily leukotriene receptor antagonist in the treatment of chronic asthma; a multicenter randomized, double blind trial. *Arch Intern Med*. 1998;158:1213-20.
36. Walker MJA. Drug names and drug classification systems. In: Page CP, Curtis MJ, Sutter MC, Walker MJ, Hoffman JR, eds. *Integrated Pharmacology*. 2nd ed. Philadelphia: Mosby; 2002:11-16.
37. Asperheim MK. *Pharmacology: An Introductory Text*. 8th ed. Philadelphia: WB Saunders; 1996.

PHARMACODYNAMICS: MECHANISM OF ACTION

TARGETS FOR DRUG ACTION

Sites of drug action may include receptors, ion channels, transport molecules, and enzymes that catalyze chemical reactions. A receptor is sometimes considered to be any target for a drug, or it can be a specific protein that exists in the phospholipid cell membrane, delineated from the other targets (Figure 2-1). However, in general, the sites for drug action include binding sites on proteins that undergo a conformational change in the presence of ligand (drug) to initiate a cascade of events leading to the drug's action. Additionally, structural proteins such as tubulin or tumor DNA can become drug targets simply by being destroyed by chemotherapeutic agents. In the case of microbial or parasitic infections, some structure on the invading organism becomes the target of drug therapy.

Receptor Types

Four receptor superfamilies have been identified: ion channel–linked receptors (ligand gated and voltage gated), G-protein–coupled receptors, DNA-coupled receptors, and kinase-linked receptors (Figure 2-2).[1] All except the intracellular DNA-coupled receptor are transmembrane receptors in that they contain receptors responding to ligands outside the cell but contain structural proteins that link this region to the intracellular domain.

Ion channels, also known as *inotropic receptors*, are membrane receptors coupled directly to an ion channel.[2,3] Structurally, they are transmembrane proteins arranged around a central aqueous channel (pore). The channel opens in response to a ligand or a voltage change (nerve impulse) in the membrane, allowing the selective transfer of ions from a greater concentration to a lesser concentration. Ion specificity is determined by the structural configuration of the amino acids (pore size) and the charge on the molecule. Both the charge and size of the pore vary for each type of ion channel. Common ion channels include sodium (Na^+) and calcium (Ca^{2+}) channels in which these cations diffuse into the cell, causing a depolarization, and potassium (K^+) channels in which the cytosol becomes more negative as the ion flows out of the cell (Figure 2-3). Several different subtypes exist for each of these main types of channels; however, they all share a property for quick activation, meaning channel opening in a millisecond timescale.[4]

Ligand-gated channels also consist of protein subunits surrounding a central pore. Examples include the nicotinic acetylcholine, γ-aminobutyric acid ($GABA_A$), glycine, and serotonin receptors.[5-7] For these channels, opening of the pore depends on binding of the neurotransmitters to one of the peptide subunits. The nicotinic acetylcholine receptor consists of five transmembrane subunits with two binding sites for the neurotransmitter.[8] When two

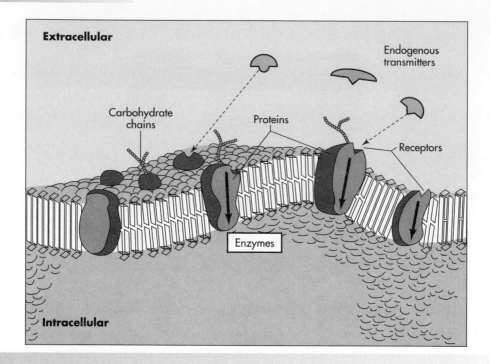

Figure 2-1

Proteins embedded in cell membranes generally extend further on both the extracellular and intracellular sides. Attached to the proteins on the extracellular side are carbohydrate (glycosylation) chains. Also shown on the extracellular side of some of the proteins are receptor sites to which endogenous transmitter compounds bind. Arrows indicate the direction of communication to the other side of the membrane. (From Brody TM, Larner J, Minneman KP, eds. *Human Pharmacology: Molecular to Clinical.* Philadelphia: Mosby; 1998.)

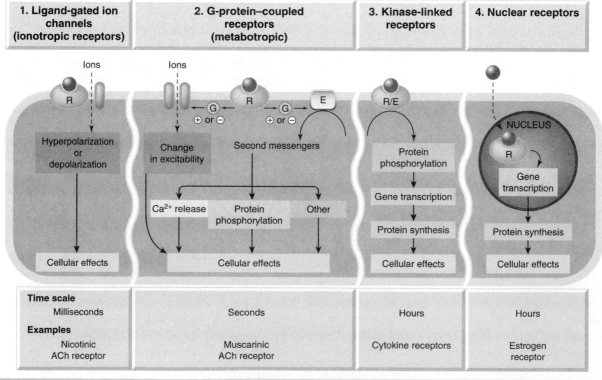

Figure 2-2

Types of receptor-effector linkage. *R,* Receptor; *G,* G-protein; *E,* enzyme; *ACh,* acetylcholine. (From Rang HP, Dale MM, Ritter JM, Gardner P. *Pharmacology.* 5th ed. New York: Churchill Livingstone; 2003.)

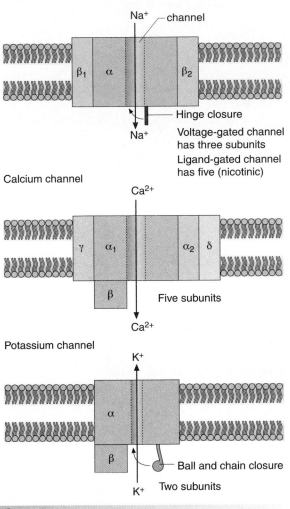

Sodium channel

Na⁺ — channel

β₁ α β₂

Hinge closure

Na⁺

Voltage-gated channel has three subunits

Ligand-gated channel has five (nicotinic)

Calcium channel

Ca²⁺

γ α₁ α₂ δ

β Five subunits

Ca²⁺

Potassium channel

K⁺

α

β Ball and chain closure

K⁺ Two subunits

Figure 2-3

Typical membrane ion channels. (The different subunits (α, β, γ) in different channels are not the same peptide sequences.) Ions diffuse down their concentration gradients when the channel is open. Two types of inactivation of open channels have been described (hinged and ball and chain), which involve an intracellular loop of the channel. (From Waller DG, Renwick AG, Hillier K. *Medical Pharmacology Therapeutics.* New York: WB Saunders; 2001.)

acetylcholine molecules bind to these sites, channel opening is triggered (Figure 2-4). As with voltage-gated channels, channel opening is a millisecond event because the ligand becomes rapidly degraded. The patch-clamp technique developed by Neher and Sakmann is a way to measure the ion flow that occurs through the channel during opening.[9] A tight

seal is formed between a micropipette containing an electrode and a cell membrane (Figure 2-5). When the cell is exposed to a neurotransmitter or to a voltage change, the pipette is able to measure the current passing through a single channel. Many drugs are tested in this manner to determine their effects on specific ion channels. This has become a very important tool in the drug discovery process because there is evidence to support ion-channel mutations in a number of diseases (e.g., cystic fibrosis, long QT syndrome, and several types of myopathies).[10] In addition, targeting ion channels for treatment in cardiovascular and neurodegenerative diseases has become common.[11,12] Examples of drugs that bind to ion channels include vasodilator drugs that inhibit the opening of L-type calcium channels in cardiac and smooth muscles and the benzodiazepine tranquilizers that bind to the GABA$_A$ receptor.

G-protein–linked receptors consist of a trans-membrane receptor coupled to an intracellular system by a guanosine-binding protein (G-protein).[2,13,14] The actual receptor crosses the membrane seven times, with the outer loops containing the active site for ligand binding (Figure 2-6). The inner loops are involved in the signaling of the G-protein. Once the appropriate ligand or drug binds to the extracellular side, a conformational change occurs in the three-dimensional structure of the receptor that activates the G-protein, which then activates other effectors such as ion channels and enzymes. G-proteins are heterotrimers consisting of three protein subunits, α-, β-, and γ-subunits (Figure 2-7). Once activated, the α-subunit binds guanosine triphosphate (GTP) and loses its affinity for the βγ-subunit (joined sub-unit). The α-subunit bound to GTP dissociates from the βγ-subunit, and each exerts its influence on a second messenger system. There are several different types of G-proteins, the functions of which are determined by the type of α-subunit[15] (Figure 2-8). G_s stimulates the membrane-bound adenylate cyclase to produce cyclic adenosine monophosphate (cAMP); G_i inhibits the formation of cAMP; and G_q activates phospholipase C, which in turn increases intracellular concentrations of calcium. The ultimate effects may be seen on enzyme activity, contractile proteins, ion channels, and cytokine production.[16] Examples of receptors that are linked to G-proteins include subtypes of the muscarinic acetylcholine receptor, dopamine receptor, and norepinephrine receptor, as well as a variety of hormone receptors.[16]

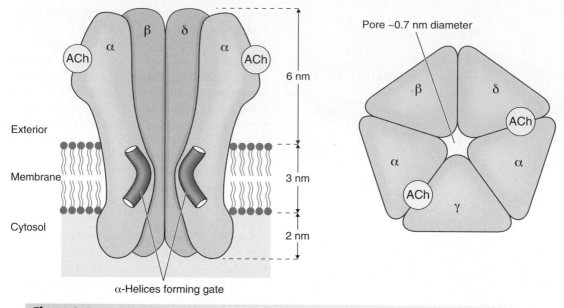

Figure 2-4

Structure of the nicotinic acetylcholine *(ACh)* receptor (a typical ligand-gated ion channel) in side-view *(left)* and plane-view *(right)*. The five receptor subunits (α, β, γ, σ) form a cluster surrounding a central transmembrane pore, the lining of which is formed by the M2 helical segments of each subunit. These contain a preponderance of negatively charged amino acids, which makes the pore cation selective. There are two acetylcholine-binding sites in the extracellular portion of the receptor, at the interface between the α- and the adjoining subunits. When acetylcholine binds, the kinked α-helices swing out of the way, thus opening the channel pore. (Based on Unwin 1993, 1995.) (From Rang HP, Dale MM, Ritter JM, Gardner P. *Pharmacology.* 5th ed. New York: Churchill Livingstone; 2003.)

In addition, G-protein–linked receptors function as targets for drugs for approximately 30 currently available medications including montelukast (Singulair), losartan (Cozaar), and loratadine (Claritin).[17] It is expected that therapeutic intervention with these receptors will have a major impact on a variety of diseases in the future.

DNA-coupled receptors are intracellular receptors that stimulate gene transcription, leading to the synthesis of proteins and enzymes.[18] Because most are located intracellularly in the nucleus, the ligands must be lipophilic to facilitate crossing the cell membrane. Many of the ligands that activate this type of receptor are steroid hormones including estrogen, progesterone, cortisol, and thyroid hormone.[16] Each receptor contains two highly conserved regions, one for binding to DNA and the other for binding to the hormone. When the hormone binds to the receptor on the nuclear membrane, it interacts with a hormone response element on the genome to either activate or depress gene expression. If gene expression is activated, an increase in RNA polymerase activity is detected within a few minutes. The result is altered protein synthesis. Mineralocorticoids act at these receptors to stimulate the production of new carrier proteins involved in transport of ions through the kidney tubules.[19]

The last type of receptor to be discussed is the kinase-linked receptor (Figure 2-9). Kinase-linked receptors have a single transmembrane helical region with a larger extracellular domain for ligand binding. The size of the extracellular region is related to the size of the endogenous ligand, an example of which is the insulin molecule. Insulin binding produces a dimerization, that is, a linkage of two kinase receptors that then phosphorylate each other. The autophosphorylation of the tyrosine amino acids further provides strong binding sites for other intracellular proteins. These intracellular proteins vary, depending on the receptor involved, but are usually related to cell division and growth, with the final product being transcription of genes.[16,20]

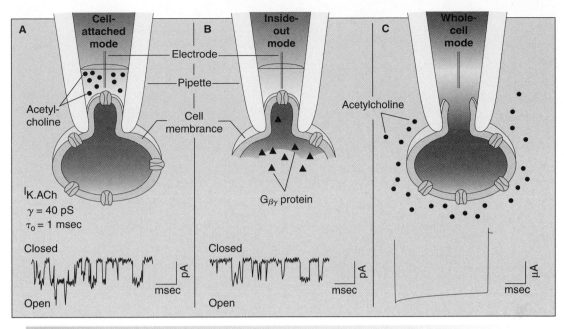

Figure 2-5

Patch-Clamp measurement of ion-channel activity, with the acetylcholine-sensitive potassium channel (I_{KACh}) used as an example. In the "cell-attached" mode (Panel A), a pipette is pressed tightly against the cell membrane, suction is applied, and a tight seal is formed between the pipette and the membrane. The seal ensures that the pipette captures the current flowing through the channel. In the cell-attached membrane patch, the intracellular contents remain undisturbed. Here, acetylcholine in the pipette activates the I_{KACh}, which has a characteristic open time (τ_o) of 1 and a conductance (γ) of 40 picosiemens. In the inside-out mode (Panel B), after a cell-attached patch has been formed, the pipette is pulled away from the cell, ripping off a patch of membrane that forms an enclosed vesicle. The brief exposure to air disrupts only the free hemisphere of the membrane, leaving the formerly intracellular surface of the membrane exposed to the bath. Now the milieu of the intracellular surface of the channels can be altered. In this figure, adding purified $G_{\beta\gamma}$ protein to the exposed cytoplasmic surface activates the I_{KACh}. In the whole-cell mode (Panel C), after a cell-attached patch has been formed, a pulse of suction disrupts the membrane circumscribed by the pipette, making the entire intracellular space accessible to the pipette. Instead of disrupting the patch by suction, a pore-forming molecule, such as amphotericin B or nystatin, can be incorporated into the intact patch, allowing ions access to the interior of the cell but maintaining a barrier to larger molecules. In the figure, the net current (I_{KACh}) after the application of acetylcholine is shown. (Redrawn from Ackerman MJ, Clapham DE. Ion channels: basic science and clinical disease. *N Engl J Med.* 1997;336:1575-1586.)

Other Sites of Drug Action

In addition to the receptors discussed previously, drugs may bind to several other specific sites. In the kidney tubules, in particular, specific cell membrane ion pumps and carrier proteins act as sites of drug action. Many diuretics bind to Na^+ transporters in the renal tubules to block reabsorption of sodium. If Na^+ is not reabsorbed, water is lost (excreted), and plasma volume is decreased, resulting in a lowering of blood pressure.[16] Digoxin binds to the Na^+/K^+-adenosine triphosphatase pump in cardiac tissue to

inhibit it, ultimately resulting in greater contractility of the ventricles.[21]

Enzymes represent another target for drugs. Drugs that bind to acetylcholinesterase to inactivate it have been developed. This allows active acetylcholine to remain at the synaptic cleft longer to activate the neuromuscular junction. Drugs used in the treatment of myasthenia gravis work in this manner.[22]

Other targets for drugs include molecular targets that are not part of human cells. Some antibiotics bind to the bacterial ribosome and not to the similar

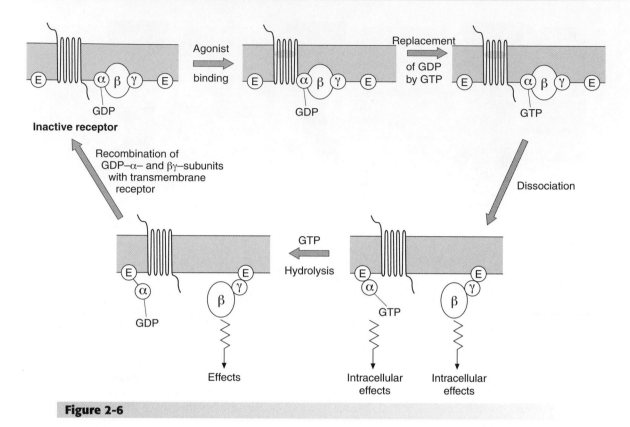

Figure 2-6

The functioning of G-protein subunits. Ligand binding results in replacement of guanosine diphosphate *(GDP)* on the α-subunit by guanosine triphospahte *(GTP)* and this is followed by dissociation of the α- and βγ-subunits, which affect a range of intracellular systems (shown as *E* on the figure) such as second messenger systems (e.g. adenylate cyclase and phospholipase C), other enzymes and ion channels. Hydrolysis of GTP inactivates the α-subunit, which then reforms the inactive transmembrane receptor. (From Waller DG, Renwick AG, Hillier K. *Medical Pharmacology Therapeutics.* New York: WB Saunders; 2001.)

organelle in humans. The same is true for antiviral agents in that they bind to viral DNA and RNA but not necessarily to the human nucleotides.[23]

DRUG-RECEPTOR INTERACTIONS

The binding of drugs to receptors has a certain **specificity** and **selectivity**. Drugs that act on only one type of receptor are considered specific for that receptor. For example, norepinephrine is specific for binding only to a sympathetic adrenergic receptor and not to a parasympathetic cholinergic receptor.[24] However, norepinephrine is not selective for only one subtype of adrenergic receptor. The β-adrenoceptor blocker propranolol is also specific for β-receptors but is not selective because it can bind both β_1- and β_2-adrenoceptors. Metoprolol, another β-adrenoceptor blocker, is selective in that it will bind preferentially

to β_1- and not β_2-receptors. However, as the concentration of a nonselective drug is increased, it will begin to bind to all subtypes of receptors. These concepts of specificity and selectivity are important because the more specific and selective a drug is, the more targeted the therapeutic approach can be. In addition, selective drugs tend to have fewer adverse effects than nonselective drugs.

Agonists and Antagonists

The strength of binding of a drug to a receptor can be illustrated both quantitatively and qualitatively. Drug binding experiments in which a radioactive ligand is used can be performed to measure binding affinity.[25] In these experiments, varying concentrations of the radioactive drug are incubated with the tissue containing the receptor of interest. The

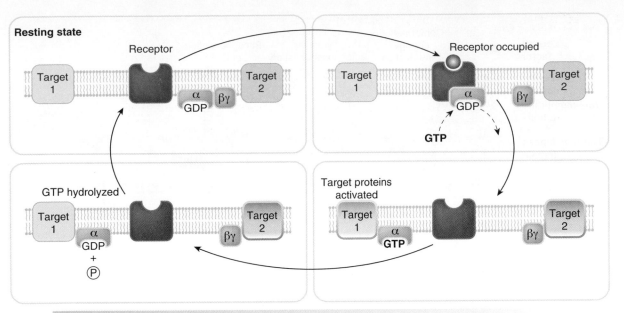

Figure 2-7

The function of the G-protein. The G-protein consists of three subunits (α, β, γ), which are anchored to the membrane through attached lipid residues. Coupling of the α-subunit to an agonist-occupied receptor causes the bound guanosine diphosphate *(GDP)* to exchange with intracellular guanosine triphosphate *(GTP);* the α-GTP complex then dissociates from the receptor and from the βγ-subunit complex and interacts with a target protein (target 1, which may be an enzyme such as adenylate cyclase or an ion channel). The βγ-complex may also activate a target protein (target 2). The guanosine triphosphatase (GTPase) activity of the α-subunit is increased when the target protein is bound, leading to hydrolysis of the bound GTP to GDP, whereupon the α-subunit reunites with the βγ-complex. The activated state of the target proteins is shown in color. (From Rang HP, Dale MM, Ritter JM, Gardner P. *Pharmacology.* 5th ed. New York: Churchill Livingstone; 2003.)

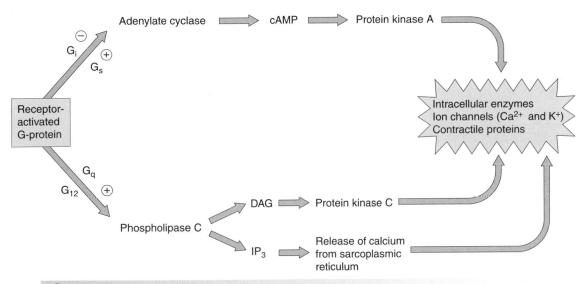

Figure 2-8

The intracellular consequences of receptor activation and G-protein dissociation. The G-proteins affect the second messenger systems and the changes in cAMP, cGMP, diacylglycerol *(DAG),* and inositol trisphosphate *(IP$_3$)* produce a number of intracellular changes directly, indirectly via actions on protein kinases (which change the activities of other proteins by phosphorylation), or by actions on ion channels, which alter the internal environment. (From Waller DG, Renwick AG, Hillier K. *Medical Pharmacology Therapeutics.* New York: WB Saunders; 2001.)

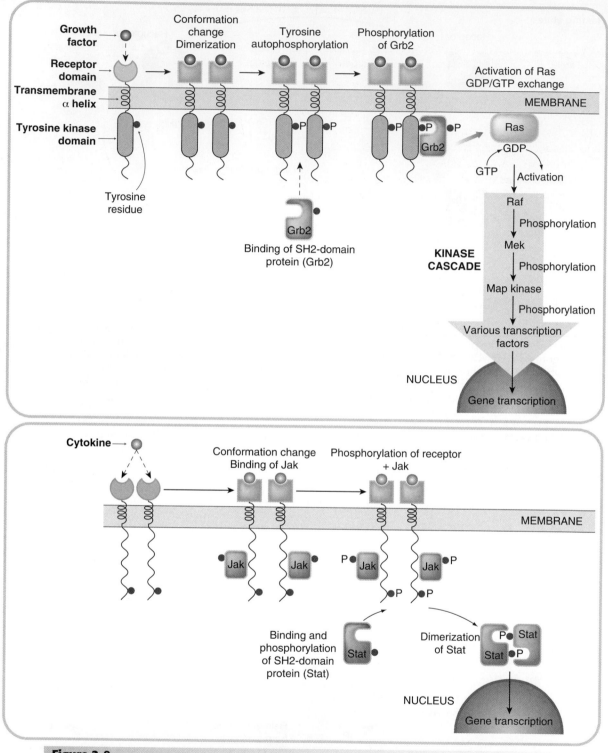

Figure 2-9

Transduction mechanisms of kinase-linked receptors. The first step following agonist binding is dimerization, which leads to autophosphorylation of the intracellular domain of each receptor. SH2 domain proteins then bind to the phosphorylated receptor and are themselves phosphorylated. Two well-characterized pathways are shown. **A,** The growth factor (Ras/Raf/MAP kinase) pathway; **B,** The cytokine (Jak/Stat) pathway. Several other pathways exist, and these phosphorylation cascades interact with components of G-protein systems. (From Rang HP, Dale MM, Ritter JM, Gardner P. *Pharmacology.* 5th ed. New York: Churchill Livingstone; 2003.)

tissue is then removed and analyzed for its radio-activity. A binding curve that shows the relationship between concentration and the amount of drug bound is then created. If two drugs are incubated with the receptor of interest, they may compete for occupation in the same receptor. In this case, each drug will reduce the binding affinity of the other drug. The first drug may be called the *agonist* in that it binds to the receptor and produces a change that triggers a response.[26] When the second drug is added, it may compete for receptor occupation with the first drug by blocking its access to the receptor and therefore its response and so may be labeled as the *antagonist*. Strictly speaking, however, an antagonist is defined as a ligand that binds to the receptor but does not cause the usual conformational change in the receptor. The effect of a reversible binding antagonist **(competitive antagonist)** can be overcome by using greater concentrations of the agonist, but the effect of a **noncompetitive antagonist** cannot be reversed by an additional concentration of an agonist. Noncompetitive antagonists block receptors permanently. In our example, the second drug might be a true antagonist or actually turn out to be a **partial agonist**. The partial agonist is a drug that might demonstrate both agonist and antagonist properties toward a receptor. At low concentrations it will trigger a response, but at high concentrations it will compete with the natural ligand by physically preventing access of that ligand to its receptor; therefore only a partial or submaximal response will be attained.

Dose-Response Curves

When a drug is administered to a patient, a certain response will occur. As the target cells become exposed to increasing concentrations of the drug, increasing numbers of receptors become activated, and the magnitude of the response increases. If we continue to increase the dose of the drug, the response grows until there is a maximal response. At this point, further increases in drug concentration produce no further response. Pharmacologists demonstrate this "drug receptor theory" by graphing a **dose-response curve** (Figure 2-10).[27]

In the dose-response curve, by convention, the dose is plotted on the x-axis and the response is plotted on the y-axis. These curves resemble rectangular hyperbolas. The plateau portion of this curve represents the **Emax** or the maximum response

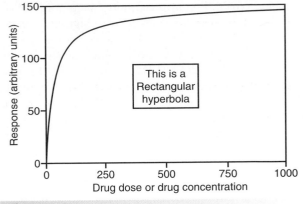

Figure 2-10

A typical dose-response curve. (Redrawn from Luty J, Harrison P. *Basic and Clinical Pharmacology Made Memorable.* Philadelphia: Churchill Livingstone; 1997.)

that can occur despite infinite concentrations.[28] The Emax is also a measure of drug **efficacy** or strength of the response. If two drugs that occupy the same proportion of receptors are compared, the drug with the higher Emax represents the one with greater efficacy, that is, greater maximal response. Full agonists produce a maximal response, but partial agonists produce only a submaximal response.

Because drugs produce responses over a wide range of doses, dose-response curves are usually transformed into log–dose-response curves by determining the logarithm of the dose (Figure 2-11).[28]

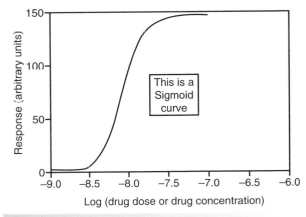

Figure 2-11

A typical log–dose-response curve. (Redrawn from Luty J, Harrison P. *Basic and Clinical Pharmacology Made Memorable.* Philadelphia: Churchill Livingstone; 1997.)

The new curve then approximates a sigmoid curve. The Emax is still obvious on the sigmoid curve, and the linear portion of this curve makes it easy to determine other parameters such as the **Kd** or median effective dose **(ED50).** The Kd is the dose that produces one half of the expected maximum, Emax, or the dose that produces 50% of the expected response. For the purposes of this book, Kd and ED_{50} can be viewed as representing the same concept. The Kd and ED_{50} are measures of potency. Potency is a measure of binding affinity. The more potent a drug is, the lower is the concentration needed to produce a certain response. When dose-response curves for two drugs are compared, the one with the lower Kd is the more potent drug (Figure 2-12).

The log–dose-response curve can also be used to display the concepts of competitive and non-competitive antagonists and partial agonists (Figures 2-13 and 2-14).[28] Competitive antagonists compete with the agonists for available receptors and make the agonists look less potent (shift of the log–dose-response curve to the right). Non-competitive antagonists cannot be displaced from the receptor and will block agonist effects permanently, thus reducing the Emax. Log–dose-response curves for the partial agonist look similar to those for the noncompetitive antagonist in that Emax is lowered.

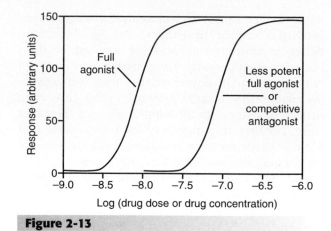

Figure 2-13

Log–dose-response curves. (Redrawn from Luty J, Harrison P. *Basic and Clinical Pharmacology Made Memorable.* Philadelphia: Churchill Livingstone; 1997.)

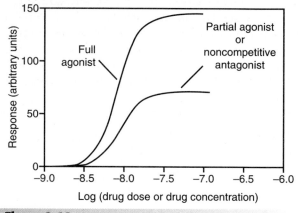

Figure 2-14

Log–dose-response curves. (Redrawn from Luty J, Harrison P. *Basic and Clinical Pharmacology Made Memorable.* Philadelphia: Churchill Livingstone; 1997.)

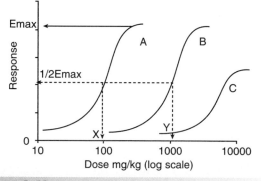

Figure 2-12

Graded dose-response curves for three drugs differing in affinity and maximal efficacies. The doses indicated by X and Y represent the dose of drug required to cause 50% of that drug's maximal effect. Drug A is about 10 times more potent than Drug B. Drug A and Drug B have greater efficacies than Drug C. (Redrawn from Flynn EJ. Pharmacodynamic and pharmacokinetic principles of pharmacology. *J Neurol Phys Ther.* 2003;27:94.)

DRUG SAFETY

Data obtained from studies examining dose-response relationships may be manipulated to reflect how drugs affect populations in terms of efficacy and safety. Pooling drug responses across many subjects and evaluating the final outcomes in terms of effectiveness help determine how safe a drug is expected to be. Quantal dose-response curves for effectiveness and for toxic effects are used to determine a therapeutic and safety index.

Quantal Dose-Response Curves

Dose-response curves represent graded responses to a drug taken by a single subject or by many subjects from a single population. A **quantal dose-response** curve is a variation on the dose-response curve that is used to examine discrete outcomes instead of a gradation of responses.[27,28] These curves are used to assess outcomes in heterogeneous populations and also help to assess the safety of drugs. Typically, two curves are established. The first is used to examine the beneficial effects of the drug, and the second, to examine the toxic or lethal effects of the drug. An example is a drug that is used to treat migraines. Increasing doses of drug are given to subjects to stop the headache, not just lessen the pain. For each dose, the number of subjects cured by the drug is recorded. One milligram of the drug may cure four subjects. Five milligrams may cure an additional six subjects. Ten milligrams may cure 12 more subjects. Additional amounts of the drug are given until all the subjects (100%) are relieved of headache (Figure 2-15). This bell-shaped curve can then be re-plotted as a cumulative percentage responding (y-axis) versus dose (x-axis). The second curve is determined by repeating the experiment, but this time, with greater drug concentrations. The outcome in this case is an unwanted effect, possibly death (theoretically only). The ED_{50} is determined for the first curve but for the curve representing unwanted effects, the lethal dose that kills 50% of the subjects taking the drug (LD_{50}) is determined. The bell-shaped curves are transformed into sigmoid curves and then graphed together on the same x- and y-axes, and the ED_{50} and LD_{50} are compared (Figure 2-16). If the two curves are far apart from each other, then the drug is considered relatively safe. This means that a much greater amount of the drug would have to be taken to kill the patient than to help the patient. Pharmacologists may also determine the toxic dose at 50% (TD_{50}), the dose that produces adverse effects as opposed to lethal effects in half of the population, so that the doses producing side effects are known.

Therapeutic Index

The **therapeutic index** (TI) describes the distance between a quantal dose-response curve for a desired effect and a quantal dose-response curve for the undesired drug effect. It is calculated as the ratio

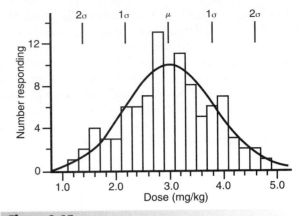

Figure 2-15

Quantal effects. Typical set of data after administration of increasing doses of drug to a group of subjects and observation of minimum dose at which each subject responds. Data shown are for 100 subjects; dose increased in 0.2 mg/kg of body weight increments. Mean (μ) (and median) dose is 3.0 mg/kg. Results plotted as histogram (bar graph) showing number responding to each dose; smooth curve is normal distribution function calculated for μ of 3.0 and $\bar{v}$ of 0.8. (Redrawn from Brody TM, Larner J, Minneman KP, eds. *Human Pharmacology: Molecular to Clinical.* Philadelphia: Mosby; 1998.)

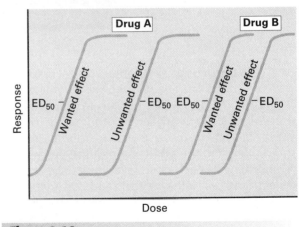

Figure 2-16

Dose-response curves for two hypothetical drugs. Drug X: the dose that brings out the maximum wanted effect is less than the lowest dose that produces the unwanted effect. The ratio ED50 (unwanted effect)/ED50 (wanted effect) indicates that drug X has a large therapeutic index; it is thus highly selective in its wanted action. Drug Y causes unwanted effects at doses well below those which produce its maximum benefit. The ratio ED50 (unwanted effect)/ED50 (wanted effect) indicates that the drug has a small therapeutic index; it is thus nonselective. (From Bennett PN, Brown MJ, eds. *Clinical Pharmacology.* 9th ed. New York: Churchill Livingstone; 2003:37-40.)

of the LD_{50} to the ED_{50}. The greater this value, the less lethal is the drug. Some drugs have very low TIs (e.g., lithium and digoxin).[29, 30] Patients taking drugs with low TIs, less than 2.5, must be monitored for adverse reactions.[31] Because it is likely that adverse events will occur, a "defined target plasma concentration" is used to determine proper dosing instead of some observable or toxic event.[31] An additional parameter, called the *safety margin*, is calculated as the ratio of the LD_{01} (dose that kills 1% of the subjects) to the ED_{99} (dose that is effective in 99% of the subjects). The safety margin is a more conservative measure of safety than the TI.

These measures of safety have some specific limitations. First, patients respond individually to medications. The TI does not take into consideration other drugs that a patient may be taking that could lead to a drug-drug interaction. Second, it is not always easy to decide on a measure of effectiveness. Patients and the medical community may not share the same definition of what is effective. Patients may want complete cessation of their migraine headaches, whereas physicians may interpret the drug as being successful if a patient is able to return to work even if some discomfort is still present. Third, data from toxicity studies come from experiments with animals, and thus the findings cannot be readily applied to the human population. Some social and economic factors also diminish the significance of the TI. Patient compliance issues such as failure to take prescribed medications as specified and borrowing or taking friends' drugs that are expired or issued at different doses are factors that may render a drug that is presumed to be safe, dangerous.

New methods are now being explored to help quantify the benefits and risks associated with drug use. One method is called the *number-needed-to-treat (NNT)*.[25] This method calculates the number of patients that must be exposed to a drug for one patient to experience the desired effect. It is hoped that this method will take into consideration individual variations among patients and provide a more realistic measure of drug safety, at least one that can be more easily explained to patients.

ACTIVITIES 2

■ 1. Constructing a quantal dose response curve. Groups of mice will receive varying doses of a drug used to lower heart rate. Some of the mice will have bradycardia, and some of the mice will have excessive bradycardia leading to death. Refer to the table and plot the percentage responding at each dose level for its therapeutic effect and its lethal effect and calculate the therapeutic index. Discuss whether the drug is safe. Describe a situation in which the therapeutic index may be misleading.

Dose (mg/kg)	Bradycardia	Death
1	0%	0%
2	3%	0%
3	13%	0%
4	45%	3%
5	80%	23%
6	100%	68%
7	100%	100%
8	100%	100%

■ 2. Discuss the difference between a medication's mechanism of action and its therapeutic effect.

References

1. Triggle DJ. Pharmacological receptors: a century of discovery—and more. *Pharm Acta Helv.* 2000;74:79-84.
2. Hille B. *Ionic Channels of Excitable Membranes.* Sunderland, Mass: Sinauer Associates Inc.; 1992.
3. Catterall WA. From ionic currents to molecular mechanisms: the structure and function of voltage-gated sodium channels. *Neuron.* 2000;26:13-25.
4. Lim PO, MacFayden RJ, Clarkson PBM, MacDonald TM. Impaired exercise tolerance in hypertensive patients. *Ann Intern Med.* 1996;124:41-55.
5. Bormann J. The 'ABC' of GABA receptors. *Trends Pharmacol Sci.* 2000;21:16-19.
6. Changeux J. Chemical signaling in the brain. *Sci Am.* 1993:58-62.
7. Macdonald RL, Olsen RW. GABA$_A$ receptor channels. *Annu Rev Neurosci.* 1994;17:569-602.
8. Unwin N. Acetylcholine receptor channel imaged in the open state. *Nature.* 1995;373:37-43.
9 Hamill OP, Neher ME, Sakmann B, Sigworth FJ. Improved patch-clamp techniques for high resolution current recording from cells and cell-free membrane patches. *Pflugers Arch.* 1981;391:85-100.
10. Ackerman MJ, Clapham DE. Ion channels: basic science and clinical disease. *N Engl J Med.* 1997;336:1575-1586.
11. Leonardi A, Sironi G, Motta G. Receptors in cardiovascular disease: review and introduction. *Pharm Acta Helv.* 2000;74:157-161.
12. Gualtieri F. Cholinergic receptors and neurodegenerative diseases. *Pharm Acta Helv.* 2000;74:85-89.
13. Hescheler J, Schultz G. Heterotrimeric G-proteins involved in the modulation of voltage-dependent calcium channels of neuroendocrine cells. *Ann NY Acad Sci.* 1994;733:306-312.
14. Wickman KD, Clapham DE. G-protein regulation of ion channels. *Curr Opin Neurobiol.* 1995;5:278-285.
15. Degtiar VE, Wittig B, Schultz G, Kalkbrenner F. A specific G(o) heterotrimer couples somatostatin receptors to voltage-gated calcium channels in RINm5F cells. *FEBS Lett.* 1996;380:137-141.
16. Waller DG, Renwick AG, Hillier K. *Medical Pharmacology Therapeutics.* New York: WB Saunders; 2001.
17. Wise A, Gearing K, Rees S. Target validation of G-protein coupled receptors. *Drug Discov Today.* 2002;7:235-246.
18. Bourguet W, Germain P, Gronemeyer H. Nuclear receptor ligand-binding domains: three-dimensional structures, molecular interactions and pharmacological implications. *Trends Pharmacol Sci.* 2000;21:381-388.
19. Rang HP, Dale MM, Ritter JM, Moore JL. *Pharmacology.* 5th ed. New York: Churchill Livingstone; 2003.
20. Bakheit AMO, Thilmann AF, Ward AB, et al. A randomized, double-blind, placebo-controlled, dose-ranging study to compare the efficacy and safety of three doses of botulinum toxin type A (Dysport) with placebo in upper limb spasticity after stroke. *Stroke.* 2000;31:2402-2406.
21. Akera T, Brody TM. Drugs to treat heart failure: cardiac glycosides. In: Brody TM, Larner J, Minneman KP, eds. *Human Pharmacology: Molecular to Clinical.* Philadelphia: Mosby; 1998:213-226.
22. Vincent A, Palace J, Hilton-Jones D. Myasthenia gravis. *Lancet.* 2001;357:2122-2128.
23. Thielman NM, Neu HC. Principles of antimicrobial use. In: Brody MJ, Larner J, Minneman KP, eds. *Human Pharmacology: Molecular to Clinical.* Philadelphia: Mosby; 1998:641-654.
24. Brody MJ, Garrison JC. Sites of action: receptors. In: Brody MJ, Larner J, Minneman KP, eds. *Human Pharmacology: Molecular to Clinical.* Philadelphia: Mosby; 1998:9-26.
25. Rang HP, Dale MM, Ritter JM, Gardner P. *Pharmacology.* 4th ed. New York: Churchill Livingstone; 2001.
26. Bennett PN, Brown MJ. General pharmacology. In: Bennett PN, Brown MJ, eds. *Clinical Pharmacology.* 9th ed. New York: Churchill Livingstone; 2003:37-40.
27. Pratt WB, Taylor P. *Principles of Drug Actions: The Basis of Pharmacology.* New York: Churchill Livingstone; 1992.
28. Brody MJ. Concentration-response relationships. In: Brody MJ, Larner J, Minneman KP, eds. *Human Pharmacology: Molecular to Clinical.* Philadelphia: Mosby; 1998:27-33.
29. Simard M, Gumbiner B, Lee A, Lewis H, Norman D. Lithium carbonate intoxication. a case report and review of the literature. *Arch Intern Med.* 1989;149:36-46.
30. Brody TM. Introduction and definitions. In: Brody TM, Larner J, Minneman KP, eds. *Human Pharmacology: Molecular to Clinical.* Philadelphia: Mosby; 1998:3-8.
31. Somogyi A. Clinical pharmacokinetics and dosing schedules. In: Brody TM, Larner J, Minneman KP, eds. *Human Pharmacology: Molecular to Clinical.* Philadelphia: Mosby; 1998:47-64.

CHAPTER 3

PHARMACOKINETICS AND DRUG DOSING

WHAT IS PHARMACOKINETICS?

Strictly defined, *pharmacokinetics* refers to the rate at which drug concentrations accumulate in and are eliminated from various organs of the body. It is what the body does to the drug, and in the liberal sense, encompasses how a drug is absorbed, distributed, metabolized, and ultimately eliminated from the body.[1] This chapter examines pharmacokinetics in the broad sense and includes discussion of the movement of drugs across cell membranes, routes of administration, and volume of distribution, as well as the more literal definition of *pharmacokinetics*—breakdown reactions and elimination. Each of these concepts may be explained both physiologically and mathematically. The mathematical description of pharmacokinetics determines the dosing schedules but because of the complex nature of the equations, our discussion on this topic will be simplified.

MOVEMENT OF DRUGS ACROSS CELL MEMBRANES

As drugs move from their site of administration to their target tissue, they cross many biological barriers. These barriers or cell membranes are commonly bilayers of lipid molecules with hydrophilic regions on the outside and inside layers of the membrane and a hydrophobic region between the two layers.[2] Lipid-soluble molecules are able to diffuse readily into cells across this membrane. Water-filled channels are also found, through which water-soluble substances of small size may cross. In addition, special proteins called *carrier proteins* that allow passage of specific substances are interspersed throughout the membrane. Depending on the location, more or less of these water-soluble channels and carrier proteins exist; for example, the jejunum contains many channels and carriers, whereas the urinary bladder has few.

Drugs cross membranes in four main ways: (1) **pinocytosis**, (2) **diffusion** through the water-filled channels or specialized ion channels, (3) carrier-mediated processes that include **facilitated diffusion** or **active transport**, and (4) **passive diffusion** through the lipid membrane (Figure 3-1).[3] The method of pinocytosis has limited usefulness for drug transport at this time because it is primarily concerned with the uptake of macromolecules. However, certain drugs have been incorporated into a lipid vesicle or liposome, necessitating the use of this method for drug transfer.[3-5] Passage of drugs through ion channels occurs for very small molecules such as therapeutic ions (e.g., lithium and radioactive iodide).[2,6] If such small molecules pass through the water-filled pores, they must be water-soluble. The impetus for drug transfer for this process is a concentration gradient. Carrier-mediated processes are involved in movement of drugs across the blood-brain barrier, the gastrointestinal (GI) epithelium, and the renal tubules. This method involves a transmembrane protein that binds to a drug, changes conformation (shape), and then releases the molecule on the other side of the membrane. When this process is passive, it is called *facilitated diffusion*. The drug in this case must resemble a natural ligand and travel from an area of high concentration to one of low

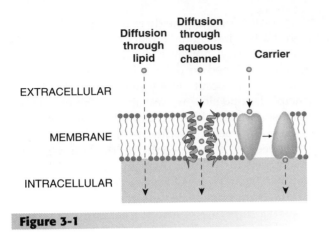

Figure 3-1

Routes by which solutes can traverse cell membranes. (Molecules can also cross cellular barriers by pinocytosis.) (From Rang HP, Dale MM, Ritter JM, Moore, PK. *Pharmacology.* 5th ed. New York: Churchill Livingstone; 2003.)

concentration. Levodopa, a drug used for the treatment of Parkinson's disease, is transferred through the duodenum and jejunum and across the blood-brain barrier by facilitated diffusion by means of a large neutral amino acid–specific carrier system.[7] In the renal tubules, many drugs act by binding to carrier proteins.[8] When binding is strong, the molecule is released slowly; therefore the actual drug action is to block carrier function. Many diuretics act in this manner and prevent the reabsorption of sodium.[9] When a drug requires transport against a concentration gradient, energy is required and it is called *active transport.*

Passive Diffusion of Drugs Across Lipid Membranes

Passive diffusion down a concentration gradient is the primary method by which drugs cross membranes.[10] Nonpolar neutral molecules dissolve easily in lipids and therefore traverse cell membranes without difficulty. Fick's law describes this passive diffusion as a function of the concentration difference across the membrane, the thickness of the membrane, and the permeability coefficient, P. The greater the concentration difference between the two sides of the membrane, the greater will be the rate of diffusion. In addition, the thicker the membrane, the more slowly the drug will cross.

The permeability coefficient is unique to each drug and depends on certain physicochemical

factors such as its lipid solubility and degree of ionization. Lipid solubility is determined by the molecule's **partition coefficient**.[11] There is a close correlation between the partition coefficient and the compound's solubility, and this correlation is an important factor in determining the drug's rate of absorption and elimination. Thiopental is a sedative-hypnotic agent that is used as an anesthetic. It has an effective partition coefficient value of 2000.[11] This drug is extremely soluble in lipids, allowing for rapid diffusion across the lipid-rich blood-brain barrier to produce a quick loss of consciousness (within seconds). Pentobarbital is also a sedative-hypnotic agent that has a coefficient of 42. It is less lipid soluble and therefore diffuses into the brain at a slower rate than thiopental. It has been used for its preanesthetic effect of reducing anxiety and facilitating anesthesia induction when given along with other barbiturates. Barbital, another sedative-hypnotic agent, has a coefficient value of 1.1. This drug is much less membrane soluble than either thiopental or pentobarbital, and thus diffusion is slower. It was prescribed for people who could fall asleep but had trouble staying asleep. Barbital and pentobarbital are rarely used now for sleep disturbances or anxiety because of their addictive quality, but the issue of lipid solubility is well illustrated by these drugs.

Even if a drug is lipid soluble, its molecular weight may preclude absorption from the GI tract. Molecules of drugs such as insulin are simply too large to pass through the GI mucosa; therefore these drugs must be administered by injection.[12]

Many drugs are weak acids or bases and therefore can exist in both an unionized (electrically neutral) and ionized (either a positive or negative charge) form. The problem is that ionized molecules have very low lipid solubility. However, the degree of ionization depends on the pH of the local environment and the negative logarithm of the acid ionization constant (pK_a) of the compound.[1] In an acidic environment such as the stomach, weak acids will exist in an uncharged or neutral state (Figure 3-2). Thus drugs like aspirin that are acidic will be absorbed from this area. However, in the intestine where the pH is greater, the compound would tend to give off hydrogen and thus exist in an ionized state. In the stomach, basic drugs will more likely exist in a charged form but be neutral in the intestine. The loss of protons in the small intestine will increase the percentage of neutral molecules

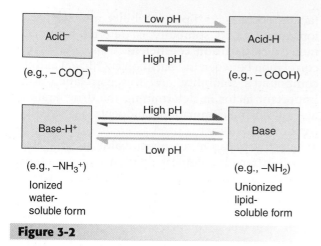

Figure 3-2

The effect of pH on drug ionization. (From Waller DG, Renwick AG, Hillier K. *Medical Pharmacology and Therapeutics.* New York: WB Saunders; 2002.)

and thus aid in drug absorption into the circulation. However, in the intestine, neutrality is not the only parameter influencing absorption, because the very large surface area for absorption is also a determining factor in how a drug gets through the mucosal surface.

DRUG ABSORPTION AND ROUTES OF ADMINISTRATION

Drug absorption is the process by which the drug is transferred from its site of administration to the systemic circulation.[2] The efficiency and ease of this process depends on the physicochemical properties of drugs as discussed previously but also depends on route of administration including oral, intravenous (IV), intramuscular, inhalation, sublingual, subcutaneous, and topical applications.

Absorption from the Gastrointestinal Tract

Oral administration of drugs with absorption occurring from the GI tract is the most convenient and most favored route of administration by patients. Medicines that are absorbed in this manner are dispensed in tablet, capsule, or syrup form. However, a number of factors make this method one of the most complex ways of giving medications.

The drug formulation influences the rate of absorption because the tablet or capsule must disintegrate, releasing the drug into the GI contents before absorption can take place.[2] Most tablets will dissolve quickly; however, some formulations are specially designed to delay disintegration so that absorption can occur slowly over time. This is the principle behind slow-release agents. Tablets coated with a semipermeable membrane will demonstrate delayed absorption. Additionally, tablets may be formulated to dissolve only in the intestines to prevent gastric irritation. Aspirin coated in an acid-insoluble layer (enteric-coated) delays absorption until the drug reaches the intestine.

Gastric emptying is also influential on the rate at which drugs are absorbed. If gastric emptying is hastened, then the drug will be delivered to the small intestine more quickly and enhance absorption. Co-administration of cholinomimetic agents (drugs that stimulate the parasympathetic system) will speed gastric emptying.[2] However, excessive motility will decrease absorption. The presence of food in the GI tract tends to delay absorption, although there are exceptions (e.g., propranolol) that undergo greater absorption with food, probably as a result of increased splanchnic blood flow after a meal.[2]

Breakdown of drugs may occur in the GI tract before or during absorption. The intestinal lumen and wall contain many enzymes such as monoamine oxidase and L-aromatic amino acid decarboxylase, CYP3A, which are responsible for the breakdown of many drugs.[2] In addition, the GI bacteria and the very acidic environment of the stomach contribute to reduced absorption. Penicillin G is unstable in the low pH of the stomach, and therefore very large oral doses would need to be given to patients if this were the preferred route of administration. Instead, this drug is administered intravenously.[13] Because there is loss of the drug in the GI tract before absorption, only a fraction of the given oral dose actually enters the systemic circulation. The term to describe this fraction is **bioavailability**. Bioavailability refers to the percentage of drug that makes it into the systemic circulation from the site of administration, taking into consideration early degradation. It is more of a conceptual image than an exact percentage because bioavailability is variable and may be altered by the local pH, intestinal motility, and presence of food. However, drugs that typically exhibit low bioavailability are either given by injection or administered to the patient with special instructions. Alendronate is a drug that reduces bone absorption, commonly given to postmenopausal women with osteoporosis. This drug is only 1% to 10% bioavailable, and for this reason, patients are asked to take the drug on an empty stomach, 30 minutes before eating.[14] When a drug is administered intravenously, 100% of it is bioavailable because all of it enters the systemic circulation.

Even if a compound makes it through the intestinal wall into the portal circulation, a significant amount of drug may undergo metabolism in the liver before it ever arrives at the target organ. This is referred to as *first-pass metabolism* or *first-pass elimination*.[2] When a drug is administered orally, its first stop after the GI tract is the liver. Because the liver is considered the primary organ of drug metabolism, some of the drug is degraded before it makes its entrance systemically. In fact, every time the drug cycles through the liver, approximately 20% is potentially metabolized because that is the percentage of cardiac output that enters the organ.[15] First-pass metabolism can be avoided if a drug is administered by any route other than the oral route (e.g., through a topical patch, intranasal administration, or IV infusion).

Enteral Drug Administration

Enteral administration refers to drugs being administered anywhere along the GI tract. This includes **oral**, **sublingual**, and **rectal administration**. However, some pharmacologists do not consider sublingual and rectal administration to be enteral because both methods avoid intestinal absorption.[15] Sublingual absorption refers to passage of drug through the buccal or sublingual mucosa. The classic example is sublingual nitroglycerin, which is placed under the tongue and absorbed rapidly into the venous drainage from the mouth to enter the superior vena cava within 1 to 3 minutes.[16] However, the patient must be able to tolerate the taste and also the irritation to the mucous membranes.

Rectal drugs take the form of solutions, suspensions, or suppositories. The rectal mucosa is rich in blood and lymph vessels and offers absorption free from first-pass metabolism. An advantage of this route of administration is that it can be used for a patient who is vomiting or experiencing motion sickness or migraine. It is also a good choice for a patient who cannot swallow or for a child who is uncooperative. The disadvantage is that rectal absorption is inconsistent.

Parenteral Drug Administration

Parenteral administration refers to administration of drugs in any manner other than through the GI tract; however, some pharmacologists exclude topical and inhalation administration from this category.[17] The parenteral route can then be considered the route that requires some type of injection including **IV**, **subcutaneous**, **intramuscular**, **epidural**, and **intrathecal** injections. Absorption from all but the IV method occurs by passive diffusion along the drug's concentration gradient but is limited by the density of absorbing capillaries and the solubility of the drug in the interstitial fluid. IV administration of drugs avoids the absorption phase because the correct concentration of medication is injected immediately into the blood. However, the major disadvantage to this method is that if the wrong amount of drug is injected, there is no recourse. Pumping the stomach or administering an emetic drug will not change the outcome of an overdose given intravenously. However, to avoid a catastrophe, it is recommended that IV injections be performed slowly, preferably over a period of 1 to 2 minutes. The circulation time between the antecubital vein and the brain is about 10 to 15 seconds, so if a sudden loss of consciousness occurs, presumably the infusion can be stopped before the complete dose enters the circulation.[11] In addition, there is the risk of local venous thrombosis with prolonged infusion and infection at the site of an IV catheter.

A subcutaneous injection is when the drug is given under the skin into the fat or connective tissue. This method is effective only for drugs that are nonirritating to the tissues. It is a useful method for self-administration, but if repeated injections are given at one site, lipoatrophy may occur. This is particularly true for insulin injections.[18] In addition, absorption may be variable because the rate may be slowed by immobilization of the limb or cooling of the area causing vasoconstriction. In contrast, heating and massage of an area that has received an injection will facilitate absorption of a drug.[19] Thus caution is necessary when physical therapy heat modalities are used near an area of the body that has been injected.

An intramuscular injection is drug administration by injection directly into skeletal muscle. Because muscles have greater blood flow, absorption is more rapid than for subcutaneous injections. The disadvantage to this method is that injection into an exercising muscle must be avoided because the increase in blood flow with activity will hasten absorption. In addition, this method is painful and often difficult to self-administer. Rapid absorption, particularly of insulin, could lead to fatal hypoglycemia.[20]

Intrathecal injections use the cerebrospinal fluid for drug transport. An intrathecal injection is given directly into the spinal subarachnoid space, facilitating drug entry into the central nervous system. Epidural injections deliver drug within the spinal column but outside the dura. Other parenteral routes include intraarticular (delivery into a synovial cavity), intraosseous (delivery into the bone marrow), intraarterial (delivery into an artery), and intraperitoneal (delivery into the peritoneal cavity). There are also implanted delivery systems, which consist of a pump and drug reservoir implanted in the belly. Insulin, morphine, and baclofen may be delivered in this manner.[18,21,22]

Other Routes of Drug Administration

The lungs have a large surface area and an extensive capillary network, which is excellent for drug absorption.[2] Inhaled anesthetics can be rapidly taken up into the circulation and distributed to the brain for quick induction of sleep. In addition, drugs such as bronchodilators that are used to stop an asthma attack can be inhaled directly into the bronchiole tubules, the target tissue, for effective treatment.

Topical applications of drugs are useful for the treatment of skin, ear, nose, and eye disorders. The advantage of this method is treatment without a systemic effect, although if the agent is applied in a great enough concentration, these effects will occur.

Special transdermal delivery systems have been engineered with a "rate-controlling membrane" specifically to introduce drug through the skin into the circulation and bypass the liver.[15] Scopolamine skin patches for the prevention of motion sickness and fentanyl skin patches for the treatment of pain are examples. Transdermal systems are also used to administer estrogens and nitroglycerin.

Exercise and Absorption

Neither the effects of exercise on pharmacological action nor the impact of administration on the body's response to exercise and exercise performance have been well studied for many drugs. It is not typical to assess the impact of exercise during clinical trials; hence, data on dosing with exercise do not become apparent until after the drug has been approved. Antibiotic-induced Achilles tendinopathy specifically associated with ciprofloxacin did not receive attention until years after the drug was out of clinical trials.[23,24]

Data on exercise studies are presented throughout this text as individual drugs are considered. However, a few points regarding absorption can be discussed at this time. Exercise does appear to affect drug absorption, but this is variable. Theoretically, exercise should reduce absorption of orally administered drugs because the increased kinetic movement of a drug across the GI mucosa (increased tissue heat during exercise will increase kinetic molecular movement) may be offset by a reduction in splanchnic blood flow. However, research has not supported this notion. In a study of 10 patients with Parkinson's disease receiving levodopa, absorption was decreased in five patients, increased in three patients, and unchanged in two patients during cycling exercise.[25] In another study, blood levodopa levels were related to unified Parkinson's disease rating scales with and without exercise in 10 patients with the disease.[26] This study revealed that exercise begun at 1 hour after levodopa ingestion did not influence motor scores or plasma level of the drug, indicating that absorption was not affected. Yet another study on levodopa indicated improved absorption after 2 hours of cycling exercise in 12 patients with Parkinson's disease.[27] Therefore at least for levodopa, we cannot state with any certainty the effect of exercise on absorption of this drug. Exercise, however, was shown to reduce midazolam (an anxiolytic agent) absorption in six healthy volunteers after 50 minutes of treadmill running.[28] Therefore the effect of exercise on absorption of orally administered drugs is variable and probably depends on exercise intensity and mode, fitness of the patient, drug properties, and presence or absence of any other medical condition.

Other reports in the literature indicate that exercise has no significant effect on the absorption of oral drugs but does increase absorption from intramuscular, subcutaneous, transdermal, and inhalation sites of administration.[29] Intramuscular, subcutaneous, and transdermal preparations will show increased absorption when applied near an exercising muscle, and absorption may be delayed if preparations are applied far away from an exercising muscle because of the shift in blood flow toward the exercising limb. This is particularly important for insulin-dependent diabetics to understand because, as mentioned previously, a sudden increase in insulin absorption may cause fatal hypoglycemia.[20] Injection sites must be far from the exercising tissues. Increased skin temperature and skin hydration occurring with exercise may be helpful for the patient with a transdermal nitroglycerin patch, especially if the patient experiences angina with activity. However, there is also the risk that exercise-induced vasodilation will lead to hypotension and syncope because of more rapid absorption.[30]

DISTRIBUTION OF DRUGS

Once a drug enters the systemic circulation, it is distributed throughout the body. This begins the second phase of pharmacokinetics called *distribution*.[3] The drug may be distributed to different parts of the body, interstitial and intracellular fluids, and extravascular tissues. The rate at which this occurs depends on a variety of factors including organ blood flow, degree of drug ionization in the different compartments, the binding to plasma proteins, molecular weight, lipid solubility, and any local metabolism that takes place at any tissue other than the target organ.

If a drug is given intravenously, the initial distribution is related to blood flow. The brain, heart, liver, and kidneys are among the most highly perfused organs and therefore receive most of the drug soon after it is administered.[1] Distribution to the muscle, skin, and fat takes longer, and the drug may not reach equilibration for several hours in these tissues (Figure 3-3). Agents that are very lipid soluble are initially distributed to the brain first and then slowly diffuse out into the body to reach other lipid tissues. Later, the drug may diffuse out of the fat and back into the brain. This produces the hungover feeling that patients experience after awakening from anesthesia. Patients who have the same body mass but more fat tissue may need to have their dose adjusted for very lipid-soluble medications because at one time there may be more drug in the fat tissue than free drug available to act at the target tissue. At some later time, however, the drug will diffuse back into the circulation, prolonging some of its effects.

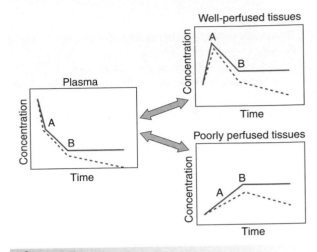

Figure 3-3

A simplified scheme for the redistribution of drugs between tissues. The initial decrease in plasma concentrations results from uptake into well-perfused tissues, which essentially reaches equilibrium at point A. Between points A and B, the drug continues to enter poorly perfused tissues, which results in a decrease in the concentrations in both plasma and well-perfused tissues. At point B, all tissues are in equilibrium. The scheme has been simplified by representing the phases as discreet linear steps and also by the omission of any removal process. The presence of a removal process would produce a parallel decrease in all tissues from point B (shown as ------). (From Waller DG, Renwick AG, Hillier K. *Medical Pharmacology and Therapeutics.* New York: WB Saunders; 2002.)

Binding to Plasma Proteins

Distribution also depends on the presence of plasma proteins. Albumin is a plasma protein that binds particularly to acidic drugs. Once a drug binds to albumin, it is temporarily unable to interact with the target tissue, because only free drug can produce a response. Drugs that bind to plasma proteins tend to have more drug-drug interactions because of competition for binding sites. In addition, proteins act as drug depots. Warfarin, an anticoagulant, binds readily to albumin. If a second drug that also exhibits strong binding to albumin is taken, the warfarin will be displaced, and a greater than normal amount of drug will be suddenly free to act on its target tissue, causing the patient to hemorrhage.[31]

Many basic drugs bind to α_1-acid glycoprotein. Unfortunately, the concentration of this globulin is variable and increases with age, inflammation, and

Table 3-1

Examples of Drugs that Undergo Extensive Plasma Protein Binding and May Show Therapeutically Important Interactions	
Bound to Albumin	**Bound to α_1-Acid Glycoprotein**
Clofibrate	Chlorpromazine
Digitoxin	Propranolol
Furosemide (frusemide)	Quinidine
Ibuprofen	Tricyclics
Indometacin (indomethacin)	Lidocaine
Phenytoin	
Salicylates	
Sulfonamides	
Thiazides	
Tolbutamide	
Warfarin	

From Waller DG, Renwick AG, Hillier K. *Medical Pharmacology and Therapeutics.* New York: WB Saunders; 2002.

other illnesses. Table 3-1 presents examples of drugs that show extensive binding to plasma proteins.

The presence of disease may alter the protein binding of many drugs. In cirrhosis of the liver, hypoalbuminemia will exist, leaving more drugs in their free, unbound state to exert harmful influences.[1] Therefore it is important that drug dose be adjusted in the presence of chronic illness.

Blood-Brain and Placental Barriers

Lipid-soluble drugs, such as the anesthetic agent thiopental, easily pass into the brain.[31] However, water-soluble drugs have a very difficult time entering this organ. This fact has led to the concept of a blood-brain barrier. Many areas of the brain have tight junctions between capillary endothelial cells and fewer and smaller aqueous pores available for drug diffusion. The only way for a water-soluble drug to enter the brain is via a specific carrier or injection into the cerebrospinal fluid.

The placenta is much less of a barrier than the brain. It is essentially assumed that all drugs cross over from the maternal circulation to the fetus, although not all drugs exert harmful influences.

Drug diffusion, however, is delayed as a result of limited placental blood flow. This means that if a woman receives a drug during pregnancy, the drug would not be detected in the fetal circulation for several minutes. The mother then can receive drugs just before delivery without crossover to the baby.

METABOLISM

Metabolism, also called *biotransformation,* is the third phase of pharmacokinetics and refers to how a drug is inactivated and prepared for elimination.[31] This phase primarily takes place in the liver with the goal of decreasing the drug's pharmacological activity and lipid solubility. Reducing lipid solubility is crucial to this process because the compound must be polar to be excreted via the kidney tubules. If this were not the case, the compound would be reabsorbed back into the circulation and be redistributed to target tissues. Drug metabolism involves two processes that usually occur sequentially and are labeled **phase I** and **phase II** reactions (Figure 3-4).

Phase I Metabolism

Phase I reactions are catabolic and involve oxidation, reduction, or hydrolysis reactions, with oxidation occurring most frequently. Most of these reactions are catalyzed by a group of enzymes known as the cytochrome P450 monooxygenases.[32] Several hundred isoforms of these enzymes are found primarily in the liver, although they are active in the lungs, kidneys, and GI tract as well. A specific nomenclature has been developed to help identify these P450 enzymes, beginning with the capital letters *CYP*. The next few numbers indicate the isoform family, subfamily, and gene product (Table 3-2).

Although the goal of metabolism is to inactivate a drug, sometimes a more active metabolite is created. A good example of this is the sedative diazepam, which converts to desmethyldiazepam during phase I reactions and increases the overall duration of drug activity.[33] Some drugs are administered in a prodrug form, which is then converted into the active substance only after it interacts with the enzymes.

A variety of individual variations in P450 enzymes influence drug development and therapeutics. Differences between species limit the types

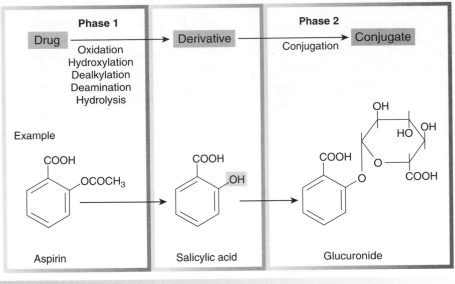

Figure 3-4

The two phases of drug metabolism. (From Rang HP, Dale MM, Ritter JM, Moore, PK. *Pharmacology.* 5th ed. New York: Churchill Livingstone; 2003.)

Table 3-2

Examples of Common Drugs That Are Substrates for P450 Isoenzymes	
Isoenzyme P450	**Drug**
CYP1A1	Theophylline
CYP1A2	Caffeine, paracetamol, tacrine, theophylline
CYP2A6	Methoxyflurane
CYP2C8	Taxol
CYP2C9	Ibuprofen, phenytoin, tolbutamide, warfarin
CYP2C19	Omeprazole
CYP2D6	Clozapine, codeine, debrisoquine, metoprolol
CYP2E1	Alcohol, enflurane, halothane
CYP3A4/5	Cyclosporine, losartan, nifedipine, terfenadine

From Pichard L, et al. Predictability of drug metabolism from in vitro studies. In: Alván G, Balant LP, Bechtel PR, Boobis AR, Gram LF, Paintaud G, Pithan K, eds. *COST B1 Conference on Variability and Specificity in Drug Metabolism.* Luxembourg: European Commission; 1995:45-46.

of animals that can be used for testing. There are also differences in these enzymes among the human population, resulting in variations in response to drugs.[34,35] In addition, enzyme inhibitors and inducers in the environment and diet may have huge effects on therapeutic outcomes. For example, cigarette smoke and cruciferous vegetables (e.g., broccoli and cabbage) are inducers of these enzymes. Essentially, this means that the activity of the microsomal enzymes is increased, which in turn hastens drug metabolism. Grapefruit juice acts to inhibit the P450 enzymes, which in turn inhibit drug metabolism.[36] The risk in this case is that plasma levels of the drug will increase and might reach a toxic level. In addition, sometimes two drugs will compete for the same P450 enzyme and slow the rate of metabolism for one or both drugs, which is also considered enzyme inhibition. This will result in higher than normal drug plasma levels, producing an adverse event. Some drugs, such as phenobarbital, when given on a long-term basis, can induce their own metabolism, producing drug tolerance.[37] Tolerance is defined as needing increasing amounts of a drug to produce an effect. Patients presenting with variations in their P450 enzymes are referred to as either "fast metabolizers" or "slow metabolizers."

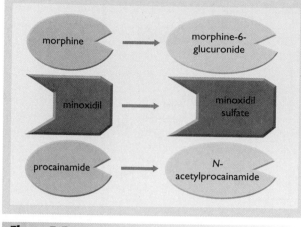

Figure 3-5

Examples of conjugations that result in the production of active drug metabolites. (From Page C, Curtis MJ, Sutter MC, Walker MJ, Hoffman BB, eds. *Integrated Pharmacology*. 2nd ed. 2002. Philadelphia: Mosby; 2002.)

Phase II Metabolism

In phase II, the drug undergoes conjugation reactions.[1] Hydrophilic groups such as glucuronic acid, glutathione, acetate, and sulfate groups become attached to the drug molecule. In general, these reactions inactivate the compound and make it less lipid soluble; however, there are some exceptions (Figure 3-5).

DRUG ELIMINATION

Drugs are eliminated from the body by a variety of routes. Elimination in fluids occurs through urine, breast milk, saliva, tears, and sweat.[15] Drugs can also be eliminated through the GI tract in the feces and expelled in exhaled air through the lungs. Renal and fecal excretion are the most common ways in which drugs are excreted from the body.

Renal Excretion

Many drug molecules undergo glomerular filtration to enter the tubular fluid. In addition, a small amount of drug may be secreted into the tubular fluid by nonselective carriers, especially if glomerular filtration is compromised, as it is in renal diseases. If a compound is sufficiently polar, it remains in the tubular fluid and is excreted with urine. However, lipid-soluble compounds in the tubular fluid are

often reabsorbed back into the circulation for another go-around at metabolism.

The degree of drug ionization also influences renal excretion. Basic drugs will become ionized in the acidic urine and will be readily excreted. Acidic drugs will become neutral in this environment and will be subject to reabsorption. However, the urine can be artificially alkalinized with oral or parenteral doses of bicarbonate to facilitate excretion in an overdose situation.[2]

Fecal Excretion

Uptake of drug into the hepatocytes and elimination in bile is the favored route of elimination for large-molecular-weight compounds.[15] Once a drug has entered the intestine with the bile fluids, it will be eliminated in feces. Enterohepatic recycling may occur if the drug escapes once again to the portal vein (Figure 3-6).

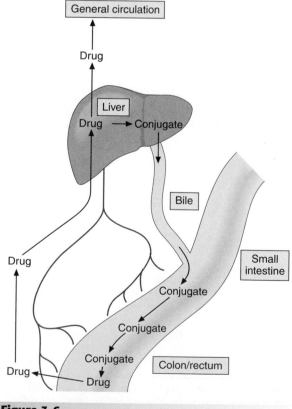

Figure 3-6

Enterohepatic circulation of drugs. (From Waller DG, Renwick AG, Hillier K. *Medical Pharmacology and Therapeutics*. New York: WB Saunders; 2002.)

MATHEMATICAL BASIS OF PHARMACOKINETICS

It is important clinically to determine the time required for drug effects to be displayed, the time course of drug action, and the concentrations of the drug in a variety of body compartments to determine the proper dosing schedule. For this determination, two models have been developed.[1] The first assumes that the body is a single uniform compartment and that a drug, when administered, is immediately distributed equally throughout the space. This model can be used to demonstrate elimination of an IV drug. A graph of the plasma drug concentration versus time shows that the elimination rate is proportional to the plasma concentration and results in an exponential loss described by a specific rate constant (Figure 3-7). The slope of this line is equal to the rate constant 2.303. The number 2.303 comes from conversion of the natural logarithm of plasma concentration into the logarithm to a base 10. The mathematical formulas that describe this elimination of drug determine how long it takes for the drug at some initial concentration to be eliminated from the body. The concentration of drug at any time after dosing depends on its clearance,

which is equal to clearance by metabolism and clearance by renal excretion. The problem with using a one-compartment model for describing drug elimination is that it does not take into account elimination of drug from other body compartments that takes longer. Additionally, this model does not take into consideration incomplete absorption of an orally administered drug. Often, there are two phases of elimination, a fast one, followed by a slow decline in drug concentration (Figure 3-8). The initial

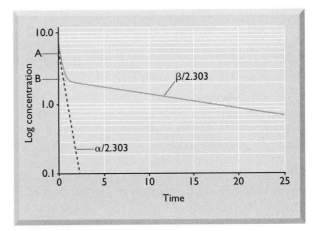

Figure 3-8

A plot of log plasma drug concentration versus time for a two-compartment open model after an intravenous bolus dose. The terminal disposition rate is β and not k_{el}, and the decreasing plasma concentration with time reflects a more complex relationship between drug distribution and elimination. The initial more rapid decline in circulating drug concentration (α) primarily reflects redistribution of the drug to the peripheral compartment (V_p) plus a modest component of elimination. The terminal, apparently linear, phase of plasma concentration versus time is a composite of drug elimination buffered by drug returning from V_p to the central compartment in which the drug distributes rapidly (V_p) to decrease the apparent rate of drug removal from the blood plasma. The phase is therefore referred to as the β phase. Extrapolation back to time zero provides an intercept (B). The extrapolated values of β are subtracted from the observed concentrations of drug at the same time after the dose and the residual values are plotted. A linear regression through these residual data points provides a slope (α) and a time zero intercept (A), that reflect a drug distribution into V_p. If the discrepancy between β and k_{el} is large, a greater error will arise from assuming that a one-compartment model is valid. (From Page C, Curtis MJ, Sutter MC, Walker MJ, Hoffman BB, eds. *Integrated Pharmacology*. 2nd ed. 2002. Philadelphia: Mosby; 2002.)

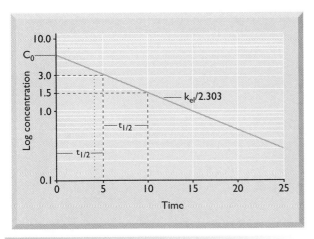

Figure 3-7

A graph of the log of the plasma drug concentration versus time with a one-compartment open pharmacokinetic model for drug disposition after an intravenous dose. Extrapolation of the line (slope is k_{el}) to time 'zero' results in an estimate of the initial drug concentration (C_0) in the compartment if distribution were instantaneous. (From Page C, Curtis MJ, Sutter MC, Walker MJ, Hoffman BB, eds. *Integrated Pharmacology*. 2nd ed. 2002. Philadelphia: Mosby; 2002.)

rapid decline in drug concentration corresponds with drug leaving the plasma compartment and being redistributed to the peripheral compartment, fat, muscle, and other tissues. The slower elimination phase corresponds to drug being eliminated from the body and also being redistributed back into the central or plasma compartment. This is a much more complicated analysis that takes into account redistribution of drug in and out of different tissues and compartments.

First-Order Elimination

A noncompartmental model has also been developed; it resembles the one-compartment model but examines the area under the curve in a plasma concentration versus time graph (Figure 3-9).[1] The curve is analyzed and subjected to equations that determine the time in which predictable amounts of drug are eliminated. This analysis has been used to determine that for most drugs, the rate of elimination is proportionate to the concentration. This principle is called *first-order elimination.*

Drugs with first-order elimination have a characteristic **half-life of elimination ($t_{1/2}$)** in that 50% of the drug is lost per unit of time.[31] If a patient is taking a drug with a $t_{1/2}$ of 4 hours and 10,000 units of the drug are given initially, then in 4 hours, the plasma concentration will be equal to 5000 units. In another 4 hours, the concentration will be down to 2500

units, and in 4 more hours (total of 12 hours since drug administration), the plasma concentration will be down to 1250 units.

First-Order Elimination and Dosing

Appropriate dosing must take into consideration the level of drug necessary to produce an effective response versus the level of drug that produces toxic effects. Usually, the dose given to patients is the one necessary to produce a response. However, because elimination is always going on, it takes time for the drug level to reach **steady state**, that is, when the amount excreted in a specified period is equal to the amount of drug administered. Steady state is usually achieved within 4 or 5 half-lives (Figure 3-10).[17] Therefore a drug with a $t_{1/2}$ of 6 hours will reach its steady state in approximately 24 to 30 hours. If this waiting period is unacceptable, then the effective response may be achieved earlier with a loading dose. The maintenance dose then reflects plasma clearance and the desired time interval between doses. In general, a drug with a $t_{1/2}$ of 6 to 12 hours can be given in repeated doses every 6 to 12 hours. A drug with a longer $t_{1/2}$ can be dosed only once a day, which is the desired amount. If the $t_{1/2}$ is short, 3 hours or less, the drug would have to be given more frequently than is compatible

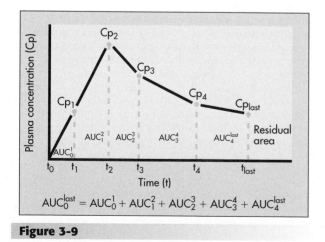

$$AUC_0^{last} = AUC_0^1 + AUC_1^2 + AUC_2^3 + AUC_3^4 + AUC_4^{last}$$

Figure 3-9

Plot of plasma concentration-time data points. Area under the curve between successive data points can be circulated by the linear trapezoidal method. (From Brody TM, Larner J, Minneman KP. *Human Pharmacology: Molecular to Clinical.* 3rd ed. Philadelphia: Mosby; 1998.)

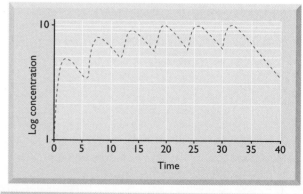

Figure 3-10

Graph of log plasma concentration versus time for a drug administered by mouth every 6 hours for six doses when the drug's terminal disposition half-life is 6 hours. The effective steady state occurs 24 to 30 hours (4 to 5 half-lives) after starting the drug. (From Page C, Curtis MJ, Sutter MC, Walker MJ, Hoffman BB, eds. *Integrated Pharmacology.* 2nd ed. 2002. Philadelphia: Mosby; 2002.)

with patient compliance and instead should be given by continuous IV infusion. Another option is development of a modified-release formulation so that the frequency of dosing can be reduced.

Zero-Order Elimination

For a few drugs, such as ethanol, phenytoin, and aspirin, elimination does not follow the patterns discussed earlier. These drugs demonstrate a linear loss in which a constant amount of the drug is lost per unit of time as opposed to being based on a percentage of plasma concentration.[17] In other words, elimination is independent of concentration.

FACTORS AFFECTING PHARMACOKINETICS

Clinicians have long noted that patients demonstrate great variability in response to identical drug treatments. To understand where these individual responses come from, we need to discuss factors that affect pharmacokinetics and dynamics such as genetics, age, environmental factors, and the presence of other disease processes.

Changes in Pharmacokinetics with Age

The incidence of adverse drug reactions increases with age.[38] Some reasons include the fact that elderly patients take many more drugs than their younger counterparts. The more drugs one takes, the greater is the likelihood of either a drug-drug interaction or an interaction with one or more other disease states. Competition for the P450 enzymes may slow metabolism, leaving a higher level of active drug in the system. In addition, the serum albumin concentration decreases with age, resulting in increases in free drug concentration. Lean body mass also decreases with age, and this will affect how certain drugs are distributed, particularly fat-soluble drugs. Additionally, renal and liver function may be reduced, slowing down drug elimination and prolonging the $t_{1/2}$. All of these factors would lead to greater than expected levels of active drug. This is particularly problematic for drugs with narrow therapeutic margins. On the other hand, reduced blood flow to the GI tract may limit overall absorption, but this is not viewed as being very significant.[15]

Although most of the changes in the elderly patient affect the kinetics of drug action, some pharmacodynamic changes also occur with aging. Elderly patients appear to be more sensitive to drugs, in part because of changes in drug-receptor interactions. Changes in receptor number or sensitivity, or even changes in signal transduction, may be to blame.[38] Specifically, elderly patients react more profoundly to sedative-hypnotics and analgesic medications.[10] These drugs are likely to produce sedation, respiratory depression, and confusion. Changes in the blood-brain barrier may allow these drugs to enter the central nervous system more easily. In addition, baroreceptor sensitivity is reduced, leading to orthostatic hypotension with these drugs, as well as with drugs for hypertension. As a result of all these changes, an elderly patient can be expected to have many more adverse drug events than a younger patient. Every drug has a risk/benefit ratio, and this ratio becomes greater with age.

Changes in Pharmacokinetics Caused by Genetics

Inherited factors may cause different responses to drugs. Single genes tend to control the production of enzymes. Gene mutations are inheritable, leading to abnormal enzymes producing increased, decreased, or completely unexpected responses to drugs. Pharmacogenetics is the study of drug responses that are produced by genes. Some inheritable conditions causing adverse drug responses include abnormal metabolism caused by defective oxidation or acetylation. The acetylation process assigns an amide group ($-NH_2$) to the drug to make it more polar. Approximately 90% of Japanese people are rapid acetylators, whereas only 50% of westerners are rapid acetylators.[15] Slow acetylators tend to have more adverse reactions than fast acetylators.

Another significant genetic defect affecting drug response is a cholinesterase deficiency.[39] Succinylcholine is a neuromuscular blocking agent that is used to induce paralysis during some major surgical procedures. The action of this drug is terminated by the enzyme cholinesterase. Affected individuals may produce so little cholinesterase that metabolism of succinylcholine is slowed and the patient requires assisted ventilation for a while after the surgery is over.

Some other heritable conditions causing a reduced drug response include resistance to the anticoagulants heparin and warfarin and resistance to vitamin D.[15]

Changes in Pharmacokinetics with Disease

As discussed previously, diseases of the liver and kidneys have profound effects on the $t_{1/2}$.[1] Metabolism and elimination are reduced, leaving active drug around longer. In addition, other illnesses such as viral infections reduce the activity of the P450 enzymes, also producing a longer $t_{1/2}$. Perhaps, however, the greatest problem associated with the presence of multiple disease processes and drug action is the fact that multiple drugs may be needed. Administration of multiple drugs increases the risk for drug-drug interactions, either because of competition for P450 enzymes or competing responses to different drugs. An example of a competing drug response occurs when a patient taking a diuretic for hypertension is also prescribed a nonsteroidal anti-inflammatory drug (NSAID) for arthritis. This occurrence is unfortunately common among the elderly. The NSAID blocks production of prostaglandins (pain-mediating substances) in the periphery and also blocks their production in the kidneys. However, prostaglandins are needed in the kidneys for maintaining adequate renal perfusion. The result of this interaction is diminished excretion from the kidneys, producing increased blood volume, which in turn raises blood pressure.

Changes in Pharmacokinetics with Exercise

Exercise affects a number of factors involved in drug pharmacokinetics including vascular flow, pH, temperature, GI function, metabolism, and excretion.[40] The drug propranolol can be used to illustrate the changes that occur with exercise.

Exercise has been shown to affect the pharmacokinetics of propranolol.[41] This drug is a β-adrenergic blocker that reduces blood pressure by blocking access of catecholamines to β-receptors in the heart. The net effect is to lower heart rate and contractility, which in turn reduces blood pressure. Propranolol is quite lipophilic and also shows high first-pass metabolism. In a study performed on healthy volunteers, propranolol was administered before prolonged exercise (25 minutes) at 70% Workload maximum (Wmax) on a cycle ergometer and during a 10-minute exercise period at 50% Wmax. Plasma concentrations of propranolol were determined at rest, during exercise, and during recovery. Oral propranolol was given for 1 week before testing with the more strenuous exercise protocol but was given intravenously by continuous infusion during testing with the light exercise protocol. Plasma concentrations of propranolol were significantly increased in both tests. However, after corrections were made for changes in the plasma volume (lost fluid) during exercise, drug elevation in plasma was only significant during exhaustive exercise, the protocol that required oral administration of propranolol. The increase in plasma level above the pre-exercise level suggests better absorption, changes in the volume of distribution (reduced drug in peripheral compartments), or reduced drug clearance. Because propranolol normally undergoes significant first-pass metabolism, we can speculate that during exhaustive exercise with oral dosing, hepatic blood flow is reduced, resulting in a smaller first-pass effect. This is a more plausible explanation when the results are compared with the IV study in which there was no first-pass effect and plasma concentration was not elevated. However, the irreconcilable findings between the two studies could also have been due to the difference in exercise. Increases in lactic acid production and a lowering of pH during the high-intensity exercise could be responsible for an increase in lipid solubility, and hence, better absorption through the GI tract. This better absorption combined with diminished blood flow to the liver in vigorous exercise are reasonable explanations for the greater plasma level. Changes in metabolism and excretion were ruled out because comparisons with another β-blocker, atenolol, did not show any change in plasma concentration during exercise performed with the IV drug. In addition, the atenolol concentration was not affected by the vigorous exercise with oral dosing, suggesting that it was the degree of ionization associated with pH changes with exercise that produced the elevated propranolol level. Drug-receptor changes were also ruled out because there was no change in concentration with atenolol, which interacts with the same receptors as propranolol. One other explanation proposed was that because propranolol binds to skeletal muscles, it is conceivable that greater muscle perfusion is responsible for a "washout of drug" from this area.

This rather lengthy discussion regarding the pharmacokinetics of propranolol with exercise was designed to illustrate the complexities that researchers face when performing drug-exercise studies. In fact, these studies are not done with most drugs, leaving the physical therapist without guidance. Many variables appear to be involved in pharmacokinetics—including type and intensity of exercise, route of administration, dosing schedule, issues regarding methods of separating the processes of metabolism from those of elimination, and examination of what is happening at the target organ and receptor levels. In addition, this study was performed with healthy subjects, which may provide an entirely different result than if it were conducted with patients with hypertension, given the changes in vascular tone and perfusion that occur in subjects who have high blood pressure. The challenge exists to design a series of studies to explore the interactions of drugs with exercise and to apply this method consistently to test a variety of different drugs, particularly those that are likely to be given to patients desiring exercise.

ACTIVITIES 3

■ 1. List chemical and physiological variables of drugs affecting pharmacokinetics and explain which enhance and which interfere with the process.

■ 2. You are treating a 70-year-old man for wrist drop caused by radial nerve dysfunction. The patient also has a host of other medical problems related to alcoholic liver disease: anemia, thrombocytopenia, jaundice, and hypo-albuminemia. How is each phase of pharmacokinetics influenced by the patient's medical condition? What should be done to ensure that the patient does not experience any adverse drug reactions?

■ 3. Interview a relative, neighbor, or patient who is over 65 years old regarding his or her medication use. Please list all prescribed and over-the-counter medicines (use generic names), including herbals, that have been taken within the past 6 months. Ask your subject about side effects, number of pills he or she takes per day, and compliance. Discuss your findings with other students to determine the 10 drugs most commonly used by this age group.

References

1. Sitar DS. Pharmacokinetic and other factors influencing drug action. In: Page C, Curtis MJ, Sutter MC, Walker MJ, Hoffman BB, eds. *Integrated Pharmacology*. Philadelphia: Mosby; 2002:39-55.
2. Rang HP, Dale MM, Ritter JM, Moore JL. *Pharmacology*. New York: Churchill Livingstone; 2003.
3. Waller DG, Renwick AG, Hillier K. *Medical Pharmacology and Therapeutics*. New York: WB Saunders; 2001.
4. Fasano A. Innovative strategies for the oral delivery of drugs and peptides. *Trends Biotechnol*. 1998;16:152-157.
5. Chonn A, Cullis PR. Recent advances in liposomal drug-delivery systems. *Curr Opin Biotechnol*. 1995;6:698-708.
6. Sachs GS, Renshaw PF, Lafer B, et al. Variability of brain lithium levels during maintenance treatment: a magnetic resonance spectroscopy study. *Biol Psychiatry*. 1995;38:422-428.
7. MDS Evidence-Based Assessment Project. Levodopa. *Mov Disord*. 2002;17:S23-S37.
8. Somogyi A. Renal transport of drugs: specificity and molecular mechanisms. *Clin Exp Pharmacol Physiol*. 1996;23:986-989.
9. Bowmer CJ, Yates MS. Drugs and the renal system. In: Clive CP, Curtis MJ, Sutter MC, Walker MJ, Hoffman BB, eds. *Integrated Pharmacology*. Philadelphia: Mosby; 2002:343-360.
10. Flynn EJ. Pharmacodynamic & pharmacokinetic principles of pharmacology & drug therapy. *J Neurol Phys Ther*. 2003;27:93-100.
11. Pratt WB. The entry, distribution, and elimination of drugs. In: Pratt WB, Taylor P, eds. *Principles of Drug Actions: The Basis of Pharmacology*. New York: Churchill Livingstone; 1990:201-296.
12. Skyler JS, Cefalu WT, Kourides IA, et al. Efficacy of inhaled human insulin in type 1 diabetes mellitus: a randomised proof-of-concept study. *Lancet*. 2001;357:331-335.

13. Shafran SD. Drugs and bacteria. In: Page C, Curtis MJ, Sutter MC, Walker MJ, Hoffman BB, eds. *Integrated Pharmacology*. Philadelphia: Mosby; 2002:111-136.

14. Wade JP. Drugs and the musculoskeletal system. In: Page C, Curtis MJ, Sutter MC, Walker MJ, Hoffman JR, eds. *Integrated Pharmacology*. Philadelphia: Mosby; 2002:437-454.

15. Bennett PN, Brown MJ. General pharmacology. In: Bennett PN, Brown MJ, eds. *Clinical Pharmacology*. New York: Churchill Livingstone; 2003:37-40.

16. Salerno E. *Pharmacology for Health Professionals*. New York: Mosby; 1999:11-21.

17. Somogyi A. Clinical pharmacokinetics and dosing schedules. In: Brody TM, Larner J, Minneman KP, eds. *Human Pharmacology: Molecular to Clinical*. Philadelphia: Mosby; 1998:47-64.

18. Margolis S, Saudek CD. *The Johns Hopkins White Papers on Diabetes*. Baltimore: Johns Hopkins Medical Institutions; 2002:1-62.

19. Linde B, MD. Dissociation of insulin absorption and blood flow during massage of a subcutaneous injection site. *Diabetes Care*. 1986;9:570-574.

20. Koivisto VA, Felig P. Effects of leg exercise on insulin absorption in diabetic patients. *N Engl J Med*. 1978; 298:79-83.

21. Ballantyne JC, Carr DB, Chalmers TC, Dear KBG, Angelillo IF, Mosteller F. Postoperative patient-controlled analgesia: meta-analyses of initial randomized control trials. *J Clin Anesth*. 1993;5:182-193.

22. Barry MJ, Albright AL, Shultz BL. Intrathecal baclofen therapy and the role of the physical therapist. *Pediatr Phys Ther*. 2000;12:77-86.

23. Reents S. *Sport and Exercise Pharmacology*. Champaign, Ill: Human Kinetics; 2000.

24. Greene BL. Physical therapist management of fluoroquinolone-induced Achilles tendinopathy. *Phys Ther*. 2002;82:1224-31.

25. Carter JH, Nutt JG, Woodward WR. The effect of exercise on levodopa absorption. *Neurology*. 1992;42:2042-2045.

26. Goetz CG, Thelen JA, MacLeod CM, Carvey PM, Bartley EA, Stebbins, GT. Blood levodopa levels and unified Parkinson's disease rating scale function: with and without exercise. *Neurology*. 1993;43:1040-1042.

27. Reuter I, Harder S, Engelhardt M, Bass H. The effect of exercise on pharmacokinetics and pharmacodynamics of levodopa. *Mov Disord*. 2000;15:862-868.

28. Stromberg C, Vanakoski J, Olkkola KT, Lindqvist A, Seppala T. Exercise alters the pharmacokinetics of midazolam. *Clin Pharmacol Ther*. 1992;51:527-532.

29. Khazaeinia T, Ramsey AA, Tam YK. The effects of exercise on the pharmacokinetics of drugs. *J Pharmacol Pharmaceut Sci*. 2000;3:292-302.

30. Vanakoski J, Seppala T. Heat exposure and drugs. A review of the effects of hyperthermia on pharmaco-kinetics. *Clin Pharmacokinet*. 1998;34:311-322.

31. Hollenberg PF, Brody TM. Absorption, distribution, metabolism, and elimination. In: Brody MJ, Larner J, Minneman KP, eds. *Human Pharmacology: Molecular to Clinical*. Philadelphia: Mosby; 1998:35-46.

32. Cupp MJ, Tracy TS. Cytochrome P450: new nomen-clature and clinical implications. *Am Fam Physician*. 1998;57:107-116.

33. Rech RH. Drugs to treat anxieties and related disorders. In: Brody MJ, Larner J, Minneman KP, eds. *Human Pharmacology: Molecular to Clinical*. Philadelphia: Mosby; 1998:365-372.

34. Lin JH, Lu AYH. Interindividual variability in inhibition and induction of cytochrome P450 enzymes. *Annu Rev Pharmacol Toxicol*. 2001;41:535-567.

35. Park BK, Kitteringham NR, Pirmohamed M, Tucker GT. Relevance of induction of human drug-metabolizing enzymes: pharmacological and toxicological implications. *Br J Clin Pharmacol*. 1996;41:477-491.

36. Kane GC, Lipsky JJ. Drug-grapefruit juice interactions. *Mayo Clin Proc*. 2000;75:933-942.

37. Sueyoshi T, Negishi M. Phenobarbital response elements of cytochrome P450 genes and nuclear receptors. *Annu Rev Pharmacol Toxicol*. 2001;41:123-143.

38. Hughes SG. Prescribing of the elderly patient: why do we need to exercise caution? *Br J Clin Pharmocol*. 1998; 46:531-533.

39. Ries CR, Quastel DMJ. Drug use in anesthesia and critical care. In: Page C, Curtis MJ, Sutter MC, Walker MJ, Hoffman BB, eds. *Integrated Pharmacology*. Philadelphia: Mosby; 2002:547-563.

40. van Baak MA. Influence of exercise on the pharmaco-kinetics of drugs. *Clin Pharmacokinet*. 1990;19:32-43.

41. van Baak MA, Mooij JMV, Schiffers PMH. Exercise and the pharmacokinetics of propranolol, verapamil, and atenolol. *Eur J Clin Pharmacol*. 1992;43:547-550.

CHAPTER 4

ADVERSE DRUG REACTIONS

RISK/BENEFIT RATIO

As mentioned in the previous chapter, every drug has a risk/benefit ratio, and this ratio increases as a patient ages.[1] However, the risks are not only experienced by the elderly but also pose a threat to people of all ages. These risks may result from drug-drug interactions, food-drug interactions, patient-related factors, allergic reactions, and side effects from the medications caused by their pharmacodynamic properties.

CLASSIFICATION OF ADVERSE DRUG REACTIONS

Adverse drug reactions (ADRs) are defined by the World Health Organization as any unintended or unwanted effects of a drug that may occur at acceptable dose levels.[2] This is a rather exclusionary definition because it does not include human errors in drug administration and patient compliance issues. Nevertheless, as defined here, the numbers of ADRs are astounding. A meta-analysis of 39 prospective studies, beginning in 1964 and ending in 1996, revealed that serious ADRs occurred in 6.7% of hospitalized patients.[2] This figure represents patients who were already hospitalized for a different reason and experienced their ADRs in the hospital, as well as patients who were admitted solely because of an ADR. This figure includes serious ADRs only, ones for which hospitalization was necessary and death may have been a final outcome. Specifically, in 1994, ADRs were among the six leading causes of death. According to this

information, it is estimated that 1 in 10 hospital admissions is drug related. If we include ADRs caused by human error and compliance issues, ADRs grow to an even more alarming number.

Criticism of this study included the fact that some of the numbers were taken from large tertiary care hospitals that attract the more seriously ill patients, the ones more likely to have an ADR.[3] However, the number of ADRs is clearly too high and greater than previously thought. One reason is that hospitals may not recognize all adverse events unless specifically looking for them. Chart reviews are not practical on an every-case basis, and even if an adverse event is discovered, the possibility of a lawsuit is a powerful disincentive for the hospital to report the incident. Reporting of an ADR today remains voluntary. The only mandatory reports come from the pharmaceutical companies, either during the clinical trial period or during postmarketing surveillance, if an event has been spontaneously communicated to the company.

Definitions

The term *side effects* has traditionally been reserved for minor effects of drugs, and the term **adverse reaction** has been used to label the serious effects of drugs at therapeutic doses.[4] **Adverse event,** however, refers to a negative outcome that occurs while a patient is taking a drug but does not imply causality as does the term *adverse reaction.* For purposes of this book, the phrases "adverse drug events" and "adverse drug reactions" will be used interchangeably and will include the major and minor drug effects. *Toxicity* refers to an adverse drug event that occurs at a high dose, although carcinogenicity (causing cancer) and teratogenicity (causing fetal damage) are special cases of toxicity.[5]

MedWatch

In recent years, governmental agencies have taken some steps to reduce the numbers of ADRs. In 1993 the Food and Drug Administration (FDA) introduced MedWatch, an online voluntary reporting site for adverse events.[6,7] The main goal of this website is to provide a way for physicians and other health care workers to submit suspicions of drug side effects and to make it easier to distribute this information to both the public and professionals. This website consists of five sections: What's New in the Past Two Weeks; Safety Information (product recalls and safety alerts); Medical Product Reporting; Continuing Education, offering continuing education units in clinical therapeutics and recognition of drug-induced diseases; and a section for voluntarily reporting a suspected adverse reaction. This last section is particularly important because clinical studies, performed on a limited number of subjects, often miss a number of ADRs that only show up when the drug is taken on a large-scale basis. Even with this website, it is estimated that adverse events remain underreported.

Once the FDA receives a negative report, it assigns a group of safety evaluators to explore more fully the potential risk involved with the drug. These evaluators search patient databases and review the drug's history in clinical trials to determine whether other adverse reports exist and to identify any common trends. In addition, it is necessary to establish a causal relationship between the drug and the adverse event and to assign a possible physiological reason for the event. These evaluators look at other drugs in the same class, as well as dose-response relationships to prove association.

The ultimate action by the FDA depends on the seriousness of the adverse event and the number of events recognized. The agency might require the drug maker to inform prescribers about the hazard and add a boxed warning label to the drug's packaging. In addition, the FDA may require patient information materials to accompany every prescription. Recently, the FDA has required some drug manufacturers to add boxed warnings or to strengthen the warning labels on certain drugs.

These changes were required as a result of reports of myocarditis with an antipsychotic drug, clozapine; fluid retention leading to congestive heart failure with the diabetic drugs rosiglitazone and pioglitazone; and liver damage with the antifungal drug terbinafine.[7] In addition, the FDA has withdrawn several drugs from the market including phenylpropanolamine, an ingredient in many cough and diet pills, because of its association with hemorrhagic stroke, and cerivastatin, an anticholesterol drug that causes rhabdomyolysis.

Alphabetical Classification of Adverse Drug Events

Adverse reactions may be classified into a number of different categories by using an alphabetical classification system (Table 4-1).[5,8] An augmented response (A) is a dose-related response. This response is related to the pharmacological action of the drug, and it is usually predictable. Examples include a hypoglycemic reaction associated with insulin and hemorrhage caused by the anticoagulant warfarin. This type of reaction is managed by reducing or withholding the dose. Bizarre effects (B) are non–dose-related and unpredictable. An anaphylactic reaction to penicillin and liver toxicity associated with inhaled anesthetic agents fall into this category. These effects are managed by eliminating use of the drug and avoiding it in the future. Category C responses are chronic effects related to dose and time. These events occur during prolonged administration or as the result of a cumulative dose. Examples include movement disorders that occur with antipsychotics and suppression of the hypothalamic-pituitary-adrenal axis by steroids. Management consists of reduction of the dose or withdrawal. Delayed effects (D) are carcinogenic, secondary cancers that occur years after use of chemotherapy agents. The last category is (E), end-of-treatment effects. Abrupt withdrawal from many drugs can lead to adverse events. A good example of this is opiate withdrawal. Management includes reintroduction of the drug and then slow withdrawal.

A simpler classification system, and the one more commonly used, consists of the following categories: Adverse Drug Events type A, which include dose-related reactions; Adverse Drug Events type B, idiosyncratic or unpredictable reactions: and Adverse Drug Withdrawal Events.[9]

Table 4-1

Alphabetical Classification of Adverse Drug Effects			
Type	**Type of Effect**	**Definition**	**Examples**
A	Augmented pharmacologic effects	Adverse effects that are known to occur from the pharmacology of drug and are dose related. They are seldom fatal and relatively common.	Hypoglycemia caused by insulin injection Bradycardia caused by β adrenoceptor antagonists Hemorrhage caused by anticoagulants
B	Bizarre effects	Adverse effects that occur unpredictably and often have a high rate of morbidity and mortality. They are uncommon.	Anaphylaxis caused by penicillin Acute hepatic necrosis caused by halothane Bone marrow suppression by chloramphenicol
C	Chronic effects	Adverse effects that occur only during prolonged treatment and not with single doses.	Iatrogenic Cushing's syndrome with prednisolone Orofacial dyskinesia caused by phenothiazine tranquilizers Colonic dysfunction caused by laxatives
D	Delayed effects	Adverse effects that occur remote from treatment, either in the children of treated patients or in patients themselves years after treatment.	Second cancers in those treated with alkylating agents for Hodgkin's disease Craniofacial malformations in infants whose mothers have taken isotretinoin Clear-cell carcinoma of the vagina in the daughters of women who took diethylstilbestrol during pregnancy
E	End-of-treatment effects	Adverse effects that occur when a drug is stopped, especially when it is stopped suddenly (so called withdrawal effects)	Unstable angina after β adrenoceptor antagonists are suddenly stopped Adrenocortical insufficiency after glucocorticosteroids such as prednisolone are stopped Withdrawal seizures when anticonvulsants such as phenobarbital or phenytoin are stopped

From Page C, Curtis MJ, Sutter MC, Walker MJ, Hoffman BB, eds. *Integrated Pharmacology*. 2nd ed. 2002. Philadelphia: Mosby; 2002.

DRUG-DRUG INTERACTIONS

A drug-drug interaction occurs when a second drug is added to a first drug, resulting in a diminished response,[4] or when the combined effect of the two drugs is additive or synergistic.[10] Drug interactions may be beneficial or harmful. An example of a desired drug-drug interaction is the combination of two pain medications so that pain is controlled better than when either drug is used alone, producing an additive response. Synergistic interactions result from combining two drugs to produce a response greater than the sum of the drugs. Examples include combining a diuretic and a β-adrenergic blocking agent to lower blood pressure.[11] Another example is the HIV cocktail, a combination of two or more antiviral drugs that attack the virus at a variety of steps in its replication process.[12] A harmful synergistic reaction occurs when a sedative is combined with either alcohol or an analgesic. Both of these combinations produce excessive central nervous system (CNS) depression.[13]

Antagonistic drug relationships result in a combined effect that is less than the response produced by each drug alone.[4] Some of these relationships are beneficial, such as when naloxone is given to reverse an opiate overdose or when flumazenil is used to treat a benzodiazepine overdose. These drugs are competitive antagonists. However, many antagonistic relationships are not desirable. When an aspirin-type drug is added to a diuretic for hypertension, the diuretic becomes less effective.[14] The aspirin inhibits prostaglandin production in the kidneys, and prostaglandin synthesis is important for maintaining renal perfusion and appropriate resorption and secretion of ions.

Pharmacokinetic and Pharmacodynamic Basis for Drug-Drug Interactions

Pharmacokinetic reasons for drug interactions include many of the issues discussed in the previous chapter. Slowing of gastrointestinal (GI) motility by drugs such as opioids and tricyclic antidepressants (the antimuscarinic effects) may increase absorption of other drugs. Laxatives, which increase GI motility, have the opposite effect by allowing less time for absorption.

Interactions during distribution occur with drugs that readily bind to plasma proteins. The antiseizure drugs, sodium valproate and phenytoin, interact when valproate causes phenytoin to displace from albumin and also inhibits metabolism of phenytoin.[15]

Enzyme inhibition and enzyme induction produce interactions that occur during metabolism. For example, birth control pills are metabolized more quickly when phenytoin is administered, leading to a diminished contraceptive effect and a possible pregnancy.[4] See Tables 4-2 and 4-3 for additional examples of enzyme- inducing and enzyme-inhibiting drugs.

The process of renal excretion is not free from drug interactions. A helpful interaction is the use of probenecid to compete with renal transport of penicillin and other antibiotics into the tubular fluid.[16] This is a useful method of prolonging the action of antibiotics for the treatment of certain infections.

FOOD-DRUG INTERACTIONS

The co-administration of certain drugs with acidic beverages such as Coca-Cola Classic and Pepsi, which have a pH under 3 can alter absorption of some drugs.[17] A weak base administered with these drinks will cause ionization of the drug and diminish

Table 4-2

Examples of Drugs that Inhibit Drug-Metabolizing Enzymes

Drugs Inhibiting Enzyme Action	Drugs with Metabolism Affected
Allopurinol	Mercaptopurine, azathioprine
Chloramphenicol	Phenytoin
Cimetidine	Amiodarone, phenytoin, pethidine
Ciprofloxacin	Theophylline
Corticosteroids	Tricyclic antidepressants, cyclophosphamide
Ciprofloxacin	Theophylline
Disulfiram	Warfarin
Erythromycin	Cyclosporine, theophylline
Monoamine oxidase inhibitors	Pethidine
Ritonavir	Saquinavir

From Rang HP, Dale MM, Ritter JM, Moore, PK. *Pharmacology*. 5th ed. New York: Churchill Livingstone; 2003.

Table 4-3

Examples of Drugs that Induce Drug Metabolizing Enzymes

Drugs Inhibiting Enzyme Action	Drugs with Metabolism Affected
Phenobarbital Rifampicin Griseofulvin Phenytoin Ethalol Carbamazepine	Warfarin Oral contraceptives Corticosteroids Cyclosporine Drugs listed in left-hand column will also be affected

From Rang HP, Dale MM, Ritter JM, Moore, PK. *Pharmacology*. 5th ed. New York: Churchill Livingstone; 2003.

The Q-T interval normally varies physiologically with the heart rate; this is corrected for by calculating a corrected Q-T interval (Q-Tc) by dividing by the square root of the R-R interval.

absorption. In addition, because the cytochrome P450 enzymes are also involved in the metabolism of food and food can induce or inhibit these enzymes, it is easy to understand why certain combinations of food and drugs should be avoided. Grapefruit juice, unlike other citrus juices, is a well-known inhibitor of these enzymes and therefore increases the bioavailability of many drugs (e.g., cyclosporine, diltiazem, and felodipine).[18,19] Repeated exposure to grapefruit juice not only inhibits the enzymes but also inhibits the expression of the genes that control their production. Therefore grapefruit juice should be avoided entirely when these drugs are taken. In other cases of nutrient-drug interactions, ingestion of the food and administration of the drug need only be separated for a few hours.

Another problem occurs with enteral feeding tubes, because a number of formulas have been implicated in drug-nutrient interactions. Absorption of warfarin, tetracycline, and phenytoin is decreased when these drugs are administered with enteral feedings. Chelation reactions in which divalent cations and drug molecules bind to each other are particularly problematic.[19] The macronutrients in enteral feedings, especially protein, may also reduce bioavailability. Certain drugs, such as phenytoin, may bind to the plastic tubing, thus reducing bioavailability.[19] The location of drug delivery can also influence drug absorption. A drug that requires an acidic environment for activation will show diminished efficacy if it is administered with tube feedings into the distal portion of the small intestine.

The management of drug-nutrient interactions becomes clear once the mechanism of the reaction is understood.[19] If interactions occur as a result of mixing the feeding formulas with the drug, formulas can be withheld for at least 2 hours before or after drug administration. If the issue is drug binding to the plastic tubing, the tubes can be flushed with saline solution. However, most of the interactions involving metabolism cannot be stopped by a time separation, so the interacting nutrient will need to be avoided.

DRUG ALLERGY AND DRUG-INDUCED ILLNESSES

Drug allergies or hypersensitivities range from mild presentations (urticaria) to very severe life-threatening events (anaphylaxis). For a drug to produce a reaction, it must have antigenic effects and stimulate antibody formation or the formation of sensitized T lymphocytes, which is immune related. It is estimated that up to one third of all ADRs are attributed to drug allergy.[20] In most instances of allergy, the drug combines with some protein and forms a complex that has antigenic activity. The synthesis of antibodies may take 1 to 2 weeks. When the patient is re-exposed to the drug, manifestations of the allergy develop. Specifically, drug allergies are classified into four types, although classifying a drug into a specific category can present a challenge.[21]

Type I (Anaphylactic Reactions)

Anaphylaxis is the most severe allergic reaction. It involves the skin and pulmonary and cardiovascular systems, producing cardiovascular and respiratory collapse. The mechanism of this reaction is degranulation of mast cells and/or basophils after exposure to a specific antigen in sensitized individuals. In general, immunoglobin (Ig) E antibodies are formed and attach to basophils and circulating mast cells in connective tissue, skin, and mucous membranes during the initial exposure. On re-administration of the antigen, the basophils and mast cells release large amounts of histamine, resulting in bronchoconstriction, peripheral vasodilation, increased vascular permeability, and increased mucus production. Specifically, this results in some of the following signs and symptoms:[22]

Neurological—dizziness, weakness, seizures
Ocular—pruritus, lacrimation, edema around the eyes
Upper airway—nasal congestion, hoarseness, stridor, laryngeal edema, cough, obstruction
Lower airway—dyspnea, tachypnea, cyanosis, bronchospasm, accessory muscle use to assist respiration, respiratory arrest
Cardiac—tachycardia, hypotension, arrhythmias, myocardial infarction, cardiac arrest
Skin—flushing, erythema, pruritus, angioedema, urticaria, maculopapular rash
GI—nausea, vomiting, diarrhea

These symptoms generally occur within minutes after antigen exposure but may still occur up to 1 hour later. This reaction may have two phases. In about 20% of cases, the initial symptom presentation is followed by a second phase of reactivity 10 hours later.[22] The condition is treated initially with parenteral epinephrine, the establishment of an airway, and supplemental oxygen. Histamine blockers (diphenhydramine and ranitidine) are also given once the patient's condition has stabilized, followed by administration of steroids to prevent the second phase of the reaction. Prevention strategies include use of self-injectable epinephrine and wearing a medical alert bracelet. Certain drug desensitization protocols (e.g., for penicillin) have also been used, but if the patient can avoid the offending agent, that is recommended.[21] In addition, the patient must be instructed to avoid drugs that exhibit cross-reactivity with the offending agent.

Type II (Cytotoxic Reaction)

In a type II reaction, the antigen adheres to the target cell. Antibodies (IgG and IgM) are formed and attach to the target tissue with subsequent antigen-antibody complex formation and activation of complement.[10] This complex then begins to destroy the target tissue. Essentially, the drug combines with a protein that the body no longer recognizes as self. Drugs known to produce this reaction include penicillin, cephalosporins, salicylates, and phenytoin. This reaction takes some time (several days to a week) as the levels of IgG and IgM increase and begin to attach to red blood cells, platelets, and basophils. The clinical manifestations include fever, arthralgia, rash, splenomegaly, and lymph node enlargement. This group of symptoms is known as *a serum sickness-like reaction,* but when there is specific internal organ involvement, it is referred to as *drug hypersensitivity syndrome* (multiorgan dysfunction).[23] More severe manifestations may include hemolytic anemia, glomerulonephritis, thrombocytopenia, and leukopenia. The reaction is self-limiting within several days to weeks after the drug is discontinued.

Type III (Autoimmune Reaction)

A type III reaction is a complex-mediated hypersensitivity reaction in which the body has difficulty eliminating antigen-antibody complexes. These complexes attach to normal tissue and activate a cascade, creating an inflammatory response. This same mechanism governs autoimmune disorders such as lupus and rheumatoid arthritis. Manifestations include serum sickness, glomerulonephritis, vasculitis, and pulmonary disorders.[4] Drug-induced lupus may be caused by isoniazid, methyldopa,

or chlorpromazine.[23] Once the drug has been discontinued, the lupus resolves in 4 to 6 weeks.

Type IV (Cell-Mediated Hypersensitivity)

A type IV reaction is mediated through T lymphocytes as opposed to antibodies. The response is a local or tissue reaction such as contact dermatitis.[4]

Clinical Manifestations of Drug-Induced Reactions

Urticarial rashes constitute an eruption of wheals that itch. The reaction may be general but is usually worse around an area in which a drug has been injected or applied topically. The reaction can also occur with oral administration. Along with angioedema, urticaria is seen in type I and III reactions.[4] Angioedema refers to edema of the lips and face. Nonurticarial rashes are seen in type I, II, and IV reactions. This category can include severe skin disorders such as exfoliative dermatitis and Stevens-Johnson syndrome in which lesions involve both the oral and anogenital mucosa along with systemic symptoms of fever, headache, arthralgia, and conjunctivitis.[10] Exudative lesions are present. Drugs that have produced these skin disorders include carbamazepine, phenytoin, penicillin, and sulfonamides. These conditions respond to epinephrine, antihistamines, and steroids.

Other drug-induced disorders include diseases of the lymphoid tissues, ocular toxicity, hepatotoxicity, ototoxicity, pulmonary toxicity, and nephrotoxicity.[10] Infectious mononucleosis, when present with a maculopapular rash, is probably an allergic reaction. Erythromycin and penicillins may cause this reaction. Pulmonary reactions such as asthma are seen in type I reactions, but pulmonary fibrosis may be seen in a type III reaction. Blood disorders such as thrombocytopenia, granulocytopenia, and aplastic anemia are seen in type II reactions. Medications may even, at times, affect the ears, producing dizziness, hearing loss, and balance difficulties. Antibiotics that have reduced clearance from the kidneys accumulate in other tissues such as the cranial nerves. Hepatotoxicity producing increased transaminase levels, jaundice, and pruritus can be a type II reaction but can also be present as a general adverse reaction because the liver is susceptible to both parenchymal hepatic damage and bile channel injury by the chemicals processed there. Lastly, various kinds of nephropathy may develop as a result of an immune response to drugs.

Diagnostic Tests for Drug Allergy

For determining whether a reaction is drug related, a number of diagnostic tests may be helpful. General lab tests such as liver function tests, determination of blood urea nitrogen and creatinine levels, and complete blood counts are useful; and a chest x-ray film can be obtained to determine the organs involved in the reaction. In addition, some more specific tests such as determination of antinuclear antibodies (for drug-induced lupus) and a urine histamine test (for anaphylaxis) may be performed. When mast cells are involved, tryptase, a protease that is contained in mast cell granules, is a useful biochemical marker.[21]

Skin tests for large polypeptides such as insulin and streptokinase are available and measure IgE-mediated reactions to determine whether the agent can be given again safely. However, the tools available are limited because we do not completely under-stand drug allergy and the different mechanisms involved.[21] Skin patch testing may show no evidence of IgE antibodies, which can mean either that they are not present or that they are present in amounts too small to be detected. However, even a very low, undetectable concentration can cause a reaction. The antigenic component of the skin test may not be the one that necessarily triggers a reaction in all patients allergic to the same agent.

OTHER CAUSES OF ADVERSE DRUG REACTIONS

Many factors can be responsible for individual variations in how patients respond to drugs. We have already discussed some issues regarding age and the presence of disease, particularly of the liver and kidneys, that affect drug metabolism. Genetic polymorphisms of drug receptors and P450 enzymes are also responsible for ADRs. In fact, any of the factors that alter pharmacokinetics or pharmacodynamics could be responsible for adverse drug events.

ACTIVITIES 4

■ 1. You are treating a patient for lateral epicondylitis. During today's session, you notice a red rash over the lateral aspect of the involved elbow. The patient tells you that she is using an herbal cream designed to reduce pain, which was purchased from a general nutrition store. Outline some questions you should ask to help determine whether this rash is a drug-induced disorder.

■ 2. Your patient is taking an anticoagulant (warfarin) for recurrent thrombophlebitis. She has also been taking aspirin for arthritic pain. Discuss the implications of combining these two drugs. Should they be given together? What are the ramifications for physical therapy intervention if they are taken together?

■ 3. You suspect an adverse drug reaction in a patient you are treating. List some sources for drug safety that you can consult to verify your suspicion.

References

1. Chutka DS, Evans JM, Fleming KC, Mikkelson KG. Drug prescribing for elderly patients. *Mayo Clin Proc.* 1995; 70:685-693.
2. Lazarou J, Pomeranz BH, Corey PN. Incidence of adverse drug reactions in hospitalized patients. *JAMA.* 1998; 279:1200-1205.
3. Bates DW. Drugs and adverse drug reactions. How worried should we be? *JAMA.* 1998;279:1216-1217.
4. Bennett PN, Brown MJ. General pharmacology. In: Bennett PN, Brown MJ, eds. *Clinical Pharmacology.* New York: Churchill Livingstone; 2003:37-40.
5. Edwards IR, Aronson JK. Adverse drug reactions: definitions, diagnosis, and management. *Lancet.* 2000; 356:1255-1259.
6. Food and Drug Administration. MedWatch: The FDA Safety information and Adverse Event Reporting Program. Available at: http://www.fda.gov/medwatch. Accessed June 24, 2003.
7. Ahmad SR. Adverse drug event monitoring at the Food and Drug Administration. *J Gen Intern Med.* 2003; 18:57-60.
8. Ferner R, Mann RD. Drug safety and pharmacovigilance. In: Page C, Curtis MJ, Sutter MC, Walker MJ, Hoffman BB, eds. *Integrated Pharmacology.* Philadelphia: Mosby; 2002:73-81.
9. Bates DW, Leape L. Adverse drug reactions. In: Carruthers SG, Hoffman BB, Melmon KL, Nierenberg DW, eds. *Melmon and Morrelli's Clinical Pharmacology.* New York: McGraw-Hill; 2000;1223-1256.
10. Kuhn M. *Pharmacotherapeutics: A Nursing Process Approach.* Philadelphia: FA Davis; 1998.
11. Curtis MJ, Pugsley MK. Drugs and the cardiovascular system. In: Page C, Curtis MJ, Sutter MC, Walker MJ, Hoffman BB, eds. *Integrated Pharmacology.* Philadelphia: Mosby; 2002: 361-414.
12. Aoki FY, Rosser S. Drugs and viruses. In: Page C, Curtis MJ, Sutter MC, Walker MJ, Hoffman BB, eds. *Integrated Pharmacology.* Philadelphia: Mosby; 2002:91-110.
13. Abramowicz M, ed. *The Medical Letter Handbook of Adverse Drug Interactions.* New Rochelle, NY: The Medical Letter, Inc.; 1999.
14. Dedier J, Stampfer M, Hankinson S, Willett W, Speizer F, Curhan G. Nonnarcotic analgesic use and the risk of hypertension in US women. *Hypertension.* 2002;40: 604-608.
15. Beydoun A, Passaro EA. Appropriate use of medications for seizures. *Postgrad Med.* 2002;111:69-82.
16. Spina SP, Dillon EC. Effect of chronic probenecid therapy on cefazolin serum concentrations. *Ann Pharmacother.* 2003;37:621-624.
17. Aria N, Kauffman CL. Current therapy: important drug interactions and reactions in dermatology. *Dermatol Clin.* 2003;21:207-215.
18. Christensen H, Asberg A, Holmboe AB, Berg KJ. Coadministration of grapefruit juice increases systemic exposure of diltiazem in healthy volunteers. *Eur J Clin Pharmacol.* 2002;58:515-520.
19. Lingtak-Neander C. Drug-nutrient interaction in clinical nutrition. *Curr Opin Clin Nutr Metab Care.* 2002;5:327-332.
20. Thong BY, Leong KP, Tang CY, Chng HH. Drug allergy in a general hospital: results of a novel prospective inpatient reporting system. *Ann Allergy Asthma Immunol.* 2003;90:342-347.
21. Gruchalla RS. Drug allergy. *J Allergy Clin Immunol.* 2003; 11:S548-S559.
22. Ellis AK, Day JH. Diagnosis and management of anaphylaxis. *CMAJ.* 2003;169:307-312.
23. Knowles SR, Uetrecht J, Shear NH. Idiosyncratic drug reactions: the reactive metabolite syndromes. *Lancet.* 2000;356:1587-1591.

Autonomic and Cardiovascular Pharmacology

CHAPTER 5

DRUGS ACTING ON THE AUTONOMIC NERVOUS SYSTEM

AUTONOMIC NERVOUS SYSTEM

The autonomic nervous system (ANS) is divided into two main anatomical divisions, the sympathetic nervous system (SNS) and the parasympathetic system (PNS). Some authors, however, include the enteric nervous system as a third division, describing the intrinsic nerve plexuses of the gastrointestinal (GI) tract.[1] The enteric system is closely aligned to the other two divisions with interconnections between them. The ANS is responsible for many involuntary functions such as contraction and relaxation of smooth muscle, exocrine and some endocrine secretions, heart rate and contractility, blood pressure, and digestion.

Anatomy and Physiology of the Autonomic Nervous System

The most significant anatomical difference between the ANS and the somatic system is that the ANS requires two neurons in sequence, whereas the somatic system uses a single motor neuron to relay information from the central nervous system (CNS) to the skeletal muscles. The two neurons comprising the autonomic pathway are known as the *preganglionic* and *postganglionic neurons.*

The preganglionic sympathetic fibers originate with their cell bodies in the lateral horn of the gray matter of the thoracic and lumbar segments (from T1 to L2) (Figure 5-1).[2] Hence, it is also called *the thoracolumbar system.* The fibers leave the spinal cord in the spinal nerves and then synapse in the paravertebral chain of the sympathetic ganglia lying bilaterally on either side of the spinal cord. The short preganglionic fiber then synapses on the cell body of the postganglionic fiber and rejoins some of the spinal nerves to reach their destination. Nerves for the abdominal and pelvic viscera have their cell bodies in unpaired prevertebral ganglia in the abdomen.

In the SNS the postganglionic neuron is long, extending to the glands and viscera, but the opposite is true for the PNS (Figure 5-2).[3] The preganglionic fibers originate in the cranial area of the spinal cord and travel a long distance to synapse in ganglia on or near their effector organs. The cranial nerves containing PNS fibers include the oculomotor, facial, glossopharyngeal, and vagus nerves. Input destined for the pelvic and abdominal viscera emerge from the sacral area and also traverse a significant distance to reach their ganglia. Thus the postganglionic fibers for the PNS are rather short compared with the postganglionic fibers for the SNS.

The adrenal medulla is a part of the SNS but provides an exception to the two-neuron rule.[4,5] It receives preganglionic fibers but lacks postganglionic neurons. Instead, it influences the target organs by secreting epinephrine, also known as *adrenaline,* directly into the blood.

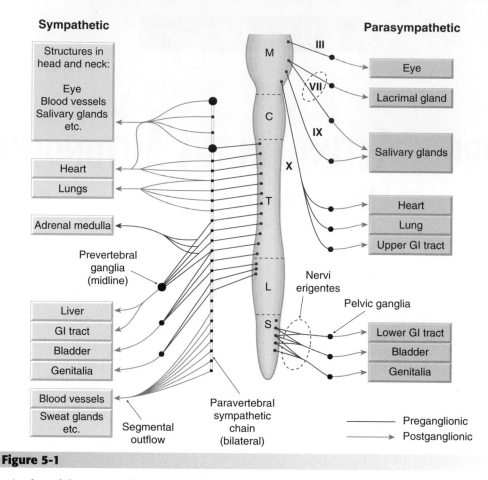

Figure 5-1

Basic plan of the mammalian autonomic nervous system. *M*, Medullary; *C*, cervical; *T*, thoracic; *L*, lumbar; *S*, sacral; *GI*, gastrointestinal. (From Rang HP, Dale MM, Ritter JM, Moore PK. *Pharmacology.* 5th ed. New York: Churchill Livingstone; 2003.)

Neurotransmitters for the Autonomic Nervous System

The preganglionic neurotransmitter for both the sympathetic and parasympathetic systems is acetylcholine (ACh).[2] When released, ACh binds to nicotinic receptors on the postganglionic cell. However, the neurotransmitter for the postganglionic neuron for each system is different. The postganglionic neuron for the sympathetic system is norepinephrine, also known as *noradrenaline.* At the target organ, norepinephrine interacts with the adrenergic receptors. Release occurs when depolarization of the nerve terminal opens calcium channels in the terminal membrane. Calcium flowing into the terminal triggers fusion and release of the synaptic vesicle containing norepinephrine. The action of norepinephrine is terminated by reuptake into the neuron and is either stored in vesicles again or is metabolized by monoamine oxidase in the mitochondria. Norepinephrine can also diffuse away from the receptor into extraneuronal cells and then can be inactivated by another enzyme, catechol-*O*-methyl-transferase (Figure 5-2).

Catecholamines are a group of chemicals that all contain a benzene ring with two hydroxyl groups and an amine side chain.[2] The natural endogenous catecholamines are norepinephrine, epinephrine, and dopamine. The precursor for the synthesis of norepinephrine and all the catecholamines is the amino acid tyrosine, which is acted on by several enzymes in the nerve terminal to form dopamine and then norepinephrine (Figure 5-3). In the adrenal medulla, the norepinephrine is further converted to epinephrine.

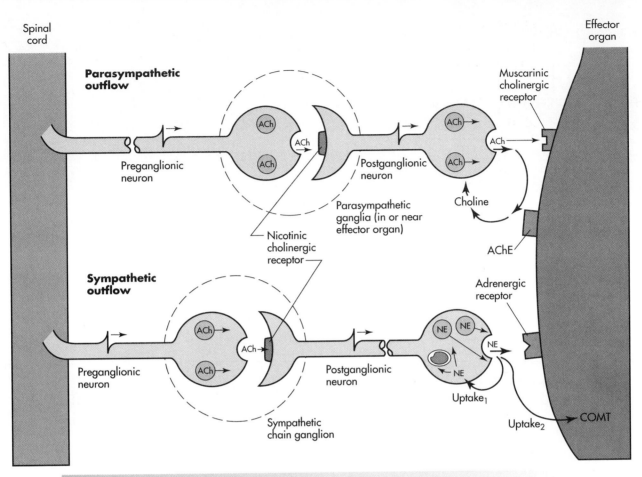

Figure 5-2

Neurochemical transmission in the parasympathetic divisions of the peripheral autonomic nervous system. The neurotransmitter liberated in both parasympathetic and sympathetic ganglia is acetylcholine *(ACh)*, which is released upon the arrival of an action potential to the preganglionic nerve terminal. ACh liberated from preganglionic neurons in the parasympathetic and sympathetic ganglia diffuses across the synaptic cleft to interact with nicotinic cholinergic receptors on cell bodies of the postganglionic neurons. The interaction of ACh with ganglionic cholinergic receptors results in the generation and propagation of action potentials that elicit the release of neurotransmitter at the postganglionic nerve terminal (neuroeffector junction). The neurotransmitter liberated from postganglionic parasympathetic nerves is ACh, which diffuses across the synaptic cleft and activates muscarinic cholinergic receptors on the effector organ. The liberated ACh is rapidly metabolized by acetylcholinesterase *(AChE)* into choline. Choline is taken up into the parasympathetic nerve terminal and used to resynthesize ACh, which is subsequently stored. A similar process occurs at the postganglionic sympathetic neuroeffector junction, except that the neurotransmitter released is norepinephrine *(NE)*, which diffuses across the neuroeffector junction to stimulate the adrenergic receptors and elicit the end-organ response. Most of the liberated NE is taken back up into the sympathetic nerve terminal *(uptake$_1$)* and is either stored in the adrenergic storage vehicles or is metabolized by monoamine oxidase *(MAO)* located in the mitochondria. A smaller amount of the liberated NE may diffuse away from the adrenergic receptors and be accumulated by extraneuronal cells *(uptake$_2$)*, after which it may be metabolized by catechol-*O*-methyltransferase *(COMT)*. (From Brody TM, Larner J, Minneman KP. *Human Pharmacology: Molecular to Clinical*. 3rd ed. Philadelphia: Mosby; 1998.)

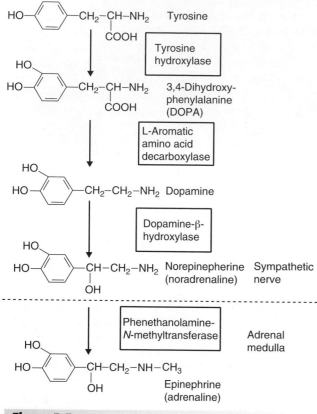

Figure 5-3

Steps in the enzymatic biosynthesis of the catecholamines dopamine, norepinephrine (noradrenaline), and epinephrine (adrenaline). The enzymes involved in each catalytic step are enclosed in boxes. The first three enzymatic steps occur in postganglionic sympathetic nerve terminals, leading to the synthesis of norepinephrine, and all four enzymatic steps occur in the adrenal medulla, resulting in the synthesis of epinephrine. (From Brody TM, Larner J, Minneman KP. *Human Pharmacology: Molecular to Clinical.* 3rd ed. Philadelphia: Mosby; 1998.)

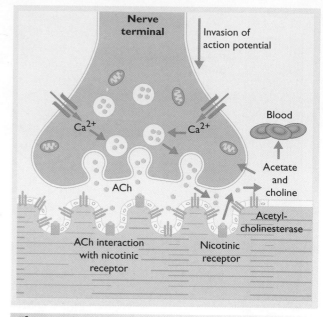

Figure 5-4

Action potential–induced release of the neurotransmitter acetylcholine *(ACh)* and its metabolism at the neuromuscular junction. (From Page C, Curtis MJ, Sutter MC, Walker MJ, Hoffman BB, eds. *Integrated Pharmacology.* 2nd ed. 2002. Philadelphia: Mosby; 2002.)

ACh is the neurotransmitter for the postganglionic neuron of the parasympathetic system.[2] Release of neurotransmitter from the PNS is quite similar to release from the SNS. An action potential passes down an axon to the terminal, resulting in a change in membrane potential. This voltage change triggers the influx of calcium into the cell, triggering the fusion of a vesicle to the cell membrane and release of ACh into the synaptic cleft. The neurotransmitter diffuses across the cleft and either binds to the muscarinic receptor or is inactivated by the enzyme acetylcholinesterase (AChE), splitting ACh into acetate and choline (Figure 5-4). Choline is then taken back into the neuron by a special choline transport system.

Receptors for the Autonomic Nervous System

There are three main types of nicotinic ACh receptors: those located on the neuromuscular junction of skeletal muscle, ganglionic receptors responsible for communication between preganglionic and postganglionic fibers of the sympathetic and parasympathetic systems, and CNS-type receptors widely dispersed throughout the neural system.[6,7] All nicotinic receptors consist of five protein subunits and contain two binding sites for ACh that need to be filled for the channel to open.

The adrenergic receptors are divided primarily into alpha (α) and beta (β) receptors, and each of these receptor types is subdivided further. There are two main α adrenoceptors, α_1 and α_2 and three β adrenoceptors, β_1, β_2, and β_3.[1,8] All of these receptors are G-protein–linked receptors but have different second messengers. α_1-Receptors increase phospholipase C, which stimulates release of intracellular calcium. These receptors function to produce constriction of blood vessels and bronchi and to relax the GI tract and the genitourinary (GU) tract; α_2 receptors decrease cyclic adenosine monophosphate formation and inhibit calcium release, which reduces sympathetic activity by acting as an autoreceptor; and the three β receptors stimulate cyclic adenosine monophosphate formation and produce increases in cardiac rate and contractility, bronchodilation, and lipolysis. Dopamine (D) receptors are another subclass of adrenoceptors. D_1 receptors are located on renal vascular smooth muscle and mediate vasodilation of the renal artery. D_2 receptors are found on presynaptic nerve terminals. Other types of dopamine receptors also exist in the CNS.

The muscarinic receptors are divided into six distinct types, M_1 to M_6, although types M_4 to M_6 have not been fully characterized.[1,9] M_1 is found mainly in the CNS and has excitatory effects. Diminished ability to up-regulate during adrenergic neuron loss in Alzheimer's disease has led to speculation that the progressive decline in cognition may be caused in part by problems with this receptor.[10] Muscarinic receptors are also thought to modulate dopaminergic neurotransmission, and therefore M_1-agonists might be helpful in treating the overactive dopaminergic transmission that occurs in schizophrenia.[11] M_1 receptors are also located in the GI tract and are involved with secretion of gastric acid after vagal stimulation during a meal. M_2 receptors are located in the heart and produce an increase in potassium (K^+) conductance and block calcium channels, reducing heart rate and contractility. These receptors are also located in the CNS and produce neural inhibition. M_3 receptors are primarily located in the glands and smooth muscle. Release of glandular secretions such as saliva, bronchial secretions, and sweat result from stimulation of M_3 receptors. GI smooth muscle contraction is also a function of M_3 receptor stimulation. M_3 receptors produce vasodilation of vascular smooth muscle by producing the release of nitric oxide from endothelial cells. M_2 and M_3 receptors are also located in the bladder.

Functions of the Autonomic Nervous System and Specific Innervations

The SNS mediates a fight-or-flight response, and the PNS tends to place the body in a more calm state. However, some authors state that there is no generalization that can be used to explain whether the SNS or PNS causes excitation or inhibition.[2]

The SNS response is triggered by direct sympathetic stimulation of the effector organs and by stimulation of the adrenal medulla to release epinephrine and norepinephrine into the circulation. This system functions as a "unit," producing a set of reactions that occur together. The SNS functions to dilate the pupils, increase heart rate and contractility, raise serum glucose level for energy, dilate the bronchioles, increase skeletal blood flow, and relax the GI and GU tracts.[3] Blood is shunted from the GI system and skin to the muscles by constriction of the arterioles and dilation of the muscular vasculature. We can remember these actions by thinking that in a fight-or-flight response, a human being needs to see better (pupil dilation), breathe better (bronchodilate), and get blood to the muscles (increase cardiac output) but does not need to look for a rest room (limited GI and GU activity). Some specific innervations and their receptors associated with the sympathetic system include the following[12]:

1. Contraction of the iris radial muscle causing mydriasis: α_1
2. Pilomotor reflex: α_1
3. Prostate contraction: α_1
4. Vasoconstriction of vascular smooth muscle: α_1
5. Adrenergic inhibition: α_2
6. Increased heart rate and contractility: β_1
7. Renin secretion: β_1
8. Skeletal muscle blood vessel dilation, bronchiole dilation, uterine relaxation, gluconeogenesis: β_2
9. Glycogenolysis: α_1 and β_2
10. Bladder wall relaxation and detrusor relaxation: β_2; trigone contraction: α_1 (net effect is decreased urination)
11. Decreased GI motility: α_2 and β_2

The PNS functions to conserve energy and is involved in rest and digestion. Some specific innervations associated with the PNS include the following[12]:

1. Contraction of the circular muscle of the eye, causing miosis
2. Decreased rate and contractility of the heart via the vagus nerve
3. Constriction of the trachea and bronchioles
4. Increased muscle motility and tone of the GI tract
5. Bladder wall contraction, detrusor contraction, and trigone relaxation, resulting in urination

Table 5-1

The Main Effects of the Autonomic Nervous System

Organ	Sympathetic Effect	Adrenergic Receptor Type	Parasympathetic Effect	Cholinergic Receptor Type
HEART				
Sinoatrial node	Rate ↑	β_1	Rate ↓	M_2
Atrial muscle	Force ↑	β_1	Force ↓	M_2
Atrioventricular node	Automaticity ↑	β_1	Conduction velocity ↓ Atrioventricular block	M_2
Ventricular muscle	Automaticity ↑ Force ↑	β_1	No effect	M_2
BLOOD VESSELS				
Arterioles				
Coronary	Constriction	α		
Muscle	Dilatation	β_2	No effect	
Viscera	Constriction	α	No effect	
Skin	Constriction	α	No effect	
Brain	Constriction	α	No effect	
Erectile tissue	Constriction	α	Dilatation	? M_3
Salivary gland	Constriction	α	Dilatation	? M_3
Veins	Constriction	α	No effect	
	Dilatation	β_2	No effect	
VISCERA				
Bronchi				
Smooth muscle	No sympathetic innervation, but dilated by circulating epinephrine	β_2	Constriction	M_3
Glands	No effect		Secretion	M_3
Gastrointestinal tract				
Smooth muscle	Motility ↓	$\alpha_1, \alpha_2, \beta_2$	Motility ↑	M_3
Sphincters	Constriction	α_2, β_2	Dilatation	M_3
Glands	No effect		Secretion	M_3
			Gastric acid secretion	M_1
Uterus				
Pregnant	Constriction	α	Variable	
Nonpregnant	Relaxation	β_2		
MALE SEX ORGANS	Ejaculation	α	Erection	? M_3

From Rang HP, Dale MM, Ritter JM, Moore, PK. *Pharmacology.* 5th ed. New York: Churchill Livingstone; 2003.
Transmitters other than acetylcholine and norepinephrine contribute to many of these responses.   *Continued*

6. Release of endothelial-derived relaxing factor in response to stimulation of muscarinic receptors, resulting in relaxation of vascular smooth muscle (vasodilation)

See Table 5-1 for more specific innervations.

Many organs are innervated by both the sympathetic and parasympathetic systems, and most of the time they have opposing effects. However, exceptions do exist because both systems perform similar secretory functions and increase salivation.

Table 5-1

The Main Effects of the Autonomic Nervous System—cont'd				
Organ	Sympathetic Effect	Adrenergic Receptor Type	Parasympathetic Effect	Cholinergic Receptor Type
EYE				
Pupil	Dilatation	α	Constriction	M_3
Ciliary muscle	Relaxation (slight)	β	Constriction	M_3
SKIN				
Sweat glands	Secretion (mainly cholinergic)	α	No effect	
Pilomotor	Piloerection	α	No effect	
SALIVARY GLANDS	Secretion	α, β	Secretion	M_3
LACRIMAL GLANDS	No effect		Secretion	M_3
KIDNEY	Renin secretion	β_2	No effect	
LIVER	Glycogenolysis Gluconeogenesis	α, β_2	No effect	

Also, some organs are innervated by only one system. The sweat glands and most blood vessels receive only sympathetic input, and the bronchial smooth muscle has only parasympathetic innervation. However, the bronchioles are extremely sensitive to circulating catecholamines because they contain β_2 receptors.[3]

Enteric Nervous System

The enteric nervous system controls exocrine and endocrine functions of the GI tract and motility, microcirculation, and immune and inflammatory processes.[1,13] It can function independently from the CNS, although it maintains connections to the brain via the SNS and PNS. It contains two major plexuses: the myenteric plexus, which innervates the two muscle layers of the entire gut and the secretory portion of the mucosa with extensions to the gallbladder and pancreas and the submucous plexus in the small intestine, which innervates the muscularis mucosa, glandular epithelium, and submucosal blood vessels. A similar plexus is found in the gallbladder, pancreas, cystic duct, and common bile duct.

The neurotransmitters involved in the enteric system were originally thought to include only ACh and serotonin. However, recent research has shown that adenosine triphosphate, γ-aminobutyric acid, substance P, vasoactive intestinal polypeptide, nitric oxide, and a variety of other peptides are active in this system.[13] The stimulatory motor neurons use ACh and substance P as their main neurotransmitters, whereas the inhibitory motor neurons contain vasoactive intestinal polypeptide and nitric oxide. Connections to these nerves include parasympathetic motor pathways through the vagus nerve that innervate the motor and secretomotor functions of the upper GI tract and the sacral nerves that control the distal colon and rectum. Post-ganglionic sympathetic fibers containing vasoactive intestinal polypeptide target the secretomotor neurons, submucosal blood vessels, and the GI sphincters. Sensory information is carried through the vagus and splanchnic nerves.

Problems with the enteric nervous system have been implicated in a number of GI disorders.[13] Severe vomiting with chemotherapy has been linked to excessive serotonin release by damaged mucosal enterochromaffin cells. High levels of serotonin activate receptors on the vagal primary afferents that extend to the vomiting center in the brainstem. Defective enteric neurons can cause a slowing of intestinal propulsion, leading to bowel obstruction. Another example is achalasia, difficulty swallowing, which is related to a loss of inhibitory myenteric neurons innervating the lower esophageal sphincter. This sphincter is tonically contracted and fails to let food cross into the stomach. Drugs that act on the nervous system to help normalize motility and secretions have been developed.

Nonadrenergic, Noncholinergic System of the Autonomic Nervous System

ACh and norepinephrine are not the only neurotransmitters associated with the ANS. It has been demonstrated that nonadrenergic, noncholinergic transmission can occur from the neurons that were thought to contain only the usual sympathetic and parasympathetic transmitters.[1] Apparently, other neurotransmitters, nitric oxide, vasoactive intestinal peptide, adenosine triphosphate, and neuropeptide Y can exist side by side with ACh and norepinephrine and be secreted by the same neuron. This complicates drug development because some drugs designed to facilitate or block the ANS would also have to exert action on these other transmitters.

DRUGS THAT MIMIC THE PARASYMPATHETIC NERVOUS SYSTEM

Drugs that affect the PNS are divided into two categories: those that act directly on the cholinergic (muscarinic) receptors and those that act indirectly by inhibiting the enzyme AChE. AChE rapidly hydrolyzes ACh in the synaptic cleft by cleaving ACh to acetate and choline. Inhibitors of AChE stimulate cholinergic action by prolonging the lifetime of ACh.

Clinical Applications for Muscarinic Agonists

Drugs that mimic the actions of the PNS are used to reduce intraocular pressure in glaucoma, to increase the motility of the GI tract in paralytic ileus, to increase tone of the detrusor muscle for the treatment of urinary retention, and to improve cognition in Alzheimer's disease. Discussion of the drugs for the GI system and for Alzheimer's disease is included in later chapters.

Effects on the Eye

Parasympathetic input to the eye contracts both the constrictor pupillae and the ciliary muscles.[14] Contraction of this muscle allows the lens to accommodate for near vision. The constrictor pupillae muscle runs circumferentially around the iris, and when it contracts, produces miosis (Figure 5-5). The ciliary muscle relaxes the suspensory ligaments, allowing the lens to bulge and adjusting the curvature of the lens, which reduces its focal length.

Aqueous humor is normally secreted slowly and continuously from the ciliary body. The fluid drains through the canal of Schlemm. However, in acute glaucoma, the canal of Schlemm becomes blocked by a dilated pupil, and the fluid cannot drain. The intraocular pressure is raised, which damages the eye and can lead to blindness. Pupil constriction under these circumstances can improve drainage by moving the pupil away from the pathway for aqueous humor, allowing the fluid to drain into the canal.

Effects on Myasthenia Gravis

Myasthenia gravis is an autoimmune disorder caused by antibodies specific for the nicotinic ACh receptor at the neuromuscular junction.[15,16] Patients demonstrate muscle weakness and easy fatigability, being unable to sustain muscular contractions. Areas of involvement may include the eyelids, extraocular muscles, extremities, diaphragm, and neck extensor muscles.[4] Occasionally, however, the disease may only manifest itself by drooping eyelids (ptosis). Diagnosis is made by using sensitive electromyography and by administering a short-acting intravenous drug (edrophonium) to prolong the effects of ACh at the junction. A positive test result for the disease consists of a rapid (within 2 minutes) but short-lived improvement (less than 5 minutes) in muscle strength. Dynamometer testing and lung vital capacity testing are used to monitor strength.[4] Other treatments for myasthenia gravis include immunosuppressant drugs such as azathioprine, cyclosporine, and prednisone. These drugs are covered in later chapters.

Effects on the Neuromuscular Junction

In addition to improving strength in some neuromuscular junction disorders, muscarinic agonists can

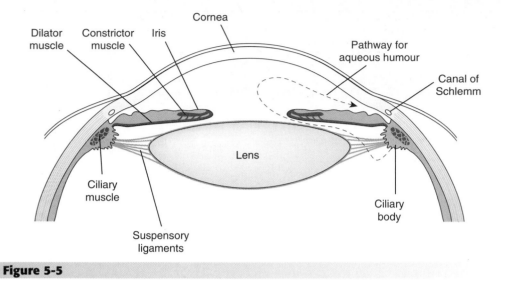

Figure 5-5

The anterior chamber of the eye, showing the pathway for secretion and drainage of the aqueous humor. (From Rang HP, Dale MM, Ritter JM, Moore, PK. *Pharmacology.* 5th ed. New York: Churchill Livingstone; 2003.)

be used to reverse muscle paralysis during surgical procedures.[14] Blocking of the neuromuscular junction is often used along with anesthesia in delicate procedures in which movement is contraindicated. Paralytic agents, or curare-like drugs (e.g., pancuronium), used to block the neuromuscular junction will occasionally produce an excessively long paralysis. Drugs that inhibit AChE can be used to terminate the action of these neuromuscular blockers. They may also be used to reverse an anticholinergic overdose.

Direct-Acting Muscarinic Agonists

Direct-acting agonists bind directly to the muscarinic receptors, functioning just like ACh, to mimic the actions of the PNS (Table 5-2). Pilocarpine and bethanechol are the two most commonly used direct-acting agents. Pilocarpine is applied topically to the cornea to produce miosis in acute glaucoma.[17] The duration of action is 24 hours. With topical application, there is a reduced chance of the drug producing a systemic adverse effect. Pilocarpine is also used for the treatment of xerostomia (dry mouth) in Sjögren's syndrome and after radiation therapy for head and neck cancers.[18,19]

Bethanechol stimulates the PNS with a particular selectivity for the detrusor muscle in the bladder (see discussion of the physiology and function of

the bladder) and the smooth muscle of the GI tract. It is used to treat urinary retention or to reduce urethral resistance in detrusor-trigone dyssynergia. It is particularly useful for postpartum or postoperative urine retention. In the GI tract, the drug stimulates gastric motility and restores peristaltic activity in a paralytic ileus.[14] It may also be used in the treatment of reflux esophagitis.[20] Unlike ACh, it is not inactivated by AChE and therefore has a longer duration of action than the endogenous transmitter. It is available in an oral form and as a subcutaneous injection. With the oral formulation, onset of action is within 30 to 90 minutes and duration of action may last up to 6 hours.[12]

Indirect-Acting Muscarinic Stimulants

Indirect-acting muscarinic stimulants act by inhibiting AChE to prolong the action of ACh. There are actually two types of cholinesterases that are seen in the body, AChE and butyrylcholinesterase (plasma cholinesterase located at nonneuronal sites). Both of these enzymes produce a very rapid breakdown of ACh, 10^4 molecules of ACh in 1 second by a single enzyme.[21] The drugs appear to inhibit both forms of the enzyme with equal potency.

In general, the indirect-acting agents fall into three categories: short-acting anticholinesterases,

Text continued on p. 64

Table 5-2

Summary of Drugs that Affect Noradrenergic Transmission

Type	Drug*	Main Action	Uses/Function	Unwanted Effects	Pharmacokinetic Aspects	Notes
SYMPATHOMIMETIC (directly acting)	Norepinephrine[†]	α/β-Agonist	Not used clinically. Transmitter at postganglionic sympathetic neurons, and in CNS. Hormone of adrenal medulla	Hypertension, vasoconstriction, tachycardia (or reflex bradycardia), ventricular dysrhythmias	Poorly absorbed by mouth. Rapid removal by tissues. Metabolized by MAO and COMT. Plasma $t_{1/2}$ ~ 2 min Given IM or SC. As norepinephrine	
	Epinephrine[†]	α/β-Agonist	Asthma (emergency treatment), anaphylactic shock, cardiac arrest. Added to local anaesthetic solutions. Main hormone of adrenal medulla.	As norepinephrine		
	Isoprenaline	β-Agonist (nonselective)	Asthma (obsolete). Not an endogenous substance	Tachycardia, dysrhythmias	Some tissue uptake, followed by inactivation (COMT) Plasma $t_{1/2}$ ~ 2 h Plasma $t_{1/2}$ ~ 2 min Given IV	Now replaced by salbutamol in treatment of asthma.
	Dobutamine	β₁-Agonist (nonselective)	Cardiogenic shock	Dysrhythmias		
	Salbutamol	β₂-Agonist	Asthma, premature labor	Tachycardia, dysrhythmias, tremor; peripheral vasodilatation	Given orally or by aerosol Mainly excreted unchanged Plasma $t_{1/2}$ ~ 4 h	
	Salmeterol	β₂-Agonist	Asthma	As salbutamol	Given by aerosol Long acting	Formoterol is similar.
	Terbutaline	β₂-Agonist	Asthma	As salbutamol	Poorly absorbed orally Given by aerosol Mainly excreted unchanged Plasma $t_{1/2}$ ~ 4 h	

From Rang HP, Dale MM, Ritter JM, Moore, PK. *Pharmacology.* 5th ed. New York: Churchill Livingstone; 2003.

NA, Noradrenaline; *MAO,* monoamine oxidase; *CNS,* central nervous system; *COMT,* catechol-O-methyltransferase; *IM,* intramuscular; *SC,* subcutaneous; *IV,* intravenous; $t_{1/2}$, half-life.

*For chemical structures, see Hardman et al (2001).

[†]Note that norepinephrine and epinephrine are the recommended drug names for noradrenaline and adrenaline, respectively.

Continued

	Drug	Type/Mechanism	Uses	Adverse effects	Pharmacokinetics	Notes
SYMPATHOMIMETIC (directly acting) —cont'd	Clenbuterol	β_2-Agonist	"Anabolic" action to increase muscle strength	As salbutamol	Active orally; long acting	Illicit use in sports.
	Phenylephrine	α_1-Agonist	Nasal decongestion	Hypertension, reflex bradycardia	Given intranasally Metabolized by MAO Short plasma $t_{1/2}$	
	Methoxamine	α-Agonist (nonselective)	Nasal decongestion	as phenylephrine	Given intranasally Plasma $t_{1/2} \sim 1$ h	
	Clonidine	α_2-Partial agonist	Hypertension, migraine	Drowsiness, orthostatic hypotension, edema and weight gain, rebound hypertension	Well absorbed orally Excreted unchanged and as conjugate Plasma $t_{1/2} \sim 12$ h	
SYMPATHOMIMETIC (indirectly acting)	Tyramine	NA release	No clinical uses; present in various foods	As norepinephrine	Normally destroyed by MAO in gut; does not enter brain	
	Amphetamine	NA release, MAO inhibitor, uptake 1 inhibitor, CNS stimulant	Used as CNS stimulant in narcolepsy, also (paradoxically) in hyperactive children Appetite suppressant Drug of abuse	Hypertension, tachycardia, insomnia Acute psychosis with overdose Dependence	Well absorbed orally Penetrates freely into brain Excreted unchanged in urine Plasma $t_{1/2} \sim 12$ h, depending on urine flow and pH	Methylphenidate is similar.
	Ephedrine	NA release, β-agonist, weak CNS stimulant	Nasal decongestion	As amphetamine, but less pronounced	Similar to amphetamine	Contraindicated if MAO inhibitors are given.
ADRENOCEPTOR ANTAGONISTS	Phenoxybenzamine	α-Antagonist (nonselective, irreversible) Uptake 1 inhibitor	Pheochromocytoma	Hypotension, flushing tachycardia, nasal congestion, impotence	Absorbed orally Plasma $t_{1/2} \sim 12$ h	Action outlasts presence of drug in plasma because of covalent binding to receptor.
	Phentolamine	α-Antagonist (nonselective), vasodilator	Rarely used	As phenoxybenzamine	Usually given IV Metabolized by liver Plasma $t_{1/2} \sim 2$ h	Tolazoline is similar.
	Prazosin	α_1-Antagonist	Hypertension	As phenoxybenzamine	Absorbed orally Metabolized by liver Plasma $t_{1/2} \sim 4$ h	Doxazosin and terazosin are similar but longer acting. *Continued*

Table 5-2

Summary of Drugs that Affect Noradrenergic Transmission—cont'd

Type	Drug*	Main Action	Uses/Function	Unwanted Effects	Pharmacokinetic Aspects	Notes
ADRENOCEPTOR ANTAGONISTS —cont'd	Tamsulosin	α_1-Antagonist ("uroselective")	Prostatic hyperplasia	Failure of ejaculation	Absorbed orally Plasma $t_{1/2}$ ~ 5 h	Selective for α_{1A}-adrenoceptor.
	Yohimbine	α_2-Antagonist	Not used clinically; claimed to be aphrodisiac	Excitement, hypertension	Absorbed orally Metabolized by liver Plasma $t_{1/2}$ ~ 4 h	Idazoxan is similar.
	Propranolol	β-Antagonist (nonselective)	Angina, hypertension, cardiac dysrhythmias, anxiety tremor, glaucoma	Bronchoconstriction, cardiac failure, cold extremities, fatigue and depression, hypoglycemia	Absorbed orally Extensive first-pass metabolism About 90% bound to plasma protein Plasma $t_{1/2}$ ~ 4 h	Timolol is similar and used mainly to treat glaucoma.
	Alprenolol	β-Antagonist (nonselective) (partial agonist)	As propranolol	As propranolol	Absorbed orally Metabolized by liver Plasma $t_{1/2}$ ~ 4 h	Oxprenolol and pindolol are similar.
	Practolol	β_1-Antagonist	Hypertension, angina, dysrhythmias	As propranolol, also oculomucocutaneous syndrome	Absorbed orally Excreted unchanged in urine Plasma $t_{1/2}$ ~ 4 h	Withdrawn from clinical use.
	Metoprolol	β_1-antagonist	Angina, hypertension, dysrhythmias	As propranolol, less risk of bronchoconstriction	Absorbed orally Mainly metabolized in liver Plasma $t_{1/2}$ ~ 3 h	Atenolol is similar with a longer half-life.
	Butoxamine	β_2-antagonist, weak α-agonist	No clinical uses			
	Labetalol	α/β-Antagonist	Hypertension in pregnancy	Postural hypotension, bronchoconstriction	Absorbed orally; conjugated in liver Plasma $t_{1/2}$ ~ 4 h	
	Carvedilol	α/β-Antagonist	Heart failure	As for other β-blockers Exacerbation of heart failure Renal failure	Absorbed orally $t_{1/2}$ ~ 10 h	Additional actions may contribute to clinical benefit.

Continued

Category	Drug	Mechanism	Clinical use	Unwanted effects	Pharmacokinetic aspects	Notes
DRUGS AFFECTING NORADRENALINE SYNTHESIS	α-Methyl-p-tyrosine, Carbidopa	Inhibits tyrosine hydroxylase; Inhibits DOPA decarboxylase	Occasionally used in pheochromocytoma; Used as adjunct to levodopa to prevent peripheral effects	Hypotension, sedation	Absorbed orally; does not enter brain	
	Methyldopa	False transmitter precursor	Hypertension in pregnancy	Hypotension, drowsiness, diarrhea, impotence, hypersensitivity reactions	Absorbed slowly by mouth; Excreted unchanged or as conjugate. Plasma $t_{1/2} \sim 6$ h	
	Reserpine	Depletes NA stores by inhibiting vesicular uptake of NA	Hypertension (obsolete)	As methyldopa. Also depression, parkinsonism. gynecomastia	Poorly absorbed orally; Slowly metabolized; Plasma $t_{1/2} \sim 100$ h; Excreted in milk	Antihypertensive effect develops slowly and persists when drug is stopped.
DRUGS AFFECTING NORADRENALINE RELEASE	Guanethidine	Inhibits NA release; also causes NA depletion and can damage NA neurons irreversibly	Hypertension (obsolete)	As methyldopa. Hypertension on first administration	Poorly absorbed orally; Mainly excreted unchanged in urine; Plasma $t_{1/2} \sim 100$ h	Action prevented by uptake 1 inhibitors. Bethanidine and debrisoquin are similar.
DRUGS AFFECTING NORADRENALINE UPTAKE	Imipramine	Blocks uptake 1; also has atropine-like action	Depression	Atropine-like side effects. Cardiac dysrhythmias in overdose	Well absorbed orally 95% bound to plasma protein; Converted active metabolite (desmethyl-imipramine); Plasma $t_{1/2} \sim 4$ h; Well absorbed orally	Desipramine and amitriptyline are similar.
	Cocaine	Local anesthetic; blocks uptake 1 CNS stimulant	Rarely used local anesthetic. Major drug of abuse	Hypertension, excitement, convulsions, dependence	Well absorbed orally	

medium-duration anticholinesterases, and irreversible anticholinesterases. Edrophonium is a very short-acting compound used to help diagnose myasthenia gravis. Neostigmine and pyridostigmine are medium-duration anticholinesterases. In fact, pyridostigmine is the treatment of choice for patients with mild myasthenia gravis because it has greater bioavailability and a half-life of 4 hours.[21,22]

Irreversible anticholinesterases contain an organic group; hence, they are called *organophosphate compounds*. These are agents that have been developed into war gases (sarin) and insecticides (malathion). These bind to AChE irreversibly, producing weakness and sensory loss. Depolarizing neuromuscular blockade occurs in which the muscle initially contracts but is quickly followed by a phase of nondepolarizing blockade with marked muscle weakness because there is no longer free ACh to act on the muscle junction.[14] Other signs are those that are related to muscarinic excess and include miosis, sweating, salivation, bronchial constriction, vomiting, and diarrhea. Death may occur as result of paralysis of the respiratory muscles and excessive bronchial secretions.[19] These agents are highly lipid soluble and are rapidly absorbed through the mucous membranes and even through intact skin. Because these compounds are absorbed rapidly through the cuticles of insects, they are used in agriculture.

Therapeutic Concerns with Direct-Acting and Indirect-Acting Muscarinic Agents

Direct-acting and indirect-acting muscarinic agents can produce significant cardiovascular effects, including bradycardia and decreased cardiac output.[1] The reduction in cardiac output results from a decrease in contractility, particularly in the atria, caused by relative denseness of the muscarinic receptors in this area. Therapists must monitor heart rate and notify the physician if the resting heart rate drops below 60 beats/min. Further dosing may be contraindicated, but the physician will make this determination.

Another adverse effect that may occur with these drugs is a generalized vasodilation, producing a marked decrease in blood pressure. Nitric oxide and endothelial-derived relaxing factor mediate this effect.[1]

Smooth muscle in the lungs and GI tract are also affected by excess muscarinic activity. This produces abdominal pain, diarrhea, vomiting, frequent urination, bronchoconstriction, and increased secretions (increased sweating and salivation). These drugs are thus contraindicated for anyone with a history of allergy and asthma. Urinary incontinence, placing the patient at risk for integumentary issues and causing the inconvenience of having to visit the bathroom frequently, presents additional problems that need to be addressed.

MUSCARINIC ANTAGONISTS

Drugs that block the muscarinic receptors are often labeled as parasympatholytic because they block the action of parasympathetic nerve activity. They all function as competitive antagonists of Ach.

Clinical Application for Antimuscarinic (Anticholinergic) Drugs

Antimuscarinic drugs are used to treat motion sickness, relieve symptoms of Parkinson's disease, dilate pupils for an ocular exam, reduce motility of the GI and GU tracts, and dilate the airways.[23] In addition, because they reduce secretions, they can be used preoperatively to prevent excessive salivation and reduce bronchiole tract secretions associated with anesthesia.

Anticholinergic Drugs

Atropine is the prototypic anticholinergic agent. It is both a central and a peripheral cholinergic antagonist, although it appears to have little effect at the nicotinic receptor sites, so the autonomic ganglia are not usually affected unless high doses are given.[1] The same is true for the nicotinic receptors at the neuromuscular junction. Atropine is primarily used to produce mydriasis in the eye for an ocular exam and as an adjunct to anesthesia to reduce respiratory secretions. However, atropine can produce a variety of effects because of the large number of parasympathetic cholinergic nerves that exist within the body, limiting the drug's usefulness.

Scopolamine is another anticholinergic drug. It has an effect similar to that of atropine but produces greater CNS depression causing drowsiness, memory loss, and sleep. Its primary use is to prevent motion sickness and vertigo caused by depression of vestibular function.[24] It is available in a parenteral preparation as an adjunct to anesthesia and in a transdermal form for prevention of motion sickness. The patch is applied behind the ear for 3 days, preferably 4 hours before a trip begins.

Synthetic anticholinergics, such as dicyclomine and glycopyrrolate, have been formulated to act more selectively on the GI tract and thus have been used for the treatment of irritable bowel syndrome.

Ipratropium is an inhaled anticholinergic agent, available alone or in combination with albuterol (a β_2-agonist), for the treatment of bronchospasm related to asthma and other chronic obstructive lung diseases.[25,26] Because this drug is inhaled directly into lung tissue rather than administered orally, there are fewer systemic effects compared with the other anticholinergic agents. Dry mouth and pharyngeal irritation are the major complaints with ipratropium, but it can also increase intraocular pressure in patients with glaucoma. Tiotropium is a new long-acting anticholinergic drug with duration of 24 hours, enabling once-a-day dosing.[27]

Therapeutic Concerns with Anticholinergic Drugs

At low doses, atropine affects the salivary glands, producing dry mouth; larger doses block accommodation of the eyes, causing blurred vision. Vagal effects become blocked as the drug level increases, producing tachycardia and diminished bronchial secretions and sweating. Parasympathetic tone to the gut and the urinary tract is blocked, producing constipation and urinary retention. In fact, after surgery, many patients complain that they have the sensation that they must urinate but are unable to relax the sphincter to produce a flow. At still higher doses, effects on the CNS include restlessness, confusion, hallucinations, and coma.[12]

Most patients seen in physical therapy will not be receiving anticholinergic drugs, at least on a long-term basis. However, many drugs, particularly the mood-altering medications, have anticholinergic adverse effects, and these need to be recognized. Most patients complain about sedation and fatigue, which reduces exercise capacity. Two other concerns include increased heart rate and the inability to cool oneself (especially in young children and the elderly).[12] Vital signs, including the patient's tem-

perature, should be monitored frequently, particularly if there is a history of cardiac issues.

DRUGS AFFECTING THE SYMPATHETIC (ADRENERGIC) NERVOUS SYSTEM

Drugs that mimic the SNS are labeled *sympathomimetic* (Table 5-2). They are designed to either facilitate norepinephrine and epinephrine release or to activate the adrenergic receptors. See Figure 5-6 for a diagram of a noradrenergic nerve terminal showing sites of drug action. Specifically, sympathomimetic drugs constrict arterioles to reduce bleeding, slow diffusion of local anesthetics, decongest mucous membranes, and raise blood pressure in shock and hypotensive states.[28]

Pharmacologic Effects of Catecholamines

Cardiac Effects

The catecholamines produce a significant increase in myocardial contractility (positive inotropic effect) and a significant increase in heart rate (positive chronotropic effect).[29] Both of these factors improve cardiac output because Heart Rate × Stroke Volume = Cardiac Output. The increase in contractility results from an increase in calcium influx into cardiac fibers. The increase in heart rate is produced by increasing the rate of membrane depolarization in the sinus node. Catecholamines also hasten cardiac conduction. Atrioventricular conduction improves, so some physicians will use catecholamines to treat heart block.

Vascular Effects

Vascular effects with these drugs vary because the net effect depends on the dose given.[28] At low doses, epinephrine will decrease peripheral vascular resistance via β_2 receptor–mediated dilation of skeletal muscle blood vessels. At higher doses, α_1 receptor influence balances the β_2 receptor influence, and at even higher doses, α_1 receptor influence predominates, producing vasoconstriction (elevated peripheral vascular resistance) and hypertension. However, the idea that there are sympathetic vasodilator nerves to the skeletal muscle has recently been challenged.[30] The skeletal dilator response may actually be α_2 receptors linked to

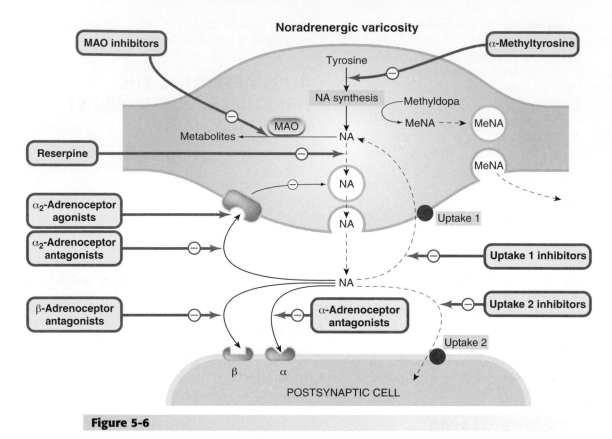

Figure 5-6

Generalized diagram of a noradrenergic nerve terminal showing sites of drug action. Action of indirectly acting sympathomimetic drugs is not shown. *NA*, Noradrenaline; *MAO*, monoamine oxides; *MeNA*, methylnoradrenaline. (From Rang HP, Dale MM, Ritter JM, Moore, PK. *Pharmacology.* 5th ed. New York: Churchill Livingstone; 2003.)

nitric oxide production, which relaxes endothelium in isolated blood vessels.[31] Norepinephrine produces predominantly an α effect at all doses, elevating blood pressure.

Central Nervous System Effects
The natural catecholamines are relatively polar, and therefore they do not enter the CNS easily.[1] However, in larger doses they are still capable of producing anxiety, tremors, and headaches. The noncatecholamine adrenergic agonists such as phenylephrine, ephedrine, and amphetamine have greater lipid solubility and produce more CNS effects.

Nonvascular Smooth Muscle Effects
Catecholamines are capable of relaxing the smooth muscle of the GI tract, reducing the strength of intestinal peristalsis.[28] In the bladder, epinephrine

will cause urinary retention by trigone sphincter constriction and detrusor relaxation. In the lungs, bronchial smooth muscle dilates in response to catecholamines acting on β_2 receptors.

Effects on Nerve Terminals
α_2 Receptors are present presynaptically on cholinergic and adrenergic nerve terminals. These are autoreceptors that act to inhibit neurotransmitter release. Clinically, they have primarily been used to reduce sympathetic outflow as a treatment for hypertension but are also being used as analgesics and for reducing spasticity.[32,33]

Metabolic Effects
Epinephrine acts to increase blood glucose and fatty acid level to supply the needed energy for activity. Insulin secretion is inhibited, and glycogenolysis and gluconeogenesis are enhanced.[28]

Direct-Acting Nonselective Adrenergic Agents

Three catecholamines occur naturally in the human body: norepinephrine, epinephrine, and dopamine. Norepinephrine and epinephrine interact directly with α and β receptors. Even though dopamine is the precursor of both norepinephrine and epinephrine, it is also a neurotransmitter, binding to and affecting dopamine receptors, as well as α and β receptors.

As mentioned previously, epinephrine has effects on all α and β receptors, but the net effect depends on the dose. Epinephrine activates β_1 receptors to increase the strength and rate of cardiac contractions; on β_2 receptors to relax bronchiole smooth muscle, activate glycogenolysis in the liver, and dilate skeletal muscle blood vessels; and on β_3 receptors to activate lipolysis in fat cells. Epinephrine activates α_1 receptors to constrict vascular smooth muscle and also on α_2 receptors presynaptically. The net effect is that epinephrine is a potent vasoconstrictor and a cardiac stimulant, although in some cases, a drop in peripheral vascular resistance is seen, producing a fall in diastolic pressure.[34]

Epinephrine is predominantly used in the emergency department to treat anaphylactic or cardiogenic shock.[35] Therapists may find this drug in the form of Ana-Guard or an EpiPen in the homes of patients at risk for anaphylaxis. Pressor-type drugs are critical during cardiopulmonary resuscitation to stimulate heart contraction, raise arterial pressure, and redistribute blood flow to important organs, with peripheral α receptor stimulation being the crucial component.[34] Epinephrine is also used to treat acute exacerbations of asthma and has a role in the treatment of allergy to relieve bronchospasm and decrease pulmonary congestion by constricting the nasal mucosal blood vessels. Small amounts of epinephrine are given along with local anesthetics to reduce circulation to the site of injection, thus preventing diffusion of the anesthetic. This is a common practice in dentistry because it prolongs the effect of the anesthetic agent.

Epinephrine is given by inhalation or by subcutaneous injection. It has a rapid onset, within 6 to 15 minutes if given by injection; sooner, if given by inhalation. The duration of action is 1 to 3 hours. In cases of severe asthma or shock, the doses may be repeated.

Norepinephrine activates α_1-adrenergic receptors to a greater extent than α_2 and β_1 receptors. It has little effect on β_2 receptors.[28] Increases in peripheral resistance and both diastolic and systolic blood pressure occur. Cardiac output does not increase as much as it does with a comparable dose of epinephrine because the vascular resistance increases so much. In addition, heart rate may not increase as much as one would expect because there are compensatory vagal reflexes in response to the elevated blood pressure. These vagal reflexes overcome the chronotropic effects, but the positive inotropic effects on the heart remain.

Dopamine, the immediate precursor of norepinephrine, activates α and β receptors and D_1 and D_2 dopaminergic receptors. These dopamine receptors exist in the renal vascular beds, and activation produces vasodilation of renal and splanchnic arterioles. At low doses, dopamine stimulates β_1 receptors, producing inotropic and chronotropic effects; but at very high doses, α receptors are stimulated, causing vascular vasoconstriction. Dopamine has been the drug of choice for the treatment of shock in renal failure because it raises blood pressure by increasing heart rate and contractility and at the same time facilitates perfusion of the kidneys.

Indirect-Acting Adrenergic Agents: Sympatholytic and Sympathomimetic

The indirect adrenergic agents are drugs that affect norepinephrine storage and release. Reserpine was traditionally used to treat mental disorders and hypertension. It is rarely used today except for research, but its mechanism of action is interesting. At low concentrations, reserpine blocks uptake of norepinephrine into the synaptic vesicles. Norepinephrine then accumulates inside the cytoplasm of the nerve where it is degraded by monoamine oxidase acting to deplete the neurotransmitter. Norepinephrine neuron-blocking drugs, such as guanethidine and bretylium, inhibit release of the neurotransmitter from the sympathetic nerve terminal. Like reserpine, these drugs are rarely used today except for experimental purposes. Essentially, these are sympatholytic drugs.

Indirect-acting sympathomimetic drugs include ephedrine and amphetamine. They are structurally related to norepinephrine but have weaker actions on the adrenergic receptors. Amphetamine is taken up into the nerve terminal by the norepinephrine uptake mechanism and enters the vesicles in exchange for norepinephrine, which is then freed to act on the postsynaptic receptors. It also blocks the action of monoamine oxidase, which in itself raises catecholamine levels. So the net effect is enhanced release of norepinephrine, producing an increase in blood pressure and cardiac contractility. Amphetamine readily enters the CNS where it facilitates the release of dopamine, producing euphoria. It also produces increased alertness, decreased fatigue, decreased appetite, and a marked increase in sympathetic activity. Some forms of the drug have been used in the treatment of narcolepsy and attention deficit disorder and are currently being studied in patients with brain injury for the purpose of improving motor and cognitive performance.[36,37]

Ephedrine was introduced to the West in 1924 from China. It is now made synthetically and can be found in many herbal medications under the name *ma-huang*. It is an orally active sympathomimetic with a longer duration of action than epinephrine, but it has a milder effect. It facilitates the release of norepinephrine, activates adrenergic receptors, and easily enters the CNS. It increases systolic and diastolic blood pressure and increases cardiac contractility. It is capable of producing effects similar to those of amphetamine.

α-Agonists

Phenylephrine is a drug that is used topically to produce mydriasis and nasal decongestion by constricting the mucosal blood vessels. It is a direct-acting synthetic adrenergic drug that primarily stimulates α_1 receptors and produces hypertension. It is found in many over-the-counter cold preparations.

Clonidine, unlike phenylephrine, lowers blood pressure. It reduces sympathetic tone by activating the α_2 receptor peripherally and in the CNS.[32] This drug is reviewed more fully in the cardiac chapters.

β-Agonists

β-Agonists are either nonselective (stimulate both β_1 and β_2 receptors) or are selective for either receptor. Isoproterenol is a potent nonselective β-agonist with positive chronotropic and inotropic

actions. It is primarily used to increase contractility of the heart during congestive heart failure. Dobutamine is a β_1-selective agonist that increases cardiac contractility without any β_2 effects. It is also used to treat shock or acute congestive heart failure and is used to induce stress to the heart as an alternative to exercise for patients undergoing myocardial perfusion studies.[38] In home care, dobutamine is used for severe congestive heart failure to prolong life while a patient waits for a heart transplant. Both isoproterenol and dobutamine are administered parenterally.

Selective β-agonists, such as terbutaline and salmeterol, are used in the treatment of asthma and other obstructive lung diseases. In addition, because β_2 receptors relax uterine contractions in a pregnant uterus, they have been instrumental in stopping premature labor and prolonging gestation.[39] The β_2-agonist drugs are covered more extensively in the pulmonary chapter.

Drugs Used to Treat Shock

For more than 60 years, epinephrine has been the primary drug used as a vasopressor during cardiac arrest. However, the evidence supporting its efficacy has been largely anecdotal.[34] In recent randomized controlled studies, epinephrine has been compared with placebo and with other vasopressors in both animals and humans; the findings suggest that some other drugs might be more effective during resuscitation. Research in this area has been ethically difficult to perform because drugs are crucial to recovery from cardiac standstill, so comparison with placebo is not always an option. In addition, standardizing doses of the drugs while someone is in the throws of cardiac arrest is not easy because the drugs are injected rapidly and without regard for some pharmacokinetic variables that influence bioavailability such as the volume of intravenous tubing or site of injection. In addition, some decrement in concentration occurs with storage of this drug.[40] The challenge is to restore cardiac contractions and increase blood pressure while maintaining cerebral and renal perfusion. Many times, cardiac function returns, but postresuscitation problems occur. There is concern about epinephrine's ability to revive patients after prolonged arrest, which has resulted in irreversible brain damage. Other concerns include the risks of severe hypertension and epinephrine overdose.

Laboratory evidence indicates that α-adrenergic agents might be extremely useful in cardiac arrest. Phenylephrine has the ability to increase aortic pressure without extreme myocardial excitation, which is particularly useful in cardiac arrest with ventricular fibrillation.[34,41] A comparison between phenylephrine and epinephrine showed no difference in overall rate of successful resuscitation, but further studies are needed before this drug becomes part of standard practice.[41]

Vasopressin, also known as *antidiuretic hormone*, is a vasoactive peptide that also acts on vasopressin receptors (V1-receptors), leading to contraction of vascular smooth muscle cells. Several animal studies show greater vital organ blood flow during resuscitation with this drug compared with epinephrine.[42] However, further study is needed before use of this drug replaces 60 years of experience with epinephrine. The current guidelines for resuscitation in adult patients recommend using either vasopressin or epinephrine.[34] However, dobutamine can be used when cardiac contractility is the primary requirement, and dopamine can be used in renal failure. Occasionally, norepinephrine is used when vasoconstriction is top priority, as might be the case in septic shock.[43]

α- and β-Adrenergic Blockers

Because α- and β-adrenergic blockers are largely used to lower blood pressure and reduce angina, they are covered in the cardiac chapters.

Therapeutic Concerns with Sympathomimetics

With the exception of the β$_2$-agonists used in the treatment of pulmonary disease, physical therapists will have little contact with patients taking sympathomimetic drugs. This is in part due to their use for the treatment of shock in the emergency department. However, because a significant number of over-the-counter cold remedies contain phenylephrine, therapists should be alert to the cardiac side effects of these medications. Given that one of the primary functions of the sympathetic system is to increase heart rate and contractility and peripheral resistance, these drugs increase the overall workload of the heart and have the potential to induce hypertension, cardiac arrhythmias, and angina, even at the lower doses contained in nasal decongestants and cold

tablets.[44,45] Other adverse effects have included cerebral hemorrhage, seizures, and deaths, particularly among ephedra users.[46] The Food and Drug Administration has taken steps to eliminate ephedra from weight loss products and herbal remedies because of the high numbers of adverse events.[47] Use of any of the products should be contraindicated for patients with hypertension, hyperthyroidism, ischemic heart disease, arrhythmias, and cerebrovascular insufficiency.

PHYSIOLOGY AND FUNCTION OF THE BLADDER

Bladder anatomy and innervation will be briefly reviewed because drugs that act on the SNS or PNS are used to treat bladder dysfunction. The lower urinary tract includes the detrusor muscle, trigone, and the urethra. The detrusor muscle receives a dominating cholinergic innervation and when it contracts, opens the bladder to produce emptying. This muscle also has β$_2$ receptors, which when stimulated, allow the bladder to relax and fill. The trigone (sphincter) and urethra have α$_1$ receptor input. Therefore sympathetic stimulation keeps the bladder from emptying. The urethra also contains striated muscle that forms the external urethral sphincter and is under voluntary control.

Anticholinergics, such as oxybutynin and tolterodine, have an antispasmodic effect on the lower urinary tract. These are potent antimuscarinics that suppress detrusor reflex contractions and increase bladder capacity in patients who have incontinence issues.

However, in elderly patients, these drugs can exacerbate existing conditions such as dry mouth, constipation, tachycardia, glaucoma, gastroesophageal reflux, and dementia.[48] None of the currently available drugs selectively block only the M$_2$ and M$_3$ receptors of the bladder.[49] In addition, some studies reveal only minimal improvements in urinary function with only one instance of leakage in less than 48 hours.[50] New drug delivery systems, such as an oxybutynin-impregnated ring implanted intravaginally, may enhance effectiveness.[51]

Other types of bladder dysfunction may also be improved with medications. Patients with bladder retention problems may be treated with cholinergic agonists such as bethanechol.[14] Those who have a tonically active trigone (inability to relax the sphincter) may be given an α–blocker such as phenoxybenzamine to facilitate flow, whereas α-agonists are used for patients with low urethral closure pressure. Calcium channel blockers can increase bladder capacity and decrease leakage in detrusor hyperactivity. This classification of drugs is discussed in Chapter 6.

ACTIVITIES 5

■ 1. Drugs that mimic the PNS may produce bradycardia and urinary and fecal incontinence. What is the impact that these adverse effects have on the patient and also on physical therapy intervention? What suggestions do you have for the patients taking these drugs to help minimize possible adverse effects?

■ 2. Interview a relative, neighbor, or patient who is over 65 years old regarding his or her medication use. Please list all prescription and over-the-counter medicines (use generic names) that have been taken within the past 6 months.

Ask your subject about side effects, number of pills he or she takes per day, and compliance. Look up the side effects and determine whether any are considered "anticholinergic." Discuss the impact that these effects have on the elderly population and how they may affect physical therapy intervention.

■ 3. Compare and contrast norepinephrine, phenylephrine, and isoproterenol (a β_1-agonist) in terms of their effects on systolic and diastolic blood pressure and heart rate.

References

1. Rang HP, Dale MM, Ritter JM, Moore JL. *Pharmacology.* 5th ed. New York: Churchill Livingstone; 2003.
2. Guyton AC, Hall JE. *Textbook of Medical Physiology.* 10th ed. Philadelphia: WB Saunders Company; 2000.
3. Katzung BG. Introduction to autonomic pharmacology. In: Katzung BG, ed. *Basic & Clinical Pharmacology.* 8th ed. New York: McGraw-Hill; 2001:75-91.
4. Kerwin R, Travis MJ, Page C, et al. Drugs and the nervous system. In: Page C, Curtis MJ, Sutter MC, Walker MJ, Hoffman BB, eds. *Integrated Pharmacology.* 2nd ed. Philadelphia: Mosby; 2002:219-280.
5. Wong DL. Why is the adrenal adrenergic? *Endocr Pathol.* 2003;14(1):25-36.
6. McGehee DS, Role LW. Physiological diversity of nicotinic acetylcholine receptors expressed by vertebrate neurons. *Ann Rev Physiol.* 1995;57:521-546.
7. Wonnacott S. Presynaptic nicotinic Ach receptors. *Trends Neurosci.* 1997;20(2):92-98.
8. Insel PA. Adrenergic receptors: evolving concepts and clinical implications. *N Engl J Med.* 1996;334(9):580-585.
9. Eglen RM, Choppin A, Dillon MP, Hegde S. Muscarinic receptor ligands and their therapeutic potential. *Curr Opin Chem Biol.* 1999;3:426-432.
10. Terry AV, Buccafusco JJ. The cholinergic hypothesis of age and Alzheimer's disease–related cognitive deficits: recent challenges and their implications for novel drug development. *J Pharmacol Exp Ther.* 2003;306(3):821-827.
11. Bymaster FP, Felder C, Ahmed S, McKinzie D. Muscarinic receptors as a target for drugs treating schizophrenia. *Curr Drug Targets CNS Neurol Disord.* 2002;1(2):163-181.
12. Salerno E. *Pharmacology for Health Professionals.* New York: Mosby; 1999.
13. Goyal RK, Hirano I. Mechanisms of disease: the enteric nervous system. *N Engl J Med.* 1996;334(17):1106-1115.
14. Pappano AJ. Cholinoceptor-activating and cholinesterase-inhibiting drugs. In: Katzung BG, ed. *Basic & Clinical Pharmacology.* 8th ed. New York: McGraw-Hill; 2001: 92-106.
15. Vincent A, Palace J, Hilton-Jones D. Myasthenia gravis. *Lancet.* 2001;357:2122-2128.
16. Nicolle MW. Myasthenia gravis. In: Carruthers SG, Hoffman BB, Melmon KL, Nierenberg DW, eds. *Melmon and Morrelli's Clinical Pharmacology.* 4th ed. New York: McGraw Hill; 2000:460-479.
17. Schuman JS. Short- and long-term safety of glaucoma drugs. *Expert Opin Drug Saf.* 2002;1(2):181-194.
18. Nieuw Amerongen AV, Veerman EC. Current therapies for xerostomia and salivary gland hypofunction associated with cancer therapies. *Support Care Cancer.* 2003;11(4):226-231.
19. O'Shaughnessy KM. Cholinergic and antimuscarinic (anticholinergic) mechanisms and drugs. In: Bennett PN, Brown MJ, eds. *Clinical Pharmacology.* 9th ed. Philadelphia: Churchill Livingstone; 2003:433-446.
20. Orenstein SR. Management of supraesophageal complications of gastroesophageal reflux disease in infants and children. *Am J Med.* 2000;108(suppl 4a):139S-143S.
21. Ehlert FJ. Drugs affecting the parasympathetic nervous system and autonomic ganglia. In: Brody MJ, Larner J, Minneman KP, eds. *Human Pharmacology: Molecular to Clinical.* 3rd ed. Philadelphia: Mosby; 1998:101-118.

22. Massey JM. Treatment of acquired myasthenia gravis. *Neurology.* 1997;48(suppl 5):S46-S51.
23. Pappano AJ, Katzung BG. Cholinoceptor-blocking drugs. In: Katzung BG, ed. *Basic & Clinical Pharmacology.* 8th ed. New York: McGraw-Hill; 2001:107-119.
24. Zuccaro TA. Pharmacological management of vertigo. *J Neurol Phys Ther.* 2003;27(3):118-121.
25. Drugs for asthma. *Med Lett Drugs Ther.* 1999;41(1044): 5-102.
26. Higgins JC. The 'crashing astigmatic.' *Am Fam Physician.* 2003;67(5):997-1004.
27. Panning CA, DeBisschop M. Tiotropium: an inhaled, long-acting anticholinergic drug for chronic obstructive pulmonary disease. *Pharmacotherapy.* 2003;23(2):183-189.
28. Hoffman BB. Adrenoceptor-activating and other sympathomimetic drugs. In: Katzung BG, ed. *Basic & Clinical Pharmacology.* 8th ed. New York: McGraw-Hill; 2001:120-137.
29. Post SR, Hammond HK, Insel PA. β-Adrenergic receptors and receptor signaling in heart failure. *Ann Rev Pharmacol Toxicol.* 1999;39:343-360.
30. Joyner MJ, Dietz NM. Sympathetic vasodilation in human muscle. *Acta Physiol Scand.* 2003;177(3):329-336.
31. Vanhoutte P. Endothelial adrenoceptors. *J Cardiovasc Pharmacol.* 2001;38(5):796-808.
32. Gavras I, Manolis AJ, Gavras H. The alpha2-adrenergic receptors in hypertension and heart failure: experimental and clinical studies. *J Hypertens.* 2001;19(12):2115-2124.
33. Remy-Neris O, Denys P, Bussel B. Intrathecal clonidine for controlling spastic hypertonia. *Phys Med Rehabil Clin N Am.* 2001;12(4):939-951.
34. Paradis NA, Wenzel V, Southall J. Pressor drugs in the treatment of cardiac arrest. *Cardiol Clin.* 2002;20(1):61-78.
35. Ellis AK, Day JH. Diagnosis and management of anaphylaxis. *CMAJ.* 2003;169(4):307-312.
36. Flanagan SR, Kane L, Rhoades D. Pharmacological modification of recovery following brain injury. *J Neurol Phys Ther.* 2003;27(3):129-137.
37. Goldstein LB. Neuropharmacology of TBI-induced plasticity. *Brain Inj.* 2003;17(8):685-694.
38. Elhendy A, Bax JJ, Poldermans D. Dobutamine stress myocardial perfusion imaging in coronary artery disease. *J Nucl Med.* 2001;43(12):1634-1646.
39. Berkman ND, Thorp JM, Lohr KN, et al. Tocolytic treatment for the management of preterm labor: a review of the evidence. *Am J Obstet Gynecol.* 2003;188(6):1648-1659.
40. Bonhome L, Benhamou D, Comoy E, Preaux N. Stability of epinephrine in alkalinized solutions. *Ann Emerg Med.* 1990;19(11):1242-1244.
41. Silfvast T, Saarnivaara L, Kinnunen A, et al. Comparison of adrenaline and phenylephrine in out-of-hospital cardiopulmonary resuscitation: a double-blind study. *Acta Anaesthesiol Scand.* 1985;29(6):610-613.
42. Wenzel V, Volker MD, Lindner KH, et al. Repeated administration of vasopressin but not epinephrine maintains coronary perfusion pressure after early and late administration during prolonged cardiopulmonary resuscitation in pigs. *Circulation.* 1999;99(10):1379-1384.
43. Bennett PN, Brown MJ. General pharmacology. In: Bennett PN, Brown MJ, eds. *Clinical Pharmacology.* 9th ed. New York: Churchill Livingstone; 2003:37-40.
44. Wortsman J. Role of epinephrine in acute stress. *Endocrinol Metab Clin N Am.* 2002;31(1):79-106.
45. Esler M, Rumantir M, Kaye D, et al. Sympathetic nerve biology in essential hypertension. *Clin Exp Pharmacol Physiol.* 2001;28(12):986-989.
46. Bent S, Tiedt TN, Odden MC, Shlipak MG. The relative safety of ephedra compared with other herbal products. *Ann Intern Med.* 2003;138(6):468-471.
47. Statement for the Record of the American Medical Association Re: Dangers of Dietary Supplement Ephedra. 2002. Available at: http://www.senate.gov/~gov_affairs/100802davis.htm. Accessed October 22, 2003.
48. Ouslander JG. Geriatric considerations in the diagnosis and management of overactive bladder. *Urology.* 2002;60(suppl5A):50-55.
49. Chapple CR, Yamanishi T, Chess-Williams R. Muscarinic receptor subtypes and management of the overactive bladder. *Urology.* 2002;60(suppl 5A):82-89.
50. Hervison P, Hay-Smith J, Ellis G, Moore K. Effectiveness of anticholinergic drugs compared with placebo in the treatment of overactive bladder: systematic review. *BMJ.* 2003;326:841-848.
51. Gupta S, Sathyan G, Mori T. New perspectives on the overactive bladder: pharmacokinetics and bioavailability. *Urology.* 2002;60(suppl 5A):78-81.

CHAPTER 6

ANTIHYPERTENSIVE AGENTS

HYPERTENSION

Hypertension is a leading cause of cardiovascular morbidity and mortality. There are some recognizable causes for high blood pressure, but in most cases there is no definitive etiology. This type of hypertension is referred to as *primary* or *essential hypertension.* Secondary hypertension is more easily understood because it is produced by a specific cause, such as an adrenal tumor secreting epinephrine, head trauma, or renal artery stenosis. However, more than 90% of patients with high blood pressure have primary hypertension.[1] It is suspected that environmental factors such as stress, poor diet, smoking, and obesity predispose individuals to hypertension. Specifically, it is thought that these factors produce an increase in sympathetic activity.[2,3] The increase in sympathetic output produces excitatory effects on the heart and peripheral vasculature to increase blood pressure. Cardiac output is increased and adaptive changes begin to occur in the vasculature. The vessels become less compliant and more reactive to pressor substances such as norepinephrine and angiotensin II. Persistent hypertension leads to hypertrophy of the left ventricle and also of the media layer of resistance vessels, leading to narrowing of the lumen.[1] In later stages of hypertension, cardiac output may return to normal, but increased vascular resistance remains.

PHYSIOLOGY AND PATHOPHYSIOLOGY OF BLOOD PRESSURE

The two main equations that describe how some hemodynamic variables influence blood pressure are as follows:

Cardiac output = Heart rate × Stroke volume

Mean arterial pressure = Cardiac output × Peripheral resistance

The first equation describes cardiac output as a function of heart rate and stroke volume. Increased cardiac output is a function of increased heart rate, increased contractility, or both.[4,5] As rate and contractility increase, so does the amount of blood that is pumped out of the heart each minute (cardiac output). Venous return (preload) also increases cardiac output unless the heart is so damaged that it cannot accommodate the additional flow (Frank-Starling Law).[6] Heart rate, stroke volume, and venous return can all be increased by the sympathetic nervous system.

The second equation describes the relationship between cardiac output and blood pressure. This equation is analogous to Ohm's law in which V = IR (voltage = current × resistance), except hemodynamically, *V* is related to pressure in the vasculature, I is blood flow, and R is resistance in the artery that impedes flow.[7,8] See Figure 6-1 for a summary of factors involved in blood pressure control.

We have several pharmacological means of controlling blood pressure through these equations. There are drugs that block the sympathetic system to reduce heart rate through β receptors. This in turn will reduce cardiac output and arterial pressure. Drugs can also decrease stroke volume by decreasing contractility. This alteration will also decrease the blood pressure. Diameter of blood vessels can be increased, resulting in a lowering of peripheral resistance and a reduced blood pressure. Reducing overall plasma volume with diuretics is also a way to decrease the pressure because there will be a concomitant reduction in stroke volume.

Control of Blood Pressure Through Baroreceptors and Chemoreceptors

The body makes an effort to maintain blood pressure within a narrow range to allow for adequate organ perfusion but also to make sure that pressure does not rise to a level at which it becomes injurious to the arterials. Quick adjustments in pressure can be made through the baroreceptor reflex.[5] Afferent nerves located in the walls of the internal carotid arteries and aortic arch are stimulated by high pressure via stretch. Impulses are then transmitted to the medullary cardiovascular control center to inhibit central sympathetic discharge. If a fall in pressure is detected, these same neurons send fewer impulses to this vasomotor center. This will initiate an increased sympathetic output, resulting in vasoconstriction and increased cardiac output to raise pressure.

Peripheral chemoreceptors also play a role in regulation of blood pressure.[5] They are located in the carotid body (between the external and internal carotid arteries) and the aortic bodies (under the concavity of the aortic arch). These organelles are sensitive to the arterial blood gases, P_{O_2}, P_{CO_2}, and pH. An increase in carbon dioxide or a drop in pH or P_{O_2} triggers an increase in afferent firing to the medulla. The hypoxia and high P_{CO_2} stimulate respiration to improve oxygenation. This increase in ventilation helps to blow off the carbon dioxide, raising the pH, which is actually inhibitory to the cardioinhibitory center and results in tachycardia. A high P_{CO_2} acting on the central chemoreceptor area produces an increase in sympathetic output, which results in a generalized vasoconstriction.

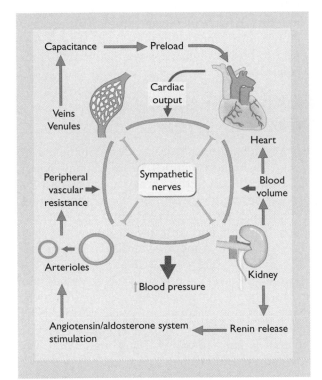

Figure 6-1

Factors involved in blood pressure control. Determinants of blood pressure are cardiac output, determined by heart rate and stroke volume. Cardiac output depends on the amount of blood returning to the heart, which in turn depends on vein and venule capacitance (preload) and blood volume (under the control of the kidneys). Peripheral vascular resistance is determined by the arterioles. (From Page C, Curtis MJ, Sutter MC, Walker MJ, Hoffman BB, eds. *Integrated Pharmacology.* 2nd ed. 2002. Philadelphia: Mosby; 2002.)

Vascular Endothelium and Intermediate Control of Blood Pressure

The vascular endothelium contains the plasma within a specific compartment and is also a source of many chemical mediators that affect blood pressure. These agents affect release of intracellular calcium (Ca^{2+}), leading to the contraction or relaxation of the vascular smooth muscle. Prostaglandins are derivatives of arachidonic acid released from damaged endothelial cells after they have been acted on by the cyclooxygenase enzyme. Prostacyclin (PGI_2) and prostaglandin E_2 (PGE_2) tend to be strong vasodilators. PGI_2 also inhibits platelet aggregation, and PGE_2 inhibits release of norepinephrine from sympathetic nerve terminals. Other prostaglandins are endothelium-derived contracting factors, specifically thromboxane A_2. Cyclooxygenase inhibitors such as aspirin can prevent this vasoconstrictor response.

Endothelium-derived relaxing factor, also known as *nitric oxide*, is released continuously, producing vasodilator tone and relaxation of vascular smooth muscle. It also inhibits the adaptive changes and the vascular smooth muscle cell proliferation that stiffens the arteries. Inhibition of platelet adhesion and aggregation is another function and very important in preventing thrombosis. Additionally, many vasodilator substances, such as bradykinin and even acetylcholine, act by producing nitric oxide. Currently, several mediators of nitric oxide are being studied for their effectiveness in relaxing vascular tone.

Several peptides are also secreted by the endothelium. These include C natriuretic peptide, endothelium-derived hyperpolarizing factor, and adrenomedulin—all of which are vasodilators.[9] Natriuretic peptides also cause diuresis, decrease aldosterone release, decrease cell growth in the vascular wall, and inhibit the renin-angiotensin system (see the following section).[10] Vasoconstrictive peptides include angiotensin-converting enzyme (ACE) and endothelin. ACE exists on the surface of endothelial cells, especially of the lungs, and is extremely important in producing angiotensin II, a powerful vasoconstrictor. Endothelins are responsible for extremely strong vasoconstriction that is long lasting as well.[11] Several endothelin inhibitors and endothelin-receptor blockers are being studied.[10]

Renin-Angiotensin System and Long-Term Control of Blood Pressure

The renin-angiotensin system works in concert with the sympathetic nervous system, producing very potent vasoconstriction. It also is responsible for the stimulation of aldosterone release, which enhances the reabsorption of sodium (Na^+) and the secretion of hydrogen (H^+) from the renal tubules, resulting in a rise in plasma volume. Renin is an enzyme secreted by the kidney juxtaglomerular apparatus, which is located in the distal convoluted tubule. It is secreted in response to diminished renal perfusion or a decrease in Na^+ concentration. Flow may be reduced because of fluid loss (dehydration or bleeding), or the kidney may sense decreased flow caused by an atherosclerotic renal artery or a sympathetically vasoconstricted artery.

Renin converts angiotensinogen (secreted by the liver) to angiotensin I, which is subsequently converted to angiotensin II with the help of ACE in the lungs (Figure 6-2). As mentioned previously, angiotensin II is a very powerful vasoconstrictor (40 times as potent as norepinephrine in elevating blood pressure).[12] Other enzymes further cleave angiotensin II into angiotensin III and IV but appear to be somewhat less vasoactive than angiotensin II.

Prostaglandins and Renal Function

The prostaglandins that are produced in the kidneys affect the hemodynamics of the renal system. PGE_2 is produced in the kidney medulla, and PGI_2 comes from the glomeruli. Prostaglandin synthesis is stimulated by ischemia, trauma, angiotensin II, catecholamines, and antidiuretic hormone. When these sympathomimetic chemicals are around, PGE_2 and PGI_2 are produced and counteract the vasoconstrictive effect on the kidneys. Vasodilation, particularly of the renal artery, is maintained to ensure that the kidneys are well perfused. The significance of the renal prostaglandins becomes apparent when patients with cirrhosis of the liver, heart failure, nephritic syndrome, or hypertension take nonsteroidal antiinflammatory drugs (NSAIDs), which inhibit prostaglandin synthesis. Under these conditions, NSAIDs can produce renal failure and exacerbate hypertension or cardiac failure.[13]

Classification of Blood Pressure

The seventh report of the Joint National Committee on Prevention, Detection, Evaluation, and Treatment of High Blood Pressure (JNC 7) provides new guidelines for the classification and management of blood pressure (Table 6-1).[14] Normal blood pressure is classified as a systolic reading <120 mm Hg and a

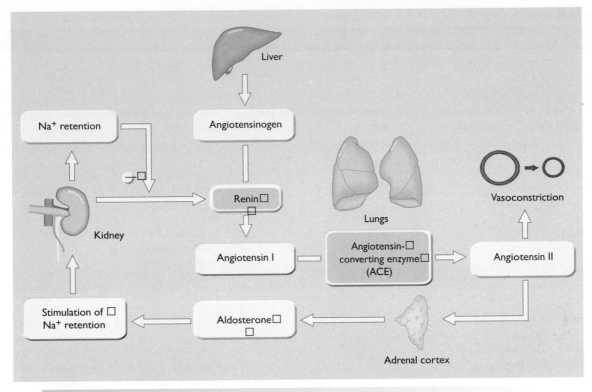

Figure 6-2

Renin-angiotensin-aldosterone system. Release of renin stimulates conversion of angiotensinogen (from the liver) to angiotensin I, which in turn is converted to angiotensin II under the influence of angiotensin-converting enzyme. Angiotensin II leads to vasoconstriction, release of aldosterone (adrenal cortex), and Na$^+$ retention. The latter increases blood pressure but reduces renin release, so the system is a homeostatic process. (From Page C, Curtis MJ, Sutter MC, Walker MJ, Hoffman BB, eds. *Integrated Pharmacology.* 2nd ed. 2002. Philadelphia: Mosby; 2002.)

diastolic reading <80 mm Hg. The JNC 7 also introduced a new classification labeled *prehypertension* with a systolic reading between 120 and 139 mm Hg or diastolic reading between 80 and 89 mm Hg. At this stage no antihypertensive drug is recommended, but patients are encouraged to follow a healthy lifestyle. The prehypertension stage is followed by stage 1 hypertension with a systolic reading between 140 and 159 mm Hg or a diastolic reading between 90 and 99 mm Hg. Monotherapy with diuretics is recommended at this time. Patients with a systolic reading of 160 mm Hg or above or a diastolic reading of 100 mm Hg or above will require two or more antihypertensive drugs to control blood pressure. This report stresses tighter controls on blood pressure than previous reports, especially for patients with diabetes or chronic kidney disease, with the recommendation that their blood pressure be less than 130/80 mm Hg.

Nondrug treatment for hypertension is always the first choice for therapy and includes exercise, reduction in weight, restriction of salt intake, cessation of smoking, and a reduction in alcohol intake.[1] When these steps are not successful, a variety of drugs can be used to reduce blood pressure. The major categories include diuretics, sympatholytics, direct-acting vasodilators, calcium antagonists, and renin-angiotensin inhibitors. Specific actions include regulating electrolyte and fluid level through the kidney tubules, altering rate and contractility of the heart, dilating arterioles, inhibiting angiotensin II production, and reducing central sympathetic output.

DIURETICS

In general, diuretics result in an increased excretion of Na$^+$ and water by the kidneys. However, the

Table 6-1

Classification and Management of Blood Pressure for Adults Aged 18 Years or Older

BP Classification	Systolic BP, mm Hg*		Diastolic BP, mm Hg*	Lifestyle Modification	Management* — Initial Drug Therapy Without Compelling Indications	With Compelling Indications
Normal	<120	and	<80	Encourage	—	—
Prehypertension	120-139	or	80-89	Yes	No antihypertensive drug indicated	Drug(s) for the compelling indications[†]
Stage 1 hypertension	140-159	or	90-99	Yes	Thiazide-type diuretics for most; may consider ACE inhibitor, ARB, β-blocker, CCB, or combination	Drug(s) for the compelling indications. Other anti-hypertensive drugs (diuretics, ACE inhibitor, ARB, β-blocker, CCB) as needed
Stage 2 hypertension	≥160	or	≥100	Yes	Two-drug combination for most (usually thiazide-type diuretic and ACE inhibitor or ARB or β-blocker or CCB)[‡]	Drug(s) for the compelling indications. Other anti-hypertensive drugs (diuretics, ACE inhibitor, ARB, β blocker, CCB) as needed

From Classification and management of blood pressure in adults aged 18 years or older: the 7th report of the Joint National Committee on Prevention, Detection, Evaluation, and Treatment of High Blood Pressure. *JAMA.* 2003;289:2560-2572.
ACE, Angiotensin-converting enzyme; *ARB,* angiotensin receptor blocker; *BP,* blood pressure; *CCB,* calcium channel blocker.
*Treatment determined by highest BP category.
[†]Treat patients with chronic kidney disease or diabetes to BP goal of less than 130/80 mm Hg.
[‡]Initial combined therapy should be used cautiously in those at risk for orthostatic hypotension.

manner in which diuretics reduce blood pressure has not been clearly defined. It is assumed that they reduce pressure by reducing plasma volume. However, in general, their action as antihypertensive agents is poorly related to their diuretic activity.[1] Loop diuretics are moderate antihypertensive drugs but strong diuretics. Thiazide diuretics are powerful antihypertensive agents but moderate diuretics. There are three major classifications of diuretic drugs, named according to their location of action.

Loop Diuretics

Loop diuretics are often used along with other diuretics in cases of salt and water overload. Specific conditions include pulmonary edema, congestive heart failure, ascites caused by liver failure, hypercalcemia, and renal failure. They are often combined with thiazide diuretics in the treatment of hypertension.

The mechanisms of action of the loop diuretics include inhibiting the $Na^+/K^+/2Cl^-$ cotransporter on the luminal membrane of the ascending loop of

Henle, blocking reabsorption of these electrolytes from the tubular fluid (Figure 6-3).[15] When this cotransporter is working, it creates a hypertonic interstitial segment in the kidney medulla, which provides the osmotic pressure needed for reabsorption of water from the collecting tubules. When the transporter is blocked by drug, the luminal fluid stays hypertonic, facilitating water loss into the tubules. A greater concentration of Na^+ in the lumen then facilitates the loss of H^+ and potassium (K^+) via exchange with Na^+ in the distal portion of the nephron.

Intravenous loop diuretics produce a short-term vasodilation secondary to facilitating release of prostaglandins.[15] This is the mechanism of action responsible for almost immediate relief in acute pulmonary edema before any diuresis has begun. Venodilation produced by the prostaglandins decreases cardiac preload, resulting in a fall in pulmonary artery wedge pressure and a decrease in symptoms.

The prototypic loop diuretic is furosemide. Some other examples are bumetanide and ethacrynic acid, which are easily absorbed from the gastrointestinal tract (>80%); absorption of furosemide is only 50%.[15] Because they are strongly bound to plasma proteins, they are not freely filtered through the glomerulus. They reach their site of action by being actively transported into the proximal convoluted tubule. Their onset of action is approximately 1 hour with duration from 3 to 6 hours. In renal disease, less drug reaches the proximal convoluted tubule, so larger doses need to be administered.

Loop diuretics are useful in the treatment of hypercalcemia because less solute is reabsorbed.[15] However, they should not be given to patients who are prone to renal stones because greater calcium excretion in the tubules can lead to precipitation.

Adverse drug reactions (ADRs) associated with loop diuretics include dehydration, hypokalemia, hyponatremia, hypocalcemia, ototoxicity, hyperglycemia, and increased levels of low-density lipoproteins (LDLs).[16] Hypokalemia and metabolic alkalosis from H^+ loss can occur, so supplemental K^+ or K^+-sparing diuretics are often given along with these drugs. The ototoxicity is associated with loss of cochlear hair cells but is not fully understood.[15] This ADR is more common at high doses, when given by rapid intravenous injection, in patients with renal disease, and when used in combination with other ototoxic drugs.

Thiazide Diuretics

The thiazide diuretics are the prime diuretics used to reduce blood pressure. They are also given along with loop diuretics in cases of congestive heart failure and severe edema. They are the diuretics of choice for patients who are prone to renal calculi.

These drugs inhibit the Na^+/Cl^- cotransporter on the luminal membrane of the distal convoluted tubule and proximal collecting duct (Figure 6-4).[15] Less Na^+ intracellularly enhances the Na^+/Ca^{2+} pump located on the basolateral cell membrane, facilitating calcium reabsorption. These drugs also enhance K^+ excretion in the collecting duct. These drugs then promote Na^+ and K^+ excretion and reabsorption of Ca^{2+}.

Hydrochlorothiazide is the prototypic thiazide diuretic. It is well absorbed through the gastrointestinal tract after oral administration and is actively secreted into the tubules. The maximum effect occurs in about 4 hours, with duration of action between 8 and 12 hours.

ADRs are similar to those of the loop diuretics, except that the thiazides may cause hypercalcemia. K^+ loss is also a significant problem.

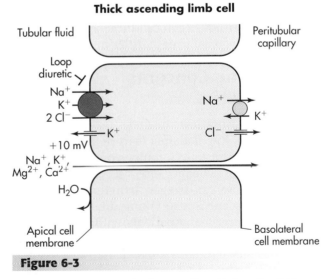

Thick ascending limb cell

Figure 6-3

Cellular transport by thick ascending limb cells. Cell model for ion transport by thick ascending limb. This segment, also referred to as the *diluting segment,* is impermeable to water, and thus the tubular lumen concentration of ions decreases. (From Brody TM, Larner J, Minneman KP. *Human Pharmacology: Molecular to Clinical.* 3rd ed. Philadelphia: Mosby; 1998.)

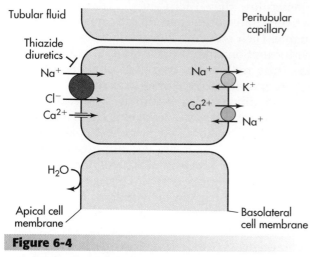

Figure 6-4

Cellular transport by distal convoluted tubule cells. Cell model for a distal convoluted tubule cell. As in the case for the thick ascending limb, this segment is relatively impermeable to water. (From Brody TM, Larner J, Minneman KP. *Human Pharmacology: Molecular to Clinical.* 3rd ed. Philadelphia: Mosby; 1998.)

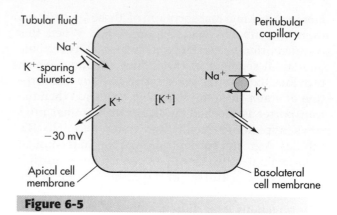

Figure 6-5

Cellular transport by principle cells of the collecting tubule. The principal cell contains both Na^+ and K^+ channels in the apical cell membrane. The Na^+ channel in the apical cell membrane depolarizes the cell membrane and thus provides an asymmetrical transepithelial voltage profile that favors K^+ secretion. (From Brody TM, Larner J, Minneman KP. *Human Pharmacology: Molecular to Clinical.* 3rd ed. Philadelphia: Mosby; 1998.)

Potassium-Sparing Diuretics

Potassium-sparing diuretics act in the collecting tubule to inhibit Na^+ reabsorption and K^+ excretion.[15] The Na^+ channel in the principal cell depolarizes the cell, creating a positive charge that repels K^+. Some of the K^+-sparing agents block this depolarization so K^+ is not excreted into the tubular fluid (Figure 6-5). Other drugs that fall within this category block the aldosterone receptor; this explains their usefulness in patients with mineralocorticoid-producing tumors, adrenal hyperplasia, cirrhosis, and congestive heart failure in which there is excessive aldosterone. However, because many of these drugs depend on excess aldosterone being present, they are not that useful in the treatment of primary hypertension. In primary hypertension, they are used for their ability to prevent K^+ deficiency secondary to loss with loop or thiazide diuretics. However, according to some authors, the rationale for using the K^+-sparing drugs with the thiazide drugs is in error because only about 5% of patients taking the thiazide diuretics lose too much K^+.[15]

Spironolactone blocks the receptor for aldosterone, but triamterene and amiloride are not dependent on excess aldosterone.[15] They are all absorbed reasonably well from the gastrointestinal tract, but they have vastly different half-lives. Triamterene is short acting and must be administered two times per day.

Hyperkalemia is the most common ADR, but nausea, lethargy, and mental confusion may also occur. In addition, because spironolactone resembles adrenal sex steroids, it can produce gynecomastia in males and menstrual irregularities in females.

Therapeutic Concerns with Diuretics

In general, diuretics produce fluid depletion, hyponatremia, hypokalemia (except the K^+-sparing drugs), and orthostatic hypotension. Of particular concern is the K^+ level because a K^+ value that is too high or too low can trigger arrhythmias, particularly if the patient is also taking digitalis for heart failure.[16] Because many patients with hypertension have cardiac disease, this is a special concern. Signs and symptoms of hypokalemia include an abnormal electrocardiogram (ECG) reading (flattened T waves), nausea, muscle weakness and fatigue, leg cramps, polyuria, hypotension, excessive sweating, and mental status changes. If hypokalemia is present, the patient may be given a K^+ supplement or encouraged to eat foods rich in K^+ such as apricots, bananas, raisins, and oranges. However, one concern is the need to consume a large number of calories to obtain a small amount of K^+. Hyperkalemia presents with ECG changes (elevated T waves), as well as nausea, diarrhea, hyperreflexia progressing to weakness, numbness, and anuria. Syncope may be present in both cases if arrhythmias are present. Cardiac arrest can also occur in both conditions. Frequent monitoring of K^+ levels is recommended for all new patients, and monthly monitoring is necessary for patients who have been taking the drug on a long-term basis.

Another issue with the diuretics is that they produce hyperglycemia and abnormally affect lipids. This is of some concern because many patients who have hypertension also have diabetes and high cholesterol and triglyceride levels.[16] In terms of lipid levels, studies conducted for less than 1 year show an increase in total cholesterol levels, especially LDL (15%) and triglyceride levels (23%). These percentages may significantly increase cardiovascular mortality. However, some longer-lasting studies (1 year) indicate that lipoprotein levels are not significantly affected.[17] As with all studies, careful scrutiny of the data is imperative for interpretation. Interpretation of cholesterol levels must be analyzed in terms of the subgroup of patients showing the elevated levels, and more specifically, the subgroup responding with elevated lipid levels. Premenopausal women do not show elevated levels, but postmenopausal women seem to be subject to this increase in lipid levels. It has also been pointed out that successful adherence to a low-fat diet may negate the effects of thiazides on cholesterol. Because the findings have not been convincing, the controversy over whether the elevated cholesterol levels are significant across the population lingers.[18,19]

Treatment of hypertension, especially with the thiazide diuretics, produces elevated glucose levels and glucose intolerance. In 4736 patients treated with a thiazide diuretic for 1 year, there was a significant increase in fasting blood sugar levels.[20] However, the percentage of patients newly diagnosed with diabetes during 3 years of drug administration was not significant. Because close control of glucose is imperative to decreasing side effects of the disease, the use of diuretics for patients with diabetes remains controversial. At present, it is suggested that patients prone to diabetes and those who already have the disease should avoid diuretics entirely.[21]

Side effects of diuretics have direct ramifications for physical therapy practice. Patients with diuretic-induced hypokalemia may experience muscle weakness or cramping. These drugs can also cause orthostatic hypotension, increasing the risk of falls.[22,23] The therapist must instruct the patient to perform leg extensions, ankle pumps, or other exercises before rising from a chair or bed. Avoiding sudden changes in position is also important. To monitor for dehydration, the therapist must check the patient for skin turgor, temperature, and moisture (including mucous membranes).[24] Any signs of dehydration must be reported immediately to the physician. The therapist should also monitor the patient for arrhythmias by checking the pulse for any irregularities. Elderly patients who are already having problems with urinary incontinence may find this problem worsening when taking diuretics, and frequent urination may interrupt therapy. Also, the therapist should be aware of the reduced exercise capacity during periods of fluid loss. During exercise, patients with hypertension taking thiazide diuretics will show an attenuated increase in blood pressure and a reduced stroke volume.[25] Heart rate response to exercise appears to be normal in these patients.

Because many patients taking diuretics are also taking NSAIDs for arthritis, it is good medical practice and good physical therapy practice to reduce patients' dependence on these drugs. The NSAIDs cause Na^+ retention and a decrease in renal perfusion, as described previously, and this combination makes the diuretics less effective. We can offer our patients a variety of modalities, assistive devices, and intervention techniques to reduce pain and inflammation associated with arthritis. An incentive for physicians to employ or consult with physical therapists is that their interventions can reduce the patient's dependence on potentially harmful pharmaceutical agents.

β ADRENOCEPTOR BLOCKERS

β Adrenoceptor blockers (antagonists) are primarily used to treat cardiovascular dysfunction. Specifically, they are used to reduce hypertension, angina, and arrhythmias and to increase survival after myocardial infarction. These drugs are also used for the treatment of glaucoma, thyrotoxicosis, anxiety, migraines, and benign essential tremors.

β-Blockers are competitive antagonists of β adrenoceptors (Figure 6-6). They reduce heart rate and contractility, resulting in a reduction in cardiac

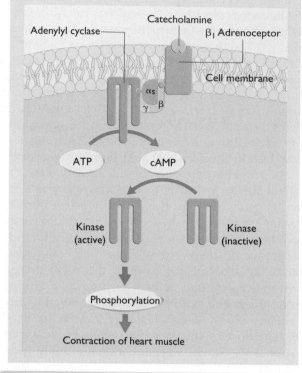

Figure 6-6

Molecular mechanism of action of β_1 adrenoceptor antagonists. Stimulation of β_1 adrenoceptors by catecholamines leads to activation of adenylyl cyclase and an elevation of cyclic adenosine monophosphate. This process is inhibited by β_1 adrenoceptor antagonists. (From Page C, Curtis MJ, Sutter MC, Walker MJ, Hoffman BB, eds. *Integrated Pharmacology.* 2nd ed. 2002. Philadelphia: Mosby; 2002.)

output and blood pressure. These drugs also exert a central inhibitory effect on sympathetic activity, reducing peripheral vascular resistance. However, their most profound effect in terms of reducing blood pressure has to do with the blockade of renin release from the kidneys. The result is a reduction in circulating angiotensin II and aldosterone, producing a vasodilatory effect.

β-Blockers are either selective or nonselective for β adrenoceptors. The nonselective antagonists will block β_1 and β_2 adrenoceptors. The selective agents will block only β_1 receptors, but this selectivity is lost at high doses. Propranolol is the prototypic nonselective agent. Atenolol and metoprolol are selective β_1 adrenoceptor antagonists. The main difference between the two is that the nonselective agents will block the β_2 receptors in the bronchioles and will also block the β_2 receptors in skeletal muscle vasculature.

β-Blockers with Intrinsic Sympathomimetic Activity

Pindolol is a partial agonist at the β_1 receptor and therefore is said to have intrinsic sympathomimetic activity. It inhibits excess β_1 receptor activity when the sympathetic system is stimulated, reducing blood pressure but with less reduction in resting heart rate than the other β-blockers. Pindolol stimulates the β receptor but at the same time blocks entrance of the more potent endogenous catecholamines. This is quite useful for the patient who tends to have bradycardia or for the patient who is receiving additional cardiac meds such as antiarrhythmic drugs, which slow the heart rate by widening the QT interval.[26] This drug should not be given to a patient who has already had a myocardial infarction or has angina.

Therapeutic Concerns with β-Blockers

Adverse effects of β-blockers are related to their receptor-blocking action. Blockade of β receptors eliminates β_2 receptor–activated vasodilation. A reflex increase in peripheral vasoconstriction may also occur as a result of the drug-induced hypotension. Both of these factors may contribute to some peripheral vasoconstriction in certain susceptible persons, such as patients with Raynaud's disease.

Blocking β_2 receptors in the lungs also leads to bronchoconstriction. In patients with normal lung function, these drugs have little effect, but in patients with obstructive disease, they can be fatal. Bradycardia progressing to heart block is another adverse effect that may occur because β receptors on the nodal tissue are blocked. At rest, these drugs may only produce small depressions in heart rate or cardiac output; however, during exercise, these values are depressed enough to reduce exercise capacity. Excessive depression of heart rate and contractility will also exacerbate congestive heart failure. Abrupt withdrawal of a β-blocker will trigger dangerous arrhythmias, angina, and even myocardial infarction.

β-Blockers have several noncardiac-related adverse effects. Blocking β_2 receptors will decrease glycogenolysis and glucagon secretion. This is particularly worrisome in patients with diabetes because these drugs impair recovery from and mask the symptoms of hypoglycemia. It has also been reported that β-blockers may promote the development of type 2 diabetes in patients with hypertension.[27-30] Additional adverse effects include fatigue, dizziness, depression, sexual dysfunction, and an increase in LDL levels. In particular, there is an increase in the number of smaller and denser LDL particles, which penetrate more easily into the vascular intima, causing damage.[31-33] Although β-blockers have been shown to reduce the mortality rate and incidence of reinfarction in patients recovering from myocardial infarction, their role in prevention of primary infarcts has been modest.[34] Some speculate that the reason for this is the abnormality in lipid levels that occurs with these drugs. The significance of the increase in lipid levels with these drugs is currently being debated.[17,19]

Renal perfusion is also reduced with β-blockers because they block prostaglandin-mediated vasodilation of the renal arteries. This does not appear to be a significant problem except in cases of renal failure or when a patient is taking an NSAID along with the β-blocker.

In physical therapy, patients must be watched for signs that congestive heart failure is developing. The physical therapist should note whether the patient is experiencing dyspnea, peripheral edema, increased weight, rales, jugular vein distension, or decreased urine output. Vital signs should be obtained frequently, particularly before the patient's next drug dose. The physician should be notified if systolic blood pressure falls below 90 mm Hg or if the pulse is below 60 beats/min. Dosing would not typically be recommended with these vital signs.

α ADRENOCEPTOR BLOCKERS

α-Blockers reduce sympathetic tone of the blood vessels, allowing vasodilation and a subsequent decrease in peripheral vascular resistance.[12] They are used in the treatment of pheochromocytoma (an epinephrine-secreting tumor), complex regional pain syndromes, and Raynaud's disease because they improve circulation. In addition, they are used to prevent autonomic hyperreflexia in patients with spinal cord injury and to improve urine flow in patients with benign prostatic hyperplasia.[35]

Phenoxybenzamine is a nonselective α-blocker because it binds to both α_1 and α_2 receptors.[12] It irreversibly binds to the receptor, so it has a long duration of action, approximately 24 hours. The body must synthesize new receptors for the drug action to be terminated. It is used to induce vasodilation in some pain syndromes in which the vasculature is constricted. It is not useful in hypertension because norepinephrine can still act on the β_1 receptors of the heart to increase blood pressure. Also blocking of α_2 receptors produces unrestricted norepinephrine release because the autoreceptors are blocked.

Prazosin, terazosin, and doxazosin are selective α_1-blockers (Figure 6-7). (Note the similar ending *azosin.*) These drugs are primarily used to lower peripheral vascular resistance, thus lowering blood pressure. They dilate both resistance and capacitance vessels. Unlike β-blockers, they have been shown to lower LDL and triglyceride levels, and they only minimally affect cardiac output and renal blood flow.[1] Therefore they do not produce any long-term tachycardia or increased renin release. However, in the short term, reflex tachycardia could be a problem.

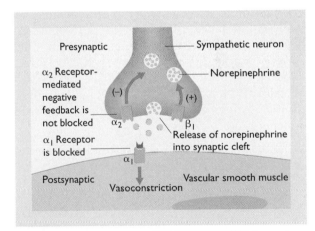

Figure 6-7

Antagonism at postsynaptic α_1 adrenoceptors. Prazosin (α_1 antagonist) prevents vasoconstriction by norepinephrine. Further effects of norepinephrine are reduced by a feedback mechanism since presynaptic α_2 adrenoceptors are not blocked by prazosin and so the α_2 adrenoceptors can be occupied by norepinephrine, thereby activating a negative feedback pathway. (From Page C, Curtis MJ, Sutter MC, Walker MJ, Hoffman BB, eds. *Integrated Pharmacology.* 2nd ed. 2002. Philadelphia: Mosby; 2002.)

Therapeutic Concerns with α-Blockers

Adverse effects of α-blockers include postural hypotension, nasal stuffiness, reflex tachycardia, and arrhythmias. The increased heart rate and arrhythmias are the result of activation of the baroreceptor reflex and the α_2 blockade as explained previously. When a decrease in blood pressure is detected, a reflex increase in heart rate occurs through the baroreceptors. This can produce angina in a patient who has poor cardiac perfusion and may be a reason for the increased incidence of heart failure during treatment with α-blockers compared with treatment with other antihypertensive agents.[36]

The selective α_1-blockers may produce a significant drop in blood pressure, especially with the first dose. This is called *first-dose syncope*.[1] This effect may be minimized by starting with one half the usual dose and dosing at bedtime. Assisted ambulation may be necessary when this drug is first administered, especially when it is given to elderly patients.

DUAL α- AND β-BLOCKERS

Dual α- and β-blockers are helpful in reducing hypertension in patients who experience increased peripheral resistance while taking the pure β-blockers. Labetalol and carvedilol are nonselective α_1- and β_1- receptor antagonists.[1] The ratio of β blockade to α blockade is 10:1 for carvedilol and 4:1 for labetalol. Labetalol also has some intrinsic sympathomimetic activity.[35] Adverse effects are similar to those of β-blockers and α-blockers.

CENTRAL ACTING α_2-AGONISTS

The centrally acting α_2 adrenoceptor agonists are primarily used to reduce blood pressure. Clonidine is the prototypic drug in this category, and it stimulates the autoinhibitory effects of norepinephrine on the sympathetic system.[12] Its action is particularly directed at the vasomotor center in the brain. This leads to a reduction of arteriolar tone, and with long-term use, a reduction in heart rate and cardiac output; however, there is less of a reduction in blood pressure than when the sympathetic system is blocked peripherally.[35]

The problem with these drugs is that they are very sedating. They also produce dry mouth, orthostatic hypotension, impotence, and galactorrhea. In addition, diffuse parenchymal injury to the liver and hemolytic anemia have been reported with some of these drugs. A rapid return of hypertension with tachycardia and restlessness is noted when the medication is withdrawn abruptly. Clonidine is now available as a transdermal preparation. The patch is changed every 7 days, providing good control of blood pressure with less sedation.[37] However, skin irritation has been reported.

VASODILATORS

Within the classification of vasodilators are the direct vasodilators—hydralazine, minoxidil, nitroprusside, and fenoldopam—and the calcium channel blockers.

Direct Vasodilators

Direct vasodilators dilate the arterioles by acting directly on the vascular smooth muscle as opposed to acting through adrenergic receptors. They are often used for the treatment of hypertensive emergencies when diastolic blood pressure is over 120 mm Hg or medical conditions such as hypertensive encephalopathy, dissecting aortic aneurysm, and pulmonary edema. Hydralazine and minoxidil are examples of direct vasodilators. Minoxidil is a more effective vasodilator and is useful if the patient also has renal failure; however, it is rarely used because of its side effects. It works by opening an ion channel called the *ATP-sensitive K^+ channel*. When this channel is opened, K^+ leaves the cell, leading to hyperpolarization. The more negative potential then reduces influx of Ca^{2+} through the L-type Ca^{2+} channel.

Sodium nitroprusside produces marked arterial and venous dilation, reducing cardiac preload and afterload. It spontaneously breaks down to nitric oxide when entering smooth muscle cells. The nitric oxide activates guanylyl cyclase, which then increases cyclic guanosine monophosphate (cGMP) levels (Figure 6-8). Increased cGMP relaxes vascular smooth muscle. Nitroprusside is administered intravenously and produces a rapid reduction in blood pressure. Patients must be monitored carefully to make sure that hypoperfusion of organs does not occur while blood pressure is falling. Sodium nitroprusside is sensitive to light and degrades easily so it must be made fresh before it is given to the patient. It also has a short duration of action and

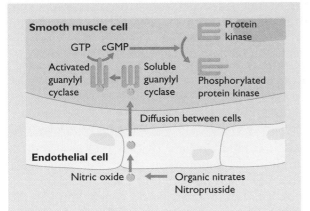

Figure 6-8

Molecular and cellular mechanisms of action of nitrate and nitrite vasodilators. The product, phosphorylated protein kinase, causes vascular smooth muscle relaxation by phosphorylating (and inactivating) myosin light chain kinase. (From Page C, Curtis MJ, Sutter MC, Walker MJ, Hoffman BB, eds. *Integrated Pharmacology*. 2nd ed. 2002. Philadelphia: Mosby; 2002.)

is metabolized in red blood cells with the liberation of cyanide. Toxicity is related to accumulation of cyanide, which may occur with prolonged administration (1 week or more).

Fenoldopam is a new drug for hypertensive emergencies that primarily dilates peripheral arterioles and also acts as a diuretic in the kidneys by increasing renal blood flow.[38] It is a parenteral agent that acts rapidly. So far, it appears to be the ideal drug with wider applications because it does not cause bradycardia like the parenteral β-blockers and can therefore be used in the treatment of congestive heart failure.[39] The drug is also renal protective and does not trigger an increase in renin release. It is as effective as nitroprusside without the elevated cyanide levels.

Therapeutic Concerns with the Direct Vasodilators

Direct vasodilators produce reflex tachycardia, leading to arrhythmias, angina, or myocardial infarction. Vasodilators also increase renin levels and Na$^+$ retention, but both of these side effects may be blocked by concomitant use of a β-blocker and a diuretic. Other side effects include nausea, dizziness, and sweating. Because these drugs are likely to be administered in the emergency department, there are no obvious implications for physical therapy.

Calcium Channel Blockers

Like β-blockers, calcium channel blockers are used for many cardiovascular indications. They are used to treat angina, arrhythmias, and hypertension. They are particularly useful for patients with conditions that may contraindicate the use of β-blockers such as asthma, diabetes, and peripheral vascular disease. The mechanism of action in hypertension is blockade of calcium influx into arterial smooth muscle, producing vasodilation and a decrease peripheral resistance.

There are three classes of calcium channel blockers, each with different properties and indications. Dihydropyridines have stronger affinity for vascular calcium channels than for calcium channels in the heart. Therefore they reduce arteriolar tone with less effect on cardiac conduction. Examples include nifedipine, nicardipine, and amlodipine. The diphenyl alkylamine verapamil primarily affects the heart, and the benzodiazepine diltiazem affects both the vasculature and the heart. Both verapamil and diltiazem depress cardiac activity, produce conduction problems, and are negative inotropic agents. Verapamil can be especially problematic because it can produce atrioventricular nodal block and is contraindicated in congestive heart failure.

There have been some problems with the calcium channel blockers. Two meta-analyses have revealed a higher risk of coronary artery disease and congestive heart failure with these drugs compared with ACE inhibitors (see the following section), β-blockers, and diuretics.[40,41] There was also a higher risk of myocardial infarction with a calcium channel blocker compared with an ACE inhibitor in patients with diabetes and hypertension.[42] Although this is still under debate, short-acting nifedipine has been linked to sudden death.[43,44] Long-duration calcium channel blockers have been recommended as a better way to attain smooth blood pressure control for chronic hypertension. The short-acting agent is used in the emergency department for a hypertensive crisis.

Therapeutic Concerns with Calcium Channel Blockers

Calcium channel blockers tend to produce a throbbing headache, dizziness, hypotension, bradycardia (verapamil and diltiazem), reflex tachycardia (nifedipine), sweating, tremor, flushing, and constipation. The combination of a β-blocker and verapamil is contraindicated because of the negative inotropic effects, and verapamil alone is contraindicated in congestive heart failure.

ACE INHIBITORS AND ACE RECEPTOR BLOCKERS

ACE inhibitors and ACE receptor blockers are effective in reducing hypertension and reducing afterload in congestive heart failure; they are particularly recommended for patients who have diabetes along with cardiovascular disease.

ACE Inhibitors

The ACE inhibitors block the action of ACE, reducing angiotensin II synthesis. Angiotensin II contributes to the development of hypertension by constricting arterioles and stimulating aldosterone release, which in turn stimulates Na^+ reabsorption from the kidney tubules. So by blocking this synthesis, the ACE inhibitors produce vasodilation and diuresis. These drugs also slow bradykinin inactivation, again resulting in vasodilation. Long-term use of these drugs is associated with recovery of angiotensin II levels, even though blood pressure remains low. This suggests that some other mechanism might be partly responsible for their antihypertensive effects.

The ACE inhibitors are especially useful for patients with congestive heart failure because they do not depress cardiac function. In addition, they do not adversely affect lipid or glucose levels or heart rate. ACE inhibitors are as effective as diuretics or β-blockers; however, when an ACE inhibitor and a diuretic or β-blocker are used together, effectiveness is better than when either drug is used alone.[37] ACE inhibitors are now recommended as a first-line drug for treatment of hypertension in diabetics.[45] Studies in which ACE inhibitors are compared with calcium channel blockers in terms of progression of kidney disease in diabetes have shown that these drugs exert a renal protective response. In addition, the ACE inhibitors have been shown to reduce cardiovascular events compared with placebo in high-risk patients without a low ejection fraction.[46] Some examples of ACE inhibitors are captopril, enalapril, ramipril, and lisinopril.

Therapeutic Concerns with ACE inhibitors

Common side effects of ACE inhibitors include dry cough, rashes, hypotension, hyperkalemia, and rarely, angioedema.[35] Cough occurs because these drugs interfere with the metabolism of bradykinin in the lungs. Increased levels of this vasoactive peptide act as a pulmonary irritant. In approximately 15% of patients, this cough is so severe that the drug must be withdrawn.

ACE Receptor Blockers

ACE receptor blockers (ARBs) interfere with the binding of angiotensin II to the angiotensin receptors. They are very effective at reducing blood pressure without producing a cough. Similar to the ACE inhibitors, they have also been shown to be renal protective, delaying the development of diabetic nephropathy in patients with type II diabetes.[47,48] In addition, in patients with left ventricular hypertrophy and hypertension, an ARB, losartan, decreased cardiovascular mortality and morbidity compared with atenolol.[49,50] In trials in which losartan was compared with captopril in patients with congestive heart failure, mortality was reduced more with captopril, but this difference was not statistically significant.[51] Further comparison of the ACE inhibitors and ARBs is needed.

Therapeutic Concerns with ARBs

ARBs have relatively few side effects. As mentioned previously, they do not cause cough. The other side effects are similar to those of ACE inhibitors and include hypotension, hyperkalemia, and angioedema.

VASOPEPTIDASE INHIBITORS

Vasopeptidase inhibitors are a new class of drugs, still under study, that inhibit ACE and also neutral endopeptidase.[10] Neutral endopeptidase is found on the membrane of the renal tubules, lungs, intestine, brain, heart, and peripheral blood vessels. It is responsible for the breakdown of atrial natriuretic peptide, brain natriuretic peptide, and C-type natriuretic peptide, as well as some other peptide hormones. Because these are primarily vasodilatory peptides, inhibition of neutral endopeptidase should be beneficial for patients with hypertension and congestive heart failure.

Animal studies of omapatrilat in congestive heart failure showed a decrease in left-ventricular end-diastolic pressure and an increase in cardiac output of 40%. In a study conducted with patients with congestive heart failure, omapatrilat reduced the risk of death and hospitalization but was not more effective than enalapril.[52] However, there was a greater incidence of angioedema, particularly among black patients. Clinical studies in patients with hypertension and heart failure are ongoing and so far point to a lowering of blood pressure.[53] It is too early to comment on therapeutic concerns for this drug classification.

GUIDELINES FOR THE TREATMENT OF HYPERTENSION

The first line of treatment for hypertension consists of lifestyle changes involving diet, exercise, and cessation of smoking.[54] If these changes are not effective, monotherapy is prescribed. Thiazide diuretics or β-blockers are usually the first drugs prescribed. Both have been shown to decrease coronary events in high-risk populations. ACE inhibitors are often more expensive alternatives, although some generics are available.

When a decision regarding which drug should be prescribed is made some individual patient factors must be considered. ACE inhibitors are useful for diabetic patients and for those patients who have abnormal lipid levels, as well as for patients with heart failure.[35] β-Blockers and calcium channel blockers are good for patients who have both hypertension and angina. Race is also an issue. Black patients respond well to diuretics, and Asian patients are more sensitive to β-blockers. The elderly respond better to calcium channel blockers than to diuretics. Calcium channel blockers are not recommended as the first-line defense against hypertension because some reports suggest a greater risk of myocardial infarction occurring with the short-acting dihydropyridines than with an ACE inhibitor in patients with hypertension and diabetes. In addition, studies in which the long-acting calcium antagonists were compared with other antihypertensive agents showed them to be inferior as first-line agents in reducing blood pressure because they were associated with a higher number of cardiovascular events with the exception of stroke.[40]

Diuretics appear to the be the best tolerated antihypertensive agents.[35] The Antihypertensive and Lipid-Lowering Treatment to Prevent Heart Attack Trial (ALLHAT) compared the number of myocardial infarctions, strokes, and deaths in more than 33,000 subjects with hypertension who took chlorthalidone (a generic diuretic with action identical to the thiazide diuretics), amlodipine (a calcium channel blocker),

or lisinopril (an ACE inhibitor) for 5 years.[55] A fourth drug, doxazosin (an α-blocker), was pulled from the study early when subjects taking this drug had higher rates of stroke and other cardiovascular events. Chlorthalidone was found to lower blood pressure slightly better than the other two drugs. However, patients receiving chlorthalidone had a risk of diabetes that was between 43% and 65% higher than that of patients receiving an ACE inhibitor as a result of increased blood glucose levels during treatment. Complications in terms of cardiac events associated with diabetes were not adequately studied during the 5-year study period.[56] Although diuretics have won some accolades with this study, it is still important to consider individual patient characteristics when a medication is chosen. The diuretic may be the cheapest and most effective in lowering blood pressure, but for the elderly patient who has mobility issues, the added trips to the bathroom may be hazardous. In addition, hypokalemia may produce leg cramps or complicate cardiovascular status. So in choosing a drug, age, physical status, and the presence or absence of other medical conditions are important factors to consider.

When one drug alone is not effective, combination therapy begins. By combining drugs with different mechanisms of action, the doses of each may be reduced, and the effects are usually additive. The β-blocker–diuretic combination seems most common. β Antagonists and calcium channel blockers (dihydropyridines only) are also well tolerated, but patients must be monitored for bradycardia and emerging heart failure. The ACE inhibitors plus either a diuretic or a calcium channel blocker are other effective prescriptions. The combination of calcium blockers and diuretics, however, has not been shown to have additive effects. The Anglo-Scandinavian Cardiac Outcomes Trial (ASCOT) should help answer the question about which combination is best.[35] This ongoing study is comparing a β-blocker–diuretic combination with an ACE inhibitor plus a calcium channel blocker.

THERAPEUTIC CONCERNS WITH ANTIHYPERTENSIVE AGENTS

The physical therapist treating patients taking antihypertensive medications should be concerned about excessive lowering of blood pressure, orthostatic hypotension, and syncope. The physician should be notified if systolic blood pressure falls below 90 mm Hg or if heart rate falls below

60 beats/min. Dosing should be stopped if this occurs, but this must always be the decision of the physician, not the therapist. Patients should also be monitored for reflex tachycardia. Slow rising and ankle pumping are useful techniques to prevent falls and syncope resulting from orthostatic hypotension. Patients are particularly vulnerable during frequent bouts of voiding in the middle of the night. They should be instructed to stand near a supporting object for at least 10 seconds before walking away. If a patient begins to feel woozy, he or she can cross one leg over the other and tighten the leg muscles. This has been shown to raise blood pressure.[57] Another helpful hint is for the patient to drink water throughout the day. Being dehydrated, even by a small amount, can cause blood pressure problems. A patient with orthostatic hypotension should drink a cup of water right before assuming a standing position.[57]

Heat modalities should be avoided with those antihypertensive meds that produce arterial vasodilation. The application of heat, especially from a whirlpool bath, will produce further vasodilation, will lower blood pressure, and may cause syncope.

β-Blockers, calcium channel blockers, vasodilators, and diuretics all decrease exercise performance and have ramifications for physical therapy. Exercise produces positive chronotropic and inotropic effects, but β-blockers produce negative chronotropic and inotropic effects. β-Blockers have been shown to decrease both resting and exercise heart rates in elite athletes and in patients with hypertension, but those that have intrinsic sympathomimetic action produce less reduction in these values. Lowering of maximum oxygen consumption per unit time (Vo_2 max) also occurs, regardless of whether the β-blocker is cardioselective or has intrinsic sympathomimetic action and regardless of whether subjects have normal or high blood pressure. One reason for these negative effects on exercise performance is that β-blockers reduce lipolysis and impair glycogenolysis, reducing fuels for exercise.[58,59] The masking of hypoglycemic symptoms can also be a deleterious event for a diabetic patient. Another important point to make with regard to β-blockers is that because target heart rate is not attainable during administration of these drugs, the age-related equations to predict maximum heart rate do not apply. A training rate that is 20 beats/min greater than the resting rate can be used as a maximum, provided the patient is free of symptoms at this level.[60] β-Blockers should be reserved for those patients with coronary artery disease who are not involved in endurance activities.

With regard to diuretics, exercise potentiates the fluid and potassium loss seen with these drugs. Potassium depletion contributes to muscle fatigue, cramping, and possible arrhythmias; and fluid loss contributes to dehydration. Hypovolemia compromises venous return so heart rate increases. Thermoregulation is also compromised because blood flow is shunted away from the skin to the muscles and because peripheral arterioles vasoconstrict. A result is reduced sweating. These effects translate into reduced exercise performance. Therefore diuretics are not the best choice of drugs for the serious endurance athlete.[61]

Additional information on the effects of α_1-blockers, calcium channel blockers, and ACE inhibitors on exercise performance is available from the literature. α_1-Blockers significantly reduce Vo_2 max, maximal workload, and duration of exercise on a bicycle ergometer in well-trained athletic men with hypertension.[62] Similar results have been reported for calcium channel blockers.[63] However, ACE inhibitors have been shown to cause less reduction in some of these values and may be better tolerated in terms of side effects.[64]

In addition to exercise counseling, physical therapists can play a large role in helping patients reduce their blood pressure. Providing education on the physiology of blood pressure, encouraging patients to comply with their medication regimens, and carefully observing patients for any adverse reactions are forms of assistance that physical therapists can easily provide. Reducing blood pressure even a small amount can be helpful in reducing morbidity and mortality. A recent meta-analysis of 61 long-term studies of initially healthy individuals showed that for every 20-point increase in systolic pressure or 10-point increase in diastolic pressure, there is a doubling chance of having a fatal stroke or myocardial infarction.[65] The reverse analysis demonstrates that reducing systolic pressure by 10 points or diastolic pressure by 5 points can produce a 30% to 40% decrease in the risk of fatal myocardial infarction and stroke.

ACTIVITIES 6

■ 1. AB is a 46-year-old man who has a painful right wrist. He reports tripping over a rock while training for the New York City Marathon, landing on an outstretched hand. He has only 6 weeks left to train and does not want any lingering injuries while running the big race.

Medical History

He has a history of hypertension for which he has been taking propranolol and hydrochlorothiazide, and over the last 2 days, plenty of aspirin for the wrist pain. He denies any other illness or musculoskeletal problem.

While performing your examination, you notice that the patient appears to have some cramping in his lower extremities. When you question him about this, he states that he just ran 8 miles to your clinic. You also notice that his clothes are dry, despite the high heat and humidity outside. You continue with the examination.

Vital Signs

Blood pressure, 90/60 mm Hg; resting pulse, 110 beats/min

Wrist Exam

Mild edema on the dorsum of the right hand with limited active and passive wrist range of motion. Strength testing demonstrates weakness caused by pain in the right hand but also a 4/5 grade for biceps, triceps, wrist flexors, and extensors. Grip strength measures only 25 lb. Grip strength on the left measures 40 lb. These results were not what you expected.

The patient continues to show evidence of mild cramping, and after further questioning, the patient reports feeling weak. You are very concerned and decide to call for an ambulance.

Labs

Results of tests on blood drawn from the patient 2 hours later were as follows: sodium concentration, 122 mEq/L; potassium concentration, 2.5 mEq/L; hemoglobin level, 16 g/dL, creatinine clearance, 1.1 mg/100 mL; glucose level, 100 mg/mL.

Arterial Blood Gases

Metabolic alkalosis

Urinalysis

Positive for protein and had a high specific gravity.

Questions

a. Analyze the physical findings and lab work to determine what is abnormal.
b. What do you think is going on with this patient?
c. What type of medication changes should be made?

■ 2. A 54-year-old obese patient complains of dizziness and dyspnea while on the treadmill in your office. He reported that he fainted yesterday while he was walking briskly from his car to his office. He has been having angina associated with exercise and stress for more than 2 years and is currently taking verapamil.

Medical History

Borderline type II diabetes; angina

Vital Signs

Blood pressure, 80/60 mm Hg; pulse, 48 beats/min
The patient is transported to the emergency department.

ECG

QRS is normal, but the P-R interval is increased.

Labs

Blood urea nitrogen level is slightly elevated. Blood glucose level is 70 mg/100 mL.

Chest

Scattered wheezes noted

Questions

a. What do you think is going on with this patient? What is the immediate course of treatment?
b. What suggestions do you have for changing medications and why?
c. What can you do in physical therapy to make sure that this does not happen again?

■ 3. Research the literature and briefly review two articles that would help you decide on the best pharmacological treatment for the following patient.

A 55-year-old man with mild hypertension (155/95 mm Hg). The patient is slim and athletic (runs 3 miles, four times a week). Despite his low weight and dedication to exercise, he has high cholesterol (high-density lipoprotein level, 45 mg/100 mL; low-density lipoprotein, 270 mg/100 mL; triglyceride level, 300 mg/100 mL). What might you prescribe for the hypertension? Note that he also had symptoms of diabetes 5 years ago when he was overweight.

References

1. Curtis MJ, Pugsley MK. Drugs and the cardiovascular system. In: Page C, Curtis MJ, Sutter MC, Walker MJ, Hoffman BB, eds. *Integrated Pharmacology*. 2nd ed. Philadelphia: Mosby; 2002:361-414.
2. Wortsman J. Role of epinephrine in acute stress. *Endocrinol Metab Clin N Am*. 2002;31(1):79-106.
3. Esler M, Rumantir M, Kaye D, et al. Sympathetic nerve biology in essential hypertension. *Clin Exp Pharmacol Physiol*. 2001;28(12):986-989.
4. Boulpaep EL. Organization of the cardiovascular system. In: Boron WF, Boulpaep EL, eds. *Medical Physiology*. Philadelphia: Saunders; 2003:423-446.
5. Boulpaep EL. Regulation of arterial pressure and cardiac output. In: Boron WF, Boulpaep EL, eds. *Medical Physiology*. Philadelphia: Saunders; 2003: 534-557.
6. Weems WA, Downey JM. The mechanical activity of the heart. In: Johnson LR, ed. *Essential Medical Physiology*. New York: Raven Press; 1992:179-188.
7. Weems WA, Downey JM. Regulation of arterial pressure. In: Johnson LR, ed. *Essential Medical Physiology*. New York: Raven Press; 1992:195-204.
8. Weisbrodt NW, Downey JM. Hemodynamics. In: Johnson LR, ed. *Essential Medical Physiology*. New York: Raven Press; 1992:151-164.
9. Busse R, Edwards G, Feletou M, Fleming I, Vanhoutte P, Weston AH. EDHF: bringing the concepts together. *Trends Pharmacol Sci*. 2002;23(8):374-380.
10. Weber MA. Vasopeptidase inhibitors. *Lancet*. 2001; 358:1525-1532.
11. Kedziersk RM, Yanagisawa M. Endothelin system: the double-edged sword in health and disease. *Ann Rev Pharmacol Toxicol*. 2001;41:851-876.
12. Rang HP, Dale MM, Ritter JM, Moore JL. *Pharmacology*. 5th ed. New York: Churchill Livingstone; 2003.
13. Brater DC. Effects of nonsteroidal antiinflammatory drug on renal function: focus on cyclooxygenase-2 selective inhibition. *Am J Med*. 1999;107:65S-71S.
14. Chobanian A, Bakris G, Black H, et al. The seventh report of the Joint National Committee on Prevention, Detection, Evaluation, and Treatment of High Blood Pressure (JNC VII). *JAMA*. 2003;289:2560-2572.

15. Brater CD. Pharmacology of diuretics. *Am J Med Sci*. 2000;319(1):38-67.
16. Greenberg A. Diuretic complications. *Am J Med Sci*. 2000;319(1):10-43.
17. Lakshman MR, Reda DJ, Materson BJ, Cushman WC, Freis ED. Diuretics and beta-blockers do not have adverse effects at 1 year on plasma lipid and lipoprotein profiles in men with hypertension. *Arch Intern Med*. 1999;159:551-558.
18. Moser M. Why are physicians not prescribing diuretics more frequently in the management of hypertension? *JAMA*. 1998;279(22):1813-1816.
19. Golomb BA, Criqui MH. Antihypertensives. *Arch Intern Med*. 1999;159:535-537.
20. Savage PJ, Pressel SL, Curb D, et al. Influence of long-term, low-dose, diuretic-based, antihypertensive therapy on glucose, lipid, uric acid, and potassium levels in older men and women with isolated systolic hypertension. *Arch Intern Med*. 158(7):741-751.
21. Peters AL, Hsueh W. Antihypertensive agents in diabetic patients. *Arch Intern Med*. 1999;159:541-542.
22. Chutka DS, Evans JM, Fleming KC, Mikkelson KG. Drug prescribing for elderly patients. *Mayo Clin Proc*. 1995;70(7):685-693.
23. Evans JG. Drugs and falls in later life [editorial]. *Lancet*. 2003;361:448.
24. Goodman CC, Snyder TE. Problems affecting multiple systems. In: Goodman CC, Boissonnault WG, Fuller KS, eds. *Pathology Implications for the Physical Therapist*. 2nd ed. Philadelphia: Saunders; 2003.
25. Lim PO, MacFayden RJ, Clarkson PBM, MacDonald TM. Impaired exercise tolerance in hypertensive patients. *Ann Intern Med*. 1996;124(1):41-55.
26. Which beta-blocker? *Med Lett Drugs Ther*. 2001;43(1097): 9-11.
27. Gress TW, Nieto FJ, Shahar E, Wofford MR, Brancati FL. Hypertension and antihypertensive therapy as risk factors for type 2 diabetes mellitus: Atherosclerosis Risk in Communities Study. *N Engl J Med*. 2000; 342(13):905-912.
28. Berne C, Pollare T, Lithell H. Effects of antihypertensive treatment on insulin sensitivity with special reference to ACE inhibitors. *Diabetes Care*. 1991;14(suppl 4):39-47.

29. Pollare T, Lithell H, Selinus I, Berne C. Sensitivity to insulin during treatment with atenolol and metoprolol: a randomised, double blind study of effects on carbohydrate and lipoprotein metabolism in hypertensive patients. *BMJ.* 1989;298(6681):1152-1157.

30. Julius S, Majahalme S, Palatini P. Antihypertensive treatment of patients with diabetes and hypertension. *Am J Hypertens.* 2001;14:310S-316S.

31. Boquist S, Ruotolo G, Hellenius M-L, Danell-Toverud K, Karpe F, Hamsten A. Effects of a cardioselective beta blocker on postprandial triglyceride-rich lipoproteins, low density lipoprotein particle size and glucose-insulin homeostasis in middle-aged men with modestly increased cardiovascular risk. *Atherosclerosis.* 1998;137:391-400.

32. Roberts W. Recent studies on the effects of beta-blockers on blood lipid levels. *Am Heart J.* 1989;117:709-714.

33. Superko HR, Haskell WL, Krauss RM. Association of lipoprotein subclass distribution with use of selective and non-selective beta-blocker medications in patients with coronary heart disease. *Atherosclerosis.* 1993;101:709-714.

34. Rochon PA, Tu JV, Anderson GM, et al. Rate of heart failure and 1-year survival for older people receiving low-dose beta-blocker therapy after myocardial infarction. *Lancet.* 2000;356: 639-644.

35. Drugs for hypertension. *Treat Guidel Med Lett.* 2003; 1(6):33-40.

36. Major cardiovascular events in hypertensive patients randomized to doxazosin vs chlorthalidone: The Antihypertensive and Lipid-Lowering Treatment to Prevent Heart Attack Trial (ALLHAT). ALLHAT Collaborative Research Group. *JAMA.* 2000;283:1967-1975.

37. Benowitz NL. Antihypertensive agents. In: Katzung BG, ed. *Basic & Clinical Pharmacology.* 8th ed. New York: McGraw Hill; 2001:155-180.

38. Murphy MB, Murray C, Shorten GD. Drug therapy: fenoldopam: selective peripheral dopamine-receptor agonist for the treatment of severe hypertension. *N Engl J Med.* 2001;345(21):1548-1557.

39. Cardiovascular drugs in the ICU. *Treat Guidel Med Lett.* 2002;1(4):19-24.

40. Pahor M, Psaty BM, Alderman MH, et al. Health outcomes associated with calcium antagonists compared with other first-line antihypertensive therapies: a meta-analysis of randomised controlled trials. *Lancet.* 2000; 356:1949-1954.

41. Blood Pressure Lowering Treatment Trialist's Collaboration. Effects of ACE inhibitors, calcium antagonists, and other blood-pressure-lowering drugs: results of prospectively designed overviews of randomised trials. *Lancet.* 2000;355:1955-1964.

42. Schrier RW, Estacio RO. Additional follow-up from the ABCD Trial in patients with type 2 diabetes and hypertension. *N Engl J Med.* 2000;342(26):1969-1971.

43. Epstein M. The Calcium Antagonist Controversy: The emerging importance of drug formulation as a determinant of risk. *Am J Cardiol.* 1997;79(10A):9-19.

44. Frishman WH, Michaelson MD. Use of calcium antagonists in patients with ischemic heart disease and systematic hypertension. *Am J Cardiol.* 1997;79(10A):33-38.

45. Yusuf S, Gerstein H, Hoogwerf B, et al. Ramipril and the development of diabetes. *JAMA.* 2001;286(15):1882-1885.

46. Yusuf S. Effects of an angiotensin-converting-enzyme inhibitor, ramipril, on cardiovascular events in high-risk patients. *N Engl J Med.* 2000;342(3):145-153.

47. Lewis EJ, Hunsicker LG, Clarke WR, et al. Renoprotective effect of the angiotensin-receptor antagonist irbesartan in patients with neuropathy due to type 2 diabetes. *N Engl J Med.* 2001;345(12):851-860.

48. Brenner BM, Cooper ME, de Zeeuw D, et al. Effects of losartan on renal and cardiovascular outcomes in patients with type 2 diabetes and neuropathy. *N Engl J Med.* 2001;345(12):861-869.

49. Dahlof B, Devereux RB, Kjeldsen SE, et al. Cardiovascular morbidity and mortality in the Losartan Intervention For Endpoint reduction in hypertension study (LIFE): a randomised trial against atenolol. *Lancet.* 2002; 359:995-1003.

50. Lindholm LH, Ibsen H, Dahlof B, et al. Cardiovascular morbidity and mortality in patients with diabetes in the Losartan Intervention For Endpoint reduction in hypertension study (LIFE): a randomised trial against atenolol. *Lancet.* 2002;359:1004-1010.

51. Pitt B, Poole-Wilson PA, Segal FA, et al. Effect of losartan compared with captopril on mortality in patients with symptomatic heart failure: randomised trial—the Losartan Heart Failure Survival Study ELITE II. *Lancet.* 2000; 355:1582-1587.

52. Packer M, Califf RM, Konstam MA, et al. Comparison of omapatrilat and enalapril in patients with chronic heart failure: the omapatrilat versus enalapril randomized trial of utility in reducing events. *Circulation.* 2002;106(8):920-926.

53. Regamey F, Maillard M, Nussberger J, Brunner HR, Burnier M. Renal hemodynamic and natriuretic effects of concomitant angiotensin-converting enzyme and neutral endopeptidase inhibition in men. *Hypertension.* 2002; 40(3):266-272.

54. Appel LJ. Nonpharmacologic therapies that reduce blood pressure: a fresh perspective. *Clin Cardiol.* 1999; 22(suppl 7):1-5.

55. ALLHAT Officers and Coordinators for the ALLHAT Collaborative Research Group. The Antihypertensive and Lipid-Lowering Treatment to Prevent Heart Attack Trial: major outcomes in high-risk hypertensive patients randomized to angiotensin-converting enzyme inhibitor or calcium channel blocker vs diuretic—The Antihypertensive and Lipid-Lowering Treatment to Prevent Heart Attack Trial (ALLHAT). *JAMA.* 2002;288:2981-2997.

56. Messerli FH, Weber MA. ALLHAT: all hit or all miss? Key questions still remain. *Am J Cardiol.* 2003; 92:280-281.

57. Skerrett PJ, ed. *Tricky Forecast: Low Pressure.* Boston: Harvard Health Publications; 2003.

58. Lundborg P, Astrom H, Bengtsson C, et al. Effect of beta-adrenoceptor blockade on exercise performance and metabolism. *Clin Sci.* 1981;61:299-305.

59. van Baak MA. Hypertension, beta-adrenoceptor blocking agents and exercise. *Int J Sports Med.* 1994;15(3): 112-115.

60. Wells BG, Dipiro JT, Schwinghammer TL, Hamilton CW. *Pharmacotherapy Handbook.* 5th ed. New York: McGraw Hill; 2003.

61. Swain R, Kaplan B. Treating hypertension in active patients. *Physician and Sportsmedicine.* 1997;25(9):268-272.

62. Tomten SE, Kjeldsen SE, Nilsson S, Westheim AS. Effect of alpha 1-adrenoceptor blockade on maximal VO2 and endurance capacity in well-trained athletic hypertensive men. *Am J Hypertens.* 1994;7(7):603-608.

63. van Baak MA, Mooij JMV, Schiffers PMH. Exercise and the pharmacokinetics of propranolol, verapamil, and atenolol. *Eur J Clin Pharmacol.* 1992;43:547-550.

64. Palatini P, Bongiovi S, Mario L, Mormino A, Pessina C. Effects of ACE inhibition on endurance exercise haemodynamics in trained subjects with mild hypertension. *Eur J Pharmacol.* 1995;48:435-439.

65. Prospective Studies Collaboration. Age-specific relevance of usual blood pressure to vascular mortality: a meta-analysis of individual data for one million adults in 61 prospective studies. *Lancet.* 2002;360:1903-1913.

Drug Therapy for Coronary Atherosclerosis and Its Repercussions

ISCHEMIC HEART DISEASE

Coronary blood flow is normally closely related to myocardial oxygen consumption, both at rest and during exercise. However, there are several factors that can alter coronary flow, creating a mismatch between perfusion (supply of oxygen) and demand. Ischemic heart disease or coronary artery disease (CAD) occurs when there is a lack of oxygen to the myocardium, usually resulting from coronary artery narrowing. This ischemic disease may present as unstable angina and acute myocardial infarction (MI) with specific electrocardiographic changes, chronic stable exertional angina, or ischemia caused by a vasospasm of the coronary vessels.

PATHOPHYSIOLOGY AND TREATMENT OF ISCHEMIC HEART DISEASE AND ANGINA

Heart rate, contractility, and wall stress (intraventricular pressure, ventricular volume, and wall thickness) during systole are the major determinants of myocardial oxygen demand (MVO_2).[1] Because the heart is continuously contracting, its oxygen needs are high; the heart uses 75% of the available oxygen, even at rest. Therefore MVO_2 is a critical factor in producing ischemia because increased activity demands a greater oxygen supply (i.e., perfusion); however, this value is usually fixed as a result of disease in the coronary arteries.

An indirect method for measuring MVO_2 is to calculate the "double product" (heart rate × systolic blood pressure).[2] Because coronary blood flows during the period of diastole, oxygen delivery is related to the duration of diastole. As heart rate increases and diastole shortens, the heart's demand for oxygen also increases. Oxygen demand is also related to vascular tone. During systole, the heart must contract with a force that exceeds aortic pressure to eject blood. Therefore the higher the blood pressure, the greater is the need for oxygen.

Coronary blood flow is inversely related to the diameter of the vessel to the fourth power.[1] Therefore diameter of the lesion is a major determinant of resistance influencing coronary perfusion. A critical loss of perfusion occurs when the lesion extends across 70% to 80% of the diameter. However, lesions smaller than this may still cause problems if vasospasm is superimposed. In addition, little reserve exists for coronary flow, so that problems begin to occur as activity and exercise increase the demand for blood flow.

Abnormalities in ventricular contraction impose further burdens on the remaining heart tissue, resulting in increased MVO_2, depletion of available oxygen, and eventually, cardiac failure. Zones of reduced perfusion develop and are at risk for more ischemia, especially if the demand for oxygen is ongoing. The nonischemic areas of the heart attempt to compensate by developing more tension in an effort to maintain cardiac output, further increasing oxygen demand. In addition, the neurochemical and metabolic factors and the neural reflexes activated to reverse the diminished perfusion begin to fail. Severe coronary atherosclerosis increases the sensitivity of the coronary arteries to catecholamines and α_1 stimulation. The direct effect is vasoconstriction of the arteries both at rest and during activity, further increasing ischemia and pain. See Figure 7-1 for a summary of factors affecting the balance between oxygen supply and demand.

Even with some pharmaceutical agents that are designed to be potent arteriole dilators producing strong dilation of resistance vessels, ischemia may still continue. A fixed stenosis will greatly affect the collateral blood flow and the patient's response to activity and exercise in what has been labeled *coronary steal*. Well-perfused tissue that is able to dilate will actually "steal" blood away from areas with fixed stenosis, resulting in greater ischemia, especially if superimposed on vasospasm. Perfusion is compromised, and the vessels distal to the area of fixed stenosis collapse.

Clinical Presentation of Angina

When demand for myocardial oxygen exceeds supply, ischemia develops and produces some typical signs and symptoms, including chest pain (angina) and ST-segment depression on an electrocardiogram. Patients often complain of pressure or the sensation of a heavy weight on their chests. They may also have a burning sensation or just a feeling of tightness. Shortness of breath along with a constrictive feeling around the larynx or upper trachea may occur. The location of the pain varies and may be limited to the sternum, left shoulder and arm, lower jaw, or lower cervical and upper thoracic spine. Radiation of pain to the left arm, and occasionally to the right arm, may occur. The typical anginal pain lasts from 30 seconds to 30 minutes and can be precipitated by exercise, a cold environment, emotional factors, walking against the wind, or walking after a large meal.

There are three major recognized forms of angina: exertional (stable), variant (Prinzmetal's), and unstable angina.[3,4] Exertional or exercise-induced angina is the most frequent type seen in patients with CAD. Usually, patients with exertional angina are free of pain at rest, but when a load is imposed on the heart, as with exercise, the supply of oxygen cannot meet the demand. Pain usually occurs at some predicted level of exertion, and there is a fixed narrowing of the coronary vessels.

Prinzmetal's angina results from a coronary spasm. Symptoms can occur at rest, usually during the night or in the early morning. In contrast to stable angina, ST-segment elevation may be seen during periods of pain. Pain is not usually experienced during exertion or emotional stress, and it is not typically relieved by rest.

Unstable angina is characterized by chest pain that increases in frequency, severity, and/or duration. Pain also occurs with less and less exertion and may even be present at rest. Unstable angina is often stratified into categories according to risk of impending nonfatal or fatal MI because it often

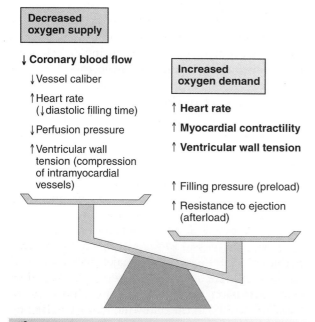

Figure 7-1

Factors affecting the balance of oxygen supply and demand in angina. (From Waller DG, Renwick AG, Hillier K. *Medical Pharmacology and Therapeutics.* New York: WB Saunders; 2001.)

occurs before an MI. Anginal episodes may occur with minimal activity, indicating a change from the predictable level of exertion that produces stable angina. Plaque rupture within the coronary artery may underlie this syndrome.

Treatment of Angina

Drug therapy for chest pain depends on the type of angina experienced. For the relief of acute anginal attacks, nitrates—particularly sublingual nitrate—are the drugs of choice.[5] Sublingual nitrate provides almost immediate relief of symptoms and may also be used to prevent an attack if administered just before activity. Patients with stable angina may be treated with a variety of drugs used on a prophylactic basis to prevent the anginal attacks. These include long-acting nitrates, β-blockers, and calcium channel blockers. Nitrates, β-blockers, calcium channel blockers, aspirin, and thrombin modulators are part of the treatment regimen for unstable angina, in addition to surgical management such as coronary artery bypass graft or percutaneous transluminal coronary artery angioplasty. The goal in this case is to reduce pain and prevent progression to an MI. Variant angina is treated with drugs that dilate the coronary arteries, including nitrates, which may be used along with a calcium channel blocker.

Nitrates

Nitrates (nitroglycerin, isosorbide dinitrate, and isosorbide mononitrate) dilate the systemic veins and arterioles, as well as the large and medium-sized coronary arteries. Veins respond to the lowest dose of nitrates, and arteries respond at higher doses.[2] Nitrates work directly on vascular smooth muscle as opposed to exerting action through a specific receptor. The exact mechanism of action is unknown, but evidence points to the liberation of nitric oxide from vascular endothelial cells and even from platelets. In addition, the nitrate itself will reduce to nitric oxide, which then combines with a thiol group in the vascular endothelium to form nitrosothiols. This then activates guanylate cyclase, leading to production of guanosine monophosphate and a subsequent reduction in the amount of intracellular calcium available for contraction.[6]

Originally, it was believed that nitrates produced a redistribution of coronary flow to ischemic areas. However, there is limited evidence to support improved cardiac perfusion in CAD.[6] Rather, the relief of angina appears to result from the nitrate's ability to reduce cardiac workload by decreasing preload and afterload. Vasodilation of venous capacitance vessels, leading to reduced venous return and a reduction in left ventricular filling pressure (preload), reduces ventricular wall tension and therefore myocardial oxygen demand. Arterial resistance vessels (mainly the large arteries) dilate, producing a reduced resistance to ventricular emptying (afterload), which also reduces oxygen demand. Coronary artery dilation may also occur, but to a limited extent. The specific beneficial effects of nitrates include decreased ventricular volume, decreased arterial pressure, decreased ejection time, decreased ventricular diastolic pressure, and vasodilation of epicardial coronary arteries. Nitroglycerin also produces a negative inotropic effect. Therefore it tends not to produce the "coronary steal phenomenon."[2]

Nitrates come in a variety of forms including intravenous (IV), sublingual, and topical preparations; a lingual spray; chewable and oral tablets; and patches. These preparations also have different durations of action: the oral and transdermal forms are the long-acting versions for controlling the frequency of anginal attacks, and the sublingual, transmucosal, and chewable tablet preparations are the short-acting, quick responders. Most patients wear the transdermal patch for 12 hours during the day and carry sublingual nitroglycerin tablets for added exertional periods. Tolerance to nitrates occurs quickly, so it is recommended that patients be free of the drug for at least 8 hours a day, preferably during sleep, to avoid this effect.[7] The patch must be placed above the elbow, preferably on the chest, for full effectiveness.

Sublingual nitroglycerin is kept in a tightly closed brown bottle that limits exposure to light. It is also kept in a glass container because it adheres to plastic surfaces.[2] It has a short shelf-life, maintaining potency for only 3 months, and any tablets that remain 90 days after the bottle is opened must be discarded. Patients are instructed to place a tablet under the tongue to dissolve, which takes 20 to 30 seconds. The drug will produce a gentle tingling or burning sensation if it is still active. If it doesn't produce this reaction, then the patient should obtain a prescription refill as soon as possible. Patients may also experience a vascular headache from meningeal artery vasodilation.

Relief of angina should occur in 1 to 2 minutes. Drug action can be hastened by sitting, leaning forward, and inhaling deeply.[5] If at the end of 5 minutes, angina is still present, the patient may take a second dose. If another 5 minutes pass and the pain is still present, the patient may take a third sublingual dose. Up to three sublingual doses may be taken within 15 minutes.[8] If pain is not relieved after three doses, then the patient may be having an MI, and transport to the hospital is warranted. Some cardiologists counsel patients to seek medical care immediately if the angina is not substantially relieved by nitroglycerin after the first dose or if the discomfort returns after administration of a single tablet.[5]

Nitroglycerin is more effective when taken at the very beginning of chest discomfort or administered 5 to 10 minutes before an activity that might precipitate an acute attack, such as physical therapy. In practice, however, this is not usually done. Patients may reserve medication for more severe episodes of pain that do not stop with cessation of activity. Others have the notion that the less often they use nitroglycerin, the less serious is their cardiac condition. It is important for patients to understand that nitroglycerin is not addictive and that it is not a narcotic or a painkiller.

Therapeutic concerns with nitrates include monitoring for reflex tachycardia, dizziness, orthostatic hypotension, and weakness. Taking precautions against falls, especially for patients with orthostatic hypotension, is warranted. Because nitrates cause vasodilation of arterioles and veins, thermal modalities that also cause vasodilation may exacerbate blood pooling in the lower extremities and lead to syncope. Long-term use of long-acting nitrates is associated with the development of abnormal hemoglobin, methemoglobin, compromising oxygen delivery.

β-Blockers

β-Blockers are frequently used as initial therapy for stable angina along with short-acting nitrates for patients with no contraindications. β-Blockers reduce myocardial oxygen demand by decreasing contractility and exertional tachycardia, which relieves angina. In patients with stable angina, the dose can be titrated to reduce resting heart rate to between 55 and 60 beats/min. The dose should also be adjusted to limit exercise heart rate to within 75% of the rate that produces chest pain.[9] These drugs should be avoided in patients with bradycardia, asthma, hypotension, and heart block.

Calcium Channel Blockers

Because calcium in cardiac and smooth muscle is a key component for initiating contraction, blocking calcium channels reduces contractility and arteriole tone. Two types of calcium channels are known to exist in the heart: the L-type and the T-type.[10] They differ in that the L-type channel produces a long and large high threshold current, whereas the T-type channel produces a short, small, and low-threshold current. They are also active during different phases of the cardiac action potential. T-type channels may contribute to diastolic depolarization (phase 4), which means that they are involved in helping the sinoatrial node reach its threshold for depolarization. L-type channels are active during the upstrokes (phase 0) of the sinoatrial and atrioventricular nodes and also during phases 1 and 2 of the Purkinje fibers, and ventricular and atrial muscle action potentials (see Chapter 8).[11] Therefore the drugs that block calcium channels reduce cardiac contractility throughout the heart (reducing oxygen demand) and decrease sinoatrial and atrioventricular nodal activity. Smooth muscle contraction is also reduced, producing vasodilation (reducing preload and afterload). The calcium channel blockers in current clinical use block only the L-type channels.

As mentioned previously, there are three types of calcium channel blockers currently on the market. They differ in their vascular selectivity, with the dihydropyridines (e.g., nifedipine and amlodipine) having a greater ratio of vascular smooth muscle effects relative to the cardiac effects compared with the phenethyl alkylamines (e.g., verapamil and bepridil) and dibenzazepines (diltiazem). Verapamil and diltiazem reduce cardiac contractility, and in higher doses, slow conduction through nodal tissue.

Calcium channel blockers are effective in reducing and preventing chest pain in stable angina associated with exercise as a result of a negative inotropic effect, which reduces myocardial oxygen demand. In addition, some of these drugs (diltiazem and nicardipine) have been shown to produce vasodilation in stenotic coronary arteries during exercise, preventing a coronary steal phenomenon.[12] However, some of the other calcium channel blockers, particularly in the dihydropyridine group, have induced this effect.

Short-acting dihydropyridines have also been used to prevent variant angina. However, there is evidence that the short-acting formulations increase the risk for MI.[13,14] The short-acting drugs can produce reflex sympathetic stimulation in response to the systemic vasodilation. In addition, use of the short-acting agents results in fluctuating drug levels, with reflex activity occurring during lower plasma levels of the drug. This sympathetic activity can produce a rather intense increase in heart rate and myocardial contractility that is not well tolerated by some patients. This effect can be avoided by giving the drug with a β-blocker or switching to the longer-acting calcium channel blockers. A large meta-analysis completed in 1999 in which 143 studies were examined indicated that β-blockers produced outcomes similar to those achieved with calcium channel blockers but with fewer adverse effects.[15] However, in many of these studies the short-acting nifedipine was used, biasing the literature against the calcium channel blocker for the treatment of angina.

Calcium channel blockers are often used along with either β-blockers or nitrates. The combination of a dihydropyridine and a β-blocker produces only a small risk of heart block, but use of verapamil or diltiazem along with a β-blocker is contraindicated because of excessive depression of cardiac function.[7]

Many investigators have attempted to compare calcium channel blockers with both β-blockers and nitrates for the treatment of stable angina. In several randomized reports, with a combined total of approximately 2000 patients, calcium channel blockers were found to be as effective as β-blockers in reducing angina and increasing exercise time.[9] Other studies show that amlodipine is as effective as isosorbide dinitrate (a long-acting nitrate) in relieving exercise-induced angina.[16]

The side effects of these drugs are extensions of their therapeutic effects.[7] The adverse effects associated with the dihydropyridines include dizziness, flushing of the skin, hypotension, reflex tachycardia, and peripheral edema. Verapamil and diltiazem can produce bradycardia, hypotension, congestive heart failure, heart block, and constipation.

Potassium Channel Openers

Nicorandil (not yet available in the United States) opens an adenosine triphosphate–sensitive potassium channel, which allows the flow of potassium out of the cell, hyperpolarizing the cell membrane.[6] The more negative membrane potential inhibits the opening of the L-type calcium channels, producing vasodilation in the systemic and coronary arteries. Because of its relatively short half-life, this drug has not been widely used. It also produces a headache and significant reflex activation of the sympathetic nervous system, as well as dizziness, nausea, and vomiting.

Therapeutic Regimens

The choice of drug or combination of drugs for the treatment of stable angina depends on the presence of coexisting medical conditions and the patient's individual response. β-Blockers and nitrates are frequently used together because the combination seems to be more effective than when each drug is used separately.[9] The β-blockers reduce the reflex tachycardia caused by the nitrates, and the nitrates reduce the bradycardia produced by the β-blockers. Nitrates are also more effective when given along with calcium channel blockers.[9]

In patients who have both mild chronic stable angina and hypertension, monotherapy with a long-acting calcium channel blocker or β-blocker may adequately control symptoms. For more moderate symptoms, the β-blocker–calcium channel blocker combination is good, but a patient may also respond well to two different calcium channel blockers, nifedipine and verapamil.

Nitrates and calcium channel blockers are effective for the treatment of variant angina. The mechanism for relief in this case is prevention of coronary artery spasm. Calcium channel blockers from all the categories can be effective for treating this condition.

THROMBOSIS AND ANTITHROMBOTIC THERAPY

Platelet aggregation and vasoconstriction initiate the hemostatic process. When endothelial cells are damaged, platelets bind to the damaged vessel through the interaction of platelet glycoprotein receptors (GP Ib/IX and GP Ia/IIb) and exposed endothelial collagen.[6] The platelet becomes activated and releases thromboxane A_2 (TXA_2), adenosine diphosphate (ADP), epinephrine, von Willebrand's factor, fibrinogen, calcium, and serotonin. These

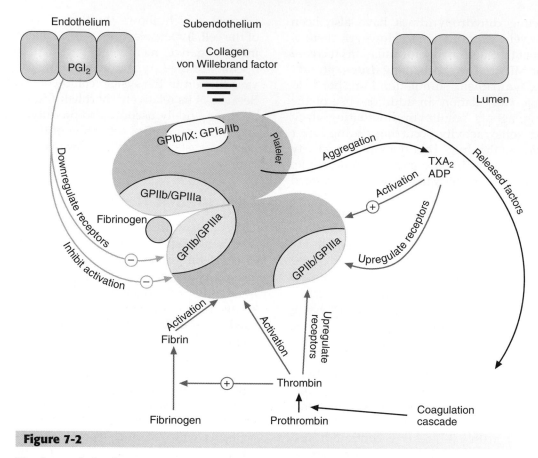

Figure 7-2

Platelets and platelet aggregation. Subendothelial macromolecules, such as collagen, interact with glycoprotein receptors *(GPIb/IX and GpIa/IIb)* on platelets, causing activation of platelets and upregulation of GPIIb/GPIIIa receptors, which are cross-linked by fibrinogen during aggregation. Synthesis of the proaggregatory thromboxane A_2 *(TXA$_2$)* and release of adenosine diphosphate *(ADP)* and 5-hydroxytryptamine occur. TXA$_2$ and thrombin cause further platelet activation and release of proaggregatory platelet contents. This leads to further upregulation of GPIIb/GPIIIa receptors. Prostacyclin *(PGI$_2$)* from endothelial cells inhibits activation and upregulation of GPIIb/GPIIIa receptors. Thrombin is generated by the action of factor Xa on prothrombin. (From Waller DG, Renwick AG, Hillier K. *Medical Pharmacology and Therapeutics.* New York: WB Saunders; 2001.)

substances activate and recruit other platelets into the growing thrombus. Similar substances are also released from the damaged vessel. Platelets furnish a surface on which clotting factors can bind and facilitate conversion of prothrombin to thrombin (factor IIa). Thrombin converts fibrinogen to insoluble fibrin, assisting in the formation of a stable, insoluble clot. The activation of the platelet leads to a conformational change in the platelet glycoprotein receptors IIb/IIIa on the cell surface. These receptors then provide binding sites for fibrinogen molecules and adhesive molecules (von Willebrand's factor, fibronectin) and other platelets

(Figure 7-2). TXA$_2$ is key in this cascade because not only does it promote platelet aggregation, it also inhibits prostacyclin (a vasodilator) and neutralizes endogenous heparin produced by the vascular endothelium, all enhancing coagulation.

The pathways that follow platelet aggregation involve a series of reactions leading to the generation of thrombin. This response to vascular injury involves many cells (platelets, leukocytes, and endothelial cells) along with the plasma blood-clotting proteins that ultimately form a fibrin clot and initiate inflammation and repair. The cascade of events leading to this final product is usually described as

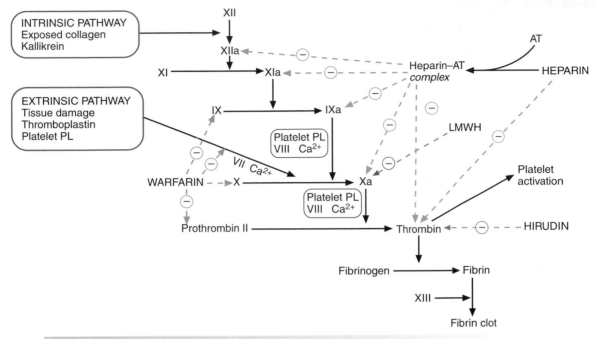

Figure 7-3

The coagulation cascade and action of anticoagulants. The complex cascade of clotting factor synthesis is initiated extrinsically by tissue damage. Activation of the clotting factors after damage requires platelet factors and calcium (Ca^{2+}). The provision of platelet products is further enhanced by the formation of thrombin, which then activates further platelets, as well as causing fibrin formation. Heparin acts at various sites in the cascade by activating the anti-clotting factor antithrombin (*AT*) and inhibiting the activating protease clotting factors shown. Low-molecular-weight heparin (*LMWH*) acts on factor Xa. Hirudin inhibits thrombin (IIa) formation. Warfarin inhibits the synthesis of the vitamin K–dependent clotting factors VII, IX, X, and II (prothrombin). Roman numerals indicate the individual clotting factors. *PL*, Platelet phospholipid. (From Waller DG, Renwick AG, Hillier K. *Medical Pharmacology and Therapeutics*. New York: WB Saunders; 2001.)

involving two distinct pathways, the extrinsic and intrinsic pathways (Figure 7-3). However, these pathways join forces to form the final common pathway, activation of factor X and subsequent conversion of prothrombin to thrombin.

The extrinsic system is initiated by the release of tissue thromboplastin (factor III) from damaged tissue.[17] A complex between this tissue factor and factor VIIa and calcium forms, followed by the sequential activation of factors VII, X, and pro-thrombin (factor II). The function of this pathway is measured by the prothrombin time or with the international normalized ratio (INR).[18]

The intrinsic pathway begins when the exposed collagen acts in conjunction with kallikrein to acti-vate factor XII to XIIa.[17] Several other factors become activated, and this pathway also joins the final common pathway. The function of this pathway is measured by the activated partial thromboplastin time (aPTT).[18]

The final common pathway involves the con-version of prothrombin into thrombin, which in turn converts fibrinogen into a stable clot. Thrombin also activates other coagulation factors to amplify its own production, as well as attracting platelets and white cells to the area of the clot. The intrinsic and extrinsic pathways are much slower than platelet aggregation and vasoconstriction.

Three categories of drugs are used to treat the various stages or conditions of thrombosis. The platelet aggregator inhibitors (aspirin, clopidogrel, ticlopidine) are used prophylactically to prevent formation of a platelet clot. Anticoagulants such as heparin and warfarin prevent extension of a clot already present, and thrombolytics lyse a clot that has recently formed.

Antiplatelet Agents

Several agents are designed to prevent platelet plugs from forming and thus can be beneficial in preventing injury from stroke and MI. These agents include aspirin, ADP receptor antagonists, and glycoprotein IIb/IIIa receptor blockers.

Aspirin

Although aspirin has been primarily recommended for unstable angina, it is also given in stable angina and in general to patients with cardiac disease to lower the risk of an MI.[9] The goal in this case is to prevent a stable thrombosis from rupturing and producing unstable angina and a subsequent MI. Aspirin inhibits the action of the cyclooxygenase enzyme, COX, to block the conversion of arachidonic acid to prostaglandin H_2, which in turn reduces production of TXA_2[7] (Figure 7-4). The reduction in TXA_2 inhibits platelet aggregation for the entire life-span of the platelet, which is approximately 8 days. Thus platelet function is diminished for this period and results in prolonged bleeding time.

A loading dose of 325 mg, followed by a daily dose of 80 mg, is recommended to reduce platelet aggregation and to help reduce the incidence of angina and MI.[19] A higher dose is needed to produce an antiinflammatory response. Chewable tablets are recommended for patients with chest pain and for those who might be having an MI. Chewed tablets will promote buccal rather than gastrointestinal (GI) absorption. Normal platelet function will return 36 hours after the last dose of the drug has been given because of the release of new platelets.[20] Aspirin reduces the incidence of death in acute MIs and also reduces the incidence of reinfarction, transient ischemic attacks, and stroke.[21,22] However, this does not completely reduce platelet activation because other pathways that enhance aggregation still exist. Aspirin may be combined with other anti-platelet agents such as ADP blockers, heparin, or warfarin for additive effects.

Adverse effects associated with aspirin include bleeding and GI irritation. Tinnitus and central nervous system toxicity occur at higher doses, and bronchoconstriction may occur in susceptible patients. In physical therapy, deep tissue work, friction massage, and vigorous mobilization are contraindicated. Patients receiving aspirin should be observed for bruising, joint swelling, blood in stools or urine, and bleeding from mucous membranes—all of which may mean the dose is

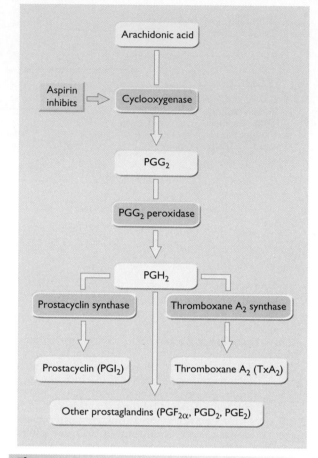

Figure 7-4

Mechanism of action of aspirin. Aspirin blocks the activity of cyclooxygenase and reduces the formation of prostacyclin and thromboxane A_2. Prostaglandin (PG) G_2, and PGH_2 are both prostaglandin cyclic endoperoxides and are unstable intermediates. (From Page C, Curtis MJ, Sutter MC, Walker MJ, Hoffman BB, eds. *Integrated Pharmacology*. 2nd ed. Philadelphia: Mosby; 2002.)

too high. See Chapter 12 for additional information on aspirin.

Adenosine Diphosphate Receptor Antagonists

Ticlopidine and clopidogrel block ADP-activated platelet aggregation, reducing the expression of the GPIIb/IIIa receptors.[23] Both are slightly more effective than aspirin in preventing recurrent stroke and transient ischemic attacks and are used separately or in combination with aspirin to prevent MI and in acute coronary syndromes without ST-segment elevation.[24] In addition, ticlopidine is used during stent placement to prevent thrombosis after percutaneous transluminal angioplasty. These drugs have an effect on bleeding similar to that of aspirin, but ticlopidine also produces neutropenia. A complete blood count is recommended 10 days after administration of the drug is started. As with aspirin, it takes 7 to 10 days for normal platelet function to return after these drugs have been discontinued.[25]

Glycoprotein IIb/IIIa Receptor Blockers

Abciximab and tirofiban are given intravenously to patients undergoing angioplasty for the prevention of acute coronary events.[26] They specifically inhibit binding of fibrin and von Willebrand's factor to the glycoprotein receptors. Platelet inhibition occurs quickly but recovers within 48 hours after the infusion is stopped. Adverse effects include bleeding, especially in the elderly and patients with low body weight.

Dipyridamole

Dipyridamole is used as a pharmacological stressor to detect myocardial ischemia in patients who cannot exercise.[6,27] It reduces the expression of the GPIIb/IIIa platelet receptors but also inhibits uptake of adenosine that is released by tissues when they are hypoxic. The excess adenosine produces vasodilation of the small resistance coronary arteries, which may already be maximally dilated. The net effect therefore is diversion of blood away from the ischemic area, producing the coronary steal phenomenon. The heart is imaged before dipyridamole administration at rest and again after drug administration by using technetium-labeled thallium to view ischemic areas.

Anticoagulant Agents

Anticoagulants are agents that prevent or delay blood coagulation by inhibiting certain clotting factors. They are available in IV, injectable, and oral forms. Usually, patients receive heparin while in the hospital but are switched over to oral warfarin before discharge.

Heparin

Heparin is a glycosaminoglycan consisting of D-glucosamine and uronic acid. The standard preparation produces a large molecule with molecular weights ranging from 5000 to 30,000 kd, with the larger molecule labeled as *unfractionated heparin*

and the smaller molecules labeled as *fractionated* or *lower molecular weight heparin* (LMWH). The varying weights of the heparin molecule affect the pharmacokinetics of the drug and make parenteral administration necessary. The higher the molecular weight, the more rapidly the drug is cleared from the circulation.

Heparin acts by binding to the circulating protein antithrombin III to activate it. This complex then neutralizes activated clotting factors. particularly factors Xa, IXa, and IIa (thrombin). Inactivation of these factors prevents the conversion of prothrombin to thrombin through the intrinsic pathway. Heparin's major effect on hemostasis is direct inhibition of thrombin, and to a lesser degree, inhibition of the other clotting factors. Unfractionated heparin has a greater effect on thrombin than the LMWHs, and only this form can inhibit platelet aggregation.

Heparin is given either intravenously or by subcutaneous injection. IV administration is preferred in emergency situations because there is a 1- to 2-hour delay in action when heparin is given subcutaneously. When given intravenously, heparin is administered by repeated bolus injections or by continuous IV infusion. Its rate of elimination is dose dependent. The half-life is 30 minutes at low doses (25 units/kg) but increases many-fold at higher doses (100 to 400 units/kg).

Heparin treatment requires close monitoring because the therapeutic index is low. The degree of anticoagulation is monitored with the aPTT, the lab test that measures the intrinsic coagulation pathway. An aPTT that is 1.5 to 2.5 the upper limit of normal (28 to 42 seconds) or 1.5 to 2.5 times the pretherapy time is desired.

Heparin is used for preventing and treating deep venous thromboembolism, pulmonary embolism (PE), and arterial thrombosis in selected cases of MI. In addition, it is used to prevent clotting in catheters and clotting that may occur after certain surgeries (e.g., hip and knee arthroplasties).

Bleeding is a common problem with heparin but can be reversed quickly by administration of protamine sulfate, which combines with heparin and inactivates it. Heparin-induced thrombocytopenia may also occur, and this disorder is paradoxically prothrombotic. Therefore frequent platelet monitoring is necessary. Osteoporosis is another side effect that may occur after long-term use (more than 3 months).

Low Molecular Weight Heparin

LMWH is obtained by fractionation or hydrolysis of the much larger heparin molecules. It has a high anti-factor Xa activity compared with heparin, which has high anti-factor IIa activity. This smaller molecule has several advantages over the unfractionated drug. The half-life is about 4 hours, much longer than that of the standard preparation. It also has greater bioavailability and a more predictable anticoagulant effect, resulting in less bleeding. The LMWHs have a limited effect on platelets, which is another reason that there is less bleeding as compared with unfractionated heparin. Dose is based on weight of the patient as opposed to laboratory monitoring, which makes home administration easier. [28,29]

LMWHs are given subcutaneously every 12 hours for up to 6 weeks after orthopedic surgery for the prevention of deep vein thrombosis (DVT). However, protocols do vary, and some patients may only receive injections until they are mobile. LMWHs are currently under study to determine their effectiveness compared with heparin for the treatment of DVT, PE, and acute MIs. Early studies show that they are just as effective as heparin for the treatment of DVT but with less bleeding tendency. [20]

Warfarin

Warfarin is an oral anticoagulant that inhibits production of a reduced form of vitamin K that is a necessary cofactor for the synthesis of several coagulation factors (factors II, IX, and X, and especially factor VII) in the liver. It is indicated for the prevention and treatment of venous thromboembolism and acute MI and in the prevention of emboli resulting from atrial fibrillation and prosthetic heart valves. [30-32]

Warfarin is highly bound to albumin (99%) in the plasma, and therefore numerous drugs and conditions interact with warfarin (Table 7-1). Some drugs that increase the activity of warfarin include antibiotics, aspirin, nonsteroidal antiinflammatory drugs, cimetidine, metronidazole, and phenytoin. Drugs that reduce its activity and lead to increased clotting include barbiturates, carbamazepine, and rifampin. Ingestion of large amounts of vegetables that contain vitamin K, such as broccoli and cauliflower, will also decrease warfarin's effectiveness.

Warfarin is metabolized by the P450 enzymes and also has a long half-life (36 to 40 hours). However, the plasma concentration of warfarin does not correlate directly with drug activity. Treatment with

Table 7-1

Drugs and Conditions Interacting with Warfarin

	Activity
Antibiotics	+
Amiodarone	+
Cimetidine	+
Clofibrate	+
Fluconazole	+
Metronidazole	+
Phenytoin	+
Barbiturates	−
Carbamazepine	−
Griseofulvin	−
Nafcillin	−
Rifampin	−
Sucralfate	−
Age	+
Biliary disease	+
Congestive heart failure	+
Hyperthyroidism	+
Hypothyroidism	−
Nephrotic syndrome	−

From Page C, Curtis MJ, Sutter MC, Walker MJ, Hoffman BB, eds. *Integrated Pharmacology.* 2nd ed. Philadelphia: Mosby; 2002.
+, Increased activity; −, decreased activity.

warfarin requires 4 to 5 days to be fully effective, partly because clotting factors are already present and active when administration is started. Therefore administration of warfarin is usually started along with heparin so that almost immediate anticoagulation is attained. After treatment is stopped, the anticoagulant effect continues until new clotting factors are synthesized.

Many patients find themselves receiving long-term warfarin therapy, and warfarin is often combined with aspirin for a superior effect. Monitoring of prothrombin time is necessary to evaluate the activity of factors II, V, VII, and X (the extrinsic coagulation pathway). Factor VII is the clotting factor that is most sensitive to vitamin K deficiency. The INR, which compares the patient's prothrombin time with a controlled value, is becoming the more accepted mode of measurement. Normally, this value is under 2. With warfarin therapy, an INR between 2.0 and 3.0 is acceptable, but any higher number indicates a much greater risk of bleeding.

Specifically, 2.0 to 2.5 is the goal for prophylaxis of DVT; 2.0 to 3.0 is the goal for thromboprophylaxis in hip and femoral surgery and for treatment of transient ischemic attacks and prevention of thromboembolism in atrial fibrillation; and 3.0 to 4.5 is the goal for prevention of recurrent DVT and thrombosis with mechanical heart valves.[6]

The major adverse effect of warfarin is bleeding. It may be treated by withdrawal of the drug and IV administration of vitamin K. Bleeding can then be controlled within 6 hours. In addition, fresh frozen plasma or clotting factors can be infused intravenously for an immediate coagulant effect.

Warfarin crosses the placenta and is highly teratogenic, producing fetal central nervous system problems and bleeding. Pregnant women with thrombosis can be treated with standard heparin or LMWH, which do not produce fetal abnormalities.

Thrombolytic Agents

Thrombolytic agents actively dissolve blood clots by promoting the conversion of plasminogen to plasmin, which in turn hydrolyzes fibrin. However, elevated levels of thrombin are released from the lysed clot, necessitating concurrent administration of aspirin or heparin. Examples of these drugs include streptokinase, urokinase, alteplase, and reteplase.

The thrombolytic agents are given intravenously or intraarterially in the emergency department. Infusions generally last for 3 to 24 hours, depending on the condition being treated. They are indicated in the initial treatment of acute peripheral vascular occlusion, DVT, PE, and acute MI. Alteplase is the only thrombolytic agent approved for acute ischemic stroke and only if therapy is initiated within 3 hours of onset. The other drugs in this category have actually been shown to increase the risk of cerebral hemorrhage and death when given to patients experiencing a stroke.

As with the other antithrombotic drugs, hemorrhage is a major side effect because the patient is placed in a general lytic state. These drugs are contraindicated in patients with internal bleeding, recent stroke, healing wounds, and metastatic cancer.

Therapeutic Concerns with Antithrombotic Drugs

Certain physical therapy interventions are contraindicated for patients who are taking anticoagulants. Débridement and rigorous manual techniques, such as deep tissue massage or chest percussions, are contraindicated. Dressing changes and wound care must be performed carefully to prevent bleeding. The patient should be observed for nosebleeds; bruising; and pain in the back, abdomen, or joints because these symptoms may indicate internal bleeding. The patient should also be asked to watch for blood in the urine or black, tar-like stools, particularly after exercise.

PHARMACOLOGICAL MANAGEMENT OF DEEP VEIN THROMBOSIS AND PULMONARY EMBOLISM

The balance between clot formation and lysis is intricately related to three factors that have been collectively labeled *Virchow's triad*.[33] The first is venous stasis, which is likely to develop from decreased velocity of blood flow, venous dilation and pooling, or venous obstruction. Venous stasis inhibits the blood's ability to dissipate locally activated clotting factors, leading to clot formation. Vessel wall injury is the second factor leading to DVT. Microtears in the vessel wall caused by distension or direct injury from a fracture, surgery, sepsis, or burn injury also damage the vessel's endothelial lining, further accelerating clotting. The lining becomes rough, causing platelet aggregation and adhesion. Even general anesthesia, by decreasing vascular tone, can disrupt the endothelial lining, increasing a patient's risk for DVT. The third factor that may be present in patients with DVT is a state of hypercoagulability. Certain medications (estrogens) and diseases (malignancies) are associated with hypercoagulability. Even surgery itself lowers fibrinolytic activity, which reaches its lowest point around the third postoperative day.[32]

Prevention of a DVT and subsequent PE begins by identifying patients at risk for these disorders. General prevention maneuvers have included mobilization, use of graduated compression elastic stockings and intermittent external compression devices, and insertion of a vena cava filter device.[33] This filter is recommended for patients when anticoagulant medications are contraindicated or for those who are at high risk for bleeding complications. The filter is inserted into the femoral vein and threaded upward to the inferior vena cava. The filter will then trap clots before they reach the heart or lungs. Obviously, this device will prevent a PE but not a DVT. For the patient who requires bed rest, ensuring that passive range-of-motion exercises are performed at least every 4 hours and that position is changed at least every 2 hours is important.

The protocol for the general surgery patient at high risk for DVT includes prophylactic subcutaneous administration of unfractionated heparin every 8 to 12 hours. However, the first dose is not administered until 6 to 12 hours after surgery and no sooner than 2 hours after placement of an epidural catheter. For the patient with a history of DVT, heparin may be given intravenously, and then the patient should be monitored with determinations of aPTT. As physicians become more comfortable with the LMWHs, less unfractionated heparin is used prophylactically in the high-risk patient. Studies demonstrate a lower incidence of bleeding and no effect on wound healing with the LMWHs as compared with the standard heparin preparation.[34] High-risk surgical patients are generally switched to warfarin and continue to receive this drug for 6 to 8 weeks.[33]

Before the use of LMWH, the traditional pharmacological approach to treating newly diagnosed DVT was to hospitalize the patient for at least 7 days. The patient would receive IV heparin, followed by subcutaneous heparin during conversion to warfarin therapy. The patient would then continue to receive the oral anticoagulant for up to 6 months.[33] LMWHs have drastically changed this protocol, at least for patients with smaller thrombi. Instead of being hospitalized, many patients can be treated on an outpatient basis.[28,35] Current guidelines (but not necessarily current practice in the United States) recommend administering LMWH at a weight-based dose of 1 mg/kg subcutaneously every 12 hours. Patients are also encouraged to remain mobile because some studies have not shown bed rest to be superior to early mobilization in preventing PEs.[36,37] It is also recommended that the patient receive warfarin immediately and report back for frequent INR monitoring (every 2 to 4 weeks). Warfarin therapy is continued for 3 to 6 months but may become a lifelong treatment if there is a history of a previous DVT.

Research into the fibrinolytic process during surgery and the development of LMWHs has also led to revisions in the pharmacological treatment of patients receiving total hip arthroplasties. Regional anesthesia is associated with a reduced risk of post-surgical DVT and PE compared with general anes-thesia. Combining this with hypotensive drugs diminishes intraoperative and postoperative blood loss. However, hypotensive agents may increase venous stasis, so hypotensive epidural anesthesia with intravenously infused epinephrine to keep blood flowing has been proposed.[32] A low dose of epinephrine can increase blood flow to the skeletal muscles of the leg, reducing the risk of thrombosis. Another change in practice has been to perform a venogram or a venous Doppler study for patients with a high risk for DVT between the fourth and seventh postoperative days. If the test result is positive, the patient can be treated with warfarin, and if it is negative, aspirin for 4 to 6 weeks can be recommended. A third change in practice is the administration of a single small dose of standard heparin intraoperatively when thrombogenesis is activated. Finding ways to shorten the duration of the procedure like heating the femoral stem to reduce the time for the prosthetic cement to polymerize, will also help reduce the incidence of DVT. In terms of pharmacological thromboprophylaxis, there continues to be controversy. Most orthopedic surgeons agree that postoperative pharmacotherapy to prevent thrombosis is necessary. However, there is no agreement on which agent should be administered (aspirin vs warfarin vs LMWHs) and how long the patient should continue to receive the drugs.[32,38,39]

PHARMACOLOGICAL MANAGEMENT OF PERIPHERAL ARTERIAL DISEASE

Systemic atherosclerosis is one of the major pathological processes leading to an atherosclerotic occlusion of the arteries to the legs, that is, peripheral arterial disease. Chronic ischemia of the legs and intermittent claudication result from atheromatous disease involving the iliac, femoral, or popliteal arteries. Clinical manifestations include claudication (pain in one or both legs, primarily in the calves, with walking that is relieved by rest), an abnormal ankle-brachial index value, ischemic ulceration or gangrene, or leg ischemia at rest.[40] Patients with peripheral arterial disease have a reduced walking ability that limits their activities of daily living.

Treatment of chronic peripheral arterial disease begins with the modification of certain risk factors: cessation of smoking and treatment of hyper-lipidemia, diabetes, and hypertension—all of which negatively affect peripheral circulation. However, treatment of these conditions does not guarantee improvement in walking distance or relief of ischemic pain. Intensive therapy with insulin and oral hypoglycemic agents was associated with a reduction in MI but not a reduction in the number of amputations associated with peripheral arterial disease in diabetics.[41,42] However, several large clinical trials have shown that lowering cholesterol was associated with a reduction in disease progression.[43,44]

The antiplatelet drugs, particularly aspirin and clopidogrel, are considered the main drugs for preventing ischemic events in patients with peripheral arterial disease. This treatment is directed toward preventing further thrombosis and progression of the disease. The Antiplatelet Trialists' Collaboration demonstrated a reduction in MIs, strokes, and deaths from vascular causes in patients with claudication who received aspirin therapy.[40] This study also showed that aspirin improved vascular graft patency in those patients who were treated with bypass surgery for their arterial disease, and low-dose aspirin has been found to be as effective as high-dose aspirin in preventing graft occlusion.

Two other drugs may produce a small effect on maximal walking ability. Pentoxifylline is a drug that improves the ability of red and white cells to squeeze through small vessels. In addition, the drug lowers plasma fibrinogen levels and has antiplatelet effects. Compared with placebo, it has been associated with a nonsignificant increase in walking distance.[40] Cilostazol is another drug that has antiaggregation effects on platelets, as well as some vasodilator effects. Its mechanism of action is not related to the antiplatelet drugs because this drug appears to interact directly with vascular smooth muscle. It has been shown to significantly increase pain-free walking distances when compared with either placebo or pentoxifylline.[45,46] However, widespread use of this drug has not yet caught on. Additional clinical trials are needed, specifically targeted to patients with intermittent claudication, which would determine the benefits of pentoxifylline and cilostazol, as well as the benefits of drugs that reduce the risk factors involved in the development of atherosclerosis on the functional impairments produced by peripheral arterial disease.

Intraarterial thrombolysis with tissue-type plasminogen activator is the treatment of choice for acute limb ischemia. Limb salvage can be achieved in about 75% of patients with thrombolytic infusion for 1 to 3 days.[6]

PHARMACOLOGICAL MANAGEMENT OF UNSTABLE ANGINA AND MYOCARDIAL INFARCTION

For unstable angina, low-dose aspirin should be administered after a loading dose if the patient has not already received aspirin therapy. This is followed by anticoagulation with IV heparin or LMWHs. A β-blocker or a heart rate–limiting calcium channel blocker may be added. The primary intervention in unstable angina that persists, despite pharmacological intervention, is coronary artery revascularization with either coronary artery bypass graft surgery or percutaneous transluminal coronary artery angioplasty, followed by insertion of a stent.[7]

The major goal in treating MIs is to improve cardiac perfusion so that ischemia and myocyte cell death is reduced. In a Q-wave MI (ruptured plaque with extensive thrombus and complete occlusion–ST-segment elevation), treatment is begun with a thrombolytic agent, aspirin, nitrates, and a β-blocker.[47,48] Another platelet aggregator inhibitor and LMWH heparin may also be administered if needed. Morphine is given to reduce pain but also because it reduces preload and afterload. Thrombolytics are effective if they are given within the first 12 hours. In a non–Q-wave MI (ruptured plaque with moderate thrombus), heparin is the drug of choice as opposed to the thrombolytics.[49] β-Blockers, aspirin, nitrates, and calcium channel blockers are also given.

After the immediate recovery from an MI, several pharmacological interventions have been used to promote survival and to prevent a secondary MI. Therapy with a moderate dose of warfarin combined with aspirin or high-dose warfarin alone has reduced the risk of reinfarction.[50] However, low-dose warfarin combined with low-dose aspirin (80 mg) is no more effective than a higher dose of aspirin (160 mg) alone.[30] Clopidogrel, along with aspirin and other medications, has recently been shown to be beneficial in terms of reducing the risk of MI and recurrent ischemia in patients who have experienced Q-wave and non–Q-wave MIs.[23,51] β–Blockers and angiotensin-converting enzyme inhibitors are associated with lower death rates after MI.[52-54]

ATHEROSCLEROSIS AND LIPID-LOWERING DRUGS

Reducing high levels of cholesterol has many positive implications for both short-term and long-term survival after an acute coronary syndrome. Specifically, lowering low-density lipoprotein (LDL) cholesterol levels has been shown to reduce the incidence of MI and stroke.[55,56]

Lipoproteins and the Atherogenesis Process

Lipids (triglycerides) and cholesterol are circulated in plasma as complexes consisting of lipid and proteins and are termed *lipoproteins.* They have been traditionally classified according to their density into chylomicrons, very-low-density lipoproteins (VLDLs), low-density lipoproteins (LDLs), and high-density lipoproteins (HDLs). Chylomicrons contain a very high concentration of triglycerides and basically transport dietary lipid to the liver, muscle, and adipose tissue. Lipoprotein lipase (located on the surface of the endothelial cells in capillaries in muscle and adipose tissue) then splits the chylomicrons, releasing free fatty acids, which can be taken up in muscle and fat. Chylomicron remnants, consisting mainly of cholesterol, are then taken up by the hepatocytes and stored, oxidized to bile acids, or released back into the plasma along with newly synthesized triglycerides as VLDL. This process is repeated as the VLDL transports the cholesterol and triglycerides to the tissue where triglycerides are removed as described previously. LDL with a large component of cholesterol is then either taken up in the tissues or liver via specific LDL receptors. However, if there is a deficiency in LDL receptors or there is excess LDL, oxidation of LDL cholesterol takes place, leading to the formation of an atheromatous plaque in the arterial walls.

HDL cholesterol is considered heart healthy. It takes up cholesterol from peripheral tissues and transfers it back to VLDL and LDL, and ultimately, to the liver. HDL can also deliver the cholesterol directly to the liver by a different mechanism. In general, a high HDL or low LDL cholesterol level is protective against heart disease.[57]

The atherogenesis process begins with endothelial dysfunction occurring with an alteration in prostacyclin and nitric oxide synthesis, causing reduced vasodilator responses.[3] Subsequent injury to this endothelium from hypertension or infection enhances monocyte attachment to the diseased endothelium. Monocytes and macrophages formed from monocytes then generate free radicals that oxidize attached LDL, resulting in oxidatively modified LDL and also in the destruction of receptors needed for normal clearance of LDL. Macrophages bind to the oxidized LDL, becoming known as *foam cells,* and migrate subendothelially, forming fatty streaks in the lining of the vessel. The fatty streaks become an atheroma when platelets and endothelial cells release cytokines and growth factors, causing the deposit of connective tissue and a general fibroproliferative inflammatory reaction. Ultimately, an atheromatous plaque, consisting of a fibrous cap of connective tissue overlying a lipid center, forms. This plaque can then rupture, providing surfacing for a thrombosis.

From this discussion, it would seem that a reduction in LDL levels would lower the risk of atherosclerosis, and in part, this is true. However, as is true with most of medicine, the story is not so simple. Sophisticated laboratory methods involving analytic ultracentrifugation or polyacrylamide gradient gel electrophoresis have delineated seven subclasses of LDL cholesterol and three subclasses of HDL cholesterol.[58,59] The subclasses are based on the size of the LDL and HDL particles. The larger the LDL and HDL particles, the less likely a person is to experience CAD and hypertension.[60] Alternately, persons with normal LDL levels but with a higher proportion being small, dense LDL particles (type IIIa+b) have a threefold higher risk for developing CAD.[58,61-63] In addition, those with this lipid profile have other health impairments including insulin resistance, hypertension, impaired HDL cholesterol transport, increased platelet aggregability, and an increased postprandial lipid level. In fact, the frequent coexistence of small LDL particles with elevated triglyceride levels and low levels of HDL has been called the *lipid triad,* and patients who have this combination of risk factors are said to have an "atherogenic lipoprotein phenotype" or metabolic syndrome.[64,65]

Leading cardiologists are proposing new standards for the measurement and diagnosis of lipoprotein disorders. The current method of delineating total, LDL, and HDL cholesterol levels along with fasting triglyceride levels is inadequate.[66] Research has shown that incorporating the LDL subclass distribution—as well as triglyceride, homocysteine, and lipoprotein (a) and (b) levels—provides the physician with more information to guide treatment toward the specific lipoprotein disorder. All of these measures are considered independent risk factors for CAD, whereas high concentrations of apolipoprotein A-1, a major protein in HDL, are associated with a lower risk of disease.[67] Unfortunately, few centers in the United States incorporate the scientific methodology needed to delineate the subclasses of LDL. However, patients can ask their cardiologists to send a blood sample to the Berkeley HeartLab (Berkeley, Calif) or LipoScience Inc (Raleigh, NC) for evaluation of their LDL subclasses.

3-Hydroxy-3-Methylglutaryl Coenzyme A Reductase Inhibitors (Statins)

The statin drugs competitively inhibit the enzyme that catalyzes the rate-limiting step in synthesis of cholesterol by the liver (Figure 7-5). The reduction in cholesterol leads to a compensatory increase in LDL receptors and increased LDL clearance. Statins also reduce the liver production of VLDL and circulating triglycerides.[68] Statins only modestly raise HDL levels, but several large clinical trials have demonstrated that they reduce risk of CAD in patients with low HDL and high LDL levels.[67,69] Six statins are currently available: atorvastatin,

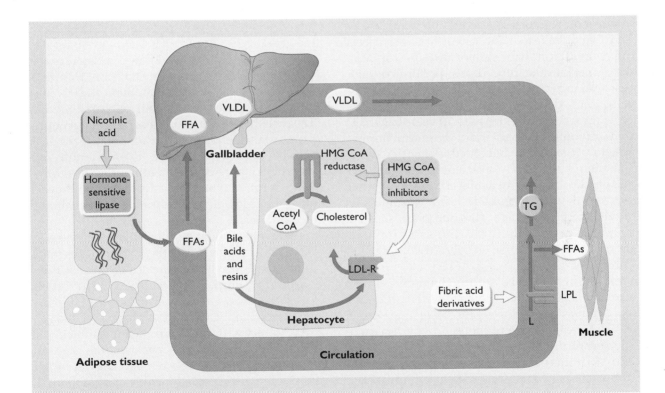

Figure 7-5

Sites of action of hypolipidemic agents. 3-Hydroxy-3-methylglutaryl coenzyme A *(HMG CoA)* reductase inhibitors lead to increased expression of low-density lipoprotein receptor (LDL-R) expression on hepatocytes and improved clearance of LDL from the plasma. Bile acid resins similarly lead to an increased LDL clearance, as well as increased cholesterol losses in bile. Fibric acid derivatives enhance lipoprotein lipase *(LPL)* action in peripheral tissues, which leads to improved clearance of triglyceride-rich particles. Nicotinic acid limits the flux of free fatty acids *(FFA)* from adipose tissue, which reduces the stimulus for hepatic very low-density lipoprotein *(VLDL)* production. When VLDL production is reduced, fewer remnant particles are available for LDL synthesis. (From Page C, Curtis MJ, Sutter MC, Walker MJ, Hoffman BB, eds. *Integrated Pharmacology.* 2nd ed. Philadelphia: Mosby; 2002.)

fluvastatin, lovastatin, pravastatin, simvastatin, and rosuvastatin.

At least three very large 5- to 6-year clinical trials carried out with patients with CAD have shown that simvastatin or pravastatin can reduce cardiac mortality, lower the incidence of stroke, and decrease mortality from all causes.[69-71] Other studies have demonstrated the benefits of the cholesterol-lowering drugs in the primary prevention of coronary disease with average total cholesterol levels but low HDL levels and in patients with hypertension but average cholesterol readings.[72-75] The most compelling evidence for the use of statins comes from a large British trial.[76] The British Heart Protection Study enlisted more than 20,000 subjects between the ages of 40 and 80 years with some risk factors for CAD, diagnosed heart disease, or stroke; but the subjects were not required to have high cholesterol levels. After 5 years, the results indicated that the subjects taking simvastatin had significantly fewer MIs, strokes, and cardiac procedures performed than subjects taking placebo. In addition, the study revealed that women benefited from the drug just as much as men, subjects older than 70 years benefited as much as younger subjects, and those with normal cholesterol levels also benefited from the drug. The results of this study also suggested that the lower the LDL cholesterol achieved, the greater the benefit, even when the LDL level was initially below the targeted value.[77] The study also showed that diabetic patients did well with simvastatin in terms of cardiac events, even when LDL levels at baseline were low.

Even though all six statins have the same mechanism of action, their potency differs. A 20-mg tablet of pravastatin reduces LDL by 24%; the same dose of atorvastatin lowers cholesterol by 46%, and the newest drug, rosuvastatin, may be the most potent.[78] In terms of efficacy, atorvastatin used to be the top reducer of LDL, but rosuvastatin may lay claim to that position now.[79] This does not imply that all patients should take either of the two most potent or efficacious drugs, because an individual may achieve his or her LDL target level with another drug that is less costly.

This discussion highlights the effectiveness of statins; however, they do have some limitations, and they are not well tolerated by all patients. Adverse effects fall into four main categories: liver abnormalities, muscle pain, interactions with drugs and food, and miscellaneous. The hepatic changes and muscle pain may occur fairly early during treatment. The liver utilizes one set of reactions to metabolize lovastatin, simvastatin, and atorvastatin and another set of reactions for fluvastatin. Still another group of reactions is used for pravastatin. Patients should have blood work done 6 weeks into treatment to monitor liver enzymes and then every 6 months thereafter. An increase in the plasma aminotransferase level to more than three times normal is seen in only 1% to 2% of patients taking statins, and full-blown symptomatic hepatitis has been rare.[67] Patients who have elevated liver enzyme levels may do well by switching to another statin.

Myalgia and muscle weakness, but not always with elevated serum creatinine phosphokinase levels, can also occur.[80,81] Reports of fatal myopathy linked to cerivastatin forced a recall of this drug from the market in August 2001. However, rarely has rhabdomyolysis or myoglobinemia been reported. The British Heart Protection Study put this problem into perspective.[76] Of more than 10,000 subjects who received simvastatin, only 49 had a myopathy. This becomes even more insignificant when compared with the placebo group, because 50 of these subjects had a myopathy. Even though muscle weakness is rare during treatment with statins, it is more common when these drugs are combined with other lipid-lowering medications (e.g., fibrates or nicotinic acid).

Statins also interact with other drugs and food. Drugs or foods that affect the liver enzymes involved in metabolism will also affect plasma statin levels. Grapefruit juice will increase blood levels of lovastatin, simvastatin, and atorvastatin; but it does not usually affect the other drugs.[78] Other drugs that interact with the statins include antacids, some antibiotics, itraconazole, cyclosporine, and many HIV antiretrovirals. The remaining adverse effects that have been reported include constipation, dizziness, GI problems, difficulty sleeping, rashes, and hair loss. There have also been some anecdotal reports of polyneuropathies with statin use.[67]

Statins are widely recommended and seem to be good medicine for anyone with a diagnosis of heart disease, a history of MI or stroke, high cholesterol levels, hypertension, diabetes, or peripheral arterial disease. Statins also have several nonlipid effects that are beneficial. Statins restore function to damaged vascular endothelium, although this may be a direct effect of lowered LDL cholesterol levels.

Other benefits include the stabilization of atherosclerotic plaques, enhanced fibrinolysis, and a reduction of inflammatory cell infiltration around atherosclerotic plaques.[6,82] There is also some evidence that statins may help counter Alzheimer's disease and vascular dementia, but further study in this area is necessary.[83] These drugs come close to being miracle drugs for patients at high risk for developing heart disease, but there are some limitations to their use. As mentioned earlier, the statins do not always sufficiently lower LDL levels, and increased doses of statins may not always continue to lower cholesterol levels.[84] In addition, they have only a modest affect on HDL levels. For patients who do not reach their target cholesterol levels with these drugs, some alternatives are available (see the following sections. Some of these alternatives can be given safely along with a statin drug.

Bile Acid–Binding Resins

Cholestyramine, colesevelam, and colestipol are bile acid–binding resins that can successfully lower LDL levels by up to 20%.[67] These are insoluble agents that bind bile salts secreted into the duodenum, thus preventing enterohepatic circulation. Bile acids are synthesized from cholesterol in the liver and secreted into the gut to aid in absorption of dietary fat. They are normally reabsorbed in the terminal ileum and sent back to the liver. Blocking bile acid reabsorption allows a compensatory increase in bile synthesis in the liver, leading to a further elimination of cholesterol. A lowered cholesterol level results in an up-regulation of LDL receptors and a more rapid clearing of LDL particles.

The primary limitation in the widespread use of these drugs is GI intolerance—extreme diarrhea in some patients and constipation in others.[6,84] Another limitation is that the taste and texture are unacceptable to many individuals. These drugs come in a powder form and are mixed with food or drink. They may also interfere with the absorption of certain drugs (e.g., digoxin, warfarin, and thyroxine), and these drugs should be administered at least 1 hour before a bile acid–binding resin is taken.

Colesevelam is the newest bile acid sequestrant and appears to have some benefits over the older drugs. This drug has less potential to interfere with other medications, and therefore it can be given simultaneously with other drugs. In addition, when it is co-administered with the statins, an additive reduction in LDL cholesterol is seen. In fact, when colesevelam was given along with simvastatin, there was a greater reduction in the LDL level than when the simvastatin dose was doubled.[85] The primary disadvantage is that colesevelam attenuates the triglyceride reduction seen with the statins.[84]

Fibrates

Bezafibrate, gemfibrozil, and ciprofibrate alter lipoprotein metabolism by activating gene transcription factors.[6,86] These factors are known as peroxisome proliferation activated receptors, and they increase lipoprotein lipase activity, enhancing the elimination of triglycerides from the lipoproteins in plasma. These drugs also enhance free fatty acid uptake by the liver by inducing a fatty acid transport protein. Fibrates also convert small LDL particles to large LDL particles. In general, triglyceride levels are lowered by 25% to 50%, and the HDL level is increased 10% to 35%.[84]

Adverse effects associated with fibrates include GI upset, increased risk of gallstones, and some drug-drug interactions with warfarin. Myositis has also been reported but occurred only when gemfibrozil was given along with a statin.[84]

Nicotinic Acid

Nicotinic acid is a B vitamin that, at elevated levels, increases HDL levels 15% to 35%, reduces LDL levels by 5% to 25%, and decreases triglyceride levels by 20% to 35%.[84] This drug reduces free fatty acid mobilization from adipocytes and ultimately leads to a reduction in LDL cholesterol levels. The fact that it has a different mechanism of action than the statins has provided a rationale for their concurrent use. Nicotinic acid plus lovastatin has been recommended for patients who continue to have high levels of triglycerides after monotherapy with a statin.[84] Adverse effects include skin flushing, pruritus, GI upset, blurred vision, fatigue, hyperuricemia, hepatic toxicity, and glucose intolerance. In general, this drug is poorly tolerated by patients.

Cholesterol Absorption Inhibitor

Ezetimibe is a new drug that inhibits intestinal absorption of cholesterol. It also keeps the cholesterol in bile from recirculating back into the liver.

It reduces LDL cholesterol levels by approximately 20% and produces modest but positive changes in other lipid markers.[87] Efficacy of ezetimibe when used alone is about equal to that of a high-dose statin, and when ezetimibe was used in combination with a statin, a 21.45% greater reduction in LDL levels was achieved compared with statin plus placebo.

The safety profile of ezetimibe is similar to that of placebo, and when given in combination with a statin, is equal to that of the statin. The only warning that has been added to the ezetimibe label relates to a risk of angioedema, but at present, the absolute number of cases is not known because this side effect was not seen in clinical trials.[88]

Ezetimibe is being marketed as monotherapy for patients who cannot tolerate statins and in combination with statins to help achieve LDL target levels. It may also be particularly useful for patients with familial hypercholesterolemia in which LDL receptors are defective.

Therapeutic Concerns with Lipid-Lowering Agents

In general, lipid-lowering drugs are safe with a low incidence of adverse effects. However, muscle soreness and rhabdomyolysis have occurred with some of the statins, particularly when they are used in combination with other lipid-lowering agents.[81] Rhabdomyolysis has also been reported when the statins are used with erythromycin and some antifungal agents. Physical therapists should question their patients about the incidence of muscle soreness that appears greater than what would be expected from physical therapy.

ACTIVITIES 7

■ 1. You are treating a 52-year-old man for chronic back pain related to a herniated disk in his lumbar area. His medical history is significant for an anterior myocardial infarction 2 years ago, and he is currently taking a β-blocker. His fasting plasma LDL level is 256 and his HDL level is 38. Both his orthopedic surgeon and cardiologist recommend exercise and weight loss to improve his functional abilities and medical status.

Questions

a. What advice would you give him?
b. What additional drugs would you recommend and why?
c. What target cholesterol levels would you aim for?
d. What adverse effects should you stay alert for during therapy?

■ 2 You are treating a 58-year-old man with adhesive capsulitis. The patient is receiving joint mobilization, passive stretching, and progressive resistive exercise. Shortly after he completes the weight lifting portion of his therapy session, he tells you that he has some chest pain. The patient has been lifting the same amount of weight for the past 2 weeks without problems. He reports that in the past he has been able to take one nitroglycerin tablet 5 minutes before activity but now he needs two tablets.

The patient has continued to smoke two packs of cigarettes each day and is concerned that his cardiac condition is worsening because of this increased need to take medication.

Vital Signs
Blood pressure, 135/80 mm Hg; pulse, 80 beats/min; respiratory rate, 18 breaths/min

Physical Exam
Height 5'8" Weight, 220 lb, Patient in no acute distress; no rales or crackles in the lungs, heart sounds are normal, no leg edema, and no jugular vein distention

You decide to end the therapy session and refer the patient to an emergency clinic.

The patient returns to the clinic in the afternoon to report his test results.

The patient has an elevated glucose level (154 mg/dL), hypercholesterolemia, and hypertriglyceridemia. Blood urea nitrogen and creatinine levels are normal, and the electrocardiogram shows no signs of ischemia or infarction.

A chest x-ray film demonstrates left ventricular hypertrophy.

Questions

a. Why does the patient have increased chest pain despite the increase in nitroglycerin?
b. What is the patient's most likely diagnosis?
c. From a pharmacological perspective, what changes need to be made?
d. Discuss why a patient may receive both warfarin and heparin at the same time.

References

1. Talbert RL. Ischemic heart disease. In: Dipiro JT, Talbert RL, Yee GC, Matzke GR, Wells BG, Posey LM, eds. *Pharmacotherapy: A Pathophysiological Approach.* 3rd ed. Stamford, Conn: Appleton & Lange; 1997:257-294.
2. Katzung BG, Chatterjees MB. Vasodilators & the treatment of angina pectoris. In: Katzung BG, ed. *Basic & Clinical Pharmacology.* 8th ed. New York: McGraw-Hill; 2001:181-199.
3. Rang HP, Dale MM, Ritter JM, Moore JL. *Pharmacology.* 5th ed. New York: Churchill Livingstone; 2003.
4. Williams SV, Fihn SD, Gibbons RJ. Guidelines for the management of patients with chronic stable angina: diagnosis and risk stratification. *Ann Intern Med.* 2001; 135(7):530-547.
5. Graboys TB, Lown B. Nitroglycerin: the "mini" wonder drug. *Circulation.* 2003;108(11):e78-e79.
6. Waller DG, Renwick AG, Hillier K. *Medical Pharmacology and Therapeutics.* New York: WB Saunders; 2001.
7. Curtis MJ, Pugsley MK. Drugs and the cardiovascular system. In: Page C, Curtis MJ, Sutter MC, Walker MJ, Hoffman BB, eds. *Integrated Pharmacology.* 2nd ed. Philadelphia: Mosby; 2002:360-414.
8. Kuhn M. *Pharmacotherapeutics: A Nursing Process Approach.* 4th ed. Philadelphia: FA Davis; 1998.
9. Fihn SD, Williams SV, Daley J, Gibbons RJ. Guidelines for the management of patients with chronic stable angina: treatment. *Ann Intern Med.* 2001;135(8 Part I):616-632.
10. Moczydlowski EG. Electrical excitability and action potentials. In: Boron WF, Boulpaep EL, eds. *Medical Physiology.* Philadelphia: Saunders; 2003:172-203.
11. Lederer WJ. Cardiac electrophysiology and the electrocardiogram. In: Boron WF, Boulpaep EL, eds. *Medical Physiology.* Philadelphia: Saunders; 2003:483-507.
12. Kaufmann PA, Mandinov L, Seiler C, Hess OM. Impact of exercise-induced coronary vasomotion on anti-ischemic therapy. *Coron Artery Dis.* 2000;11(4):363-369.
13. Frishman WH, Michaelson MD. Use of calcium antagonists in patients with ischemic heart disease and systematic hypertension. *Am J Cardiol.* 1997;79(10A):33-38.
14. Epstein M. The calcium antagonist controversy: the emerging importance of drug formulation as a determinant of risk. *Am J Cardiol.* 1997;79(10A):9-19.
15. Heidenreich PA, McDonald KM, Hastie T, et al. Meta-analysis of trials comparing β-blockers, calcium antagonists, and nitrates for stable angina. JAMA. 1999; 281(20):1927-1936.
16. Steffensen R, Melchior T, Bech J, et al. Effects of amlodipine and isosorbide dinitrate on exercise-induced and ambulatory ischemia in patients with chronic stable angina pectoris. *Cardiovasc Drugs Ther.* 1997;11:629-635.
17. Furie B, Furie BC. Molecular and cellular biology of blood coagulation. *N Engl J Med.* 1992;326(12):800-806.
18. Vaughn G. *Understanding and Evaluating Common Laboratory Tests.* Upper Saddle River, NJ: Pearson Education; 1999.
19. Hambleton J, O'Reilly RA. Drugs used in disorders of coagulation. In: Katzung BG, ed. *Basic & Clinical Pharmacology.* 8th ed. New York: McGraw Hill; 2001:564-580.
20. Hu Z. Drugs and the blood. In: Page C, Curtis MJ, Sutter MC, Walker MJ, Hoffman BB, eds. *Integrated Pharmacology.* 2nd ed. Philadelphia: Mosby; 2002:191-218.
21. Antiplatelet Trialists' Collaboration. Collaborative overview of randomised trials of antiplatelet therapy. I. Prevention of death, myocardial infarction, and stroke by prolonged antiplatelet therapy in various categories of patients. *BMJ.* 1994;308:81-106.
22. Collins R, MacMahon S, Flather M. Clinical effects of anticoagulant therapy in suspected acute myocardial infarction: systematic overview of randomised trials. *BMJ.* 1996;313:652-659.
23. CAPRIE Steering Committee. A randomised, blinded, trial of clopidogrel versus aspirin in patients at risk of ischaemic events (CAPRIE). *Lancet.* 1996;348:1329-1339.
24. The Clopidogrel in Unstable Angina to Prevent Events Trial Investigators. Effects of clopidogrel in addition to aspirin in patients with acute coronary syndromes without ST-segment elevation. *N Engl J Med.* 2001; 345(7):494-502.
25. Clopidogrel for reduction of atherosclerotic events. *Med Lett Drugs Ther.* 1998; 40 (1028):59-60.
26. Tcheng JE, Kandzari DE, Grines CL, et al. Benefits and risks of abciximab use in primary angioplasty for acute myocardial infarction: the Controlled Abciximab and Device Investigation to Lower Late Angioplasty Complications (CADILLAC) trial. *Circulation.* 2003;108(11): 1316-1323.
27. Elhendy A, Bax JJ, Poldermans D. Dobutamine stress myocardial perfusion imaging in coronary artery disease. *J Nucl Med.* 2001;43(12):1634-1646.
28. Levine M, Gent M, Hirsh J, et al. A comparison of low-molecular-weight heparin administered primarily at home with unfractionated heparin administered in the hospital for proximal deep-vein thrombosis. *N Engl J Med.* 1996;334(11):677-681.

29. Blattler W, Kreis N, Blattler IK. Practicability and quality of outpatient management of acute deep venous thrombosis. *J Vasc Surg.* 2000;32:855-860.

30. Coumadin Aspirin Reinfarction Study (CARS) Investigators. Randomised double-blind trial of fixed low-dose warfarin with aspirin after myocardial infarction. *Lancet.* 1997;350:389-396.

31. Turpie AG, Gent M, Laupacis A, et al. A comparison of aspirin with placebo in patients treated with warfarin after heart-valve replacement. *N Engl J Med.* 1993; 329:524-529.

32. Salvati EA. Multimodal prophylaxis of venous thrombosis. *Am J Orthop.* 2002;31(9 suppl):4-11.

33. Church V. Staying on guard for DVT & PE. *Nursing.* 2000; 30(2):35-42.

34. Innes GD, Dillon EC, Holmes A. Low-molecular-weight heparin in the emergency department treatment of venous thromboembolism. *J Emerg Med.* 1997;15(4): 563-566.

35. Partsch H. Bed rest versus ambulation in the initial treatment of patients with proximal deep vein thrombosis. *Curr Opin Pulm Med.* 2002;8:389-393.

36. Aschwanden M, Labs KH, Engel H, et al. Acute deep vein thrombosis: early mobilization does not increase the frequency of pulmonary embolism. *Thromb Haemost.* 2001;85:42-46.

37. Partsch H. Therapy of deep vein thrombosis with low molecular weight heparin, leg compression and immediate ambulation. *Vasa.* 2001;30:195-204.

38. Goldstein WM, Jimenez ML, Bailie DS, Wall R, Branson J. Safety of a clinical surveillance protocol with 3- and 6-week warfarin prophylaxis after total joint arthroplasty. *Orthopedics.* 2001;24(7):651-654.

39. Ragucci MV, Leali A, Moroz A, Fetto J. Comprehensive deep venous thrombosis prevention strategy after total-knee arthroplasty. *Am J Phys Med Rehabil.* 2003;82(3): 164-168.

40. Hiatt WR. Drug therapy: medical treatment of peripheral arterial disease and claudication. *N Engl J Med.* 2001; 344(21):1608-1621.

41. UK Prospective Diabetes Study (UKPDS) Group. Intensive blood-glucose control with sulphonylureas or insulin compared with conventional treatment and risk of complications in patients with type 2 diabetes. *Lancet.* 1998;352(9131):837-853.

42. The Diabetes Control and Complications Trial (DCCT). Effect of intensive diabetes management on macrovascular events and risk factors in the diabetes control and complications trial. *Am J Cardiol.* 1995;75:894-903.

43. Kroon AA, Van Asten W, Stalenhoef AF. Effect of apheresis of low-density lipoprotein on peripheral vascular disease in hypercholesterolemic patients with coronary artery disease. *Ann Intern Med.* 1996;125(12):945-954.

44. Leng GC, Price JF, Jepson RG. Lipid-lowering for lower limb atherosclerosis. *Cochrane Database Syst Rev.* 2003;3.

45. Dawson DL, Cutler BS, Hiatt WR, et al. A comparison of cilostazol and pentoxifylline for treating intermittent claudication. *Am J Med.* 2000;109(7):523-530.

46. Beebe HG, Dawson DL, Cutler BS, et al. A new pharmacological treatment for intermittent claudication: results of a randomized, multicenter trial. *Arch Intern Med.* 1999;159(17):2041-2050.

47. Arbustini E, De Servi S, Bramucci E, et al. Comparison of coronary lesions obtained by directional coronary atherectomy in unstable angina, stable angina, and restenosis after either atherectomy or angioplasty. *Am J Cardiol.* 1995;75:675-682.

48. Collin R, Peto R, Baigent C, Sleight P. Aspirin, heparin, and fibrinolytic therapy in suspected acute myocardial infarction. *N Engl J Med.* 1997;336(12):847-860.

49. Braunwald E, McCabe CH, Cannon CP, Muller JE, TIMI IIIB Investigators. An unstable angina/myocardial infarction: effects of tissue plasminogen activator and a comparison of early invasive and conservative strategies in unstable angina and non-Q-wave myocardial infarction: results of the TIMI IIIB Trial. *Circulation.* 1994; 89(4):1545-1556.

50. Hurlen M, Abdelnoor M, Smith P, Erikssen J, Arnesen H. Warfarin, aspirin, or both after myocardial infarction. *N Engl J Med.* 2002;347(13):969-974.

51. The Clopidogrel in Unstable Angina to Prevent Recurrent Events Trial Investigators. Effects of clopidogrel in addition to aspirin in patients with acute coronary syndromes without ST-segment elevation. *N Engl J Med.* 2001;345(7):494-502.

52. Rodrigues EJ, Eisenberg MJ, Pilote L. Effects of early and late administration of angiotensin-converting enzyme inhibitors on mortality after myocardial infarction. *Am J Med.* 2003;115:473-479.

53. Latini R, Staszewsky L, Maggioni AP, et al. Beneficial effects of angiotensin-converting enzyme inhibitor and nitrate association on left ventricular remodeling in patients with large acute myocardial infarction: The Delapril Remodeling after Acute Myocardial Infarction (DRAMI) trial. *Am Heart J.* 2003;146:1-8.

54. Ambrosioni E, Borghi C. Early and late angiotensin-converting enzyme inhibition after myocardial infarction: an overview of randomized clinical trials. *Am J Med.* 2003;115:503-504.

55. Ramsay LE, Haq IU, Jackson PR, Yeo WW, Pickin DM, Payne JN. Targeting lipid-lowering drug therapy for primary prevention of coronary disease: an updated Sheffield table. *Lancet.* 1996;348:387-388.

56. Aronow HD, Topol E, Roe MT, et al. Effect of lipid-lowering therapy on early mortality after acute coronary syndromes: an observational study. *Lancet.* 2001; 357:1063-1068.

57. Francis GS, ed. *Cholesterol Size, Not Just Levels, Linked with Cardiac Health.* Greenwich, Conn: Belvoir Publications; 2004.

58. Superko HR. Small, dense, low-density lipoprotein and atherosclerosis. *Curr Atheroscler Rep.* 2000;2(3):226-231.

59. Superko HR, Haskell WL, Krauss RM. Association of lipoprotein subclass distribution with use of selective and non-selective beta-blocker medications in patients with coronary heart disease. *Atherosclerosis.* 1993;101: 709-714.

60. Barzilai N, Atzmon G, Schechter C, et al. Unique lipoprotein phenotype and genotype associated with exceptional longevity. *JAMA.* 2003;290:2030-2040.

61. Superko HR. Lipoprotein subclasses and atherosclerosis. *Front Biosci.* 2001;6:D355-D365.

62. Superko HR. Small, dense low-density lipoprotein subclass pattern B: issues for the clinician. *Curr Atheroscler Rep.* 1999;1(1):50-57.

63. Superko HR, Hecht HS. Metabolic disorders contribute to subclinical coronary atherosclerosis in patients with coronary calcification. *Am J Cardiol.* 2001;88(3):260-264.

64. Grundy SM. Consensus statement: role of therapy with "statins" in patients with hypertriglyceridemia. *Am J Cardiol.* 1998;81(4A):1B-6B.

65. Expert Panel on Detection, Evaluation, and Treatment of High Blood Cholesterol in Adults. Executive summary of the third report of the National Cholesterol Education Program (NCEP) Expert Panel on Detection, Evaluation, and Treatment of High Blood Cholesterol in Adults (Adult Treatment Panel III). *JAMA.* 2001;285:2486-2497.

66. Superko HR. Hypercholesterolemia and dyslipidemia. *Curr Treat Options Cardiovasc Med.* 2000;2(2):173-187.

67. Drugs for lipid disorders. *Treat Guidel Med Lett.* 2003; 1(12):77-82.

68. Law MR, Wald NJ, Rudnicka AR. Quantifying effect of statins on low density lipoprotein cholesterol, ischaemic heart disease, and stroke: systematic review and meta-analysis. *BMJ.* 2003;326:1-7.

69. Scandinavian Simvastatin Survival Study Group. Randomised trial of cholesterol lowering in 4444 patients with coronary heart disease: The Scandinavian Simvastatin Survival Study. *Lancet.* 1994;344:1383-1389.

70. Sacks FM, Pfeffer MA, Moye LA, et al. The effect of pravastatin on coronary events after myocardial infarction in patients with average cholesterol levels. *N Engl J Med.* 1996;335:1001-1009.

71. The Long-term Intervention with Pravastatin in Ischaemic Disease (LIPID) Study Group. Prevention of cardiovascular events and death with pravastatin in patients with coronary heart disease and a broad range of initial cholesterol levels. *N Engl J Med.* 1998;339:1349-1357.

72. Shepherd J, Cobbe SM, Ford I, et al. Prevention of coronary heart disease with pravastatin in men with hypercholesterolemia. *N Engl J Med.* 1995;333:1301-1307.

73. Downs JR, Clearfield M, Weis S, et al. Primary prevention of acute coronary events with lovastatin in men and women with average cholesterol levels: results of AFCAPS/TexCAPS. *JAMA.* 1998;279:1615-1622.

74. Ridker PM, Rifai N, Pfeffer MA, et al. Inflammation, pravastatin, and the risk of coronary events after myocardial infarction in patients with average cholesterol levels. Cholesterol and Recurrent Events (CARE) investigators. *Circulation.* 1998;98(9):839-844.

75. Sever PS, Dahlof B, Poulter NR, et al. Prevention of coronary and stroke events with atorvastatin in hypertensive patients who have average or lower-than-average cholesterol concentrations, in the Anglo-Scandinavian Cardiac Outcomes Trial-Lipid Lowering Arm (ASCOT-LLA): a multicentre randomised controlled trial. *Lancet.* 2003;361:1149-1158.

76. Heart Protection Study Collaborative Group. MRC/BHF heart protection study of cholesterol lowering with simvastatin in 20536 high-risk individuals: a randomised placebo-controlled trial. *Lancet.* 2002;360:7-22.

77. Ballantyne CM. Current and future aims of lipid-lowering therapy: changing paradigms and lessons from the heart protection study on standards of efficacy and safety. *Am J Cardiol.* 2003;92(4, suppl 2):3-9.

78. Lee TH, ed. *Choose the Statin That's Right for You.* Boston, Mass: Harvard Health Publications; 2003.

79. Jones PH, Davidson MH, Stein EA, et al. Comparison of the efficacy and safety of rosuvastatin versus atorvastatin, simvastatin, and pravastatin across doses (STELLAR Trial). *Am J Cardiol.* 2003;92:152-160.

80. Wenisch C, Krause R, Fladerer P, Menjawi IE, Pohanka E. Acute rhabdomyolysis after atorvastatin and fusidic acid therapy. *Am J Med.* 2000;109(1):78-80.

81. Duell P, Connor W, Illingworth D. Rhabdomyolysis after taking atorvastatin with gemfibrozil. *Am J Cardiol.* 1998; 81:368-369.

82. Ridker PM, Rifai N, Clearfield M, et al. Measurement of C-reactive protein for the targeting of statin therapy in the primary prevention of acute coronary events. *N Engl J Med.* 2001;344(26):1959-1965.

83. Jick H, Zornberg GL, Jick S, Seshadri S, Drachman DA. Statins and the risk of dementia. *Lancet.* 2000;356: 1627-1631.

84. Thompson PD. What's new in lipid management? *Pharmacotherapy.* 2003;23(9):34S-40S.

85. Knapp HH, Schrott H, Ma P. Effectiveness of colesevelam hydrochloride in decreasing LDL cholesterol in patients with primary hypercholesterolemia. *Am J Med.* 2001; 110:352-360.

86. Staels B, Dallongeville J, Auwerx J, Schoonjans K, Leitersdorf E, Fruchart JC. Mechanism of action of fibrates on lipid and lipoprotein metabolism. *Circulation.* 1998;98(19):2088-2093.

87. Bruckert E, Giral P, Tellier P. Perspectives in cholesterol-lowering therapy: the role of ezetimibe, a new selective inhibitor of intestinal cholesterol absorption. *Circulation.* 2003;107:3124-3128.

88. Neal RC, Jones PH. Lipid-lowering: can ezetimibe help close the treatment gap? *Cleve Clin J Med.* 2003; 70(9):777-783.

CHAPTER 8

DRUG THERAPY FOR CONGESTIVE HEART FAILURE AND CARDIAC ARRHYTHMIAS

DRUG TREATMENT FOR CONGESTIVE HEART DISEASE

Congestive heart failure (CHF) refers to the inability of the heart to pump sufficient cardiac output to maintain healthy tissue and to meet the body's physiological needs. The most common diseases or conditions that lead to the development of CHF include cardiomyopathy, myocardial ischemia and infarction, hypertension, valvular disease, congenital heart disease, and coronary artery disease.[1] Structural changes, either from the loss of cardiac myocytes in cardiomyopathy or from infarction, lead to reduced cardiac contractility. Excessive afterload from hypertension or aortic stenosis produces cardiac hypertrophy, and valvular defects (regurgitation) and tachycardia reduce stroke volume. Both cardiac hypertrophy and reduced stroke volume lead to the syndrome of heart failure.

In the early stages, the heart compensates for diminished cardiac output with tachycardia and increased contractility by means of myocardial hypertrophy. However, these compensations increase cardiac workload, which further compromises pumping. The sympathetic system is activated to improve contractility, but the catecholamines produce vasoconstriction. The kidneys, sensing diminished perfusion begin to increase their secretion of renin, leading to release of angiotensin II and aldosterone. Water retention, increased blood pressure, and increased preload result. These neurohumoral compensations in response to the low blood pressure and diminished renal perfusion produce heart failure (Figure 8-1). As preload increases, more blood enters the heart, resulting in increased end-diastolic pressure, and cardiac dilation begins to occur. Angiotensin II also promotes arterial vasoconstriction and increased afterload. This cycle continues until the ventricles can no longer pump and perfusion to the major organs is impaired.

CHF tends to develop from reduced left ventricular systolic contractility, also known as systolic heart failure, as explained previously, but it can also result from impaired diastolic relaxation (diastolic heart failure). When the left ventricle fails to relax appropriately, volume to accommodate the venous return is limited. This also leads to pulmonary venous congestion and reduced cardiac output.[2]

CHF has been artificially divided into left ventricular heart failure and right ventricular failure, although they tend to occur together. Symptoms of left ventricular heart failure include reduced cardiac output and blood pressure, resulting in the backflow of fluid into the pulmonary system. Right ventricular heart failure results in the backflow of fluid into the venous circulation, resulting in peripheral edema. The overall clinical presentation may include dyspnea, cyanosis, orthopnea, peripheral edema, ascites, and fatigue. The American College of Cardiology (ACC) and the American Heart Association (AHA) define

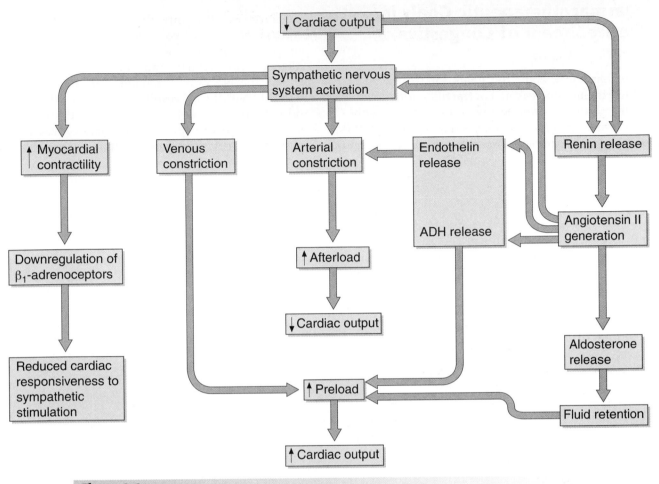

Figure 8-1

Neurohumoral consequences of heart failure. The increase in preload can improve cardiac performance in the mildly impaired heart but will lead to edema if cardiac function is significantly reduced, since the increased preload cannot restore a normal stroke volume. The increased afterload will put additional strain on the failing heart and can further decrease cardiac output. These effects are compounded by down-regulation of cardiac β_1 adrenoceptors. *ADH,* Antidiuretic hormone. (From Waller DG, Renwick AG, Hillier K. *Medical Pharmacology and Therapeutics.* New York: WB Saunders; 2001.)

heart failure caused by systolic dysfunction as a left ventricular ejection fraction <40%.[3]

CHF is a very serious syndrome that requires intensive pharmacological intervention. It is a progressive disorder, which in its severe form induces major physical limitations. There are 550,000 new cases of CHF diagnosed each year, and annual mortality is more than 50,000.[4] Patients who have symptoms during activity tend to have a 2-year mortality of 20%, and those who experience symptoms at rest have a 1-year mortality of 80%.[2] Death tends to result from progressive heart failure or from arrhythmias. The New York Heart Association (NYHA) along with the ACC and the AHA have classified CHF according to the functional limitations it produces.[4] The NYHA Classification is as follows: class I, no symptoms with ordinary physical activity; class II, symptoms on ordinary exertion; class III, symptoms on minimal exertion with marked limitation of physical activity; and class IV, symptoms at rest. At present, there has been no attempt to associate these functional limitations with objective measurements such as ventricular ejection fraction.

Pharmacotherapeutic Goals in the Treatment of Congestive Heart Failure

The pharmacotherapeutic goals for treating heart failure include increasing contractility with positive inotropic drugs (cardiac glycosides and phosphodiesterase inhibitors), decreasing congestion and edema with diuretics, and decreasing preload and afterload with a vasodilator and/or an angiotensin-converting (ACE) inhibitor.

Cardiac Glycosides

Digitalis glycosides are positive inotropic agents that enhance cardiac contractility by increasing the availability of free intracellular calcium (Ca^{2+}) to interact with contractile proteins.[1] Specifically, these drugs inhibit the Na^+/K^+-ATPase pump on the cardiac cell membrane (Figure 8-2). This pump is normally responsible for maintaining low intracellular sodium (Na^+) and high intracellular potassium (K^+)

concentrations. It pumps three Na^+ ions out of the cell in exchange for two K^+ ions into the cell. If the pump is inhibited, the high Na^+ concentration enhances intracellular transport of Ca^{2+} into the cell via the Na^+/Ca^{2+} exchange mechanism. This elevated level of Ca^{2+} results in greater contractility and therefore greater cardiac output and improved circulation. These changes reduce sympathetic activity and reduce angiotensin II and renin levels.

Digitalis has effects on the kidneys and the parasympathetic system separate from its effects on the Na^+/K^+-ATPase pump. It enhances delivery of Na^+ to the distal tubules of the kidneys, producing diuresis, and it activates the parasympathetic system with resultant increased vagal tone, which produces an antiarrhythmic effect. When atrial fibrillation coexists with heart failure, digitalis use is clearly indicated because digitalis reduces ventricular response rates.[5] However, its use in heart failure in the absence of atrial fibrillation is becoming more difficult to justify because of its adverse effects.

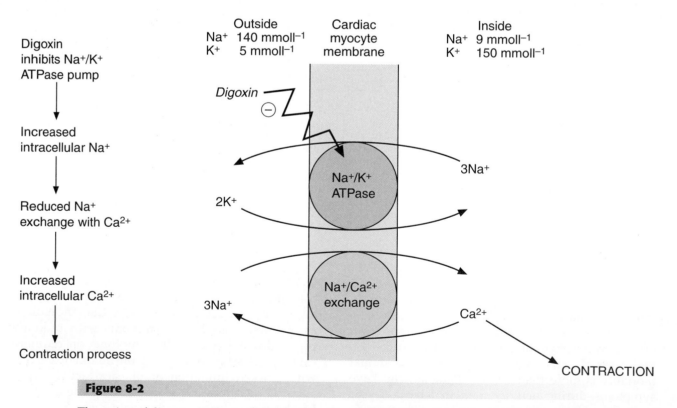

Figure 8-2

The action of digoxin on the cardiac myocyte. (From Waller DG, Renwick AG, Hillier K. *Medical Pharmacology and Therapeutics.* New York: WB Saunders; 2001.)

The Digoxin Investigators Group studied more than 6800 patients without atrial fibrillation to determine whether digoxin reduced all-cause mortality.[6] After follow-up for 37 months, there was a significant reduction, 28%, in hospital admissions for progressing heart failure but a reduction of only 6% in total hospital admissions. In addition, there were no reductions in all-cause mortality during this period. Because digitalis produces significant side effects and does not seem to lower the mortality rate, controversy over its continued use exists, at least for patients without fibrillation.[7]

The cardiac glycosides have a low therapeutic index because both therapeutic and toxic actions result from elevated cytoplasmic calcium levels.[2] High intracellular Ca^{2+} precipitates arrhythmias. Arrhythmias may also result from cardiac K^+ loss and hypokalemia, especially when these drugs are given with diuretics. Additional side effects result from gastric irritation and stimulation of the chemoreceptor trigger zone, resulting in nausea, vomiting, and diarrhea. Other effects include central nervous system disturbances such as headaches, dizziness, visual disturbances, and hallucinations. Digitalis toxicity may occur, resulting in bradycardia. Treatment entails drug withdrawal, K^+ supplementation, and administration of atropine for the sinus bradycardia. Careful monitoring of serum electrolyte and cardiac glycoside blood levels is needed.

Phosphodiesterase Inhibitors

Milrinone and amrinone are inhibitors of phosphodiesterase III found in cardiac and smooth muscle. When this enzyme is blocked, there is an increase in intracellular cyclic adenosine monophosphate, which through a cascade of events, forces the release of Ca^{2+} stores.[2] Cardiac contractility is improved, and elevated cyclic adenosine monophosphate levels in the arterial and venous smooth muscle result in marked vasodilation.

These drugs are not widely used because long-term administration with the oral formulation has been associated with increased mortality.[2] However, they are still given intravenously for short periods. Adverse effects include nausea and vomiting, tachycardia, and serious arrhythmias.

Diuretics

Diuretics are essential in the treatment of patients with CHF and lung congestion or peripheral edema.

Short-term studies have shown that diuretics decrease fluid retention and improve exercise capacity, but diuretics have not been shown to decrease mortality or slow the progression of the disease.[4] Often, patients will receive a thiazide and a loop diuretic together, and doses are adjusted frequently as the urine output and patient's weight changes. It is important for the patient to keep a daily weight record because this allows for more accurate dose adjustments to prevent severe volume overload.[8]

Although diuretics are necessary to improve the clinical presentation in CHF, specific attention should be directed toward preventing hypotension, electrolyte imbalances, activation of the neurohormonal compensatory mechanisms, and hypokalemia and hyperkalemia.[5]

β-Blockers

β-Blockers have been considered to be contraindicated for patients with CHF because they slow heart rate and decrease contractility.[4] However, several large clinical trials have shown that cardioselective β-blockers have some benefit for patients whose conditions have been stabilized with a diuretic and an ACE inhibitor. The Cardiac Insufficiency Bisoprolol Study II evaluated 2647 symptomatic patients who had NYHA class III or IV CHF and who had an ejection fraction of less than 35%.[9] There was a 42% reduction in mortality and a significant reduction in hospital admissions in the bisoprolol group. Treatment effects were independent of the severity of heart failure. Even though the patients were functionally quite impaired, they were medically stable. In addition, the mean age of the patients was 61 years, much younger than the patients with CHF seen in clinical practice.

Another study demonstrated that metoprolol improved the ejection fraction at rest and during exercise and decreased mortality among patients with mild-moderate heart failure (NYHA functional class II-III) who were taking ACE inhibitors.[10] The patients had CHF from either ischemic heart disease or idiopathic dilated cardiomyopathy, but both groups responded equally well to the β-blocker. Studies with carvedilol further substantiate a role for β-blockers in the treatment of CHF.[4,11] In fact, the beneficial effects of carvedilol, metoprolol, and bisoprolol on mortality and morbidity appear similar, regardless of the severity of CHF.[12]

Possible explanations for the usefulness of β-blockers in the treatment of CHF include the following: depression of the neurohumoral response to diminished cardiac output, antiarrhythmic properties of the drugs, and reduction of workload on the damaged myocardium. Most patients are now treated with β-blockers, but the dose is kept low initially, followed by a slow doubling every 2 to 4 weeks, until the target dose is reached.[5] Patients must also be selected carefully; those with edema are excluded from receiving a β-blocker. Even with careful selection, a patient may initially demonstrate some deterioration, followed frequently by an improvement. Side effects to look out for are hypotension, fluid retention, worsening heart failure, and bradyarrhythmias.

Angiotensin-Converting Enzyme Inhibitors

The beneficial effects of ACE inhibitors have been so convincing that these drugs are used not only in all stages of heart failure but also in patients with a high risk for CHF before symptoms and structural changes in heart tissue develop. These drugs reduce peripheral vascular resistance (afterload) and prevent aldosterone-mediated Na^+ and fluid retention. They have been shown to slow the progression of heart failure and prolong survival.[13,14] In the landmark Cooperative North Scandinavian Enalapril Survival Study (CONSENSUS-1), enalapril produced a reduction in mortality of 40% in patients with severe heart failure (NYHA class IV). In addition, there were reductions in heart size and in the need for diuretics in these patients.[15] ACE inhibitors have also been shown to protect against atherosclerosis through an antiproliferative effect, and have an anti-migratory effect on smooth muscle cells.[11] At present, they are the first drugs prescribed for chronic CHF.[5,16]

The major adverse effects of ACE inhibitors are infrequent but may include hypotension, cough, syncope, hyperkalemia, and angioedema. Some of these may be avoided by slow titration and regular monitoring of blood pressure, electrolyte levels, and renal function.

Angiotensin-Converting Enzyme Receptor Blockers

Given the fact that ACE inhibitors have proved to be beneficial in reducing mortality in patients with CHF, it only stands to reason that ACE receptor blockers would be equally beneficial. In fact, several large clinical studies have shown this to be true. The Evaluation of Losartan In The Elderly (ELITE) trial compared losartan with captopril in 722 patients with CHF for 48 weeks.[17] The losartan group had fewer deaths and hospitalizations, as well as a 46% reduction in all-cause mortality. However, when the ELITE II trial, which was the ELITE trial extended for 2 additional years, was completed, no significant reduction in all-cause mortality was found.[18] The ELITE II trial, however, did show that ACE receptor blockers were better tolerated than ACE inhibitors. This trial also enrolled more than 3000 subjects.

The Optimal Trial in Myocardial Infarction with the Angiotensin II Antagonist Losartan (OPTIMAAL) demonstrated that losartan did not produce reduced mortality when compared with captopril, but the authors theorized that the poorer performance by losartan was due to the low dose used in the study.[19] The dose chosen for this study is the recommended starting dose for the treatment of hypertension and therefore is inadequate for patients with CHF. However, The Valsartan Heart Failure Trial demonstrated reduced mortality in patients who were either intolerant to or had never taken an ACE inhibitor, showing that these drugs are effective for patients with CHF.[20] Finally, in a recent meta-analysis investigators attempted to determine whether ACE receptor blockers reduced the number of deaths and hospitalizations among patients with CHF to a greater extent than ACE inhibitors.[21] This study failed to show any superiority of ACE blockers over ACE inhibitors but did echo the other studies in showing that an ACE blocker is more tolerable than an ACE inhibitor. However, the authors did discover that an ACE blocker given in combination with an ACE inhibitor was superior to use of the ACE inhibitor alone. Several large clinical trials are being carried out to determine whether ACE blockers have any superiority over the ACE inhibitors.

Nitrates

Nitrates reduce the myocardial oxygen requirement by dilating smooth muscle and increasing the volume of the venous vascular bed to reduce preload and ventricular filling pressure. For chronic heart failure, isosorbide dinitrate or mononitrate may be given orally, and isosorbide in either form is especially useful for patients who cannot tolerate ACE inhibitors because of hypotension or ensuing renal failure.[4,22,23]

Spironolactone

Aldosterone release is elevated in CHF, promoting Na^+ retention, K^+ loss, sympathetic activation, myocardial and vascular fibrosis, and diminished vascular compliance.[4] Spironolactone is a K^+-sparing diuretic that blocks the aldosterone receptor.[24] It is currently being recommended for use in NYHA class IV CHF, but only if renal function is preserved. In the Randomized Aldactone Evaluation Study (RALES), roughly 1600 patients with moderate to severe heart failure were examined to determine whether spironolactone added to the regimen of an ACE inhibitor and a loop diuretic with or without digitalis prolongs life. This study was discontinued early after only 24 months because of the overwhelmingly significant benefit seen with spironolactone in terms of reducing the numbers of deaths and hospitalizations among patients with CHF.[25] Low-dose spironolactone, given along with an ACE inhibitor, has been shown to be beneficial for patients with CHF and moderate to severe impairment. It is theorized that the ACE inhibitors do not depress aldosterone levels, which are elevated in heart failure, so that the actions of spironolactone are needed to alter further the neurohumoral mechanism involved in this disease. Aldosterone antagonists are also believed to play a role in vessel wall and myocardial remodeling.[26] However, because these drugs are K^+ sparing, the patients must be monitored for hyperkalemia and renal function. Additionally, aldosterone blockade has been shown to reduce vascular collagen turnover and significantly decreases the early morning rise in heart rate seen in heart failure.[27,28] Further studies are necessary to validate spironolactone's use in CHF and substantiate its regular use.

Management of Decompensated CHF

Traditionally, β-agonists, such as dobutamine, have been used to treat decompensated CHF. Although these agents are effective for improving hemodynamics and decreasing some of the symptoms associated with CHF through β receptor activation, improvement tends to be short term. Increasing β activation leads to increased cardiac workload; and ultimately, symptomatic left ventricular dysfunction

returns.[29] In addition, frequent arrhythmias and tachycardia, which can be fatal, are side effects of this treatment. Many patients become dependent on intravenous inotropic infusions despite many weaning attempts.[7] Dependence is recognized by symptomatic hypotension, recurrent congestive symptoms, and worsening renal status shortly after the inotropic therapy is discontinued. If possible, the patient is sent home, and continuous inotropic therapy is used as a bridge to the use of a left ventricular assist device, to transplantation, or to the end of life.[30]

Human B-type natriuretic peptide is a cardiac hormone that is secreted by the ventricular myocardium in response to fluid overload in CHF and offers a new therapeutic approach to decompensated failure.[29] This hormone produces cardiac vasodilation and natriuresis. It is now available as a member of a new drug classification, natriuretic peptides, and is named *nesiritide*. Nesiritide reduces preload and afterload and increases cardiac output without increasing heart rate, unlike the traditional drugs for acute decompensated failure. In addition, this drug improves the glomerular filtration rate and has a sympatholytic cardiac effect. Its big advantage over the β-agonists is that nesiritide reduces ventricular ectopy. It significantly reduced the number of ventricular tachycardic events and premature ventricular beats in a 24-hour period when compared with dobutamine.[29,31,32]

Other drugs useful for decompensated heart failure include a loop diuretic such as intravenous furosemide, which produces rapid diuresis; sublingual nitroglycerin; and oxygen in high concentrations.[2] Morphine can also be used to help relieve shortness of breath, anxiety, and pain.[33] Morphine also has a significant venodilator effect, which is helpful in reducing venous return. The patient may improve once excess fluid is removed and the β-blocker and ACE inhibitor can be restarted. See Figure 8.3 to review the pharmacological management of CHF and at what stage in the disease these drugs are introduced.

New Staging in Heart Failure and Pharmacological Intervention

The NYHA Classification has been primarily used to describe the functional limitations experienced by patients with heart failure. However, as mentioned

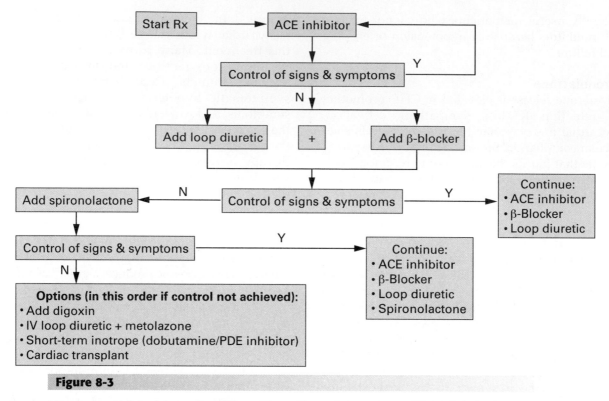

Figure 8-3

Management of chronic cardiac failure. *N*, no; *Y*, yes; *Rx*, treatment; *PDE*, phosphodiesterase. (From Bennett PN, Brown MJ, eds. *Clinical Pharmacology.* 9th ed. New York: Churchill Livingstone; 2003. Reproduced with permission from *Lancet*.)

earlier, this system does not take into consideration structural abnormalities or the risk of developing clinical heart failure. The ACC, in conjunction with the AHA, describes a new approach to classifying CHF and its therapy.[34] The ACC/AHA staging system is to be used as a complement to the NYHA classification system. It is shaped like a pyramid with stage A at the bottom (Figure 8-4). Stage A identifies the patient who is at high risk for heart failure but has no structural abnormalities or symptoms. The primary treatments at this stage are ACE inhibitors and lifestyle changes. Stage B represents the patient with a structural abnormality who has no symptoms of heart failure. The patient may, however, have left ventricular hypertrophy or a low ejection fraction. ACE inhibitors and β-blockers are the cornerstones of treatment in this phase. Patients in stage C present with symptoms of heart failure and/or a structural abnormality. Again, ACE inhibitors and β-blockers are the treatment choices, but diuretics and cardiac glycosides are used to prevent fluid congestion. Therapy with spironolactone is also initiated for patients with advanced symptoms. Nonpharmacological therapy, such as use of implantable defibrillators, may also be instituted at this time if the need arises. Patients in stage D of this classification system have CHF that is refractory to standard therapy and require intravenous administration of inotropes or nesiritide, mechanical assistance, or transplantation.

DRUG TREATMENT FOR CARDIAC ARRHYTHMIA

Arrhythmias are a result of abnormal electrical events that occur in the heart as a result of ischemia, hypoxia, excessive myocardial fiber stretch, excessive discharge or sensitivity to catecholamines, scarred

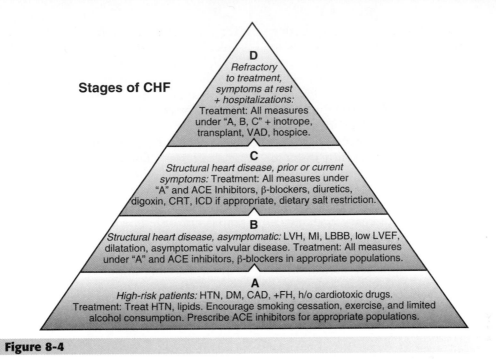

Stages of CHF

D
Refractory to treatment, symptoms at rest + hospitalizations: Treatment: All measures under "A, B, C" + inotrope, transplant, VAD, hospice.

C
Structural heart disease, prior or current symptoms: Treatment: All measures under "A" and ACE Inhibitors, β-blockers, diuretics, digoxin, CRT, ICD if appropriate, dietary salt restriction.

B
Structural heart disease, asymptomatic: LVH, MI, LBBB, low LVEF, dilatation, asymptomatic valvular disease. Treatment: All measures under "A" and ACE inhibitors, β-blockers in appropriate populations.

A
High-risk patients: HTN, DM, CAD, +FH, h/o cardiotoxic drugs. Treatment: Treat HTN, lipids. Encourage smoking cessation, exercise, and limited alcohol consumption. Prescribe ACE inhibitors for appropriate populations.

Figure 8-4

Heart failure staging pyramid. *HTN,* Hypertension; *DM,* diabetes mellitus; *CAD,* coronary artery disease; *FH,* family history; *ACE,* angiotensin-converting enzyme; *LVH,* left ventricular hypertrophy; *MI,* myocardial infarction; *LBBB,* left bundle branch block; *LVEF,* left ventricular ejection fraction; *CRT,* cardiac resynchronization therapy; *ICD,* implantable cardioverter-defibrillator; *VAD,* ventricular assist device. (Redrawn from Brozena SC, Jessup M. The new staging system for heart failure: what every primary care physician should know. *Geriatrics.* 2003;58[6]:31-36. Prepared for *Geriatrics* by Susan C Brozena, MD, FACC, and Mariell Jessup, MD, FACC.)

tissue, drug toxicity, or electrolyte imbalance.[22,35] Most arrhythmias result from disturbances in either impulse formation or impulse conduction. To understand these rhythm disturbances and how drug therapy suppresses them, we must review normal cardiac electrophysiology.

Contractility and its coordination throughout the heart are achieved by a specialized conduction system. Sinus rhythm begins with impulses originating in the sinoatrial (SA) node and conducted through the atria, the atrioventricular (AV) node, bundle of His, Purkinje fibers, and finally to the ventricles. Cardiac cells and muscle are electrically sensitive because of various voltage-gated plasma membrane channels in which ions—including Na^+, K^+ and Ca^{+2} ions—travel to control the electrical potential.[2]

Ventricular and atrial cell membranes maintain a resting membrane potential between –85 and –90 mV as a result of an unequal distribution of electrolytes (high concentration of K^+ inside the cell compared with outside the cell).[36] This gradient is maintained by the Na^+/K^+-ATPase pump, which moves three Na^+ ions outward in exchange for two K^+ ions inward. An action potential is generated when voltage-gated Na^+ channels open and entering ions depolarize the cell. This channel is referred to as the fast inward Na^+ current (I_{Na+}). If the Na^+ channel remains open for more than a few milliseconds, the channel will inactivate, and a second action potential cannot occur. This is called the *effective refractory period.* The hyperpolarizing phase of the action potential begins with the opening of different types of K^+ channels, which carry these ions in an outward direction. The slow inward Ca^{2+} current (I_{SI}) is responsible for the plateau phase of the action potential. Calcium enters the cell, balancing an outward K^+ current.

At the SA and AV nodal tissue, the resting membrane potential is more positive and tends to be unstable.[36] This instability produces firing of the SA node at a rate that is faster than in any other region of the heart. The SA nodal action potential is conducted rapidly through the atria but then delayed at the AV node because of dependence on a slow inward Ca^{2+} channel. Once the action potential enters the ventricle, it is conducted rapidly through the bundle of His, Purkinje fibers, and then ultimately through the entire ventricular mass.

Ventricular and SA node action potentials are different in shape owing to the different ion channels that produce them.[22] For the typical ventricular cell, the cardiac phases are as follows:

Phase 0 is the period of rapid depolarization in which there is a rapid influx of Na^+ ions. It occurs when the membrane potential reaches its critical firing threshold (approximately –60 mV). The inward Na^+ current becomes large enough to produce an all-or-nothing depolarization. The channel then inactivates and is closed during the plateau phase.

Phase 1 is early, brief repolarization, triggered by an outward flow of K^+ ions and Na^+ channel inactivation.

Phase 2 is the plateau phase in which the K^+ current is balanced by a slow inward Ca^{2+} flux. This K^+ current is actually a specialized current known as an inward rectifier, which means that K^+ conductance falls as the membrane becomes more depolarized. Therefore there is too little outward K^+ current to bring the potential down to resting. Thus inward Ca^{2+} current largely maintains the plateau at this point.

Ca^{2+} channels behave like Na^+ channels, but in terms of activation and inactivation, they have a slower time course.

Phase 3 is referred to as repolarization. At this point, the Ca^{2+} channels close, and the cell repolarizes as another K^+ channel opens and the ions flow out.

Phase 4 is the resting phase, but for the SA node, this phase is called *diastolic depolarization*. In the SA node, several types of ion channels open to bring the membrane potential to threshold to trigger the full action potential. This potential change is largely produced by increasing inward Ca^{2+} currents (from L-type and T-type calcium channels) during diastole. In addition, the SA node has greater susceptibility to Na^+ during this phase, even though it lacks the fast Na^+ current that characterizes phase 0 on the atrial or ventricular myocytes. Figure 8-5 shows the configuration of the action potential in different areas of the heart.

In the interval between phase 0 and the end of phase 2, the depolarizing channels become inactivated. This is also known as the absolute refractory period because the cell is unable to produce another action potential.[36] However, during phase 3, a high amplitude stimulus may open enough Na^+ channels to produce another action potential, overcoming the K^+ outward current. Thus this phase is known as the relative refractory period. The conduction of an electrical impulse is quite rapid but orderly, except in the case of disease. A localized ischemic area or tissue that has experienced a previous myocardial infarction may slow or interrupt a traveling impulse. For example, an impulse conducting down a Purkinje fiber may spread to an adjacent fiber that has failed to transmit and instead pass up it in a reverse direction. If this retrograde conduction should excite the original tissue that already transmitted the impulse, a reentrant excitation occurs.

Mechanism for Arrhythmia

Abnormal impulse generation is responsible for many arrhythmias. This may be due to an enhanced normal automatic rhythm (nodal tachycardia) or an "abnormal automaticity."[23,36,37] The pacemaker (SA) rate may be altered by shortening diastolic depolarization (increasing the slope of phase 4) through catecholamine stimulation. In addition, raising the resting diastolic potential (making it more positive) or making the threshold potential more negative will produce similar results, that is, trigger an action potential sooner. Likewise, slowing heart rate can be achieved by vagus nerve stimulation reversing the values just mentioned.

The SA node has the highest rate of spontaneous discharge (70 beats/min) and therefore controls the heart rate. If the SA node fails to initiate an electrical impulse, then the heart tissue with the next fastest rate takes over.[37] This is often the AV node, which can initiate an impulse 45 times per minute. Next in line is the His-Purkinje system at 25 discharges per minute.

Abnormal automaticity occurs when an ectopic focus develops (usually in the Purkinje fibers) that presents with a faster rate than the SA node or other potential pacemaker. This is known as ectopic pacemaker activity. This type of activity can also lead

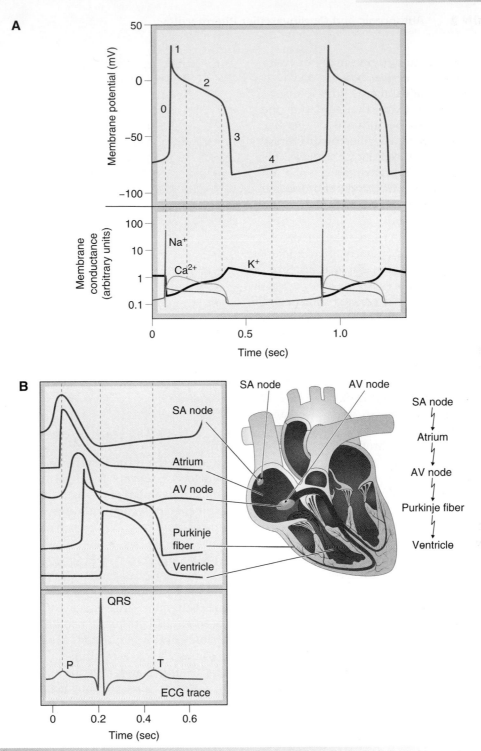

Figure 8-5

The cardiac action potential. **A,** Phases of the action potential: 0, rapid depolarization; 1, partial repolarization; 2, plateau; 3, repolarization; 4, pacemaker depolarization. The lower panel shows the accompanying changes in membrane conductance for Na^+, K^+, and Ca^{2+}.
B, Conduction of the impulse through the heart, with the corresponding electrocardiogram (ECG) trace. Note that the longest delay occurs at the atrioventricular (AV) node, where the action potential has a characteristically slow waveform. (From Rang HP, Dale MM, Ritter JM, Moore JL. *Pharmacology.* 5th ed. New York: Churchill Livingstone; 2003. **A** modified from Nobel D. *The initiation of the heart beat.* Oxford, UK: Oxford University Press; 1975.)

to another phenomenon underlying many arrhythmias called *delayed after-depolarization.*[22] Delayed afterdepolarizations occur in phase 4 in response to excess calcium release from the sarcoplasmic reticulum. They can also be induced by cardiac glycosides, norepinephrine, or phosphodiesterase inhibitors that increase intracellular Ca^{2+} levels. It is thought that excess calcium activates Na^+-Ca^{2+} exchange, which brings one Ca^{2+} ion out of the cell in exchange for transfer of three Na^+ ions into the cell, producing depolarization.

Abnormal automaticity may also be produced by early after-depolarizations.[22] Early afterdepolarizations occur during phase 2 or 3 and result from bradycardia or drugs that prolong the action potential. They may involve decreased conduction through one of the K^+ channels.

Abnormal impulse conduction refers to heart block or circus reentry movements.[22] The most common site for heart block is the AV node. First-degree block refers to slowing of the impulse through the node. Second-degree block occurs when not all the impulses from the SA node are transmitted to the ventricles, and third-degree block is when there is complete block through the AV node. In third-degree block the atria and ventricles beat independently of each other, with the ventricles beating at their intrinsically slower rate or at a rate determined by whatever pacemaker activates distal to the block.

Reentry rhythm underlies a variety of arrhythmias, and depending on the site of the reentrant circuit, can affect the atria, ventricles, or nodal tissues.[22] Basically, the reentry circuit describes a situation in which there is a partial conduction block. Normally, an impulse traveling around a ring of tissue will conduct in both directions, and the two impulses will extinguish themselves when they meet. However, if the area has ischemic damage, enough so that one impulse is blocked but the second can get through, a continuous circle of activity can occur. This is known as circus movement and occurs with a unidirectional block. Essentially, the impulse re-excites tissues that have just passed through their refractory period, but it does this over and over again (Figure 8-6). Wolff-Parkinson-White syndrome is an anatomical anomaly that consists of a ring of tissue linking the atria and ventricles, which is often a location for circus reentry arrhythmias. Treatment for this condition is directed at converting a unidirectional block into a bidirectional block or at

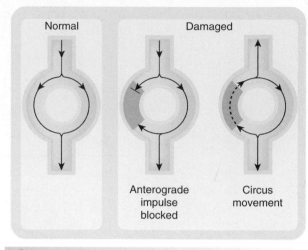

Figure 8-6

Generation of a reentrant rhythm by a damaged area of myocardium. The damaged area (dark) conducts in one direction only. This disturbs the normal pattern of conduction and permits continuous circulation of the impulse to occur. (From Rang HP, Dale MM, Ritter JM, Moore JL. *Pharmacology.* 5th ed. New York: Churchill Livingstone; 2003.)

extending the refractory period. Difficulty in treatment occurs because different components of the circus movement are mediated by different ion channel activity, necessitating use of more than one type of drug.[38]

Classification of Antiarrhythmic Drugs

The Vaughan-Williams classification system proposed in 1970 offers a useful way to discuss the various antidysrhythmic drugs.[39,40] This system classifies drugs according to their electrophysiological effects and the phase of the cardiac cycle they affect. There are four classes of drugs: class I (drugs that block Na^+ channels); class II (β-blockers); class III (drugs that prolong the cardiac action potential); and class IV (Ca^{+2} blockers).

Class I Drugs

Class I drugs act by blocking Na^+ channels, slowing the rate of rise of phase 0.[40] These drugs are also referred to as membrane-stabilizing agents. They are considered "use-dependent blockers," meaning that they bind more rapidly to open channels to block rapidly firing cells, rather than to fully repolarized channels. Thus they do not affect resting membrane potential. Class I drugs are further divided according to the duration of their effect on the action potential.[41] Class Ia drugs produce a moderate slowing of the action potential (adjunctive class III action) by blocking K^+ currents, prolonging the effective refractory period. Examples of class Ia drugs include quinidine, disopyramide, and procainamide. Quinidine is the prototypic class Ia drug.[2] In addition to its class Ia activity, quinidine has a positive inotropic effect (through a lengthening of ventricular systole) and an antimuscarinic effect. These agents are effective in suppressing premature ventricular beats, recurrent ventricular tachycardia, and reentry arrhythmias. Because it slows conduction, quinidine can block reentry by converting a unidirectional block to a bidirectional block. Adverse drug reactions include nausea, vomiting, and diarrhea. Larger doses may cause cinchonism (headache, vertigo, tinnitus, blurred vision, and disorientation). Perhaps most worrisome is that this drug and many other antiarrhythmics may exacerbate arrhythmias. Quinidine may cause not only SA and AV block but also sinus tachycardia. It is difficult to predict whether this drug will have a beneficial effect or a negative effect. Problems with this drug most definitely occur if hypokalemia is present.

Class Ib drugs block Na^+ channels minimally, slowing depolarization but also decreasing the action potential duration by shortening the refractory period and suppressing conduction.[41] Class Ib agents include lidocaine and the oral agents mexiletine and tocainide. As with class Ia drugs, use of these drugs is decreasing, although they are still used to inhibit ventricular tachycardia. Adverse effects occur primarily in the central nervous system and include drowsiness, slurred speech, paresthesias, confusion, and convulsions as the dose increases.

Class Ic drugs markedly slow phase 0 depolarization, even in healthy tissue, so conduction is slowed in all cardiac tissue, producing a prolonged depressant effect on conduction velocity and a wide QRS complex.[42] Flecainide and propafenone are class Ic agents. They are approved for treatment of refractory ventricular arrhythmias. Common adverse effects include dizziness, blurred vision, and headaches. Syncope can occur and is indicative of the proarrhythmic effects that these drugs have. Flecainide can induce life-threatening ventricular tachycardia and lead to death.[43]

Class II Drugs

Class II antiarrhythmic drugs include the β-adrenergic antagonists. These drugs depress sinus node automaticity and prolong AV nodal conduction. They are useful in treating atrial flutter and fibrillation and can also stop reentry. These are also excellent drugs for treating arrhythmias associated with exercise or any arrhythmia provoked by increased sympathetic activity.[44] The agents most commonly used for their antidysrhythmic effects include propranolol, acebutolol, and esmolol. Esmolol is a short-acting $β_1$-selective blocker used solely for the treatment of arrhythmias.[41] It is given intravenously and has a very short half-life (9 minutes), which allows it to be titrated rapidly against response.

Class III Drugs

Class III antiarrhythmic drugs prolong repolarization and the effective refractory period by blocking K^+ channels. They are considered to be the most effective antidysrhythmic agents. Amiodarone is used for the prevention and treatment of life-threatening atrial and ventricular arrhythmias. It also has some Na^+ and Ca^{2+} channel blocking abilities and binds β receptors noncompetitively. However, its usefulness is limited by its adverse effects. The list of side effects includes interstitial pulmonary fibrosis, gastrointestinal problems, blurred vision, ataxia, dizziness, liver toxicity, neuropathy, and bluish discoloration on exposed areas of the skin. Some of these may occur after only short-term use but will disappear when the drug is withdrawn. However, because of its long half-life, several months may be needed for the drug to completely clear from the body. In terms of its cardiovascular adverse effects, amiodarone may cause bradycardia, heart block, and ventricular arrhythmias. The proarrhythmic effects of the class III drugs are particularly more prevalent in the hypertrophied heart.[45] In addition, the risk of developing life-threatening arrhythmias appears to be greater within the first few days of dosing. Some physicians propose a 72-hour hospitalization when administration of these drugs is initiated to monitor patients for electrical changes.[46]

Another class III drug is sotalol.[41] This is actually a β-blocker, but it prolongs the action potential by delaying the outward K^+ current. It is not as effective as amiodarone in preventing ventricular arrhythmias but lacks some of its side effects.

Ibutilide and dofetilide are additional class III drugs that have recently been released.[41]

Class IV Drugs

Class IV drugs include the Ca^{2+} channel blockers.[2] These drugs inhibit Ca^{2+} transport through the membrane channels, resulting in depression of contractility, and in the pacemaker cells, suppression of automatic activity. Verapamil and diltiazem are most commonly used for supraventricular tachycardia and atrial fibrillation. They decrease the SA nodal rate and AV nodal conduction.

Other Antiarrhythmics

Adenosine is another antiarrhythmic agent, but it does not fall within the Vaughan-Williams classification system. It stimulates adenosine receptors in the SA and AV node, which ultimately open K^+ channels. Reentry movement is terminated by hyperpolarization and a decrease in action potential duration. Intravenous adenosine is used to stop supraventricular tachycardia. Adverse effects include bronchospasm and hypotension, which are usually not very serious because of adenosine's extremely short half-life (seconds) and the fact that this drug is not negatively inotropic like verapamil.[47]

The last antiarrhythmic to discuss is digitalis. This drug is primarily used in the treatment of CHF but is also used to control or slow ventricular rate in a supraventricular tachycardia by prolonging the AV refractory period and also by producing a parasympathomimetic effect. It loses its effectiveness during exercise as the body shifts toward more sympathetic control of heart function, so it is reserved for patients who are more sedentary.[41]

Therapeutic Concerns with Antiarrhythmic Agents

The presence of side effects such as faintness, dizziness, or visual disturbances may indicate toxic drug effects from the antiarrhythmics or additional arrhythmias. All antiarrhythmic drugs can also produce arrhythmias, and efficacy in suppressing arrhythmias is only between 30% and 60%.[48] In addition, with the exception of amiodarone, no single antiarrhythmic agent shows superiority. Proarrhythmic effects are most likely to be seen with the drugs that prolong the QT interval (i.e., the action potential) on an electrocardiogram (ECG).[49] Hypokalemia, in particular, enhances the risk.

Arrhythmias may only be detected by monitoring with an ECG. If an ECG is not available, palpation of pulses for rate and regularity may detect rhythm disturbances.

Little information is available on how these drugs affect short- and long-term–duration exercise and how exercise affects arrhythmias.[44] Many antiarrhythmics have negative inotropic effects and therefore should impair exercise performance. Exercise may also increase rhythm disturbances as a result of an increase in circulating catecholamines and render the drugs ineffective during these periods.[41] Patients are cautioned to watch for the signs of these disturbances and are also instructed not to stop exercising abruptly because this can facilitate an irregular rhythm.[50]

Treatment for Some Specific Arrhythmias

Although treatment of irregular rhythm is challenging, some effective protocols have been outlined for specific arrhythmias. Drugs, pacemakers, implantable defibrillators, and surgery may be used separately or in combination to treat a variety of arrhythmias.

Atrial Fibrillation

Atrial fibrillation is one of the most common cardiac arrhythmias.[51] It is defined as an "erratic quivering or twitching" of the atrial muscle caused by multiple ectopic atrial foci or a rapidly circulating circus movement.[52,53] There are no true P waves because the ectopic foci do not actually depolarize the atria. The AV node tends to control the impulses that produce a ventricular response; however, the ventricular rate can still be normal, slow, or very fast, and usually the QRS complex has an irregular rhythm. In patients who have a ventricular response rate lower than 100 beats/min, cardiac output is not affected. However, if the patient exercises or if the ventricular rate is greater than 100 beats/min at rest, then cardiac output is diminished and signs of heart failure may occur. Another problem with atrial fibrillation is the development of atrial thrombus caused by coagulation of blood within the atria, leading to an embolus, and ultimately, a stroke.[2]

There are several pharmacological approaches to the management of atrial fibrillation. If the ventricular response rate is normal or slightly slowed, no pharmacological management may be indicated. However, if the ventricular response rate is fast, treatment must be directed at first toward control of this rate. Intravenous verapamil or diltiazem will produce a drop in ventricular rate within minutes. Diltiazem is preferred in patients with CHF. β-Blockers can also be used to control ventricular rate. In fact, these are the drugs of choice when there are accessory electrical pathways that may become activated if the Ca^{2+} channel blockers produce a maximum slowing of AV nodal conduction.[41] In addition, they are very effective agents in thyrotoxicosis and in postoperative cardiac surgery. Esmolol is available for intravenous use, and oral β-blockers (atenolol and metoprolol) can be used for long-term rate control.[53,54]

Until recently, there had been controversy over the primary initial approach to atrial fibrillation—rate control or rhythm control.[55] However, two large studies have shown no difference in morbidity or symptoms between the two strategies.[56,57] This widens the treatment approach because trying to control rhythm with larger and larger doses of antiarrhythmic agents that have a poor benefit/risk ratio is not desirable if rate can be controlled with a safer drug.[58]

If there is only a short history of atrial fibrillation and the heart is not enlarged, the patient may benefit from cardioversion and rhythm control. Electrical conversion is the choice if treatment is urgent, or the patient can be given amiodarone for conversion in hours to days. If rhythm control can be delayed safely for a month, anticoagulation therapy with warfarin is recommended. However, long-term treatment with warfarin is considered mandatory to prevent embolic events in patients who have no contraindications to anticoagulation therapy such as history of falls or gastrointestinal bleeding or a high risk for hemorrhage.[59-61] New approaches with the antiplatelet drugs are currently being explored for efficacy in reducing embolic events in these patients.

For maintaining sinus rhythm over time, class Ia and Ic agents have been found to be helpful; however, amiodarone might still be the most effective drug.[41] For patients in whom sinus rhythm cannot be achieved with drugs, other therapies such as AV node ablation and pacemaker implantation or other implantable device–based therapy (implantable defibrillators with antitachycardia pacing) may be helpful.[62]

Atrial Flutter

Atrial flutter is a rapid series of atrial depolarizations caused by a single ectopic focus in the atria.[52] This focus depolarizes at a rate of 250 to 350 times per minute. Because the firing rate is so rapid, the P waves are called *flutter waves* and have a characteristic "sawtooth" pattern. On an ECG, the QRS complex is usually normal, but there is more than one P wave for every QRS complex. The AV node is able to block some of the impulses from the atria and helps prevent the ventricle from contracting too rapidly, so that cardiac output is not usually affected.

First-line therapy for patients with atrial flutter is radiofrequency ablation.[63] This arrhythmia responds well to this treatment because it involves a single reentrant circuit. If the patient is not a candidate for ablation, then class Ic and class III drugs are indicated.[64]

Atrioventricular Block

First-degree heart block rarely requires treatment, but any higher degree of block should be treated with intravenous atropine. This may be followed by electrical cardiac pacing. The β-agonist isoproterenol may also be given, but there is an increased risk of producing ectopic beats.[2] A permanent electrical pacemaker is usually indicated.

Junctional (Nodal) Tachycardias

Junctional tachycardias may arise from reentry circuits within the AV node.[52] Cessation of the arrhythmia can be achieved with either vagal maneuvers, such as carotid sinus massage, or adenosine. Other drugs that are effective include β-blockers, diltiazem, and verapamil. However, care must be taken to prevent AV block in cases in which there is an accessory AV pathway. Junctional tachycardias through an accessory pathway may respond well to flecainide, sotalol, or amiodarone.[2] Radiofrequency ablation is also being increasingly used for the arrhythmia.

Ventricular Tachycardia

Ventricular tachycardia is a series of premature ventricular contractions in a row.[52] It results from rapid firing by a single ventricular focus. P waves tend to be absent, and the QRS complexes are wide and bizarre. Ventricular rate is between 100 and 250 beats/min. This condition is often associated with ischemic heart disease but can also result from drugs that prolong the QT interval. Treatment consists of immediate injection with class I drugs, such as lidocaine or procainamide, or defibrillation. For recurrent ventricular tachycardia, amiodarone or sotalol may be chosen.

Torsades de pointes is a specialized form of ventricular tachycardia resulting from antiarrhythmic agents at a toxic level.[52] It is associated with a prolonged QT interval (greater than 0.5 seconds) and presents with a twisting configuration. Cardiac output is severely affected, and this rhythm either converts to ventricular fibrillation or terminates spontaneously.

Ventricular Fibrillation

Ventricular fibrillation is the most prevalent arrhythmia in acute cardiac arrest.[2] It presents as an irregular quivering of the ventricular muscle, resulting in severely diminished cardiac output. Treatment is defibrillation, followed by cardiopulmonary resuscitation. For recurrent fibrillation, suppression with sotalol or amiodarone with a β-blocker is suggested. An implantable cardioverter-defibrillator is also recommended.

ACTIVITIES 8

■ 1. AP is a 78-year-old woman who presents with a 1-week history of progressive shortness of breath (SOB). She reports the need to sleep on three pillows to breathe comfortably through the night. She also reports a 15-lb weight gain within the last month. The SOB has worsened considerably in the last 2 days so that she is unable to ambulate more than 10 feet without resting.

Medical History
CHF × 3 years, coronary artery disease (CAD) × 10 years, inferior wall myocardial infarction (MI) 1 year ago, type II diabetes × 20 years, degenerative joint disease (DJD) × 10 years

Social History
The patient lives alone. She uses a walker to ambulate throughout her house but requires a wheelchair for most outside excursions. Her daughter lives 1 hour away but visits her weekly to help with the shopping.

Medications
Lisinopril, furosemide, verapamil, warfarin, nitro patch, sublingual nitro, ibuprofen, glipizide (decreases blood glucose level in type II diabetics)

Physical Exam
Vital signs: blood pressure (BP), 135/88 mm Hg, pulse, 110 beats/min; respiratory rate (RR) 28 breaths/min; Weight, 190 lb

Neck
Mild jugular venous distension (JVD), no lymphadenopathy

Cardiac
Irregular rhythm, systolic murmur

Lungs
Crackles and wheezes noted

Extremities
Pedal edema, pedal pulses 1+ bilaterally, extremities cold to touch

Neurological Findings
Within normal limits (WNL)

Labs
Na^+ 129 mEq/L, K^+ 4.7 mEq/L, chloride 101 mEq/L, $Paco_2$ 47 mm Hg, blood urea nitrogen (BUN) 53 mg/dL, serum creatinine 2.3 mg/dL, glucose 130 mg/dL, hemoglobin 10.0 g/dL, platelets 259,000/mm³, white blood cell (WBC) count 8800/mm³, international normalized ratio (INR) 3.5

Chest X-Ray
Mild pulmonary edema and cardiomegaly

ECG
No acute ST or T wave changes

Questions

a. What signs and symptoms indicate the presence or severity of the patient's condition?

b. Could any of these problems have been caused by drug therapy?

c. What do you think is her diagnosis?

d. Would you recommend a medication change? If yes, what would you suggest and what information should be provided to the patient about her new meds?

e. Are there any physical therapy interventions to reduce this patient's dependence on medications?

■ 2. Interview a patient with CHF. Use the following questions to assess how much the patient understands about his/her condition, the medications, and his/her ability to determine when the condition is worsening.

Questions for patient

a. Do you know when your heart failure began?

b. What medications are you taking and what are they used for?

c. Do you know what side effects these drugs produce and can you differentiate between the adverse drug effects and the symptoms of heart failure?

d. How do you monitor your symptoms of heart failure and what do you do to help manage them?

Questions

a. If you were seeing this patient in the home care setting, how would you determine whether this patient's medical condition is worsening?

b. What suggestions do you have regarding how to improve this patient's understanding of CHF, as well as his/her condition?

References

1. Curtis MJ, Pugsley MK. Drugs and the cardiovascular system. In: Page C, Curtis MJ, Sutter MC, Walker MJ, Hoffman BB, eds. *Integrated Pharmacology*. 2nd ed. Philadelphia: Mosby; 2002:361-414.

2. Waller DG, Renwick AG, Hillier K. *Medical Pharmacology and Therapeutics*. New York: WB Saunders; 2001.

3. Baker DW, Chin MI I, Cinquegirani MP, et al. ACC/AHA guidelines for the evaluation and management of chronic heart failure in the adult: executive summary. *J Am Coll Card.* 2001;38(7):2101-2113.

4. DiBianco R. Update on therapy for heart failure. *Am J Med.* 2003;115:480-488.

5. Lonn E, McKelvie R. Drug treatment in heart failure. *BMJ.* 2000;320(7243):1188-1192.

6. The Digitalis Investigators Group I. The effect of digoxin on mortality and morbidity in patients with heart failure. *N Engl J Med.* 1997;336:525-533.

7. Stevenson LW. Clinical use of inotropic therapy for heart failure: looking backward or forward? Part II: chronic inotropic therapy. *Circulation.* 2003;108(4):492-497.

8. Stromberg A. Educating nurses and patients to manage heart failure. *Eur J Cardiovasc Nurs.* 2002;1:33-40.

9. CIBIS-II Investigators and Committees. The cardiac insufficiency bisoprolol study II (CIBIS-II): a randomised trial. *Lancet.* 1999;353:9-13.

10. Waagstein F, Stromblad O, Andersson B, et al. Increased exercise ejection fraction and reversed remodeling after long-term treatment with metoprolol in congestive heart failure: a randomized, stratified, double-blind, placebo-controlled trial in mild to moderate heart failure due to ischemic or idiopathic dilated cardiomyopathy. *Eur J Heart Fail.* 2003;5(5):679-691.

11. Palazzuoli A, Bruni F, Puccdetti M, Pastorelli P, Angori AL, Auteri A. Effects of carvedilol on left ventricular remodeling and systolic function in elderly patients with heart failure. *Eur J Heart Fail.* 2002; 4(6):765-770.

12. Bouzamondo A, Hulot JS, Sanchez P, Lechat P. Beta-blocker benefit according to severity of heart failure. *Eur J Heart Fail.* 2003;5(3):281-289.

13. Garg R, Yusuf S. Overview of randomized trials of angiotensin-converting enzyme inhibitors on mortality and morbidity in patients with heart failure. *JAMA.* 1995;273:1450-1456.

14. Flather MD, Yusuf S, Kober L, et al. Long-term ACE-inhibitor therapy in patients with heart failure or left-ventricular dysfunction: a systematic overview of data from individual patients. *Lancet.* 2000;355:1575-1581.

15. The CONSENSUS Trial Study Group. Effects of enalapril on mortality in severe congestive heart failure: results of the cooperative north Scandinavian Enalapril Survival Study (CONSENSUS). *N Engl J Med.* 1986;314: 1547-1552.

16. Ball S. Should all patients with heart failure now receive an ACE inhibitor? *Eur J Heart Fail.* 2001;3(6): 635-636.

17. Pitt B, Segal R, Martinez EA, et al. Randomised trial of losartan versus captopril in patients over 65 with heart failure (Evaluation of Losartan in the Elderly Study, ELITE). *Lancet.* 1997;349:747-752.

18. Pitt B, Poole-Wilson PA, Segal R, et al. Effect of losartan compared with captopril on mortality in patients with symptomatic heart failure: randomised trial: The Losartan Heart Failure Survival Study ELITE II. *Lancet.* 2000;355:1582-1587.

19. Dickstein K, Kjekshus J. Effects of losartan and captopril on mortality and morbidity in high-risk patients after acute myocardial infarction: The OPTIMAAL randomised trial. Optimal Trial in Myocardial Infarction with Angiotensin II Antagonist Losartan. *Lancet.* 2002; 360:752-760.

20. Maggioni AP, Anand I, Gottlieb SO, Latini R, Tognoni G, Cohn JN. Effects of valsartan on morbidity and mortality in patients with heart failure not receiving angiotensin-converting enzyme inhibitors. *J Am Coll Cardiol.* 2002; 40:1414-1421.

21. Jong P, Demers C, McKelvie RS, Liu PP. Angiotensin receptor blockers in heart failure: meta-analysis of randomized controlled trials. *J Am Coll Cardiol.* 2002; 39(3):463-470.

22. Rang HP, Dale MM, Ritter JM, Moore JL. *Pharmacology.* 5th ed. New York: Churchill Livingstone; 2003.

23. Bennett PN, Brown MJ. General pharmacology. In: Bennett PN, Brown MJ, eds. *Clinical Pharmacology.* 9th ed. New York: Churchill Livingstone; 2003:37-40.

24. Spironolactone for heart failure. *Med Lett Drugs Ther.* 1999; 41(1061):81-82.

25. The RALES Investigators. Effectiveness of spironolactone added to an angiotensin-converting enzyme inhibitor and a loop diuretic for severe chronic congestive heart failure (the Randomized Aldactone Evaluation Study [RALES]). *Am J Cardiol.* 1996;78:902-907.

26. Rajagopalan S, Pitt B. Aldosterone antagonists in the treatment of hypertension and target organ damage. *Curr Hypertens Rep.* 2001;3(3):240-248.

27. MacFadyen RJ, Barr CS, Struthers AD. Aldosterone blockade reduces vascular collagen turnover, improves heart rate variability and reduces early morning rise in heart rate in heart failure patients. *Cardiovasc Res.* 1997; 35(1):30-34.

28. Pitt B. Do diuretics and aldosterone receptor antagonists improve ventricular remodeling? *J Cardiac Fail.* 2002; 8(suppl 6):S491-S493.

29. Burger AJ, Horton DP, LeJemtel T, et al. Effect of nesiritide (B-type natriuretic peptide) and dobutamine on ventricular arrhythmias in the treatment of patients with acutely decompensated congestive heart failure: The PRECEDENT study. *Am Heart J.* 2002;144:1102-1108.

30. Hon JK, Yacoub MH. Bridge to recovery with the use of left ventricular assist device and clenbuterol. Ann Thorac Surg. 2003;75:S36-S41.

31. Burger AJ, Elkayam U, Neibaur MT. Comparison of the occurrence of ventricular arrhythmias in patients with acutely decompensated congestive heart failure receiving dobutamine versus nesiritide therapy. *Am J Cardiol.* 2001; 88:35-39.

32. Elkayam U, Akhter MW, Tummala P, Khan S, Singh H. Nesiritide: a new drug for the treatment of decompensated heart failure. *J Cardiovasc Pharmacol Ther.* 2002;7(3):181-194.

33. Johnson MJ, McDonagh TA, Harkness A, McKay SE, Dargie HJ. Morphine for the relief of breathlessness in patients with chronic heart failure: a pilot study. *Eur J Heart Fail.* 2002;4(6):753-756.

34. Brozena SC, Jessup M. The new staging system for heart failure: what every primary care physician should know. *Geriatrics.* 2003;58(6):31-37.

35. Oliver MF. Metabolic causes and prevention of ventricular fibrillation during acute coronary syndromes. *Am J Med.* 2002;112(4):305-311.

36. Guyton AC, Hall JE. Textbook of Medical Physiology. 10th ed. Philadelphia: WB Saunders Company; 2000.

37. Bennett PN, Brown MJ. Cardiac arrhythmia and failure. In: Bennett PN, Brown MJ, eds. *General Pharmacology.* New York: Churchill Livingstone; 2003:497-520.

38. Tsuchiya T, Okumura K, Honda T, Iwasa A, Ashikaga K. Effects of verapamil and lidocaine on two components of the re-entry circuit of verapamil-sensitive idiopathic left ventricular tachycardia. *J Am Coll Cardiol.* 2001; 37(5):1415-1421.

39. Vaughan Williams EM. Classifying antiarrhythmic actions: by facts or speculation. *J Clin Pharmacol.* 1992; 32(11):964-977.

40. Vaughan Williams EM. The relevance of cellular to clinical electrophysiology in classifying antiarrhythmic actions. *J Cardiovasc Pharmacol.* 1992;20(suppl 2):S1-S7.

41. Haugh KH. Antidysrhythmic agents at the turn of the twenty-first century. *Crit Care Nurs Clin North Am.* 2002; 14(1):53-69.

42. Kawabata M, Hirao K, Horikawa T, et al. Syncope in patients with atrial flutter during treatment with class Ic antiarrhythmic drugs. *J Electrocardiol.* 2001;34(1):65-71.

43. Echt L. Mortality and morbidity in patients receiving encainide, flecainide, or placebo. *N Engl J Med.* 1991; 324:781-788.

44. Belardinelli R. Arrhythmias during acute and chronic exercise in chronic heart failure. *Int J Cardiol.* 2003; 90(2):213-218.

45. El-Sherif N, Turitto G. Torsade de pointes. *Curr Opin Cardiol.* 2003;18(1):6-13.

46. Al-Khatib SM, Allen NM, Kramer JM, Califf RM. What clinicians should know about the QT interval. *JAMA.* 2003;289(16):2120-2127.

47. Pinter A, Dorian P. Intravenous antiarrhythmic agents. *Curr Opin Cardiol.* 2001;16:17-22.

48. Sanguinetti MC, Bennett PB. Antiarrhythmic drug target choices and screening. *Circ Res.* 2003;93:491-499.

49. Wolbrette DL. Risk of proarrhythmia with class III antiarrhythmic agents: sex-based differences and other issues. *Am J Cardiol.* 2003;91(6A):39D-44D.

50. Goodman CC. The cardiovascular system. In: Goodman CC, Boissonnault WG, Fuller KS, eds. *Pathology Implications for the Physical Therapist.* 2nd ed. Philadelphia: Saunders; 2003:367-467.

51. Aronow WS. Atrial fibrillation. *Heart Disease.* 2002; 4(2):91-101.

52. Hillegass E. Electrocardiography. In: Hillegass E, Sadowsky HS, eds. *Essentials of Cardiopulmonary Physical Therapy.* Philadelphia: Saunders; 1994:355-400.

53. Grant AO. Mechanisms of atrial fibrillation and action of drugs used in its management. *Am J Cardiol.* 1998; 82:43N-49N.

54. Snow V, Weiss M, LeFevre R, et al. Management of newly detected atrial fibrillation: recommendations from the American College of Physicians and the American Academy of Family Physicians. *Ann Intern Med.* 2003; 139(12):I32-I35.

55. Saxonhouse SJ, Curtis AB. Risks and benefits of rate control versus maintenance of sinus rhythm. *Am J Cardiol.* 2003;91(6A):27D-32D.

56. Van Gelder I, Hagens VE, Bosker HA, et al. A comparison of rate control and rhythm control in patients with recurrent persistent atrial fibrillation. *N Engl J Med.* 2002;347(23)1834-1840.

57. The Atrial Fibrillation Follow-up Investigation of Rhythm Management (AFFIRM). A comparison of rate control and rhythm control in patients with atrial fibrillation. *N Engl J Med.* 2002;347(23):1825-1833.

58. Cain ME. Atrial fibrillation: rhythm or rate control. *N Engl J Med.* 2002;347(23):1822-1823.

59. Connolly SJ. Preventing stroke in patients with atrial fibrillation: current treatments and new concepts. *Am Heart J.* 2003;145:418-423.

60. Man-Son-Hing M, Laupacis A. Balancing the risks of stroke and upper gastrointestinal tract bleeding in older patients with atrial fibrillation. *Arch Intern Med.* 2002; 162:541-550.

61. Howard PA. Guidelines for stroke prevention in patients with atrial fibrillation. *Drugs.* 1999;58(6):998-1009.

62. Maisel WH, Stevenson LW. Atrial fibrillation in heart failure: epidemiology, pathophysiology, and rationale for therapy. *Am J Cardiol.* 2003;91(6A):2D-8D.

63. Carlson MD. How to manage atrial fibrillation: an update on recent clinical trials. *Cardiol Rev.* 2001;9(2)60-69.

64. Coso FG, Delpon E. New antiarrhythmic drugs for atrial flutter and atrial fibrillation: a conceptual breakthrough at last? *Circulation.* 2002;105(3):276-278.

Treatment for Pulmonary and Gastrointestinal Disorders

CHAPTER 9

DRUG THERAPY FOR PULMONARY DISORDERS

REGULATION OF RESPIRATION AND AIRWAY SMOOTH MUSCLE TONE

The basic rhythm for respiration comes from the medullary rhythmicity center, which receives input from the pontine and higher central nervous system centers, as well as vagal afferent input from the lungs. Several chemical substances in the blood also affect the respiratory center. Peripheral control comes from carbon dioxide (CO_2) chemoreceptors in the medulla and oxygen chemoreceptors in the carotid bodies and aortic arch that respond to changes in the blood partial pressure of these substances. Respiratory rate is increased by elevated blood P_{CO_2} and lowered blood P_{O_2}. There is also some degree of voluntary control that can be superimposed on automatic breathing, implying connections between the cortex and the muscles of respiration.

Airway smooth muscle tone is influenced by a balance maintained between the parasympathetic nervous system, sympathetic nervous system, circulating catecholamines, and a third nervous pathway called *the nonadrenergic-noncholinergic system* (Figure 9-1).[1,2] The parasympathetic nervous system, acting through the vagus nerve, releases acetylcholine to interact with muscarinic receptors. There are three types of muscarinic (M) receptors involved in this system: M_1 receptors exist in the ganglia on the postsynaptic cells, which mediate the transmission of acetylcholine to nicotinic receptors; M_2

receptors are autoreceptors on the postganglionic nerves; and M_3 receptors are found on bronchial smooth muscle and glands. Stimulation of this system produces mainly bronchoconstriction in the larger airways and mucus secretion. The sympathetic nerves directly innervate blood vessels and glands to produce constriction and inhibit secretion, but they do not innervate airway smooth muscle. Instead, the sympathetic effect on bronchial smooth muscle is produced by circulating catecholamines, specifically epinephrine from the adrenal glands, which primarily activates β_2 receptors. Stimulation of these receptors relaxes smooth muscle, inhibits release of chemicals from mast cells, and increases mucociliary clearance. α Receptors also exist on the airways but appear to produce airway constriction only in diseased lungs. The nonadrenergic-noncholinergic mediators include nitric oxide, which produces relaxation of the airways, and excitatory neuropeptides such as substance P and neurokinin A. These agents produce constriction, increase vascular permeability, and increase mucus secretion.

In addition to the efferent pathways, afferent pathways also contribute to airway regulation. Specialized irritant receptors and C fibers fire off in response to inflammatory mediators to produce coughing, bronchoconstriction, and mucus secretion. Physical stimuli such as breathing in cold air can also stimulate these receptors and produce bronchoconstriction.

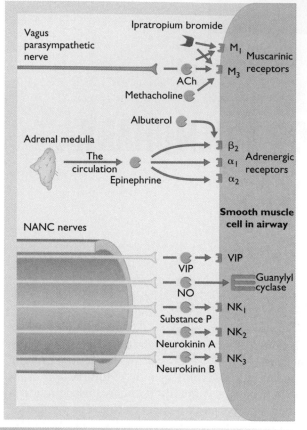

Figure 9-1

Airway smooth muscle tone and innervation. A constructor tone is provided by the vagus nerve and release of acetylcholine *(ACh)*. This is blocked by the mixed M_1/M_2 antagonist, ipratropium bromide. Methacholine challenge, to assess for asthma, activates these receptors. Epinephrine relaxes airway smooth muscle by activating β_2 receptors. This is mimicked by the therapeutic drug, albuterol. The other features of the figure, including vasoactive intestinal polypeptide *(VIP)* activation of VIP receptors, nitrergic release of nitric oxide *(NO)*, and activation of various neurokinin *(NK)* receptors, all part of the nonadrenergic noncholinergic *(NANC)* system, may represent targets for future drug development. (From Page C, Curtis AB, Sutter MC, Walker MJ, Hoffman BB, eds. *Integrated Pharmacology*. 2nd ed. Philadelphia: Mosby; 2002.)

BRONCHIAL ASTHMA

Asthma is considered to be a chronic inflammatory disorder of the airways that produces acute broncho-constriction and shortness of breath.[3,4] The bronchi become hyperreactive as a result of an inflammatory process involving a variety of stimulants including allergens, environmental chemicals, exercise, cold air, aspirin-type drugs, and viruses. Inflammatory mediators are released from mast cells, eosinophils, neutrophils, and macrophages in response to these stimuli (Figure 9-2).[5] These chemical mediators are particularly damaging to the respiratory epithelium. Histamine is released preformed so that it produces an immediate bronchial reaction, which is responsible for the abrupt onset of symptoms. A later phase also produces a more sustained bronchial reaction, resulting from arachidonic acid release from damaged cell membranes and eosinophil accumulation. Metabolites of arachidonic acid from both the cyclooxygenase (prostaglandin D_2) pathway and lipoxygenase (cysteinyl-leukotrienes C_4 and D_4) pathways produce the second or late phase of bronchoconstriction (Figure 9-3). Platelet activating factor is another mediator that is being increasingly recognized for its role in the production of asthma. These mediators interact to produce the typical signs of asthma, which include mucosal edema, mucus secretion, bronchoconstriction, and damage to the ciliated epithelium resulting in wheezing, hyper-ventilation, cough, shortness of breath, and a reduction in the forced expiratory volume in one second (FEV_1).

Asthma associated with a specific allergen is labeled as extrinsic type disease and is probably the most common form.[4] In allergic asthma T helper cells are predominantly activated, and they release cytokines, forcing the production and release of immunoglobulin E (IgE) from B cells. Interleukin-3 (IL-3), IL-4, and IL-5 are also released, becoming chemotactic for eosinophils. Again, the inflammatory mediators, histamines, leukotrienes and prosta-glandins become involved. A few hours later, eosino-phil proteins, which cause tissue damage, become the ongoing stimulus for the asthma, producing the delayed phase (Figure 9-4).

Asthma not associated with a known allergy is considered intrinsic asthma. Two other categories of asthma are exercise-induced asthma (EIA) and asthma associated with chronic obstructive pulmo-nary disease (COPD). Exercise, especially when con-ducted in cold dry air, produces bronchoconstriction in some patients. This wheeze regularly occurs within just a few minutes of exercise. As described in the following section, preventive treatment with β_2 inhalers usually works well for this type of asthma. Asthma may coexist with COPD, and if identified, must be treated somewhat differently than if COPD exists alone.

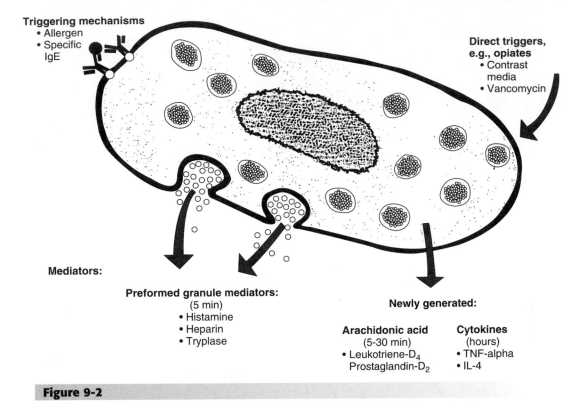

Triggering mechanisms
- Allergen
- Specific
  IgE

**Direct triggers,
e.g., opiates**
- Contrast
  media
- Vancomycin

Mediators:

Preformed granule mediators:
(5 min)
- Histamine
- Heparin
- Tryplase

Newly generated:

Arachidonic acid
(5-30 min)
- Leukotriene-D_4
  Prostaglandin-D_2

Cytokines
(hours)
- TNF-alpha
- IL-4

Figure 9-2

Mast cell mediator release. Some mediators are also produced by basophils. Tryptase can be assayed in serum or secretions as a marker of mast cell degranulation. Oral steroids control the production of newly generated mediators but have little effect on the release of preformed granule mediators. (Redrawn from Brody MJ, Larner J, Minneman KP, eds. *Human Pharmacology: Molecular to Clinical*. 3rd ed. Philadelphia: Mosby; 1998.)

Inhalation Delivery Devices

Delivery of drug to the lungs allows the medication to interact directly with the diseased tissue. This mode of administration reduces the risk of adverse effects, specifically systemic reactions, and allows for the reduction of dose compared with oral administration. Most of the inhaled drugs are administered through a pressurized metered-dose inhaler. This is an aerosol delivery system that uses a chlorofluorocarbon propellant to spray drug into the respiratory tract. The use of chlorofluorocarbons as a propellant is being phased out slowly and replaced with either no propellant or new, ozone-friendly propellants (hydrofluorocarbons).

These metered-dose inhalers are convenient and inexpensive but require some coordination and practice for effective use. Correct use requires activation of the device and a simultaneous inhalation. Children and the elderly seem to have problems maneuvering the device and coordinating the inhalation. The device containing the canister of drug is warmed to room temperature and then shaken well. The mouthpiece is held approximately 1 inch from the mouth unless a spacer is used. The patient performs a normal exhalation and then presses down on the canister while breathing in slowly for 2 to 5 seconds. The patient should hold his or her breath for up to 10 seconds if possible to allow the medicine to enter the lungs. If 2 puffs are prescribed, the patient should wait 5 minutes between inhalations. After steroids have been inhaled, the mouth must be rinsed well with mouthwash.

Metered-dose inhalers spray at high velocities, causing some of the drug particles to hit the back of the throat instead of being inhaled deeply into the lungs.[6] A spacer is a cylinder that is attached to the metered-dose inhaler, which helps capture the large high-velocity particles, allowing the slower, lower velocity drug particles to reach their target site deep

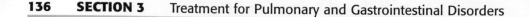

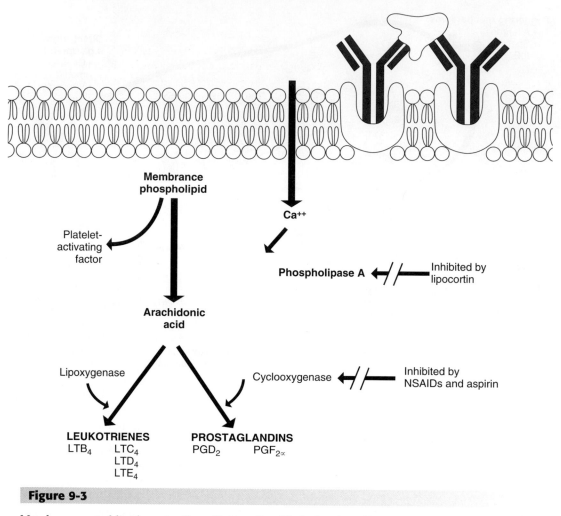

Figure 9-3

Newly generated lipid mast cell mediators. Specific leukotriene D_4-receptor antagonists are effective in the treatment of asthma. *NSAIDS,* Nonsteroidal antiinflammatory drugs. (Redrawn from Brody MJ, Larner J, Minneman KP, eds. *Human Pharmacology: Molecular to Clinical.* 3rd ed. Philadelphia: Mosby; 1998.)

in the lungs.[3,7] To reach and settle in the airways, particles must be between 2 and 6 microns. The spacer also gives the patient some extra time to coordinate slow inspiration with the ejection of the drug from the canister. Even with the spacer, only about 20% of the drug inhaled reaches the lungs.[8] Most is swallowed: some enters the systemic circulation through the gastrointestinal tract, and some is ejected with mouth rinsing. The addition of a spacer makes the device less portable, so one manufacturer has developed a collapsible spacer to be used with the inhalation device.

Dry powder inhalers or breath-activated devices are delivery devices that scatter a fine powder into the lungs by means of a brisk inhalation.[3,9] These devices are easier to coordinate than metered-dose inhalers, and some studies have shown that they are more effective.[10] However, not all patients can inhale strongly enough to use these devices, especially patients with severe airflow obstruction.[11] Also, some patients find the dry powder irritating.

The other major drug delivery system for pulmonary problems is the nebulizer. This device dispenses liquid medication in oxygen or room air so that what is inhaled is a mist of extremely fine particles.[12] Use of the nebulizer simply requires the patient to breathe through a face mask or mouthpiece so that no coordination of inspiration is

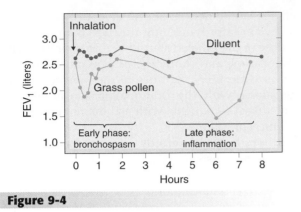

Figure 9-4

The two phases of asthma as demonstrated by the changes in the forced expiratory volume in 1 second (FEV$_1$) after inhalation of grass pollen in an allergic subject. (From Cockcroft DW. Mechanism of perennial allergic asthma. *Lancet.* 1983;[8344]2:253-256.)

required. Therefore it is often used by the elderly and very young patients. These devices require an external gas source or an electronically powered compressor.

Drug Treatment for Asthma

The drugs used to treat asthma can be divided into two categories, short-term relievers and long-term controllers. The short-term relievers are those drugs that are used during acute asthma attacks. For this reason they are also referred to as *rescue inhalers.* They include β$_2$-agonists, anticholinergics, and some sympathomimetics. The long-term controllers are those used to prevent attacks from occurring and include steroids, leukotriene modifiers, theophylline, and cromolyn.

β$_2$ Adrenoceptor Agonists

β$_2$-Agonists are the most commonly prescribed drugs for the treatment of asthma. These agents are available in metered-dose inhalers and nebulizers, as well as in tablet and injectable forms. They produce relaxation of airway smooth muscle, resulting in bronchodilation, inhibit inflammatory mediator release from mast cells, and enhance mucociliary clearance.

Two categories of β$_2$-agonists are actually used in the treatment of asthma, short-acting agents and longer-acting agents. After inhalation of the short-acting agent, action is rapid, often within 5 to

10 minutes. Maximum effect usually occurs in 30 minutes, and duration of action is 4 to 6 hours. Examples of the short-acting agents include salbutamol, albuterol, and terbutaline.

Salmeterol and formoterol are longer-acting agents that produce bronchodilation for 12 to 15 hours.[4] These drugs contain a long lipophilic side chain on the molecule that binds to the membrane near the receptor, slowing washout of the drug. These longer-acting agents are not appropriate for acute asthmatic episodes because of their delayed action, but they may be used to prevent nocturnal asthmatic attacks and provide protection for unanticipated or prolonged physical activity.

The usual dose for the short-acting β$_2$-agonists is 2 puffs every 4 to 6 hours or as needed. If a patient uses more than 1 canister per month, it probably means that he or she has inadequate control, and an adjustment on the long-term controller is needed.[13] Regular use of the short-acting agents offers no advantage over as-needed use and may actually lead to tolerance.[14]

Salmeterol and the other long-acting agents are given regularly, twice daily, and not on an as-needed basis. As mentioned earlier, they are not indicated for acute asthma attacks because they have a slow onset of action and a prolonged effect. Patients taking these drugs regularly should use a short-acting bronchodilator as needed to control acute symptoms. Long-term daily use of salmeterol has been reported to lead to tolerance, at least for EIA.[15,16] Other studies have shown that the long-term agents can decrease responsiveness to the short-acting drugs, but this is controversial.[16]

Oral β$_2$-agonists can also be given, but they are less effective, produce more adverse effects, and have a slower onset of action than the same drug given by inhalation. Oral syrup formulations are available and may be appropriate for small children with mild asthma who are unable to use an inhaler.[17] Administering the drug by a nebulizer is also an option.

Side effects of β$_2$-agonists include tremor, tachycardia, hypokalemia, and hyperglycemia.[17] Increased mortality has been reported with the overuse of β$_2$ inhalers, but this was most likely due to worsening disease rather than actual use of the drug. Less selective adrenergic agonists, such as epinephrine or isoproterenol, are more likely to produce side effects than β$_2$-selective agents, particularly cardiac arrhythmias and rebound bronchospasm.

Anticholinergic Agents

The muscarinic receptor antagonists cause bronchodilation by blocking the action of acetylcholine on airway smooth muscle. These drugs do not prevent all types of bronchospasm but are effective against asthma produced by irritant stimuli.[1] These drugs also decrease mucus secretion, which is why they are more effective for COPD than asthma.

The anticholinergic agents that may be used in asthma treatment include inhaled ipratropium, tiotropium, and oxitropium. These synthetic compounds are permanently charged, preventing significant systemic absorption after inhalation, thus minimizing side effects.[18] When inhaled, they produce maximum bronchodilation in 30 minutes with duration up to 5 hours. Ipratropium is available alone or in combination with the β_2-agonist albuterol. In general, dry mouth and pharyngeal irritation are the major side effects, but tachycardia may occur with excessive dosing. Although anticholinergic agents are primarily used in the treatment of COPD, they offer some additional efficacy in the treatment of asthma when combined with a β_2-agonist.[19]

Corticosteroids

Regular use of an inhaled corticosteroid can reduce bronchial inflammation and hyperresponsiveness in patients with persistent asthma.[17] Steroids block the release of arachidonic acid from airway epithelial cells, which in turn blocks production of prostaglandins and leukotrienes. In addition, they inhibit transcription factors for the synthesis of interleukins and tumor necrosis factor, which are involved in stimulating the immune system. Related to this action, steroids decrease the number of mast cells and eosinophils that migrate into the area and also reduce edema formation by acting on the vascular endothelium. Specifically, they reduce the number of cytokines produced by the T2 helper cells that activate eosinophils and are responsible for facilitating the production of IgE.[4]

Inhaled steroids have been the drug of choice for reducing the number of asthmatic attacks in patients who have mild to moderate persistent asthma and for those who require β_2 inhalers more than once a day. Regular use of an inhaled steroid is associated with a reduced number of deaths from asthma.[20] Examples of inhaled steroids include beclomethasone, budesonide, and fluticasone. Fluticasone is also available in combination with salmeterol.[21] In

fact, the combination of the two drugs is more effective in improving lung function than doubling the dose of the inhaled steroid.[22,23] The combination of fluticasone and salmeterol is also more effective in improving FEV_1 than use of the inhaled fluticasone along with the oral leukotriene antagonist montelukast in patients with asthma not controlled by fluticasone alone.[24]

Although oral steroids are associated with some deleterious side effects, recommended use of inhaled steroids does not pose a risk of serious toxic effects. Dysphonia and oral candidiasis are the most common occurrences because of local deposition of the drug. Use of the spacer device and diligent rinsing of the mouth after inhalation can decrease these effects. Some other side effects include a dose-dependent slowing of growth in some children and adolescents but most likely with no effect on final adult height.[25] Decreased bone density, cataract formation, suppression of the hypothalamic-pituitary-adrenal axis, and glaucoma have also been reported.[26-30]

Oral or parenteral corticosteroids are the most effective treatments for acute exacerbations of asthma that do not respond well to β_2-agonists.[17] Even when patients do respond to short-term relievers, they may still receive a 10-day course of oral steroids to help decrease symptoms and prevent relapses. Long-term daily use of oral steroids produces severe side effects including hyperglycemia, weight gain, increased blood pressure, osteoporosis, cataracts, increased susceptibility to infection, muscle wasting, central fat deposition, moon facies, purple abdominal striae, atrophic skin, capillary fragility, and neuropsychiatric disorders. Because systemic use shuts down the hypothalamic-pituitary-adrenal axis, sudden withdrawal of steroids can be fatal, since it takes time for the endogenous production of corticosteroids to resume. Corticosteroid side effects may be minimized by administering a single morning dose to correspond to the normal peak cortisol concentration that occurs in the early morning or by switching to every other day dosing.[3] The benefits and adverse effects of steroids are more fully described in Chapter 13.

Leukotriene Antagonists and Leukotriene Receptor Blockers

Leukotriene antagonists and leukotriene receptor blockers block the actions of leukotrienes, decreasing the migration of eosinophils, production of mucus, and bronchoconstriction.[31,32] They are the first new class of antiasthmatic agents in 30 years.[33] Montelukast and zafirlukast are leukotriene receptor antagonists, and zileuton inhibits synthesis of leukotrienes. These drugs have been slightly less effective than the long-acting β-agonists and inhaled steroids, but the addition of these agents permits a reduction in corticosteroid dose.[34,35] They can be used as primary monotherapy in mild persistent asthma with near-normal lung function, although a fast-acting inhaler may still be needed.[36] Occasionally, someone with moderate-severe asthma (two or more bronchoconstrictive episodes per week) will do better with these drugs than with steroids.[37]

The leukotriene blockers are given orally: montelukast is given once daily, and zafirlukast, twice daily. In several large clinical studies, they have demonstrated few adverse drug reactions.[37] The side effect profile was similar to that of placebo with complaints of gastrointestinal upset and headache.[38] Montelukast is approved for use in children 6 to 12 years old and has a safety profile equal to that found for use in adults.

Cromolyn and Nedocromil

Cromolyn and nedocromil inhibit mast cell degranulation.[3] When stimulated, mast cells release granules containing histamine, leukotrienes, and prostaglandins—all of which produce an inflammatory response. These drugs block release of these inflammatory mediators and thus decrease airway hyperresponsiveness, but they have no bronchodilating activity. They are used only for prophylaxis.

Cromolyn and nedocromil are not effective for all patients with asthma. A 4-week trial period may be necessary to determine their effectiveness. Children often respond better than adults.[4] A benefit of these drugs is that they have relatively few side effects with the exception of their bitter taste, but they are less effective than inhaled corticosteroids.[17]

Theophylline

Theophylline is a methylxanthine, a substance found in coffee, tea, and chocolate.[6] It was developed as a result of the observation that consuming great amounts of caffeine-containing beverages reduced the incidence of asthma. It acts as a phosphodiesterase inhibitor, which in turn increases intracellular cyclic adenosine monophosphate, resulting in relaxation of smooth muscle. It also has some antiinflammatory properties.

Theophylline was previously used as a long-term controller for asthma, but because of its low therapeutic index, it has largely been replaced by leukotriene antagonists.[39] The drug is still used for patients who do not respond to the standard asthma agents. In addition, it is used in the emergency department for acute and severe asthmatic attacks along with oxygen, steroids, and bronchodilators. It is occasionally used in the treatment of spinal cord injury because there is some evidence that it increases diaphragmatic strength and endurance.

Theophylline's adverse effects include nausea, vomiting, headache, insomnia, nervousness, tachycardia, and hypertension.[6] Arrhythmias may occur and signal that theophylline blood levels are too high. Frequent monitoring of blood levels is essential. Factors that affect theophylline's clearance include enzyme inhibition by other drugs (cimetidine, erythromycin), congestive heart failure, liver disease, older age, viral infection, and a high-carbohydrate diet.

Acute Severe Asthma (Status Asthmaticus)

Status asthmaticus is a life-threatening illness requiring rapid and aggressive treatment. It may occur because the airways become refractory to the β2-agonists, particularly when administered frequently within 36 to 38 hours to regain control over the airways. In addition, the mucus plugs that develop begin to impair the ability of the inhaled drugs to reach the distal airways.[3]

Immediate treatment involves administering humidified oxygen by mask plus intravenous (IV) fluids for hydration to help liquefy the mucus. Additional treatment includes oral or IV steroids, followed by a β2-agonist administered with a nebulizer. If cyanosis or bradycardia is observed or if breath sounds are absent, ipratropium and IV aminophylline (similar to theophylline) can be given. If the patient's condition is still not improving, then the intensive care unit should be notified, and a decision regarding intubation and mechanical ventilation should be made. Monitoring the patient's response to treatment includes measurement of peak expiratory flow rate, oxygen saturation, and blood gases every 15 to 30 minutes.

Exercise-Induced Asthma

EIA, also known as exercise-induced airway narrowing or exercise-induced bronchospasm, is acute airway constriction that occurs after exercise or strenuous exertion. Some patients with asthma exhibit symptoms only with exercise. EIA may also occur in 40% to 90% of patients who experience bronchoconstriction as a reaction to other triggers.[40]

There are two theories regarding the pathogenesis of EIA.[40] One theory is that inhalation of cold and dry air leads to mucosal drying and increased osmolarity, stimulating mast cell degranulation. The fact that the mast cell stabilizers (cromolyn and nedocromil) are effective in controlling EIA supports this hypothesis. The other theory is that rapid airway rewarming after exercise produces vascular congestion, increased permeability, and edema, which trigger the asthma attack. Proponents of this theory believe that the greater the difference in ambient temperature between the exercise and postexercise environments, the greater the degree of bronchoconstriction will be; however, EIA also occurs in hot, dry climates. There is a high incidence of EIA in elite athletes, so some clinicians have hypothesized that EIA in these cases may be due to airway injury from factors related to high-intensity exercise.

The clinical features of EIA include bronchospasm after at least 3 to 8 minutes of exercise and/or symptoms of cough, wheezing, dyspnea, and chest tightness. These symptoms reach their peak in about 15 minutes, and recovery generally occurs within 60 minutes. A late-phase response may also occur 4 to 6 hours after exercise. Although patients occasionally have difficulty with breathing during activity, EIA generally begins after exercise has been completed. In addition, if a person who has EIA returns to exercise soon after the symptoms subside, he or she will experience less of a problem after the second bout of exercise than after the first. This is referred to as the refractory period and generally lasts from 40 minutes to 4 hours.

EIA may be treated with or without drugs.[40,41] A high level of fitness is important in decreasing EIA because patients who exercise regularly do not demonstrate the abrupt increases in ventilation experienced by their more sedentary counterparts, which are more likely to stimulate bronchoconstriction. Swimming is often recommended over outdoor running because warm humidified air does not seem to trigger EIA. Other recommendations include warming up before exercise, covering the mouth and nose with a scarf during cold weather, and incorporating a cool-down period before ending exercise.

Pharmacological agents can also be used just before exercise to reduce the incidence of EIA.[40,41] Inhaled short-acting β_2-agonists are the most commonly used agents for this condition. They are effective in preventing symptoms if they are administered between 15 minutes and 1 hour before exercise. Duration of action is up to 4 hours. The patient is instructed to use 2 to 4 puffs of the short-acting agent 30 to 60 minutes before exercise. Patients who exercise for a prolonged period generally use a long-acting β_2-agonist such as formoterol. Formoterol has a more rapid onset of action (15 minutes) than salmeterol and is effective for up to 12 hours. It has been shown to decrease EIA after single doses, as well as with regular use.[41,42]

Inhaled cromolyn and nedocromil are also commonly used to decrease EIA.[40] They are used 10 to 20 minutes before exercise, and although they attenuate symptoms, they are less effective than the β_2-agonists.[43] Other choices include the leukotriene antagonists, which have been shown to reduce bronchoconstriction during exercise challenges.[40,44] Single doses of montelukast and zafirlukast are protective for 1 hour to 12 hours after administration, and some studies show equal effectiveness when compared with salmeterol early in the course of treatment, but after dosing for several weeks, the leukotriene antagonists demonstrated superiority.[45] Montelukast has also been shown to reduce EIA in 6- to 14-year-old children with asthma.[46] Other pharmacological agents including anticholinergic drugs, theophylline, and antihistamines have been shown to have some protection against EIA when added to a daily regimen of asthma control medications.[40] However, only certain drugs are approved for use in athletic competition by the United States and International Olympic Committees because β-agonists have the potential to be anabolic when taken in the oral form.[47-49] Although the use of these agents for increasing voluntary muscle strength holds some promise in the treatment of weakened skeletal musculature, it is doubtful that someone would want to compete against an athlete taking these agents. All inhaled corticosteroids, leukotriene antagonists, cromolyn/nedocromil, theophylline, and ipratropium are approved; but of the list of β_2-agonists, only albuterol, terbutaline, and salmeterol are approved agents. Athletes who require the use of these agents must submit clinical and laboratory values that prove the necessity of these drugs to the International Olympic Committee Medical Commission.[50]

OTHER DRUGS USEFUL IN RESPIRATORY DISORDERS

Cough, nasal congestion, and thick mucus are symptoms of respiratory disorders. For each of these indications, specific symptom reduction drugs are available.

Antitussives

These drugs are used to treat recurrent or persistent cough.[1,51] Nonspecific cough, not resulting from asthma or as a side effect of ACE inhibitors, may be triggered by mechanical or chemical stimulation of the upper respiratory tract. This stimulus is relayed to the cough center in the medulla and then to the respiratory muscles. The efferent pathway for cough involves the phrenic nerve and abrupt contraction of the intercostals muscles. Cough is necessary as a protective mechanism to expel foreign bodies or to help produce and expel mucus, but a nonproductive cough can be annoying. Peripheral cough receptors are sensitive to local anesthetics, and topical application of lidocaine is used to inhibit cough during bronchoscopy.

Drugs that suppress cough act by decreasing activity of the afferent nerves or decreasing the sensitivity of the cough center. Menthol vapor inhalation is effective in reducing sensitivity of the peripheral cough receptors. Inhalation of the menthol vapors or sucking lozenges containing menthol will decrease the need to cough. Topical anesthetics such as lidocaine, benzocaine, and bupivacaine will also reduce the sensitivity of the peripheral receptors. The opioids reduce the sensitivity of the central cough center. Codeine and hydrocodone are common ingredients in cough medicines. Narcotic preparations must be used with caution by patients with head trauma or renal or liver disease. They produce sedation, drowsiness, and constipation. Nausea and vomiting may also occur. Because overdose effects include hypotension, bradycardia, and respiratory depression, narcotics must be used with caution for patients with COPD. In addition, codeine decreases secretions in the bronchioles, thickening the sputum and producing a reduction in clearance.[4] Dextromethorphan is similar in structure and just as effective as codeine but devoid of analgesic properties.

Drugs for Rhinitis and Rhinorrhea

Rhinitis is an acute or chronic inflammation of the nasal mucosa, and rhinorrhea is the production of watery nasal secretions.[1] Both of these conditions may result from a viral infection of the nasal mucosa or an IgE-type allergy. Essentially, blood flow and vascular permeability to the mucosa are increased, resulting in fluid buildup in the nasal passages and difficulty breathing. Sympatholytic drugs that vasoconstrict the blood vessels are the major ingredients in nasal sprays. However, the major side effects of these drugs are vasoconstriction and elevated blood pressure. They can also aggravate hyperthyroidism, diabetes, glaucoma, and benign prostatic hyperplasia. This is particularly true with the oral mixtures that contain phenylephrine. Patients will develop tolerance to the topical agents, if used repeatedly, but will not usually develop tolerance to the oral decongestants.

Other treatments for rhinitis and rhinorrhea take an immunological approach.[1] Autocoids such as histamine are released as a result of an immunological reaction. Antihistamines and the local administration of glucocorticosteroids are useful in controlling disease associated with these reactions. Histamine acts on the nasal mucosa, largely on H_1 receptors. The antihistamines or H_1 receptor blockers reduce nasal congestion, mucosal irritation, and cough by reducing secretions. The first-generation H_1 antagonists, such as diphenhydramine and chlorpheniramine, were effective except that they interfered with learning and motor performance and posed a safety hazard because of the excessive somnolence they caused.[52] The newer antihistamines do not cross the blood-brain barrier and therefore produce less sedation than their older counterparts. Some examples include loratadine, cetirizine, and fexofenadine. The glucocorticosteroids that are applied topically to the nasal mucosa include triamcinolone, beclomethasone, fluticasone, and over-the-counter cromolyn—all of which are sprayed directly into the nostrils.

The leukotriene receptor antagonist montelukast has also been approved for the treatment of seasonal allergic rhinitis in adults and children.[53] It has been found to decrease symptoms more than placebo, and in one study of 460 patients, the combination of montelukast and loratadine was more effective than either drug alone. However, in a larger study of 907 subjects, the combination was found to be no better than each drug taken individually.[54] Montelukast is less effective than intranasal corticosteroids.

Mucolytics

Respiratory mucus consists of water and glyco-proteins that are cross-linked by disulphide bonds.[3] Normally only about 100 mL of fluid is produced in the respiratory tract per day, and most of this is swallowed. In disease states more mucus is produced, and it tends to be more viscous. The purpose of mucolytics is to liquefy mucus so that it can be cleared from the airway with a cough. Carbocysteine and mecysteine open disulphide bonds and reduce the viscosity of mucus. They can be given orally or by inhalation and are particularly useful in cystic fibrosis (CF). Water inhalation (breathing over a hot bowl) and use of a humidifier or vaporizer are also considered mucolytic treatments because hydration can lower viscosity.

Dornase alfa is a phosphorylated glycosylated recombinant human deoxyribonuclease that hydrolyzes DNA and is effective for airway clearance in CF.[55,56] Copious amounts of neutrophil-derived DNA accumulate in the airways in patients with CF, and DNA accumulates as a result of degenerating neutrophils. Recombinant human deoxyribonuclease I also breaks down DNA to reduce the viscosity of sputum. The most common adverse reactions associated with this treatment are upper airway irritations, including pharyngitis and laryngitis.

Respiratory Stimulants

Drugs that are used to stimulate the respiratory system are called *analeptics*.[3] They are central nervous system stimulants with very low therapeutic indexes. Doxapram increases both the rate and depth of respiration. It acts on the medullary respiratory center. Nasal intermittent positive pressure ventilation has largely replaced its use. However, it may still be used for postoperative respiratory depression and opiate overdose. Aminophylline may also be used as a respiratory stimulant when given slowly by IV infusion.

Oxygen Therapy

Oxygen therapy should be initiated whenever there is moderate or new-onset hypoxia, $PaO_2 < 50$ mm Hg.[3] Patients with chronic hypoxia may be able to maintain adequate oxygenation with a PaO_2 less than this by compensations such as increasing red blood cell mass. However, low concentrations of oxygen may still be indicated, particularly when $PaCO_2$ is increased, which is usually seen in COPD. The stimulus to breathe is the elevated CO_2, but this can be diminished in patients with chronically high CO_2 and replaced instead by a drive connected to a low oxygen level. Elevating the oxygen level therefore might remove the stimulus to breathe. High-concentration oxygen therapy is indicated when both oxygen and CO_2 levels are low, as might be seen in a patient with a pulmonary embolism, pneumonia, or myocardial infarction and early in an acute severe asthma attack. Long-term continuous oxygen therapy is given to patients with severe hypoxia and cor pulmonale caused by COPD.

CHRONIC OBSTRUCTIVE PULMONARY DISEASE

Clinical signs and symptoms of COPD include excessive production of sputum with mucus plugging, cough, increased respiratory rate, hypoventilation, hypercapnia, and hypoxia. Anatomical changes that occur include glandular hypertrophy, goblet cell metaplasia, and inflammation and fibrosis of the airways (smaller airways greater than larger airways), leading to a narrowing of the lumen and obstructive flow. Many of these changes are irreversible, which is what separates this illness from asthma. Drugs are used to improve functional abilities and to turn around the reversible component of the disease.

The therapeutic approach to COPD needs to be flexible enough to keep up with the progression of the disease. The American Thoracic Society recommends spirometry measurements to help determine the presence and severity of COPD. The ratio of FEV_1 to forced vital capacity (FVC) is used to determine airflow obstruction. An FEV_1/FVC ratio $< 70\%$ or $< 88\%$ and 89% of predicted value for men and women, respectively, along with x-ray evidence and clinical symptoms are positive for a diagnosis. Mild COPD is defined by a postbronchodilator FEV_1 of 70% to 80% or greater of predicted value; moderate

COPD, as an FEV_1 of 50% to 80% of predicted value; severe COPD, as an FEV_1 of 30% to 49% of predicted value; and very severe COPD, as an $FEV_1 < 35\%$ of predicted value.[57] During the early, largely asymptomatic phase, the therapeutic goal is to slow the loss of lung function. An important step in this process is, of course, the cessation of cigarette smoking. Behavioral approaches and nicotine replacement therapy can be helpful.[58,59] Patients should also be vaccinated with the pneumococcal vaccine and the appropriate influenza vaccine yearly.[60]

Because patients with COPD have airflow obstruction, bronchodilators are almost universally used to provide relief. Traditionally, patients have used a combination of short-acting β_2-agonists and anticholinergic drugs. Combination therapy appears to be slightly better than monotherapy with short-acting β_2-agonists in reducing exacerbations but is not superior to monotherapy with ipratropium.[60] Salbutamol and ipratropium given four times daily is the most common combination.[61] They are packaged together in a single inhaler for patient convenience. The anticholinergic compounds reduce neurogenic control of mucus, which is probably why monotherapy with ipratropium is efficacious. However, there is no evidence that either monotherapy or combination therapy slows the decline in lung function or improves survival.

The longer-acting agents, the β_2-agonists formoterol and salmeterol, and the anticholinergic agent tiotropium have recently been introduced as treatment for COPD.[61] A few clinical trials that examined FEV_1 changes over a 1-year period, exacerbation rates, and quality-of-life issues have demonstrated their efficacy over placebo and also the correspondingly shorter-acting agents. No studies have shown that the β_2-agonists or anticholinergic agents are either superior or inferior to each other. But combining a longer-acting β_2-agonist with ipratropium is more effective than combining a short-acting agent with ipratropium.[62] Hence, the practice of combining the longer-acting agent of each type of drug is catching on. However, patients must carry around two inhalers because the available long-acting β_2-agonists are given twice daily, but tiotropium is given only once, which makes combining them into a single inhaler impossible at this time.

Inhaled corticosteroids with and without long-acting β_2-agonists are also used in the treatment of COPD but are not without controversy. A subset of patients with COPD appears to respond to short-term administration of steroids with improved FEV_1 and a reduction in symptoms. However, this response is individually determined. Patients who are likely to respond are those with a history of asthma, sputum eosinophilia, and a good response to β_2-agonists.[63] The best way to determine responsiveness to steroids is with a trial. It is recommended that patients receive oral prednisone for 2 to 3 weeks.[64] If the patient responds to the prednisone, then weaning to inhaled steroids can be initiated. However, failure to respond to steroids in a baseline state does not necessarily mean that the patient will not respond during an exacerbation. Given the negative side effects associated with steroid use and the fact that several studies show that steroids have no effect on the decline of lung function, they must be used with caution.[65-67] However, a recent study has shown that the combination of fluticasone and salmeterol improved lung function and reduced the severity of shortness of breath in patients receiving this combination over a 1-year period.[68] The combination was superior to use of each drug alone. The combined use of tiotropium and the long-acting β_2-agonists is expected to be beneficial, but studies are needed to determine whether this combination is efficacious.[69]

Other treatments for COPD include antibiotics and mucolytic agents.[70] Antibiotics are often needed because the presence of copious amounts of sputum provides a fertile ground for bacterial growth. Mucolytics such as N-acetylcysteine reduce the viscosity of the mucus, but because the most effective means for mobilizing mucus from the airways is a strong cough, these patients should also receive chest physical therapy to learn how to bring up secretions to the trachea level so they can be expelled.

As COPD progresses, oxygen therapy becomes necessary to relieve hypoxemia and prolong survival.[60] Long-term administration of oxygen for at least 15 hours/day is given to patients who have hypoxemia ($PaO_2 < 60$ mm Hg, or a PaO_2 between 55 and 60 mm Hg with pulmonary hypertension or cor pulmonale) or an oxygen saturation in arterial blood (SaO_2) $< 90\%$.[57] Routine use of oxygen with less severe hypoxemia is contraindicated unless the patient has end-organ dysfunction or mental status changes because in COPD the respiratory drive is diminished and may be reduced even further if the hypoxemic drive to breathe is removed.[71]

Intubation and mechanical ventilation may be necessary during exacerbations but a noninvasive method is preferable.[6] Nasal intermittent positive pressure ventilation is the growing choice for oxygen administration in patients with COPD.

CYSTIC FIBROSIS

CF is a multisystem disease in which there is a defect in a gene on chromosome 7 that encodes a chloride channel common to epithelial cells (*CFTR*, cystic fibrosis transmembrane conductance regulator).[6,72] Failure to develop this channel affects epithelial cells lining the airways, intestines, biliary and pancreatic ducts, vas deferens, and sweat ducts. The result is that fluid secretion is diminished and what is secreted becomes more viscous, leading to plugging of ducts. There is also an up-regulation of sodium channels, particularly in the airways, leading to reabsorption of sodium. Proinflammatory pathways are also up-regulated in the airways, and bacterial killing is diminished.

Malnutrition and failure to thrive are common presentations of CF.[6] Failure of the pancreas to produce digestive enzymes leads to the inability to absorb fats and protein. Specifically, the fat-soluble vitamins A, D, E, and K cannot be absorbed.[73] The deficiency of vitamin K may lead to bleeding. Supplementation with water-miscible forms of these vitamins is necessary. In addition, pancreatic enzymes, in a microencapsulated form to improve their survival in an acid environment, are given. Drugs that inhibit acid secretion may also be administered to enhance survival of the pancreatic enzymes.

Pathophysiology at the lung appears to be due to two mechanisms, impaired secretion of chlorine (Cl^-) in serous cells of airway submucosal glands and enhanced absorption of Na^+ with subsequent hyperabsorption of electrolytes and fluids at the airway surface epithelium, leading to mucus plugging and impaired mucociliary clearance.[72] Mucus is produced in the glands but has difficulty getting out, which leads to hypertrophy of the gland. Several drugs to help correct these defective ion channels are under study. Some sodium channel blockers can block the specific type of sodium channel involved in CF (ENaC, amiloride-sensitive epithelial Na^+ channel). Amiloride is a potassium-sparing diuretic, which blocks sodium absorption in the kidney collecting duct. An aerosolized form is available for patients with CF. Benzamil is a related drug that has a longer effect on the sodium channels. Other drugs that attempt to activate an alternative calcium-activated chloride channel or activate mutant CFTRs are being tested.

Because of mucus plugging, an intense regimen for airway clearance is necessary.

In addition to the mucus plugging, the CF lung tends to harbor bacteria. Three organisms predominate: *Haemophilus influenzae*, *Staphylococcus aureus*, and *Pseudomonas aeruginosa*.[73] *P. aeruginosa* will establish itself in the lungs of approximately 80% of patients by young adulthood. Antibiotics with sensitivities for these infections are frequently given. The antibiotic should be chosen after culture of a specimen obtained from sputum or a deep throat swab. Sensitivity testing is paramount in helping to prevent antibiotic resistance. Depending on the severity of infection, oral, inhaled, or IV antibiotics may be used. Inhaled tobramycin is sometimes used every other month to help control *Pseudomonas* infections. See Chapter 21 for a more in-depth review of antibiotics.

Many patients with CF are also prescribed a β_2-agonist.[74] However, there is little evidence that these drugs are effective, and some patients may even show deterioration in lung function while taking these drugs. If the patient experiences symptomatic relief with these drugs, they can be prescribed. Theophyllines act as bronchodilators, but they also directly affect mucociliary function.[75] Despite this effect, these drugs are used only on a limited basis because of their low safety index.

Two other categories of drugs that are frequently used in the treatment of pulmonary problems are the leukotriene antagonists and steroids. Several studies have shown the presence of leukotrienes in CF, but no large study has demonstrated that the leukotriene antagonists are helpful in treating this disease. Oral steroids are being prescribed, even on a long-term basis, for many patients with CF. Given their rather extensive list of side effects, this practice is frowned upon.

Lastly, because thinning of secretions and keeping the airways open are major treatment goals in CF, mucolytic agents in combination with physical therapy are used. Postural drainage and percussion are recommended for the patient before physical activity.[76] In addition, the "flutter device" may be used to assist with mucus clearance, although this does not seem as effective as positive expiratory pressure.[77,78] The patient exhales through the device, which moves a steel ball located inside. Movement of this ball transmits a vibration into the airways, helping to mobilize secretions. The patient inhales slowly, holds his or her breath for 2 to 3 seconds, and then exhales into the stem of the device. The patient must suppress the urge to cough. This process is repeated for 5 to 10 breaths. At this point, the patient is ready for the mucus elimination process. The patient inhales slowly but fully. The breath is again held for a few seconds, and then the patient exhales forcefully through the device. This forceful elimination moves the mucus up to the mouth to be expelled by a cough. If the cough is not successful, the patient may try a "huffing" maneuver.

THERAPEUTIC CONCERNS WITH DRUGS FOR RESPIRATORY DISORDERS

Patients with respiratory illnesses will commonly receive drugs from any of the following categories: steroids, β_2-agonists, and anticholinergic agents. The therapeutic concerns are largely related to their side effects. Patients receiving the anticholinergic agents must be monitored for tachycardia, hypertension, and urinary retention. In addition, although dry mouth is seemingly a mild adverse effect associated with anticholinergic drugs, this adverse drug reaction becomes magnified with drug inhalation and pursed lip breathing. Dry mouth can produce swallowing difficulty, and over the long term, leads to an increased risk of dental caries. Caution should also be exercised when working with patients taking inhaled or oral steroids. Thrush and oral candidiasis are often seen with inhaled steroids; and bruising, osteoporosis, increased risk of infection, hypertension, hyperglycemia, and atrophy of skin and muscle are side effects of both formulations. Physical therapists must pay special attention to the strength and force of any manipulations and perform integumentary evaluations before and after the use of modalities.

The adverse effects associated β_2-agonists include tremor, tachycardia, hypokalemia, and hyperglycemia. Monitoring for angina is particularly important when patients are receiving these drugs. Adequate hydration is also necessary for all patients with thickened and copious amounts of mucus.

Patients with respiratory illnesses may experience significant dyspnea and diminished exercise tolerance related to muscle weakness, cardiac impairment, and hypoxemia. Pulmonary rehabilitation programs have been developed to address some of these impairments. Although these programs vary, they usually consist of exercise training, education, and behavior modification. Aerobic training, emphasizing endurance training, and respiratory muscle strengthening form the core of these programs. Several clinical trials have shown that these programs improve health status and increase exercise tolerance but may have little effect on mortality.[60]

In addition to demonstrating the merits of regular exercise, a few centers have started collecting data on how the bronchodilators affect exercise hemodynamics and performance.[79] Both β_2-agonists and anticholinergic drugs are expected to raise heart rate both during rest and exercise. However, studies have shown that only the β_2-agonist fenoterol, and not the anticholinergic drug oxitropium, produced increases in heart rate and a decrease in P_{AO_2} at rest. During exercise these differences were not observed, and both drugs were equally effective in attenuating exercise-induced elevations in right heart afterloads (pulmonary artery pressure, pulmonary capillary wedge pressure, and right atrial pressure). Normally, in COPD these values increase during exercise, even in the absence of cardiac disease because trapped air in the peripheral airways leads to end-expiratory positive airway pressure. Improvement in pulmonary mechanics with the bronchodilators leads to a fall of intrathoracic pressure, followed by a fall in capillary wedge pressure. A similar study also indicated that there was no difference in dyspnea scoring after walking and no difference in the distance walked in 12 minutes with either albuterol or ipratropium.[80]

Although the anticholinergics and the β_2-agonists appear equally effective during exercise, there is one drug that may improve performance beyond the individual's standard drug therapy.[81] The unlikely candidate is the opiate morphine. Patients with COPD are often limited by breathlessness because of the increased work of breathing. It is thought that morphine reduces the ventilatory drive in response to elevated CO_2, hypoxia, and exercise. The reduced respiratory effort may reduce shortness of breath. In addition, morphine produces a sedating effect that reduces anxiety. When a low dose of morphine is administered along with prochlorperazine for relief of nausea, there is a significant reduction in breathlessness along with an increase in walking distance and an increase in maximum oxygen consumption of 20%. It is significant that in addition to being used for nausea, prochlorperazine is also a "stimulant of the hypoxic response." Similar results have been reported with another opiate, dihydrocodeine.[82] However, other studies have not demonstrated an opiate effect on exercise, and given concerns regarding respiratory depression, reduced arterial oxygen saturation, and the potential for producing addiction and altering mental function, more work in this area is needed before an opiate can be recommended for improving exercise tolerance or functional abilities.

ACTIVITIES 9

■ 1. A 50-year-old woman with a history of asthma reports increasing shortness of breath (SOB) and wheezing over the past few days. She has increased the use of her inhalers to approximately six times per day. She reported disposing of her prednisone last month because she was "gaining weight."

Medical History
Asthma × 10 years, heartburn, hypertension (HTN) × 2 years

Social History
Alcohol: two beers/day, tobacco use:
1 pack/day; divorced mother of two teenagers; employed in the housekeeping department of a large city-managed hospital

Meds
Albuterol metered-dose inhaler (MDI) 2 puffs q4-6h prn, lisinopril (started 2 weeks ago), cimetidine, prednisone

Vital Signs
Blood pressure, 160/90 mm Hg; pulse, 120 beats/min; respiratory rate, 30 breaths/min; temperature, 98.7° F, weight, 150 lb

Chest
Expiratory wheezes bilaterally; chest x-ray film shows hyperinflated lungs with air trapping

Labs
Sodium concentration, 140 mEq/L; potassium concentration, 3.2 mEq/L; chloride concentration, 105 mEq/L; blood urea nitrogen level, 17 mg/dL; serum creatinine level, 1.0 mg/dL; glucose level, 110 mg/dL; hemoglobin, 14.6 g/dL; platelets, 200,000/mm^3; white blood cell (WBC) count, 7000/mm^3

FEV_1
40%

Arterial Blood Gases
Pao_2, 60 mm Hg; $Paco_2$ 50 mm Hg; pH 7.30, bicarbonate level, 25 mEq/L

Questions

a. What could have caused the patient's increased wheezing?
b. What are the immediate pharmacological goals for this patient and how should they be achieved?
c. What pharmacological interventions would you recommend for the patient after this acute exacerbation is controlled?
d. How will you monitor the efficacy and adverse effects of your treatment plan (after the acute attack subsides) and how will you address compliance issues with this patient? Why should you monitor the heart rate in this patient and what response would warrant a call to the physician?
e. This patient desires to make major lifestyle changes (i.e., lose weight, stop smoking, and exercise). What advice do you have for her regarding how to avoid exercise-induced asthma?

■ 2. A 72-year-old man has had severe COPD for the last 10 years. His FEV_1 is approximately 35% of predicted value. He is taking ipratropium, albuterol, and an inhaled corticosteroid. This patient stopped smoking 1 year ago, but his illness has progressed and he is now having dyspnea at rest. On clinical examination, he has some peripheral lower extremity edema and elevated jugular venous pressure. Lung fields are clear at this moment. Blood gases show a Pao_2 of 52 mm Hg, $Paco_2$ of 52 mm Hg, Sao_2 of 89%, and a pH of 7.32. Would oxygen therapy be recommended for this patient? What other advice should the patient receive regarding use of the three inhalers?

■ 3. A 15-year-old boy with CF has been referred to your clinic for deconditioning. He has just recovered from a severe bacterial infection and needs help developing an exercise program. Discuss what category of medications he might be receiving and also provide him with some general exercise guidelines, given his medical status.

References

1. Page CP, Hoffman BB. Drugs and the pulmonary system. In: Page C, Curtis AB, Sutter MC, Walker MJ, Hoffman BB, eds. *Integrated Pharmacology.* 2nd ed. Philadelphia: Mosby; 2002: 415-435.
2. Guyton AC, Hall JE. *Textbook of Medical Physiology.* 10th ed. Philadelphia: WB Saunders Company; 2000.
3. O'Shaughnessy KM. Respiratory system. In: Bennett PB, Brown L, eds. *General Pharmacology.* 9th ed. New York: Churchill Livingstone; 2003:549-564.
4. Rang HP, Dale MM, Ritter JM, Moore JL. *Pharmacology.* 5th ed. New York: Churchill Livingstone; 2003.
5. Barnes PJ. Pharmacology of airway smooth muscle. *Am J Respir Crit Care Med.* 1998;158(5):S123-S132.
6. Waller DG, Renwick AG, Hillier K. *Medical Pharmacology and Therapeutics.* New York: WB Saunders; 2001.
7. Kelly HW, Ahrens RC, Holmes M, et al. Evaluation of particle size distribution of salmeterol administered via metered-dose inhaler with and without valved holding chambers. *Ann Allergy Asthma Immunol.* 2001;87(6):482-487.
8. Usmani OS, Biddiscombe MF, Nightingale JA, Underwood SR, Barnes PJ. Effects of bronchodilator particle size in asthmatic patients using monodisperse aerosols. *J Appl Physiol.* 2003;95(5):2106-2112.
9. Epstein S, Maidenberg A, Hallett D, Khan K, Chapman KR. Patient handling of a dry-powder inhaler in clinical practice. *Chest.* 2001;120(5):1480-1484.
10. Golish J, Curtis-McCarthy P, McCarthy K, et al. Albuterol delivered by metered-dose inhaler (MDI), MDI with spacer, and Rotahaler device: a comparison of efficacy and safety. *J Asthma.* 1998;35(4):373-379.
11. Chapman KR, Walker L, Cluley S, Fabbri L. Improving patient compliance with asthma therapy. *Respir Med.* 2000;94(1):2-9.
12. Kelly HW. Comparison of two methods of delivering continuously nebulized albuterol. *Ann Pharmacother.* 2003;37(1):23-26.
13. Cockcroft DW, Swystun VA. Asthma control versus asthma severity. *J Allergy Clin Immunol.* 1996;98(6):1016-1018.
14. Cockcroft DW, Swystun VA. Functional antagonism: tolerance produced by inhaled beta 2 agonists. *Thorax.* 1996;51(10):1051-1056.
15. Nelson JA, Strauss L, Skowronski M, Ciufo R, Novak R, McFadden ER. Effect of long-term salmeterol treatment on exercise-induced asthma. *N Engl J Med.* 1998; 339(3):141-146.
16. Langley SJ, Masterson CM, Batty EP, Woodcock A. Bronchodilator response to salbutamol after chronic dosing with salmeterol or placebo. *Eur Respir J.* 1998; 11(5):1081-1085.
17. Drugs for asthma. *Med Lett Drugs Ther.* 1999;41(1044): 5-10.
18. O'Shaughnessy KM. Cholinergic and antimuscarinic (anticholinergic) mechanisms and drugs. In: Bennett PN, Brown MJ, eds. *Clinical Pharmacology.* 9th ed. Philadelphia: Churchill Livingstone; 2003:433-446.
19. Qureshi F, Pestian J, Davis P, Zaritsky A. Effect of nebulized ipratropium on the hospitalization rates of children with asthma. *N Engl J Med.* 1998;339(15):1030-1035.
20. Suissa S, Ernst P, Benayoun S, Baltzan M, Cai B. Low-dose inhaled corticosteroids and the prevention of death from asthma. *N Engl J Med.* 2000;343(5):332-336.
21. A combination of fluticasone and salmeterol for asthma. *Med Lett Drugs Ther.* 2001;43(1102):31-33.
22. Woolcock A. Comparison of addition of salmeterol to inhaled steroids with doubling of the dose of inhaled steroids. *Am J Respir Crit Care Med.* 1996;153:1481-1488.
23. Shrewsbury S, Pyke S, Britton M. Meta-analysis of increased dose of inhaled steroid or addition of salmeterol in symptomatic asthma (MIASMA). *BMJ.* 2000;320(7246):1368-1373.
24. Calhoun WJ, Nelson HS, Nathan RA, et al. Comparison of fluticasone propionate-salmeterol combination therapy and montelukast in patients who are symptomatic on short-acting beta(2)-agonists alone. *Am J Respir Crit Care Med.* 2001;164(5):759-763.
25. Silverstein MD, Yunginger JW, Reed CE, et al. Attained adult height after childhood asthma: effect of glucocorticoid therapy. *J Allergy Clin Immunol.* 1997;99(4): 466-474.
26. Efthimiou J, Barnes PJ. Effect of inhaled corticosteroids on bones and growth. *Eur Respir J.* 1998;11(5):1167-1177.
27. Wong CA, Walsh LJ, Smith CJ, et al. Inhaled corticosteroid use and bone-mineral density in patients with asthma. *Lancet.* 2000;355(9213):1399-1403.

28. Casale TB, Nelson HS, Stricker WE, Raff H, Newman KB. Suppression of hypothalamic-pituitary-adrenal axis activity with inhaled flunisolide and fluticasone propionate in adult asthma patients. *Ann Allergy Asthma Immunol.* 2001;87(5):379-385.

29. Barnes PJ, Pedersen S, Busse WW. Efficacy and safety of inhaled corticosteroids. *Am J Respir Crit Care Med.* 1998; 157(3):S1-S53.

30. Kelly HW, Nelson HS. Potential adverse effects of the inhaled corticosteroids. *J Allergy Clin Immunol.* 2003; 112(3):469-478.

31. Pizzichini E, Leff JA, Reiss TF, et al. Montelukast reduces airway eosinophilic inflammation in asthma: a randomized, controlled trial. *Eur Respir J.* 1999;14(1):12-18.

32. Sandrini A, Ferreira IM, Gutierrez C, Jardim JR, Zamel N, Chapman KR. Effect of montelukast on exhaled nitric oxide and nonvolatile markers of inflammation in mild asthma. *Chest.* 2003;124(4):1334-1340.

33. Barnes PJ. Anti-leukotrienes: here to stay? *Curr Opin Pharmacol.* 2003;3(3):257-263.

34. Simons FE, Villa JR, Lee BW, et al. Montelukast added to budesonide in children with persistent asthma: a randomized, double-blind, crossover study. *J Pediatr.* 2001;138(5):694-698.

35. Kavuru MS, Subramony R, Vann AR. Antileukotrienes and asthma: alternative or adjunct to inhaled steroids? *Cleve Clin J Med.* 1998;65(10):519-526.

36. Barnes PJ, Wei LX, Reiss TF, et al. Analysis of montelukast in mild persistent asthmatic patients with near-normal lung function. *Respir Med.* 2001;95(5):379-386.

37. Lipworth BJ. Leukotriene-receptor antagonists. *Lancet.* 1999;353:57-62.

38. Reiss TF. Montelukast, a once daily leukotriene receptor antagonist in the treatment of chronic asthma; a multicenter randomized, double blind trial. *Arch Intern Med.* 1998;158:1213-1220.

39. Weinberger M, Hendeles L. Drug therapy: theophylline in asthma. *N Engl J Med.* 1996;334(21):1380-1388.

40. Tan RA, Spector SL. Exercise-induced asthma: diagnosis and management. *Ann Allergy Asthma Immunol.* 2002;89:226-236.

41. Bronsky EA, Yegen U, Yeh CM, Larsen LV, Cioppa GD. Formoterol provides long-lasting protection against exercise-induced bronchospasm. *Ann Allergy Asthma Immunol.* 2002;89:407-412.

42. Formoterol (Foradil Aerolizer) for asthma. *Med Lett Drugs Ther.* 2001;43(1104):39-40.

43. Kelly KD, Spooner CH, Rowe BH. Nedocromil sodium versus sodium cromoglycate in treatment of exercise-induced bronchoconstriction: a systematic review. *Eur Respir J.* 2001;17:39-45.

44. Leff JA, Busse WW, Pearlman D, et al. Montelukast, a leukotriene-receptor antagonist, for the treatment of mild asthma and exercise-induced bronchoconstriction. *N Engl J Med.* 1998;339(3):147-152.

45. Villaran C, O'Neill SJ, Helbling A, et al. Montelukast versus salmeterol in patients with asthma and exercise-induced bronchoconstriction. Montelukast/Salmeterol Exercise Study Group. *J Allergy Clin Immunol.* 1999; 104(1):547-553.

46. Kemp JP, Dockhorn RJ, Shapiro GG, et al. Montelukast once daily inhibits exercise-induced bronchoconstriction in 6- to 14-year old children with asthma. *J Pediatr.* 1998; 133(3):424-428.

47. Martineau L, Horan MA, Rothwell NJ, Little RA. Salbutamol, a β2-adrenoceptor agonist, increases skeletal muscle strength in young men. *Clin Sci.* 1992;83:615-621.

48. van Baak MA, Mayer LH, Kempinski RE, Hartgens F. Effect of salbutamol on muscle strength and endurance performance in nonasthmatic men. *Med Sci Sports Exerc.* 2000;32(7):1300-1306.

49. Goubault C, Perault MC, Leleu E, et al. Effects of inhaled salbutamol in exercising non-asthmatic athletes. *Thorax.* 2001;56:675-679.

50. McKenzie DC, Stewart IB, Fitch KD. The asthmatic athlete, inhaled beta agonists, and performance. *Clin J Sport Med.* 2002;12(4):225-228.

51. Over-the-counter (OTC) cough remedies. *Med Lett Drugs Ther.* 2001;43(1100):23-25.

52. Drugs for allergic disorders. *Treat Guidel Med Lett.* 2003;1(15):93-100.

53. Montelukast (Singulair) for allergic rhinitis. *Med Lett Drugs Ther.* 2003;45(1152):21-22.

54. Nayak AS, Philip G, Lu S, Malice MP, Reiss TF. Efficacy and tolerability of montelukast alone or in combination with loratadine in seasonal allergic rhinitis: a multicenter, randomized, double-blind, placebo-controlled trial performed in the fall. *Ann Allergy Asthma Immunol.* 2002;88(6):592-600.

55. Harms HK, Matouk E, Tournier G, von der Hardt H, Weller PH, Romano L. Multicenter, open-label study of recombinant human DNase in cystic fibrosis patients with moderate lung disease. *Pediatr Pulmonol.* 1998;26:155-161.

56. Johnson CA, Butler SM, Konstan MW, Breen TJ, Morgan WJ. Estimating effectiveness in an observational study: a case study of dornase alfa in cystic fibrosis. *J Pediatr.* 1999;134(6):734-739.

57. Man SF, McAlister FA, Anthonisen NR, Sin DD. Contemporary management of chronic obstructive pulmonary disease. *JAMA.* 2003;290:2313-2316.

58. Fiore MC, Smith SS, Jorenby DE, Baker TB. The effectiveness of the nicotine patch for smoking cessation: a meta-analysis. *JAMA.* 1994;271(24):1940-1947.

59. Jorenby DE, Smith SS, Fiore MC, et al. Varying nicotine patch dose and type of smoking cessation counseling. *JAMA.* 1995;274(17):1347-1352.

60. Sin DD, McAlister FA, Man SF, Anthonisen NR. Contemporary management of chronic obstructive pulmonary disease. *JAMA.* 2003;290(17):2301-2312.

61. Tennant RC, Erin EM, Barnes PJ, Hansel TT. Long-acting β2-adrenoceptor agonists or tiotropium bromide for patients with COPD: is combination therapy justified? *Curr Opin Pharmacol.* 2003;3:270-276.

62. D'Urzo AD, De Salvo MC, Ramirez-Rivera A, et al. In patients with COPD, treatment with a combination of formoterol and ipratropium is more effective than a combination of salbutamol and ipratropium. *Chest.* 2001; 119:1347-1356.

63. Boushey HA. Glucocorticoid therapy for chronic obstructive pulmonary disease. *N Engl J Med.* 1999; 340(25):1990-1991.

64. Callahan CM, Dittus RS, Katz BP. Oral corticosteroid therapy for patients with stable chronic obstructive pulmonary disease. *Ann Intern Med.* 1991;114:216-223.

65. Lung Health Study Research Group. Effect of inhaled triamcinolone on the decline in pulmonary function in chronic obstructive pulmonary disease. *N Engl J Med.* 2000;343:1902-1909.

66. Burge PS, Calverley PM, Jones PW, Spencer S, Anderson JA, Maslen TK. Randomised, double blind, placebo controlled study of fluticasone propionate in patients with moderate to severe chronic obstructive pulmonary disease: the ISOLDE trial. *BMJ.* 2000; 320:1297-1303.

67. Vestbo J, Sorensen T, Lange P, Brix A, Torre P, Viskum K. Long-term effect of inhaled budesonide in mild and moderate chronic obstructive pulmonary disease: a randomised controlled trial. *Lancet.* 1999;353:1819-1823.

68. Calverley PM, Pauwels R, Vestbo J, et al. Combined salmeterol and fluticasone in the treatment of chronic obstructive pulmonary disease: a randomised controlled trial. *Lancet.* 2003;361:449-456.

69. Panning CA, DeBisschop M. Tiotropium: an inhaled, long-acting anticholinergic drug for chronic obstructive pulmonary disease. *Pharmacotherapy.* 2003;23(2):183-189.

70. Rennard SI. Chronic obstructive pulmonary disease. In: Carruthers SG, Hoffman BB, Melmon KL, Nierenberg DW, eds. *Clinical Pharmacology: Basic Principles in Therapeutics.* 4th ed. New York: McGraw-Hill; 2000.

71. Tarpy SP, Celli BR. Current concepts: long-term oxygen therapy. *N Engl J Med.* 1995;333(11):710-714.

72. Kunzelmann K, Mall M. Pharmacotherapy of the ion transport defect in cystic fibrosis. *Clin Exp Pharmacol Physiol.* 2001;28:857-867.

73. Davis PB. Cystic fibrosis. *Pediatr Rev.* 2001;22(8):257-264.

74. Bennett WD. Effect of beta-adrenergic agonists on mucociliary clearance. *J Allergy Clin Immunol.* 2002; 110(suppl 6):S291-S297.

75. Jaffe A, Balfour-Lynn IM. Treatment of severe small airways disease in children with cystic fibrosis: alternatives to corticosteroids. *Paediatr Drugs.* 2002;4(6):381-389.

76. Arens R, Gozal D, Omlin KJ, et al. Comparison of high frequency chest compression and conventional chest physiotherapy in hospitalized patients with cystic fibrosis. *Am J Respir Crit Care Med.* 1994;150(4):1154-1157.

77. McIlwaine PM, Wong LT, Peacock D, Davidson AG. Long-term comparative trial of positive expiratory pressure versus oscillating positive expiratory pressure (flutter) physiotherapy in the treatment of cystic fibrosis. *J Pediatr.* 2001;138(6):845-850.

78. Fink JB, Mahlmeister MJ. High-frequency oscillation of the airway and chest wall. *Respir Care.* 2002;47(7):797-807.

79. Saito S, Miyamoto K, Nishimura M, et al. Effects of inhaled bronchodilators on pulmonary hemodynamics at rest and during exercise in patients with COPD. *Chest.* 1999;115(2):376-382.

80. Blosser SA, Maxwell SL, Reeves-Hosche MK, Localio AR, Zwillich CW. Is an anticholinergic agent superior to a beta 2-agonist in improving dyspnea and exercise limitation in COPD? *Chest.* 1995;108:730-735.

81. Light RW, Stansbury DW, Webster JS. Effect of 30 mg of morphine alone or with promethazine or prochlorperazine on the exercise capacity of patients with COPD. *Chest.* 1996;109(4):975- 981.

82. Woodcock A, Gross ER, Gellert A, Shah S, Johnson MJ, Geddes DM. Effects of dihydrocodeine, alcohol, and caffeine on breathlessness and exercise tolerance in patients with chronic obstructive lung disease and normal blood gases. *N Engl J Med.* 1981;305(27):1611-1616.

CHAPTER 10

DRUGS FOR GASTROINTESTINAL TRACT DISORDERS

PHYSIOLOGICAL CONTROL OF DIGESTION

Control of digestion represents a multisystem effort involving neuronal and hormonal regulation. Input from all of these systems coordinates the three phases of digestion.

Neuronal Control

The gastrointestinal (GI) tract can be viewed as a long, hollow tube surrounded by strong smooth muscle that propels food from one end to the other. Most of its length consists of five layers: an inner mucosal layer, a submucosal layer, circular smooth muscle, longitudinal smooth muscle, and an outer serosal layer (peritoneum) continuous with the mesentery.[1] Two interconnected neural plexuses, which together are known as the enteric nervous system, contained within the wall of the GI tract provide neural input for smooth muscle contraction.[2] The myenteric plexus is located between the circular muscle and the longitudinal muscle layers, and the submucosal plexus is located between the mucosal layer and the circular muscle layers. Both plexuses receive preganglionic input from the parasympathetic fibers of the vagus nerve where most of the fibers are cholinergic and excitatory, although some are inhibitory. There is also parasympathetic innervation to the colon from the sacral segments of the spinal cord via the pelvic nerve. The neurons

within the plexus secrete acetylcholine (Ach) and norepinephrine, but also serotonin, purines, nitric oxide, and several peptides. The neural plexuses are concerned mainly with GI motility, but they also communicate with mechanoreceptors that monitor wall stretch and chemoreceptors that check the osmolality, pH, and chemical composition of the contents.

The sympathetic system innervates the GI tract through the thoracic ganglia and the celiac, superior mesenteric, and inferior mesenteric ganglia. Control is exerted mainly by influencing the neural activity of the plexuses. The sympathetic system controls mucus secretion, decreases motility, and increases sphincter function. This system also increases the vascular smooth muscle tone of the vessels supplying the GI tract.

Hormonal Control

The GI tract is considered an endocrine organ because it produces hormones that pass through the portal circulation into the general circulation, only to return to exert influence on their organ of origin. One of the most important hormones produced by the GI tract is gastrin. Gastrin is produced by the mucosal G cells of the gastric antrum and duodenum. Its primary function is to stimulate gastric acid secretion from the parietal cells, which aid in digestion of food, particularly in the breakdown of protein. Gastrin also increases pepsinogen (which becomes pepsin when exposed to acid, another proteolytic enzyme) secretion, increases gastric blood flow, and increases gastric smooth muscle contraction. Growth of the mucosa of the stomach and small and large intestine is facilitated by gastrin, probably as a protective mechanism against the acidity. The stimulus for gastrin production is vagal stimulation, which results from intake of amino acids, alcohol, and calcium; whereas inhibition occurs in response to excessive acidity (pH below 2.5).

Secretin is another GI hormone that is secreted by S cells in the mucosa of the duodenum and jejunum. This hormone is released and activated when chyme enters the intestine with a pH less than 3.0. Secretin stimulates the pancreas to secrete a bicarbonate-containing solution. This is responsible for increasing the pH as foodstuff enters the intestine.

Cholecystokinin is secreted from the duodenum and jejunum, particularly when products of protein digestion and fatty acids arrive in the area. This hormone stimulates contraction of the gallbladder to release its bicarbonate contents into the small intestine also stimulates the secretion of pancreatic enzymes. The pancreatic enzymes include trypsin, chymotrypsin, carboxypeptidase, and elastase. Pancreatic lipase is involved in the breakdown of triglycerides, forming micelles for easier absorption, and pancreatic amylase is the enzyme that breaks down carbohydrate.

Two other important hormones are gastric inhibitory peptide and motilin. Gastric inhibitory peptide is released from the intestinal mucosa in response to glucose and fats. It turns off gastric acid secretion in the stomach as the chyme passes into the intestine. Motilin stimulates intestinal motility.

Phases of Digestion

There are three main phases of digestion, the first of which begins even before food enters the mouth.[3] This is the cephalic or psychic neural phase. The smell, sight, or anticipation of food initiates the release of acid in the stomach. The parietal cells secrete acid to keep the pH between 1 and 4 for the denaturing of protein, the chief cells secrete pepsinogen, and the mucoid cells secrete mucus that serves to protect the surface cells of the stomach from the digestive properties of the acid and enzymes.

The next phase is called *the gastric phase*. It begins when food comes into contact with the antrum. Gastrin is released as a result of stretching. Gastrin conveys information to the upper parts of the stomach to increase secretion of gastric acid. The third phase begins when the chyme enters the duodenum and is referred to as *the intestinal phase*. During this phase the proteolytic enzyme activity in the stomach decreases and acid secretion lessens. As the food moves into the intestine, a bicarbonate solution and the pancreatic enzymes are released to further aid in digestion and absorption.

ACID-RELATED DISEASE AND ITS TREATMENT

Because the parietal cell secretes acid, it has become the target of many drugs for the treatment of acid-related disorders. The wall of the parietal cell contains three receptors, one for each of the following chemicals: Ach, histamine, and gastrin (Figure 10-1).[4] When histamine occupies the receptor, a cascade of events is initiated that results in adenosine triphosphate conversion into cyclic adenosine monophosphate, providing the energy for the proton (acid) pump. When either Ach or gastrin occupies the receptor, the signal to initiate the production of acid is the calcium ion. The proton pump is located in the parietal cell and can be blocked by histamine blockers, anticholinergic agents, and drugs called *proton pump inhibitors* (PPIs).

The pump itself transports chloride (Cl^-) into the stomach lumen along with potassium (K^+). The K^+ is then exchanged for hydrogen (H^+) from within the cell by the energy derived from the K^+/H^+-ATPase pump (Figure 10-2). The actual acid is obtained from the combination of carbon dioxide and water to yield carbonic acid, which then dissociates into H^+ and a bicarbonate ion. The enzyme that catalyzes the binding of carbon dioxide and water is called *carbonic anhydrase*. This pump is inhibited by prostaglandins E_2 and I_2, which also stimulate mucus and bicarbonate secretion.

Disease Related to Excess Acid Production

Excess acid secretion is related to several diseases of the GI tract. Gastroesophageal reflux disease (GERD) occurs when there is an upward movement of gastric contents into the esophagus.[5] This results

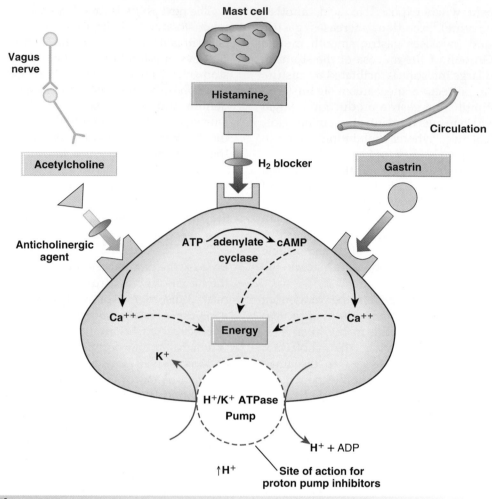

Figure 10-1

Parietal cell stimulation and secretion. *ADP,* Adenosine diphosphate; *ATP,* adenosine triphosphate; *cAMP,* cyclic adenosine monophosphate; H^+, hydrogen; H_2, histamine 2; K^+, potassium. (From Lilley LL, Harrington S, Snyder JS, eds. *Pharmacology and the Nursing Process.* 4th ed. St. Louis: Mosby; 2005.)

from a transient relaxation of the lower esophageal sphincter. It may result from gastric distension after a large meal or delayed gastric emptying and may increase in frequency when alcohol or fatty food is consumed. The refluxed material is usually returned to the stomach by means of peristaltic waves. Regular reflux produces a mucosal injury to the esophagus, resulting in hyperemia, inflammation, and heartburn. Other symptoms include belching and pain in the retrosternal or epigastric area, which may radiate to the throat, shoulder, or back. Pain usually occurs soon after eating and is exacerbated by bending at the waist, lying down, or anything that increases intraabdominal pressure such as a tight belt or waistband.

Persistent GERD can lead to Barrett's esophagus,[6] in which the esophagus displays strictures, scar tissue, spasms, and edema caused by repeated injury to the mucosa. Barrett's esophagus is associated with an increased risk of esophageal cancer.

Peptic ulcer disease describes a group of ulcerative disorders that occur in the upper GI tract (stomach and duodenum). An ulcer can affect one or all the layers of the stomach and duodenum. It may penetrate only the mucosal surface, or it can extend into the smooth muscle layers. Healing can

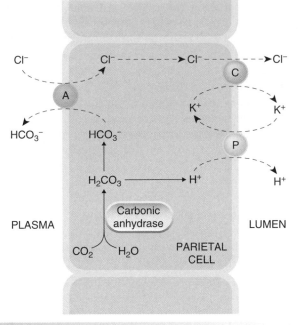

Figure 10-2

A schematic illustration of the secretion of hydrochloric acid by the gastric parietal cell. Secretion involves a proton pump *(P)*, which is an H^+/K^+-ATPase pump, a symport carrier *(C)* for potassium *(K$^+$)* and chlorine *(Cl$^-$)*, and an antiport *(A)*, which exchanges Cl^- and HCO_3^-. A Na^+/H^+ antiport at the interface with the plasma may also have a role (not shown). (From Rang HP, Dale MM, Ritter JM, Moore JL. *Pharmacology*. 5th ed. New York: Churchill Livingstone; 2003.)

occur, initially with scar tissue, and later, with a new muscle layer that is prone to further ulceration. Many cases of peptic ulcer disease result from *Helicobacter pylori* infection.[7] This is a Gram-negative bacillus that causes chronic gastritis. Gastritis and ulceration result from the host immune responses to eradicate the organism, which induces proinflammatory cytokine expression and inflammation, as well as producing a reduction in somatostatin levels.[8] Somatostatin inversely regulates gastrin production. Therefore this bacterium indirectly increases gastrin and subsequent acid release. Aspirin and nonsteroidal antiinflammatory drugs (NSAIDs) also account for many gastric and duodenal ulcers.

Pharmacological Management (Acid-Suppressive Drugs)

Antacids, histamine blockers, and PPIs are the primary drugs used to suppress gastric hyper-

acidity. They represent three distinct mechanisms of action and therefore may be used in combination for more effective treatment. Specifically, antacids can be administered along with histamine blockers, although for optimal results, the histamine blockers need to be taken at least 1 hour before the antacids.

Antacids

The use of antacids dates back to the ancient Greeks in the first century AD.[4] They would crush coral, which is calcium carbonate (the active ingredient in Tums), and use it to treat heartburn. Even though some excellent medications for acid conditions are available today, many people continue to take the over-the-counter (OTC) antacid formulations.

There are several basic preparations: aluminum-based, magnesium-based, and calcium-based. There is also a sodium bicarbonate–based solution. The mechanism of action is to neutralize the gastric acidity. However, it is also believed that the antacids enhance gastric mucosal defensive properties by stimulating secretion of mucus, prostaglandins, and bicarbonate. These actions result in a reduction of pain and an improved resistance to irritation.

Side effects of the antacids are minimal. However, the effervescent products (e.g., Alka-Seltzer) contain a great deal of sodium and should not be used regularly if a patient is on a sodium-restricted diet. Other side effects include GI disturbances. The magnesium preparations may produce diarrhea, and both aluminum and calcium preparations can produce constipation. Some drug-drug interactions can also occur with antacids. The increase in stomach pH will reduce the absorption of acidic drugs and increase the absorption of basic drugs.

Histamine 2 Receptor Antagonists

Histamine 2 (H_2) antagonists reduce stimulated acid secretion.[9] They are able to inhibit not only histamine-stimulated release but also gastrin- and Ach-stimulated acid release, inhibiting nearly 90% of all acid secretion in the stomach. These drugs also promote the healing of ulcers, but unfortunately ulcers often reappear after therapy is stopped.

The prototypic drugs in this category include cimetidine and ranitidine.[4] These drugs are available in low doses without a prescription for self-administration. Newer H_2 antagonists include nizatidine and famotidine. They are generally well tolerated but can produce diarrhea, dizziness, muscle pain, and rashes. Hypergastrinemia has also been reported. Cimetidine can cause gynecomastia because of its affinity for the androgen receptors, and this drug also inhibits the P450 enzymes. Therefore it can slow down the metabolism of several drugs, including anticoagulants and some tricyclic antidepressants. A temporary rebound in acid secretion above pretreatment levels has been reported when these drugs are abruptly withdrawn.[10,11]

Proton Pump Inhibitors

Omeprazole (now available OTC) was the first PPI on the market.[12] It irreversibly inhibits the H^+/K^+-ATPase pump, blocking the final step in acid secretion. Other drugs in this category include lansoprazole, pantoprazole, and rabeprazole.[13] The PPIs completely block all acid secretion, both basal and stimulated, from the stomach, although they have little influence on H^+ secretion in other areas. These drugs have been approved for long-term use, but there is some concern that this type of administration will produce more GI infections because an acidic environment offers some protection against invaders.

In numerous studies omeprazole has been shown to be more effective than placebo in healing duodenal ulcers; it is also superior to H_2 receptor antagonists.[12] The superiority extends to maintenance therapy as well. PPIs are superior in preventing bleeding with stress ulceration and reduce the need for further endoscopic therapy to treat upper GI bleeding. There appears to be little difference in effectiveness between the PPIs. Side effects are minimal and similar to those of placebo or H_2 receptor blockers, but there have been some reports of *Campylobacter jejuni* enteritis and fungal infections.[14,15] There have also been some reports of cardiovascular abnormalities (angina, tachycardia, palpitations), musculoskeletal pain, and respiratory effects, mostly with lansoprazole and pantoprazole.[16]

Mucosal Protectors

A few drugs that either enhance the mucosal protective mechanisms or provide a physical boundary over the surface of an ulcer are available.

Bismuth Chelate

Bismuth chelate offers numerous protective properties against an *H. pylori*–induced ulcer.[17,18] It is believed to coat the base of the ulcer, enhance prostaglandin synthesis, and increase gastric mucous epithelial cell growth. It also has a direct toxic effect on the bacillus. Blackening of the tongue and feces, as well as nausea and vomiting, are some side effects.

Sucralfate

Sucralfate is used to protect the mucosal lining in cases of active stress ulcerations and chronic peptic ulcer disease. The term *stress ulcer* refers to a GI ulceration that develops during periods of major physiological stress.[19,20] Patients who are at high risk for this ulcer include those with large surface area burns, trauma, liver failure, and acute respiratory distress syndrome and those undergoing major surgery. They appear in approximately 5% to 10% of patients receiving intensive care and result in perforation and bleeding.

Sucralfate acts locally by binding directly to the surface of the ulcer. When it is exposed to an acid environment, the drug dissociates into aluminum hydroxide (an antacid) and sulfated sucrose. The sulfated molecules attach to the ulcer, forming a protective coating over the area. The drug is also thought to stimulate prostaglandin synthesis and mucus and bicarbonate release.

One advantage of this drug is that it stays local and therefore does not interact with other drugs in the circulation. However, the drug can decrease the absorption of other medications. This interaction can be avoided by administering sucralfate separately, at least 2 hours after administration of any other agent. Side effects are minor and include constipation and nausea.

Misoprostol

Misoprostol is a synthetic prostaglandin analog.[4] It is believed to inhibit acid secretion, enhance the production of mucus and bicarbonate, and maintain blood flow to the mucosa. Diarrhea is a common side effect.

Management of *H. pylori* Infection

The presence of *H. pylori* infection leads to chronic gastritis and peptic ulcer disease and also to GERD and gastric cancer.[21] Combination therapy is the standard regimen for eradication of *H. pylori* and treatment of the associated ulcer. Because eradication of the bacterium decreases ulcer recurrence and enhances healing, antibiotics must be combined with acid-controlling drugs.[22] If *H. pylori* is not eliminated, ulcers recur in 50% to 90% of patients after antiulcer drugs are withdrawn. One of the first regimens for eliminating the microbe included bismuth triple therapy consisting of colloidal bismuth, tetracycline, and metronidazole.[23] This regimen demonstrated eradication rates above 80%. More recently, a PPI and two antibiotics (choice of clarithromycin, amoxicillin, and metronidazole) have been used, producing an eradication rate of 90%. In fact, with good compliance, the bacterium may be eliminated in as little as 1 week. Efficacy depends on twice-a-day dosing of the PPI, not on which PPI is chosen. A quadruple regimen of the classical bismuth triple therapy plus a PPI can also be used.

Management of Nonsteroidal Antiinflammatory Drug–Induced Ulcers

The increasing trend toward administering NSAIDs and aspirin has led to a greater number of cases of peptic ulcer disease than the presence of *H. pylori* infection.[24] Long-term NSAID use leads to gastritis and ulcerations, probably through blockade of prostaglandin production (see Chapter 12).[25] In some cases *H. pylori* infection is present concomitantly with an NSAID-induced ulcer. In these cases bacterial eradication alone is not adequate to prevent further bleeding.

Treatment regimens for *H. pylori* infection with NSAID use initially include the eradication of the bacterium, followed by acid suppression therapy. NSAIDs should also be discontinued if possible. If these drugs must be continued, it is imperative to have the patient continue suppression therapy, particularly with a PPI. Misoprostol, available as a single agent or in combination with diclofenac, has been approved for the prevention of NSAID-induced ulcers, but diarrhea and abdominal cramping limit its use.[26] The PPIs are now being recommended along with a gastroprotective drug when NSAIDs are needed. An alternative is to switch to the newer cyclooxygenase-2 inhibitors that are more GI friendly but may pose additional cardiac risks.

NAUSEA AND VOMITING

Vomiting is the forceful expulsion of stomach contents through the mouth. It is usually preceded by nausea and repeated contractions of the abdominal muscles (retching). Vomiting can be a protective response to the ingestion of toxic chemicals or to an overdose of drugs but may also be an annoying or disabling side effect of medication. Vomiting also accompanies many serious disease processes.

Although antiemetic drugs are quite helpful, it is important to acknowledge that even with treatment, nausea and vomiting from chemotherapy still occur in more than 50% of patients receiving strong emetogenic drugs for cancer, such as cisplatin, and in more than 40% of patients receiving mild to moderately emetogenic drugs, such as doxorubicin and cyclophosphamide.[27] Because emesis can necessitate the withdrawal of chemotherapeutic agents, it is important that antiemetic drugs be used in conjunction with the anticancer medication regimen.

Neural Mechanisms Involved in Vomiting

Two separate areas in the medulla regulate vomiting.[28,29] The chemoreceptor trigger zone (CTZ) is located on the floor of the fourth ventricle of the cerebrum. Here it is exposed to both blood and cerebrospinal fluid where it can respond to the presence of drugs and toxins. The vomiting center, located in the dorsal reticular formation of the medulla, is responsible for the integration of signals from the GI tract, pharynx, vestibular system, and the CTZ (Figure 10-3). Hypoxia of this area produces vomiting, which accounts for events that occur during a myocardial infarction or brain ischemia caused by increased intracranial pressure. Information from abdominal organs, the liver, gallbladder, and other areas is communicated to the vomiting center through visceral afferent neurons. Mechanoreceptors located in the muscular wall of the stomach and chemoreceptors located in the mucosa of the upper GI tract also send information regarding stretch and chemical make-up of the stomach to the vomiting center. The neurotransmitters involved in vomiting include dopamine, serotonin, and opioid receptors in the GI tract and CTZ and norepinephrine and Ach receptors in the vestibular center.

Antiemetic Drugs

Antiemetic drugs are mainly used to combat nausea and vomiting produced by many chemotherapy agents and illnesses related to vestibular motion. They include anticholinergic agents, antihistamines, neuroleptic agents, prokinetic drugs, serotonin

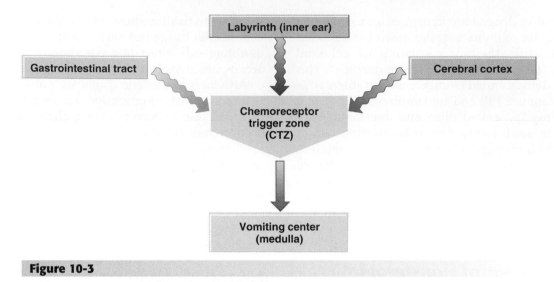

Figure 10-3

The various pathways and areas in the body that send signals to the vomiting center. (From Lilley LL, Harrington S, Snyder JS, eds. *Pharmacology and the Nursing Process*. 4th ed. St. Louis: Mosby; 2005.)

inhibitors, and tetrahydrocannabinol.[30] Steroids with or without anxiolytics may also be used.

Anticholinergics

Scopolamine is the primary anticholinergic drug used to prevent vomiting related to motion. It binds to Ach receptors on the vestibular nuclei located in the inner ear (labyrinths) and blocks the communication between this area and the vomiting center. The most common form of scopolamine is a transdermal patch with a duration of action of up to 72 hours. The patch is applied to hairless skin behind the ear at least 4 hours before travel. Side effects include dizziness, drowsiness, blurred vision, dilated pupils, dry mouth, and difficulty with urination.

Neuroleptic Drugs

Neuroleptic drugs are antipsychotic agents that block dopamine receptors in the CTZ. Many of these drugs also have anticholinergic actions. Prochlorperazine and promethazine are commonly used for preventing nausea and vomiting during or immediately after surgery. Side effects include orthostatic hypotension, tachycardia, blurred vision, dry eyes, and urinary retention. Long-term use produces extrapyramidal symptoms, akathisia, and tardive dyskinesia (see Chapter 17). Haloperidol and droperidol are commonly used for chemotherapy-induced vomiting.

Antihistamines

Cyclizine, dimenhydrinate, and diphenhydramine are H_1-blocking agents that act by inhibiting vestibular input to the CTZ.[31] Specifically, they block Ach binding to H_1 receptors in the vestibular nuclei. They are used to treat motion sickness. Dizziness and sedation are the main side effects; and therefore these drugs are not recommended for patients who will be driving.

Prokinetic Drugs

Prokinetic drugs block dopamine in the CTZ, but their primary action is to stimulate peristalsis, facilitating emptying of the stomach. Metoclopramide is used for delayed gastric emptying, GERD, and chemotherapy-related vomiting. It has both central and peripheral antiemetic effects. Side effects include sedation, diarrhea, weakness, and prolactin release—and with prolonged use—extrapyramidal signs and motor restlessness. Patients taking prokinetic drugs may also experience hypotension, hypertension, and tachycardia. Other drugs in this category include trimethobenzamide and domperidone.

Serotonin Blockers

The serotonin antagonists used to prevent emesis specifically block the serotonin receptors in the GI tract, CTZ, and vomiting center.[27] They represent one of the newest classes of drugs for the prevention of nausea and vomiting caused by cancer chemotherapy. They include dolasetron, granisetron, ondansetron, and the most recently released, palonosetron. They are equal in efficacy to a high dose of metoclopramide and can be administered in intravenous or oral formulations.[32] Side effects include headache, dizziness, and diarrhea but not extrapyramidal effects. These drugs are usually administered 30 minutes before chemotherapy and often in conjunction with a steroid (dexamethasone).

Cannabinoids

Dronabinol, a schedule II controlled substance, is a synthetic derivative of THC (delta-9-tetrahydrocannabinol) used in the treatment of chemotherapy-related emesis. It is also used as an appetite stimulant for patients with AIDS.[28] Its antiemetic effects were originally observed in patients who were using marijuana during chemotherapy. Its mechanism of action in this role is unclear, but it may possess some antiadrenergic activity and block prostaglandin synthesis. It is considered a second-line agent in the treatment of emesis because of its side effects, which include ataxia, light-headedness, blurred vision, dry mouth, weakness, tachycardia or bradycardia, and central nervous system effects such as confusion, mood changes, and anxiety.[31]

Corticosteroids

Corticosteroids are useful for decreasing emesis when mildly emetic chemotherapy drugs are administered but not with highly emetogenic agents when used alone.[30] The mechanism of action for this effect is poorly understood, but when steroids are combined with a serotonin blocker, this regimen is more effective than treatment with each drug alone. This combination is now standard practice for reducing chemotherapy-induced emesis.

Neurokinin 1 Receptor Antagonists

The category of neurokinin 1 (NK$_1$) receptor antagonists contains several compounds that are currently under study for the treatment of emesis related to chemotherapy. The focus of these drugs is to antagonize substance P.[33] Substance P binds to the tachykinin neurokinin 1 receptor and is capable of producing emesis through this mechanism. Aprepitant was recently approved by the Food and Drug Administration for use with corticosteroids and selective serotonin receptor antagonists for the treatment of acute emesis and delayed emesis (more

than 24 hours after infusion) associated with chemotherapy.[34] When taken as monotherapy, aprepitant is no more effective than the serotonin antagonists, but its usefulness is realized in combination therapy. Side effects are mild but annoying. In comparison studies, hiccups occurred in 11% of patients receiving aprepitant and 6% of patients receiving the standard regimen.

DIARRHEA

Diarrhea refers to the frequent passage of loose stools. The definition implies increased frequency, fluidity, and stool water excretion.[35] Acute diarrhea is that which appears suddenly in a previously healthy person and lasts between 3 and 14 days.[36] Frequency of defecation is three or more times per day or 200 g of stool per day, and abdominal cramping is present. Chronic diarrhea refers to diarrhea lasting more than 3 to 4 weeks in conjunction with loss of appetite, fever, nausea, weight reduction, and fatigue.

Most cases of diarrhea are due to water and electrolyte imbalances in the intestinal tract.[37] Increased secretion of electrolytes and water into the lumen, the loss of protein from the GI mucosa, and increased osmotic pressure in the intestine are all culprits. Underlying pathologic conditions associated with chronic diarrhea include irritable bowel syndrome (IBS), Crohn's disease, ulcerative colitis, bowel impaction with overflow, bacterial overgrowth, bile acid malabsorption, celiac disease, short bowel syndrome, laxative abuse, and diarrhea associated with diabetes. Other causes of fecal incontinence have to do with structural abnormalities, for example, weakness of the external anal sphincter and anorectal sensory loss, as well as use of some medications that reduce sphincter tone (anticholinergics such as tolterodine tartarate and oxybutynin and antispasticity drugs such as baclofen).[38]

Antidiarrheal Agents

Drugs that fall into the category of antidiarrheal agents include adsorbents, anticholinergics, intestinal flora modifiers, and opiates.

Adsorbents

Adsorbents coat the wall of the GI tract, bind to the diarrhea-causing bacteria, and then carry them out with the feces.[35] Examples of these agents include activated charcoal, bismuth subsalicylate, and attapulgite. The last two are commonly known as Pepto-Bismol and Kaopectate, respectively. Because bismuth subsalicylate is a salicylate similar to aspirin, it should be used with caution in children recovering from the flu or chickenpox because of the higher risk for Reye's syndrome. In addition, because it is an aspirin product, it has some of the same adverse effects, including increased bleeding time, GI bleeding, confusion associated with high doses, and hearing loss or tinnitus. The adsorbents decrease the effectiveness of many drugs, particularly digoxin, hypoglycemic drugs, and oral anticoagulants.

Anticholinergics

Anticholinergics reduce diarrhea by reducing peristalsis of the GI tract. The anticholinergic agents used for this purpose include atropine, hyoscyamine, and hyoscine.[35] They can be used in conjunction with adsorbents and opiates, but because of their side effects (Chapter 5), they are rarely the first choice for treatment.

Intestinal Flora Modifiers

Intestinal flora modifiers are bacterial products obtained from *Lactobacillus* organisms. They are normal occupants of the intestine that create an unfavorable atmosphere for the growth of certain kinds of diarrhea-causing bacteria. However, antibiotics destroy this normal flora and tip the balance in favor of the harmful bugs. *Lactobacillus acidophilus* returns the balance to normal flora and suppresses the growth of harmful organisms, and it is available as an OTC remedy.

Opiates

Several opiates act as antidiarrheal drugs: codeine, loperamide, and diphenoxylate.[37] Their mechanism of action in this venue is to decrease GI motility and propulsion. Slowing transit time increases the absorption of electrolytes and water. In addition, they can reduce pain occurring with diarrhea. Loperamide can be obtained as an OTC medication, but the others require a prescription because they cross the blood-brain barrier. The opiates can be addicting and produce respiratory depression. Side effects of the opiates include sedation, dizziness, constipation, nausea and vomiting, respiratory depression, bradycardia, hypotension, and urinary retention (see Chapter 12).

CONSTIPATION

Constipation is a movement disorder of the colon and rectum resulting in infrequent or painful defecation, hard stools, or the sense that there is incomplete evacuation. It can be a symptom of a bowel impaction or it can be due to some endocrine or neurogenic disorders. A sedentary lifestyle, a diet low in roughage or fluids, and certain medications can also be blamed. Constipation is usually managed by an improved diet, exercise, and use of laxatives. Surgical management is usually reserved for a bowel impaction, organic or structural disorders of the bowel, or cancer.

Laxatives

Nonsurgical treatment of constipation can be divided into three categories: improved fiber and fluid supplementation, increased physical activity, and pharmacological treatment. The pharmacological approach involves the use of laxatives that may act by softening the fecal consistency or increasing fecal movement through the colon and rectum. There are five basic types of laxatives and many are available as OTC medications (Figure 10-4).

Bulk-Forming Laxatives

Psyllium (Metamucil) and methylcellulose (Citrucel) act by increasing water absorption, resulting in softening and greater bulk of the intestinal contents.[35] As the fiber swells, it distends the colon. This in turn results in increased peristalsis. These are relatively safe drugs that can be used on a prolonged basis without causing dependency. They are contraindicated in patients with abdominal pain and/or nausea and vomiting and must be consumed with a full glass of water to prevent esophageal obstruction and fecal impaction.

Emollient Laxatives

Emollient laxatives are also known as fecal softeners and lubricant laxatives. Stool softeners such as docusate sodium (Colace) facilitate water and fat absorption into the stool, and the lubricant laxative, mineral oil, lubricates the fecal material and the wall of the intestine. Reabsorption of water back into the body is blocked. Side effects are minimal but can include skin rashes, decreased absorption of vitamins, and electrolyte imbalances. Staining of clothing can also occur when mineral oil is used.

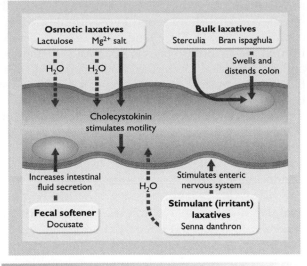

Osmotic laxatives
Lactulose   Mg^{2+} salt

Bulk laxatives
Sterculia   Bran ispaghula

Swells and distends colon

H_2O H_2O

Cholecystokinin stimulates motility

Increases intestinal fluid secretion

H_2O

Stimulates enteric nervous system

Fecal softener
Docusate

Stimulant (irritant) laxatives
Senna danthron

Figure 10-4

Mechanism of action of laxatives. Bulk laxatives absorb water, and on swelling, slowly distend the colon and increase peristaltic motility; osmotic laxatives enhance peristalsis by osmotically increasing the bowel fluid volume; stimulant (irritant) laxatives stimulate the enteric nervous system; fecal softeners increase intestinal fluid secretion. (From Page C, Curtis AB, Sutter MC, Walker MJ, Hoffman BB, eds. *Integrated Pharmacology.* 2nd ed. Philadelphia: Mosby; 2002.)

Hyperosmotic Laxatives

Hyperosmotic laxatives work primarily in the large intestine by drawing fluid into the colon. Examples include glycerin, lactulose, and polyethylene glycol. Lactulose is a synthetic sugar that is not digested in the stomach or absorbed in the small intestine. However, it is metabolized in the large intestine into a hyperosmotic solution that draws fluid into the colon. Polyethylene glycol is a laxative used before diagnostic or surgical bowel procedures, but it is also prescribed for pediatric constipation.[39] It is a very potent laxative, producing almost complete gastric emptying. Adverse events associated with these agents include abdominal bloating, rectal irritation, and electrolyte abnormalities.

Saline Laxatives

Saline laxatives, like the hyperosmotic laxatives, increase osmotic pressure by increasing water and electrolyte secretions into the small bowel.[40] What results is a very watery stool, which in turn stimulates peristalsis. Magnesium sulfate, magnesium

citrate, and sodium phosphate (Fleet Enema) are drugs within this category.

Stimulant Laxatives

Stimulant laxatives include natural extracts of plant products and also synthetic chemical agents that stimulate intestinal peristalsis.[35] Senna is a commonly used OTC stimulant. It facilitates propulsive motility of the colon by stimulating the enteric nervous system. Other examples include casanthranol and bisacodyl. Long-term administration of these products should be avoided because dependence may occur, as well as a "cathartic colon," which involves damage to the intestinal cells and progressive loss of colon function. Ultimately, the colon has reduced motility and dilation, and underlying intestinal disease is exacerbated.

IRRITABLE BOWEL SYNDROME

IBS is characterized by a constellation of symptoms including intermittent bouts of abdominal pain, bloating, diarrhea, and constipation.[41,42] In addition, several other complaints have been documented with this disorder, including sleep disturbances, depression, fibromyalgia, rheumatological findings, and genitourinary dysfunction. Two subcategories exist: diarrhea-predominant and constipation-predominant IBS, but these are rather poorly delineated.

The etiology and pathophysiology of IBS are unclear.[42] There is no biological marker, and no structural or physiological abnormalities are uniform among patients with IBS. There seems to be a genetic predisposition in some families, but in 30% of cases, patients had a preceding gastroenteric infection. Patients do share a dysregulation of intestinal motor and sensory function, with hypersensitivity of the GI tract to normal events, alterations in fluid and electrolyte balance in the bowel, and neuroendocrine disorders that contribute to impaired intestinal motility. However, it is unclear whether IBS is primarily a central nervous system disorder with changes directed toward the intestines or an intestinal disorder in which abnormal afferent information is sent to the brain.

About 70% of patients have mild disease, 25% have moderate disease, and 5% have severe disease. Psychosocial difficulties along with lifestyle impairment are the factors that motivate patients to seek medical assistance.

Treatment for Irritable Bowel Syndrome

Treatment for IBS consists mainly of agents designed to control the bouts of diarrhea and constipation. Fiber supplementation is used to reduce constipation, and antispasmodics are used to treat diarrhea.

Bulking Agents

Fiber supplementation (psyllium or methylcellulose) can provide needed bulk for some patients with IBS and predominant constipation.[43] The fiber decreases transit time through the gut, reducing bile salt concentrations in the colon. Because bile salts increase colonic contractions, this indirectly reduces pain. However, some patients with IBS may respond negatively to the fiber with increased pain and bloating. For these patients, fiber should be added slowly to the diet, and a switch to soluble fiber—found in fruits, vegetables, and legumes—should be made. Patients should consume 20 to 30 grams of fiber per day.[42]

If fiber therapy does not appear to be useful, other pharmacotherapy can be recommended; however, no single drug has been proven to be effective in the majority of cases of IBS.

Antidiarrheal Agents

Some studies on IBS have indicated that the opiate analogues, diphenoxylate and loperamide, have efficacy for the treatment of diarrhea in IBS.[44] However, in a systematic review on the management of IBS, loperamide was found to be effective but not more effective than placebo for the treatment of pain and overall symptoms.[41] Fedotozine is a peripheral kappa opioid agonist (see Chapter 12) that has demonstrated effectiveness in the management of abdominal pain and may, in the future, be approved for use in IBS.[42] It is thought to normalize hypersensitivity in IBS by acting on vagal and nonvagal peripheral nerves. Last in this category is cholestyramine, a bile acid–binding agent that is normally used to lower cholesterol levels.[42] When some bile acids are eliminated, colonic contractions are reduced.

Antispasmodics

Antispasmodics used to treat IBS include drugs that act directly on the intestinal smooth muscle, anticholinergics, and calcium channel blockers.[42]

Mebeverine directly relaxes intestinal smooth muscle, and dicyclomine and hyoscyamine are anticholinergic agents. They tend to be used on an as-needed basis before meals to avoid distention and postprandial cramping. The calcium channel blockers, verapamil and nifedipine, have also been useful for some patients to reduce pain and fecal urgency. Overall, the antispasmodics decrease pain, but according to recent meta-analyses, they may not alter the symptoms of diarrhea or constipation.[41,44]

Serotonergic Agonists and Antagonists

The serotonin receptors located on the enterochromaffin cells have a role in the initiation of peristalsis.[41] Tegaserod is a partial serotonin agonist that increases intestinal motility, facilitating transit time through the bowel. It is currently recommended for short-term use in women whose primary symptom is constipation. It is recommended for women because there were more women enrolled in the clinical studies and tegaserod has questionable efficacy in men. This drug reduces bloating and abdominal pain and improves bowel habits compared with placebo. Diarrhea is the most common side effect. The drug may be temporarily withheld when diarrhea occurs. Overall, clinical trials of tegaserod demonstrate high quality in terms of methodology and show that this drug provides significant relief of global IBS symptoms compared with placebo.[43]

The serotonin receptor is also of interest in the treatment of IBS, but only in diarrhea-predominant IBS. Alosetron is a serotonin receptor antagonist that slows transit time through the GI tract.[41,45] This drug significantly reduces symptoms compared with placebo; however, in November 2000, the drug was withdrawn from the market. This resulted from reports of ischemic colitis and severe constipation leading to several hospital admissions and seven deaths. The drug was later reintroduced in June 2002 with restricted marketing for women with diarrhea-type IBS who have not responded at all to other conventional therapies. The recommended starting dose was lowered.

Other Therapies

Because stress and depression may exacerbate the symptoms of IBS, anxiolytic agents and tricyclic antidepressants (see Chapter 16) may be used in treatment.[44] Low-dose tricyclic antidepressants have been shown to be effective in reducing pain and may be useful in diarrhea-predominant IBS. This effect is probably related to the anticholinergic effects of these drugs.

Cognitive therapy and various behavioral therapies in which patients learn how to identify and manage stressful events are currently under study.[41] In a few facilities biofeedback therapy is offered to patients with IBS. Specifically, this modality is used to help patients sense changes in rectal distention and to help them regulate bowel habits (see the following section).

THERAPEUTIC CONCERNS WITH GASTROINTESTINAL AGENTS

There are few therapeutic concerns with drugs used to treat GI disorders that influence physical therapy. However, the choice of physical therapy intervention is influenced by the specific disorder or symptoms experienced by the patient. For example, exercises performed in the supine position and those that increase intraabdominal pressure should be performed with caution in patients with GERD.[46] These choices can exacerbate acid reflux, particularly if therapy is scheduled soon after a meal. In addition, bending over at the waist can increase reflux.

The other major concern for the treatment of patients with GI problems is the presence of dehydration.[36] Significant vomiting and/or diarrhea will cause fluid loss and electrolyte imbalances. Signs and symptoms of dehydration include absence of perspiration, tearing, and salivation; elevated body temperature; postural hypotension; dry skin and mucous membranes; headache; lethargy; sunken eyes; poor capillary refill; and skin turgor. Pulse may be rapid, and blood pressure may be low. Oral rehydration with a glucose-based electrolyte solution is recommended unless the patient is severely dehydrated or comatose. In those cases, intravenous fluids will be administered. Otherwise, the patient should be encouraged to drink fluids and consume some salt, either in the form of soup or saltine crackers. Orange juice or bananas can be consumed to replace potassium.

On the other end of the spectrum, patients with constipation can be helped by physical therapy. Healthy eating and regular exercise promote good bowel habits. Moderate exercise can benefit patients with IBS and also those with colitis or Crohn's disease.[47] Exercise improves gastric emptying, but intense exercise can inhibit gastric emptying and disrupt GI absorption. In some cases GI bleeding may occur.

Therapists may also find themselves involved in the treatment of constipation caused by pelvic floor dyssynergia. Approximately 50% of patients who complain of constipation have asynergic defecation. A paradoxical increase in anal pressure during straining occurs. This condition is diagnosed by the patient's inability to expel a rectal balloon and by pelvic floor magnetic resonance imaging and evacuation scintigraphy. Biofeedback techniques, including sensory retraining and electromyography, are being investigated to help synchronize evacuation.[48,49] For sensory re-education, a water-filled balloon is inserted into the rectum. It is slowly removed while the patient concentrates on its sensation while trying to relax the anal sphincter and ease its evacuation. The electromyography training is performed with either intraluminal electrodes or surface electrodes taped to the perianal skin. The patient watches the recording while first learning to relax the pelvic floor musculature. The patient also practices straining while keeping the pelvic floor muscles relaxed.

ACTIVITIES 10

■ 1. RL is a 39-year-old woman with a history of epigastric pain. She gets relief from eating and OTC antacid tablets. She has had this pain in the past but has never had medical advice about this condition. She is a 1 pack/day smoker and works as a busy executive in New York City. She runs 6 miles daily for the physical and emotional benefits. Results of her physical exam are normal except for epigastric tenderness and bilateral chondromalacia patella, which she treats with daily aspirin.

c. What is the treatment for this condition?
d. What are the physical therapy implications?
e. What should this patient know about smoking and H_2 blockers?

■ 2. You are treating a 72-year-old woman for low back pain of unknown etiology. She also complains about constipation over the last 3 months and reports taking laxatives up to three times a day. She appears otherwise healthy, watches her weight, and exercises 3 times a week.

Questions

a. List questions you would ask regarding this patient's medical history and present symptoms.
b. What is the cause of the pain?

Questions

a. List questions you would ask regarding this patient's medical history and present symptoms.
b. Why is long-term laxative use a problem?

References

1. Porth CM. Structure and function of the gastrointestinal system. In: *Essentials of Pathophysiology*. Philadelphia: Lippincott Williams & Wilkins; 2004:459-472.
2. Goyal RK, Hirano I. Mechanisms of disease: the enteric nervous system. *N Engl J Med.* 1996;334(17):1106-1115.
3. Guyton AC, Hall JE. *Textbook of Medical Physiology.* 10th ed. Philadelphia: WB Saunders Company; 2000.
4. Lilley LL, Harrington S, Snyder JS. Acid-controlling agents. In: Lilley LL, Harrington S, Snyder JS, eds. *Pharmacology and the Nursing Process.* 4th ed. St. Louis: Mosby; 2005:841-856.
5. Orlando RC. Pathogenesis of gastroesophageal reflux disease. *Am J Med Sci.* 2003;326(5):274-278.
6. Spechler SJ. Clinical manifestations and esophageal complications of GERD. *Am J Med Sci.* 2003;326(5):279-284.
7. Walsh JH, Peterson WL. Drug therapy: the treatment of *Helicobacter pylori* infection in the management of peptic ulcer disease. *N Engl J Med.* 1995;333(15):984-991.
8. Blaser MJ, Atherton JC. *Helicobacter pylori* persistence: biology and disease. *J Clin Invest.* 2004;113(3):321-333.
9. Rang HP, Dale MM, Ritter JM, Moore JL. *Pharmacology.* 5th ed. New York: Churchill Livingstone; 2003.
10. Huang JQ, Hunt RH. Pharmacological and pharmacodynamic essentials of H2-receptor antagonists and proton pump inhibitors for the practising physician. *Best Pract Res Clin Gastroenterol.* 2001;15(3):355-370.
11. Takeuchi K, Kajimura M, Kodaira M, Lin S, Hanai H, Kaneko E. Up-regulation of H2 receptor and adenylate cyclase in rabbit parietal cells during prolonged treatment with H2-receptor antagonists. *Dig Dis Sci.* 1999;44(8):1703-1709.
12. Richardson P, Hawkey CJ, Stack WA. Proton pump inhibitors. *Drugs.* 1998;56(3):307-335.
13. Esomeprazole (Nexium). *Med Lett Drugs Ther.* 2001;43(1103):36-37.
14. Neal K, Scott HM, Slack RC, Logan RF. Omeprazole as a risk factor for *Campylobacter* gastroenteritis: case-control study. *BMJ.* 1996;312:414-415.
15. Goenka MK, Kochhar R, Chakrabarti A, et al. *Candida* overgrowth after treatment of duodenal ulcer: a comparison of cimetidine, famotidine, and omeprazole. *J Clin Gastroenterol.* 1996;23(1):7-10.
16. Der G. An overview of proton pump inhibitors. *Gastroenterol Nurs.* 2003;26(5):182-190.
17. Soll AH. Medical treatment of peptic ulcer disease: practice guidelines. *JAMA.* 1996;275(8):622-629.
18. Gilster J, Bacon K, Marlink K, Sheppard B, Deveney C, Rutten M. Bismuth subsalicylate increases intracellular Ca2+, MAP-kinase activity, and cell proliferation in normal human gastric mucous epithelial cells. *Dig Dis Sci.* 2004;49(3):370-378.
19. Porth CM. Alterations in gastrointestinal function. In: Porth CM, ed. *Essentials of Pathophysiology.* Lippincott Williams & Wilkins; 2004:473-493.
20. Spirt MJ. Stress-related mucosal disease: risk factors and prophylactic therapy. *Clin Ther.* 2004;26(2):197-213.
21. Kuipers EJ, Janssen MJR, de Boer WA. Good bugs and bad bugs: indications and therapies for *Helicobacter pylori* eradication. *Curr Opin Pharmacol.* 2003;3:480-485.
22. Gisbert JP, Khorrami S, Carballo F, Calvet X, Gene E, Dominguez-Munoz JE. *H. pylori* eradication therapy vs. antisecretory non-eradication therapy (with or without long-term maintenance antisecretory therapy) for the prevention of recurrent bleeding from peptic ulcer. *Cochrane Database Syst Rev.* 2003;4(CD004062).

23. Rauws EAJ, van der Hulst RWM. The management of *H pylori* infection: most straightforward cases can be managed in primary care with eradication treatment. *BMJ*. 1998;316(7126):162-163.

24. Sung JJ. Management of nonsteroidal anti-inflammatory drug-related peptic ulcer bleeding. *Am J Med*. 2001; 110(1A):S29-S32.

25. Price AB. Pathology of drug-associated gastrointestinal disease. *Br J Clin Pharmacol*. 2003;56(5):477-482.

26. Hawkey CJ, Langman MJS. Non-steroidal anti-inflammatory drugs: overall risks and management. Complementary roles for COX-2 inhibitors and proton pump inhibitors. *Gut*. 2003;52(4):600-608.

27. Palonosetron (Aloxi) for prevention of nausea and vomiting due to cancer chemotherapy. *Med Lett Drugs Ther*. 2004;46(1179):27-28.

28. Veyrat-Follet C, Farinotti R, Palmer JL. Physiology of chemotherapy-induced emesis and antiemetic therapy. *Drugs*. 1997;53(2):206-234.

29. Hornby PJ. Central neurocircuitry associated with emesis. *Am J Med*. 2001;111(suppl 8A):106S-112S.

30. Lilley LL, Harrington S, Snyder JS. Antiemetic and antinausea agents. In: Lilley LL, Harrington S, Snyder JS, eds. *Pharmacology and the Nursing Process*. 4th ed. St. Louis: Mosby; 2005:872-882.

31. McKenry LM, Salerno E. Drugs affecting the gastrointestinal tract. In: McKenry LM, Salerno E, eds. *Mosby's Pharmacology in Nursing*. 21st ed. St Louis: Mosby; 2003:752-786.

32. Grunberg SM, Hesketh PJ. Drug therapy: control of chemotherapy-induced emesis. *N Engl J Med*. 1993; 329(24):1790-1796.

33. Hesketh PJ. Potential role of the NK1 receptor antagonists in chemotherapy-induced nausea and vomiting. *Support Care Cancer*. 2001;9:350-354.

34. Aprepitant (Emend) for prevention of nausea and vomiting due to cancer chemotherapy. *Med Lett Drugs Ther*. 2003;45(1162):62-63.

35. Lilley LL, Harrington S, Snyder JS. Antidiarrheals and laxatives. In: Lilley LL, Harrington S, Snyder JS, eds. *Pharmacology and the Nursing Process*. 4th ed. St Louis: Mosby; 2005:857-871.

36. Thielman NM, Guerrant RL. Acute infectious diarrhea. *N Engl J Med*. 2004;350:38-47.

37. Scarlett Y. Medical management of fecal incontinence. *Gastroenterology*. 2004;126:S55-S63.

38. Rao SSC. Pathophysiology of adult fecal incontinence. *Gastroenterology*. 2004;126:S14-S22.

39. Bell EA, Wall GC. Pediatric constipation therapy using guidelines and polyethylene glycol 2250. *Ann Pharmacother*. 2004;38:686-693.

40. Lembo A, Camilleri M. Current concepts in chronic constipation. *N Engl J Med*. 2003;349(14):1360-1368.

41. Brandt LJ, Bjorkman DJ, Fennerty B, et al. Systematic review on the management of irritable bowel syndrome in North America. *Am J Gastroenterol*. 2002;97(11):S7-S26.

42. Birrer RB. Irritable bowel syndrome. *Dis Mon*. 2002; 48(2):101-144.

43. Talley N. Evaluation of drug treatment in irritable bowel syndrome. *Br J Clin Pharmacol*. 2003;56(6):362-369.

44. Mertz HR. Irritable bowel syndrome. *N Engl J Med*. 2003; 349:2136-2146.

45. Mayer EA, Bradesi S. Alosetron and irritable bowel syndrome. *Expert Opin Pharmacother*. 2003;4(11):2089-2098.

46. Goodman CC. The gastrointestinal system. In: Goodman CC, Boissonnault WG, Fuller JH, eds. *Pathology Implications for the Physical Therapist*. Philadelphia: Saunders; 2003:628-665.

47. Bi L, Triadafilopoulos G. Exercise and gastrointestinal function and disease: an evidence-based review of risks and benefits. *Clin Gastroenterol Hepatol*. 2003;1(5):345-355.

48. Bassotti G, Chistolini F, Sietchiping-Nzepa F, de Roberto G, Morelli A, Chiarioni G. Biofeedback for pelvic floor dysfunction in constipation. *BMJ*. 2004;328:393-396.

49. Stessman M. Biofeedback: its role in the treatment of chronic constipation. *Gastroenterol Nurs*. 2003;26(6):251-260.

4
SECTION

Pain Control

CHAPTER 11

❦

ANESTHETIC AGENTS

❦

TYPES OF ANESTHESIA

There are three basic categories of anesthetics: general, local, and regional. Within each category, there are different modes of administration. General anesthesia may be given by the inhaled or intravenous (IV) mode. Local anesthesia can be administered through an injection or by topical administration, and regional anesthesia involves numbing a large area of the body, as in spinal anesthesia.

GENERAL ANESTHESIA

General anesthesia produces a progressive and reversible central nervous system (CNS) depression. Many different drugs are used to induce anesthesia, each with individual characteristics and different side effects. The ideal agent must produce a loss of consciousness, analgesia, amnesia, skeletal muscle relaxation, and inhibition of sensory and autonomic reflexes and must have a rapid onset.[1] In addition, it must be nontoxic and achieve the desired effect without producing hypoxia, laryngospasm, excessive tracheobronchial secretions, or respiratory depression. However, none of the anesthetic agents available today meet these criteria. Therefore it is common practice to administer several different medications in small amounts to produce the desired effects while minimizing toxic effects. This practice is called *balanced anesthesia,* and it involves administering a combination of inhaled and IV anesthetics along with narcotics and neuromuscular blocking agents.

Induction of anesthesia involves the patient passing through different levels of CNS depression.[1] The first stage is analgesia, followed by the second stage, which is delirium. In this stage consciousness is lost, and excitement and muscle activity may be marked. Rapid respirations and vomiting may occur, and breathing is irregular. The third stage is referred to as *surgical anesthesia.* It is marked by rhythmic breathing with deep respirations. The fourth stage is medullary paralysis, characterized by respiratory and cardiovascular collapse. Blood pressure falls, pupils dilate, and spontaneous breathing ceases. Anesthesia is irreversible at this point.

In today's practice of anesthesia, these phases, as described previously, are somewhat unrecognizable. Drug-induced rapid loss of consciousness, premedication, and assisted ventilation produce a blurring of these stages. Basically, the adequacy of anesthesia is now assessed by certain respiratory and cardiovascular responses.

Premedication

Premedication, before anesthesia is induced, is administered for a variety of reasons including sedation, analgesia, antiemesis, infection control, and minimization of anesthetic side effects; disease-modifying agents may also be given to control for any adverse effects on a patient's underlying medical condition.[2] Preoperative sedation with a benzodiazepine or a barbiturate may be given 1 to 2 hours before surgery. These drugs are not only effective at reducing anxiety but also provide a certain baseline sedation that facilitates a loss of consciousness with reduced anesthesia.

The patient might also receive promethazine to combat the nausea and vomiting produced by the anesthetics. This drug is an antihistamine with antiemetic, anticholinergic, and sedative properties. Recent food in the stomach poses a risk of aspiration because the normal protective airway responses are diminished during the loss of consciousness.[2] Preoperative fasting and postponing the surgery are options, but these strategies will not always guarantee an empty stomach because opioids reduce gastric mobility, nor is this practical in an emergency. Intubation along with neuromuscular paralysis can be instituted as soon as the IV anesthesia takes effect as a means of guarding against aspiration when surgery must be performed on an emergency basis.

Antimicrobial prophylaxis (usually a single intramuscular injection within an hour of the start of surgery) can decrease the incidence of infection, particularly wound infection after certain procedures, but this benefit must be weighed against the risk of allergic reactions and the development of resistant bacteria.[3,4] It is recommended for procedures associated with high infection rates such as those involving implantation of prosthetic material, those involving the gastrointestinal tract, and those involving trauma in which the wound is already dirty. Host factors such as immunosuppression or the presence of valvular and other cardiac diseases also warrant prophylaxis. The patient who has had a long preoperative hospitalization also needs prophylaxis because he or she may have been exposed to a hospital-based resistant organism.

Patients with preexisting chronic obstructive pulmonary disease (COPD) or respiratory limitations are predisposed to experience atelectasis, pneumonia, hypoxia, and respiratory failure after surgery, particularly abdominal and thoracic surgery. Pretreatment with bronchodilators and antibiotics and chest physical therapy should be standard treatment for several days before the surgery.[2] General anesthetics decrease myocardial performance, so patients with congestive heart failure (CHF) should also receive premedication to help control cardiac symptoms.

Certain medications should be discontinued before surgery (Table 11-1).[2] Diuretics can create hypovolemia and hypokalemia, which must be corrected over several days to decrease the risk of arrhythmias during surgery. In addition, diabetic patients should have their oral diabetic drugs withheld on the morning of the procedure to prevent hypoglycemia and patients who receive insulin will be asked to reduce their dose and quite possibly will receive IV glucose. Anesthetic agents can also interact with preexisting drug therapy (Table 11-2).

Inhaled Anesthesia

Commonly used inhalation agents include nitrous oxide, halothane, methoxyflurane, isoflurane, desflurane, and sevoflurane. Nitrous oxide is used primarily during dental surgery. Inhalation agents are vaporized and mixed with oxygen and then given through a mask or endotracheal tube.[5] Once gas exchange occurs in the lungs, these drugs are circulated to the brain and other organs. From there, these drugs diffuse into fats because of their great lipid solubility. Over time, these drugs diffuse back out into the general circulation and then again into the brain. This phenomenon is responsible for the hangover feeling that many patients have the day after surgery.

The degree of anesthesia is determined by a drug's concentration in the CNS. The rate at which an effective concentration of drug reaches the brain (the rate of anesthetic induction) is related to a variety of factors including solubility of the drug, concentration of drug in the inspired air, respiratory rate and depth, blood flow to the lungs, and the loss of drug through expired air. The anesthetic agent must first transfer from the alveolar air to blood and then to the brain. The rate at which this occurs depends on the solubility of the agent in the blood. The "blood:gas partition coefficient" is an index explaining the relative affinity for the drug to blood versus air. For desflurane, sevoflurane, and nitrous oxide, this index is quite low, indicating low solubility in blood (range of 0.47 to 0.69).[2] Methoxyflurane is extremely soluble and has a much higher index of 13.[6] There is an inverse relationship between solubility in blood and the rate of increase in a drug's partial pressure or tension. When a drug of low solubility is inhaled and diffuses into arterial blood, only a few molecules are required to raise its partial pressure, and arterial tension rises quickly. However, when the drug has high solubility, more molecules dissolve in the blood before there is significant change in the partial pressure, causing the arterial tension of the gas to rise slowly. Raising the minute

Table 11-1

Drugs to be Stopped, Continued, or Started Preoperatively		
	Drugs	**Perioperative Aims**
STOP	Oral hypoglycemics	Avoid hypoglycemia and cerebral damage
	Monoamine oxidase inhibitors (MAOIs)	Avoid hypertensive crisis and hyperpyrexia
	Warfarin (e.g., for atrial difibrillation or prosthetic valve, convert to heparin and discontinue shortly before surgery)	Avoid excessive bleeding intraoperatively (with minimal increase in risk of cerebral embolism and stroke)
	Diuretics	Avoid hypovolemia and hypokalemia
CONTINUE	Opioids	Avoid preoperative pain
	Anticonvulsants	Avoid seizure
	Bronchodilators	Avoid bronchoconstriction
	Antihypertensives and cardiac drugs with exception of diuretics	Avoid hypertension, angina, congestive heart failure, arrhythmia
	Adrenocorticosteroids (increase dose)	Avoid adrenal insufficiency
	Insulin (decrease dose)	Avoid ketoacidosis
START	Histamine H_1 and H_2 receptor antagonists	Allergy prophylaxis in atopic patients
	Benzodiazepines	Provide anxiolysis and anterograde amnesia in frightened patients
	Bronchodilators (inhaled)	Avoid bronchoconstriction in patients with stable asthma
	Anticholinergics	Avoid bradycardia in young children (cardiac output depends on the heart rate)
	Adrenocorticosteroids (increase dose)	Avoid adrenal insufficiency if drug history positive in the last year
	Antacids, histamine H_1 receptor antagonists, gastric motility agents	Increase gastric pH and decrease gastric residual volume
	Antiemetics	Reduce risk of nausea and vomiting
	Heparin	Prevent deep vein thrombosis and pulmonary embolism
	Antibiotics	Prevent wound infection and subacute bacterial endocarditis

From Page C, Curtis MJ, Sutter MC, Walker MJ, Hoffman BB, eds. *Integrated Pharmacology.* 2nd ed. Philadelphia: Mosby; 2002.

ventilation and increasing the concentration of drug in the inspired air also enhance the uptake and distribution of the inhaled agent. Cardiac output or blood flow to the lungs slows induction of the anesthesia because more blood going to the lungs reduces the relative concentration of drug and necessitates a greater partial pressure to achieve anesthesia.[6]

The major route of elimination of inhaled agents is through expired air, although some agents are metabolized by the liver enzymes. How quickly elimination occurs is related to the drug's solubility. Agents that have a low solubility in blood will be the most quickly eliminated. Therefore rapid recovery occurs with nitrous oxide, and slow recovery from anesthesia occurs with methoxyflurane. The speed of onset and recovery mimic each other.

The potency of an inhaled anesthetic agent is not expressed by the kd or median effective dose (ED_{50}), but rather by the minimum alveolar concentration (MAC) that suppresses movement in response to a surgical incision in 50% of subjects.[2] It is estimated that 1.3 times the MAC will prevent movement in 95% of subjects.[7]

The mechanism of action of inhaled drugs is not completely understood. One theory is that the molecules of gas dissolve in the phospholipid bilayer

Table 11-2

Anesthetic Interactions with Preexisting Therapy

Body Location	Drug	Anesthetic Interaction
Brain	Acute alcohol intoxication	Potentiates general anesthetics
	Long-term alcohol abuse	Increases general anesthetic requirements
	Clonidine	Potentiates general anesthetics (but continue preoperatively to avoid intraoperative "rebound" hypertension because of its short half-life)
Lung	Smoking	Pulmonary injury decreases oxygen transfer and carbon monoxide decreases blood oxygen capacity
	Past use of bleomycin	High FiO_2 can precipitate adult respiratory distress syndrome
Circulation	Diuretics	Hypovolemia increases risk of hypotension and acute hypokalemia increases risk of arrhythmias during general anesthesia
	β-Adrenoceptor agonists, bronchodilators	Potentiate arrhythmias from volatile inhaled anesthetics
	β-Adrenoceptor antagonists	Potentiate myocardial depression from general anesthetics
	Ca^{2+} antagonists	Potentiate myocardial depression from general anesthetics
	Monoamine oxidase inhibitors (MAOIs)	Sympathetic stimulants or meperidine may precipitate hypertension and hyperpyrexia
	Past use of doxorubicin	Cardiomyopathy increases risk of heart failure from anesthesia
	Aminoglycosides	Potentiate nondepolarizing neuromuscular blockers

From Page C, Curtis MJ, Sutter MC, Walker MJ, Hoffman BB, eds. *Integrated Pharmacology.* 2nd ed. Philadelphia: Mosby; 2002. *FiO₂,* Fractional concentration of oxygen in inspired gas.

of the neuronal membrane, causing the membrane to expand and impeding the opening of sodium channels. However, it has been pointed out that anesthetics cause only a slight upset in the lipid membrane.[8] It is more likely that inhaled agents act differently in different neural tissues and affect a variety of specific membrane proteins and ion channels, particularly enhancing the inhibitory effects of γ-aminobutyric acid ($GABA_A$) receptors. Anesthetics also inhibit the function of excitatory receptors, including glutamate, acetylcholine (ACh), and 5-hydroxytryptamine.[9] Currently, researchers are investigating an anesthetic-sensitive potassium (K^+) channel labeled *TREK.*[10] When the inhaled drug activates this channel, neural membrane excitability becomes depressed. Anesthetics affect all parts of the nervous system, but it is thought that most of the influence takes place at the thalamus, cortex, and hippocampus, producing a lack of interest in sensory input and memory loss.

Most inhaled anesthetics have a profound effect on the cardiovascular system.[2] Most decrease arterial pressure and depress contractility, producing significant reflex tachycardia. The heart may also become sensitized to epinephrine, resulting in arrhythmias. In terms of the pulmonary system, there is a reduction in respiratory rate and mucociliary function. Responsiveness of the chemoreceptors to carbon dioxide and oxygen is reduced, which is confounded by administration of opioids. Therefore these drugs should not be used for patients with CHF or COPD. The inhaled agents also have the potential to produce hepatotoxicity and nephrotoxicity and an increase in cerebral blood flow, so they are not recommended for use in patients with increased intracranial pressure caused by head trauma or a brain tumor.

Another complication of inhaled anesthetics is malignant hyperthermia.[6] This is a genetically related condition characterized by extreme muscular rigidity, hypertension, tachycardia, and fatal hyperthermia resulting from exposure to certain anesthetic agents, particularly halothane and methoxyflurane. The pathologic condition is excessive calcium release from the sarcoplasmic reticulum. Quick administration of dantrolene (a drug that inhibits calcium release from the sarcoplasmic reticulum) may prevent a fatality.

Despite their side effects, not all of the inhaled agents produce the same level of risk. Isoflurane and desflurane have limited effects on the cardiovascular system, and because inhaled agents are never used in isolation, the addition of another type of drug may work synergistically so that the concentration of the inhaled agent may be reduced, thus diminishing the risks. A thorough assessment by the anesthesiologist is always necessary in determining the appropriate drugs for anesthesia.

Intravenous Anesthetic Agents

In recent years use of IV drugs in anesthesia has increased. The anesthetic agents that comprise the IV category are a diverse group of drugs that include barbiturates, short-acting hypnotics, opioids, benzodiazepines, and neuroleptics.[1] The IV anesthetics act as adjuncts to inhaled drugs or may be given on their own without the gaseous agents. They require no specialized equipment such as a face mask for administration and induce anesthesia very rapidly. Induction occurs as soon as the drug reaches the brain and may be faster than that achieved with some of the newer inhaled agents. The IV anesthetics—particularly thiopental, etomidate, and propofol—are the drugs of choice for induction of anesthesia. The recovery rate with many of these agents is fast enough that they may be used in short, outpatient procedures, and propofol matches the recovery time of the fastest inhaled drug.

Ultra-Short-Acting Barbiturates: Thiopental

Thiopental is a short-acting barbiturate and is one of the most commonly used agents for induction of anesthesia. Its mechanism of action is binding to the GABA-gated chloride channel, which enhances the inhibitory effect of GABA. This drug produces a more pleasing rapid induction than any of the inhaled anesthetics. After IV injection, the drug is rapidly distributed to the brain as a result of its extensive blood flow and high lipid solubility. Loss of consciousness occurs within 20 to 30 seconds. However, the blood concentration drops off rapidly by about 80% in the first 1 to 2 minutes after injection as equilibration with the brain occurs.[10] After a short period, the concentration in the brain decreases as the drug is redistributed to other tissues. This redistribution, rather than metabolism, accounts for the short duration of action. Recovery occurs within about 5 to 10 minutes, unless additional drug is injected, and after several hours, much of the thiopental in the body will have been redistributed into fat. Redistribution back into the brain occurs again and is responsible for the "hangover effect." Hepatic metabolism occurs quite slowly, so that if there is repeated administration, the drug accumulates, causing slow awakening. Therefore thiopental is not used to maintain surgical anesthesia but only for induction.

The disadvantages of thiopental include poor analgesic action and inadequate skeletal muscle relaxation, so frequently, pain medication and muscle relaxants must also be administered. In addition, as the dose increases, thiopental produces decreases in arterial blood pressure (caused by venodilation), stroke volume, heart rate, and cardiac output.[11] There is actually a narrow margin between the anesthetic dose and the dose that produces cardiovascular depression. Other adverse effects include respiratory depression, bronchospasm, laryngospasm, and reflex tachycardia if the patient experiences excessive hypotension.

Methohexital is another ultra-short-acting barbiturate.[11] It is stronger than thiopental and shorter acting. It is often used in oral surgery, fracture reduction, and during electroconvulsive therapy. This drug is less likely to produce bronchospasm, so it may be used for patients with asthma.

Etomidate

Etomidate is used for induction of anesthesia and along with other agents in balanced sedation.[10,11]

It has a larger margin of safety compared with thiopental and is associated with minimal cardiovascular and respiratory depression. Loss of consciousness occurs in seconds, and recovery occurs within 3 to 5 minutes. It is also metabolized more rapidly than the barbiturates and therefore does not produce a hangover effect. The negative aspects of this drug include lack of analgesic effect, production of involuntary movements during induction, pain on injection, and significant postoperative nausea and vomiting.

Ketamine

Ketamine is a short-acting hypnotic, nonbarbiturate agent that is related to phencyclidine, an anesthetic agent used in veterinary medicine.[12] It binds to N-methyl-D-aspartate (NMDA) receptors, inhibiting the excitatory effects of glutamate and opioid receptors. It is best suited for short diagnostic procedures or surgical procedures that do not require skeletal muscle relaxation. It is often used in burn units where patients are frequently anesthetized for dressing changes. Induction occurs in 2 to 5 minutes, and anesthesia lasts for approximately 20 minutes.[10]

Ketamine produces dissociative anesthesia characterized by catatonia, amnesia, and analgesia without loss of consciousness.[1] The mechanism of action is not fully understood, but ketamine produces a generalized sensory blockade in the higher brain centers. It produces a rapid induction with good pain control but poor muscle relaxation.

Ketamine increases the tone of skeletal, cardiac, and respiratory muscles that raise blood pressure, heart rate, and respiratory rate.[1] Ketamine also increases secretions from the salivary and bronchial glands, produces vomiting, and increases intracranial pressure. Because of its adverse effects, this drug is not recommended for patients with ischemic heart disease or COPD or those who have sustained head trauma. Another major drawback of this drug is the occurrence of "emergence reactions." Some patients will experience hallucinations or disturbing dreams as the drug wears off. Diazepam, a benzodiazepine, administered with ketamine will reduce these reactions.

Propofol

Propofol is one of the most popular IV anesthetics because it has few side effects. Induction is smooth and occurs within 40 seconds after administration. It lowers blood pressure without myocardial depression and also lowers intracranial pressure. It also acts as an antiemetic agent.[13,14] Propofol is the ideal agent for ambulatory anesthesia because it has a short duration of action without a hangover effect or significant postoperative drowsiness. It is used not only to induce anesthesia but also for maintenance of anesthesia during surgery. At lower doses it can be used to attain a state of conscious sedation, a drug-induced reduction in anxiety that allows the patient to maintain an airway and respond to verbal commands.[1,14,15] It is also administered as a sedative to critically ill patients.[16]

The major drawback to using propofol is that it offers little pain control, so an analgesic is required. In addition, it can cause lethal metabolic acidosis and skeletal myopathy, and it is occasionally associated with dystonic movements and seizure-like activity.[17,18] Benztropine can be used to treat the dystonia.

Benzodiazepines

A few members of the class of drugs known as benzodiazepines, diazepam and midazolam, are used in anesthesia practice. Midazolam is more potent than diazepam, and its onset of action when given intravenously is usually less than 2 minutes.[11] Complete recovery takes approximately 90 minutes after a single dose, so it is not used to induce or maintain anesthesia but rather as premedication. Used intravenously, it prolongs the postanesthetic recovery period but also produces anterograde amnesia, which is usually desirable. Cardiovascular side effects are uncommon at the doses used for sedation, and the associated respiratory depression is usually tolerable.

Opioid Use in Anesthesia

Optimal treatment with opioids should provide a rapid onset of analgesia and rapid recovery without postoperative pain. With large doses, general anesthesia can be achieved. At lower doses, opioids help maintain anesthesia produced by other agents. Commonly used agents include IV morphine, fentanyl, remifentanil, and sufentanil.[11]

IV opioids are not good amnesic agents and cause respiratory depression and chest wall rigidity, which may impair ventilation.[1] They also are responsible for postoperative nausea and vomiting. Naloxone is a narcotic antagonist that can rapidly reverse the respiratory depression associated with opioids.

Neuroleptanesthesia

Neuroleptanesthesia is general anesthesia produced by a combination of a neuroleptic agent (dopamine antagonist, antipsychotic) and an opioid analgesic.[1] The usual drugs are fentanyl and droperidol. Patients are neither asleep nor fully awake but are in a profound state of analgesia and will experience retrograde amnesia. Neuroleptanesthesia is used for short procedures requiring some patient cooperation. The combination of fentanyl and droperidol is given as an adjunct to other anesthetic drugs for maintenance of anesthesia. Adverse effects include bradycardia, bronchospasm, and muscle rigidity.

Adjuvants to Anesthesia

In addition to the anesthetic agents already discussed, several other types of drugs may be given during the perioperative period to augment the anesthesia process. Atropine is frequently administered to prevent bradycardia and the excessive respiratory secretions associated with many of the anesthetic agents, but it may delay voiding after surgery. There are also reports that dextromethorphan, an NMDA antagonist, can block receptor sites in the spinal cord and CNS, leading to a reduction in the amount of postoperative pain medication required.[19] Clonidine, an α_2-agonist, also reduces the need for pain medication after surgery and reduces nausea and shivering as well.

Other intraoperative agents include neuromuscular blocking agents.[2] These are required for intubation because laryngeal spasm can cause reflex closure of the vocal cords and subsequent hypoxemia. Neuromuscular blockers are also needed during abdominal and thoracic surgery to prevent reflex muscle contractions and for delicate surgeries such as microsurgery. There are two types of neuromuscular blockers: nondepolarizing blockers and depolarizing blockers. Nondepolarizing blockers are competitive antagonists of Ach at the neuromuscular junction. Examples of these are tubocurarine, pancuronium, and rocuronium. These drugs block access of Ach to its binding site without activating the receptor. Rocuronium produces its effect in 90 seconds. Partial recovery occurs in about 30 minutes. After surgery, neostigmine, an anticholinesterase agent, can be used to reverse the effects of these drugs if recovery time needs to be shortened.

Depolarizing blockers bind and depolarize the motor end plate.[2] The end plate remains depolarized throughout the procedure because the drug is only broken down by the cholinesterase in the plasma. Initially, muscle fasciculations and unsynchronized contractions occur, followed by flaccid paralysis. Succinylcholine is the only drug of this kind available, and it is very useful in facilitating endotracheal intubation. It takes effect rapidly (similar to rocuronium) and has a short plasma half-life of about 5 minutes.

Drug Selection Process for General Anesthesia

The crucial goal for all anesthesiologists is to maintain proper pain control, amnesia, and sedation for their patients undergoing surgical procedures. Current guidelines recommend propofol for short-term, same-day surgery procedures when rapid awakening is needed.[20] This may be combined with midazolam for sedation in an anxious patient and with fentanyl for pain relief. For longer procedures and procedures in which a hospital stay is dictated, induction of anesthesia is usually achieved with a barbiturate, followed by administration of an inhaled anesthetic for maintenance. Lorazepam is recommended for attaining amnesia in these longer procedures, and morphine or hydromorphone is recommended for pain control and sedation. As the dose of these types of drugs is increased, the dose of the true anesthetic can be minimized. Reversal agents are also kept on hand to correct any mishaps or lingering effects of the opioids and neuromuscular blockers.

Therapeutic Concerns with Anesthesia

When a patient returns to therapy after surgery, he or she may not be completely over the effects of anesthesia. If the physical therapist is treating the patient the day after surgery, the patient may still be confused or woozy and may show signs of neuromuscular weakness. General anesthetics depress mucociliary clearance in the airways, leading to pooling of mucus and secretions. The patient should be encouraged to cough and breathe deeply. This will help expel some of the anesthetic gases and also mobilize secretions. Proper guarding during ambulation is necessary because of lingering weakness from the anesthesia. Despite the hang-over effect, patients should be encouraged to move to help reduce abdominal distention caused by the anesthetic and muscle relaxant drugs.

REGIONAL AND LOCAL ANESTHESIA

Regional anesthesia is an alternative to general anesthesia for surgery performed on the extremities or even the lower abdomen.[10] Regional anesthesia involves the administration of a local anesthetic agent by a variety of methods including topical anesthesia, infiltration anesthesia, peripheral nerve block, IV regional block, and epidural or spinal administration. The choice of regional versus general is related to the patient's medical status and type of surgery and also the anesthesiologist's experiences and preferences. The two types of anesthesia may also be given together to reduce the need for high doses of general anesthetics. In some cases, regional anesthesia may be unsuccessful, and general anesthesia will then be necessary.

Local Anesthetic Agents

Local anesthetic agents have a similar structure consisting of a lipophilic aromatic ring and a hydrophilic tertiary amine separated by a carbon chain.[10] This link can be either an amide or an ester bond (Figure 11-1). The structural-functional way of looking at these compounds is important because this is how they are classified. The esters include cocaine, procaine, tetracaine, and benzocaine. They are rapidly metabolized by blood pseudocholinesterase, ending in the formation of para-aminobenzoic acid, a possible allergen. The amides consist of lidocaine, mepivacaine, bupivacaine, and prilocaine. These drugs are metabolized more slowly in the liver and rarely produce an allergic reaction. Procaine has a short duration of action, 20 to 45 minutes. Lidocaine has an intermediate duration, 1 to 2 hours, and bupivacaine has a long duration, lasting 3 to 6 hours. Most local anesthetics, with the exception of cocaine, cause vasodilation. Epinephrine increases the duration of action by vasoconstricting the area receiving the injection and decreasing the rate of absorption. Epinephrine is added in a ratio of 1 to 200,000 of lidocaine, which will double the anesthetic's duration of action.[21] Repeated injection will also prolong the anesthesia. A vasoconstrictor should not be used for nerve block of a finger, toe, or nose because the whole blood supply may be stopped by intense vasoconstriction in these areas.

Local anesthetic agents are weak bases and tend to remain ionized at physiological pH and at acidic pH.[10] They become neutral at high pH. Thus a local anesthetic agent needs a more basic environment to penetrate the nerve sheath and axon membrane and to reach the sodium channel where it binds. Once inside the axon, it becomes ionized again and binds to the channel. This is significant because during inflammation, the environment tends to be acidic and therefore resistant to local anesthetic agents.

Local anesthetics selectively block conduction of the small myelinated axons (A delta and C fibers) more readily than the larger fibers.[2] The mechanism of action is blockade of sodium channels. Because nociceptive input is carried on these smaller fibers, pain sensation is blocked more than other sensations such as touch and proprioception. Because they are quite large, motor axons tend to be unaffected by these agents, unless the dose injected is excessive. However, exceptions occur when the motor nerves in the large nerve trunks are located circumferentially and therefore exposed to the drug first. In this case, motor paralysis occurs before sensory loss. Local anesthetics also exhibit use-dependent blockade.[22] They block nerves that have a high firing rate as seen when A delta and C fibers transmit pain impulses.

Adverse reactions to local anesthetic drugs may occur but are rare.[2] They can result from excess drug entering the systemic circulation. If this occurs, the reaction is fairly rapid (within 10 minutes). Side effects tend to be a mixture of CNS stimulation and depressant effects. Restlessness, tremors, and confusion may progress to convulsions, then finally to CNS depression. Cardiac reactions include arrhythmias, followed by bradycardia, hypotension, and cardiac arrest. Respiratory depression can also occur. Resuscitative drugs and equipment should be kept nearby. Any tissue that depends on conduction or transmission of impulses may be affected.

The advantages of local anesthesia include quick recovery, low systemic toxicity, and action confined largely to nerve tissue. The disadvantages may include incomplete analgesia and the time it takes to achieve anesthesia.

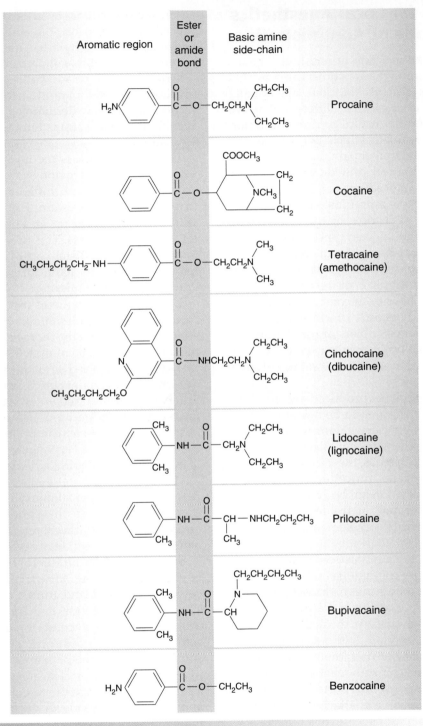

Figure 11-1

Structures of local anesthetics. The general structure of local anesthetic molecules consists of aromatic group *(left)*, ester or amide group *(shaded)*, and amine group *(right)*. Benzocaine is an exception, lacking a side-chain amino group. (From Rang HP, Dale MM, Ritter JM, Moore JL. *Pharmacology*. 5th ed. New York: Churchill Livingstone; 2003.)

Clinical Uses for Local Anesthetics and Their Mode of Administration

Nerve blocks are the injection of anesthetic agents around a nerve to numb the area innervated by that nerve. The nerves that are blocked are usually peripheral nerves or a plexus. Differential nerve blocks are particularly useful in rehabilitation medicine to help evaluate which nerves may be involved in the production of pain. In addition, this type of administration can provide pain relief for certain nonsurgical procedures such as physical therapy treatment for musculoskeletal injuries. Injection of a local anesthetic near the sympathetic stellate ganglion is a specialized type of nerve block that is used to reduce pain in chronic regional pain syndrome. The presence of analgesia, increases in skin surface temperature, and/or the appearance of Horner's syndrome have been considered by some clinicians as being diagnostic of chronic regional pain syndrome. However, others argue that to use this block diagnostically, the results need to be compared with the results of injection of saline solution in the same region.[23]

Infiltration anesthesia is produced by injecting the drug throughout the area to be numbed.[19] It is performed by injecting the drug along a prospective incision line or along the edges of a laceration to be sutured. It has been used as the primary form of pain control for several procedures, including removal of skin lesions, foreign body removal, and breast biopsies. Infiltration of the local anesthetic also reduces the need for supplemental analgesics after surgery.

Local anesthetics are administered during laparoscopic procedures by continuous infusion and are given intraarticularly during arthroscopic knee surgery.[19] Continuous infusion has also been used after digital tenolysis surgery to facilitate immediate postoperative motion without pain.[24] Use of indwelling brachial plexus catheters filled with ropivacaine left in place for pain relief after shoulder arthroscopy has also been reported.[25] In some instances, these catheters are attached to patient-controlled anesthesia pumps.[26]

Topical anesthesia is the application of drug to the skin or mucous membranes. It is often used for eye, ear, nose, and throat procedures and for rectal surgery.[22] When used in this mode, drugs should be capable of rapidly penetrating the skin or mucosa with diminished ability to flow away from the local site of pain. Cocaine penetrates well through the nasal mucosa, so it has been used for nose and throat procedures. It also has the ability to vasoconstrict, which is, in part, why it has a medium duration of action as opposed to a short duration.

Drugs can also be administered by iontophoresis or phonophoresis to produce analgesia for minor surgery (specifically dermatological procedures).[27-29] Technically, this is transdermal administration of local anesthetics.

IV regional block is the injection of drug into a vein that has been previously exsanguinated with a tourniquet.[21] After cuff inflation, the limb is raised to drain the venous system. The veins are then filled with the local anesthetic, and the cuff remains tight for at least 20 minutes. This procedure may be used to numb an entire distal part of an extremity and is frequently used in hand surgery for procedures lasting less than 45 minutes.

Epidural and intrathecal injections of local anesthetics are other modes of administration. Epidural anesthesia is used in the thoracic, lumbar, and sacral regions of the spinal column. The epidural requires that drug be injected into the space between the dura and bony canal where it can act on nerve roots. Lumbar epidurals allow for excellent pain relief for a laparotomy and are also used extensively in obstetrics. The catheter can be left in place safely for up to 7 to 10 days.[30] Hypotension is a side effect, as is the risk of developing a hematoma if the patient has been receiving lower molecular weight heparins. Permanent neurological injury has occurred during this procedure when the patient has been taking anticoagulants. Intrathecal migration of the catheter and intraneural injection are other risk factors.

Subarachnoid or intrathecal block is the injection of the drug into the subarachnoid space, usually between the third and fourth lumbar vertebrae.[31] The anesthetic solution then spreads, but where it actually ends up depends on the density of the solution and the posture of the patient. For low spinal anesthesia, the patient is placed either flat or in a Fowler's position. The anesthetic is mixed with a solution denser than the cerebrospinal fluid (CSF), and the solution tends to diffuse downward. If a higher level of anesthesia is desired, the patient can be placed in a Trendelenburg's position with the head sharply flexed. In this case the anesthetic agent will be mixed with a solution that has a lower specific gravity than the CSF so it will diffuse upward. If the solution is equal to the CSF in specific gravity, the anesthesia will act at the site of injection.

Intrathecal injections are indicated for lower abdominal procedures and procedures in the inguinal area or lower extremities.[31] Onset of action occurs within 1 to 2 minutes, and duration is between 1 and 3 hours, depending on the choice of drug. Headache appears to be the most common complaint associated with spinal blocks. This results from actual puncture of the dura, which may remain open for days to weeks after the procedure, facilitating the loss of CSF. The head pain lessens as the CSF pressure returns to normal. Hypotension may also occur.

Caudal anesthesia results from the injection of the anesthetic agent into the sacral part of the vertebral canal so that the drug infuses around the cauda equina.[31] This type of anesthesia is used in obstetric and genital surgery. The advantages of this block are reductions in headaches and less hypotension.

Therapeutic Concerns with Local Anesthetic Agents

The local anesthetic agents offer several benefits over general anesthesia. Patients experience rapid recovery without hangover symptoms, and there should be no interference with cardiovascular, respiratory, or renal function. However, the physical therapist should be aware that if he or she is seeing a patient immediately after a block, as often occurs in patients with chronic regional pain syndrome, sensation and strength will be diminished.[32] Sensory and strength testing will therefore be necessary before applying modalities or attempting motor activities. In addition, the force of any manipulation will also need to be carefully monitored because the patient will not be able to provide accurate feedback.

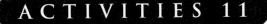

ACTIVITIES 11

■ 1. Many disease states can alter a patient's response to general anesthesia. For the following illnesses or conditions, list some interactions that might occur.
a. Alcoholism
b. Obesity
c. A pediatric surgical case
d. Elderly
e. Patients who smoke
f. Recent head trauma

2. For the following drugs, research how each affects anesthesia.
a. Steroids
b. Antibiotics
c. Antiepilepsy drugs
d. Antihypertensives
e. Psychotropic drugs
f. Oral contraceptives
g. Anticoagulants

3. Discuss the following local anesthetics in terms of the tissue affected and therapeutic use: topical, infiltration, block, spinal.

References

1. Trevor AJ, Miller RD. General anesthetics. In: Katzung BG, ed. *Basic and Clinical Pharmacology.* New York: McGraw Hill; 2001:419-435.
2. Ries CR, Quastel DMJ. Drug use in anesthesia and critical care. In: Page C, Curtis MJ, Sutter MC, Walker MJ, Hoffman BB, eds. *Integrated Pharmacology.* 2nd ed. Philadelphia: Mosby; 2002:547-563.
3. Antimicrobial prophylaxis in surgery. *Med Lett Drugs Ther.* 2001;43(1119):108.
4. Infectious Diseases Quality Improvement Organization Support Center (QIOSC). *National Surgical Infection Prevention Medicare Quality Improvement Project.* Oklahoma City, OK: Oklahoma Foundation for Medical Quality, Inc.; 2002:1-51.
5. Joshi GP. Inhalational techniques in ambulatory anesthesia. *Anesthesiol Clin North Am.* 2003;21(2):263-272.
6. Sung YF, Holtzman SG. Pain control with general anesthetics. In: Brody MJ, Larner J, Minneman KP, eds. *Human Pharmacology: Molecular to Clinical.* 3rd ed. Philadelphia: Mosby; 1998:421-434.

7. Eger E. Age, minimum alveolar anesthetic concentration, and minimum alveolar anesthetic concentration-awake. *Anesth Analg.* 2001;93(4):947-953.

8. Campagna JA, Miller KW, Forman SA. Mechanisms of actions of inhaled anesthetics. *N Engl J Med.* 2003; 348(21):2110-2124.

9. Sonner JS, Antognini JF, Dutton RC, et al. Inhaled anesthetics and immobility: mechanisms, mysteries, and minimum alveolar anesthetic concentration. *Anesth Analg.* 2003;97(3):718-740.

10. Rang HP, Dale MM, Ritter JM, Moore JL. *Pharmacology.* 5th ed. New York: Churchill Livingstone; 2003.

11. Tesniere A, Servin F. Intravenous techniques in ambulatory anesthesia. *Anesthesiol Clin North Am.* 2003; 21(2):273-288.

12. Stewart CE. Ketamine as a street drug. *Emerg Med Serv.* 2001;30(11):30, 32, 34.

13. Visser K, Hassink EA, Bonsel GJ, Moen J, Kalkman CJ. Randomized controlled trial of total intravenous anesthesia with propofol versus inhalation anesthesia with isoflurane–nitrous oxide. *Anesthesiology.* 2001; 95(3):616-626.

14. Gare M, Parail A, Milosavljevic D, Kersten J, Warltier DC, Pagel PS. Conscious sedation with midazolam or propofol does not alter left ventricular diastolic performance in patients with preexisting diastolic dysfunction: a transmitral and tissue Doppler transthoracic echocardiography study. *Anesth Analg.* 2001;93(4):865-871.

15. Byrne MF, Baillie J. Propofol for conscious sedation? *Gastroenterology.* 2002;123(1):373-375.

16. Angelini G, Ketzler JT, Coursin DB. Use of propofol and other nonbenzodiazepine sedatives in the intensive care unit. *Crit Care Clin.* 2001;17(4):863-880.

17. Short TG, Young Y. Toxicity of intravenous anaesthetics. *Best Pract Res Clin Anaesthesiol.* 2003;17(1):77-89.

18. Schramm BM, Orser BA. Dystonic reaction to propofol attenuated by benztropine (Cogentin). *Anesth Analg.* 2002;94(5):1237-1240.

19. Redmond M, Florence B, Glass P. Effective analgesic modalities for ambulatory patients. *Anesthesiol Clin North Am.* 2003;21(2):329-346.

20. Liu LL, Gropper MA. Postoperative analgesia and sedation in the adult intensive care unit: a guide to drug selection. *Drugs.* 2003;63(8):755-767.

21. Bennett PN, Brown MJ. General pharmacology. In: Bennett PN, Brown MJ, eds. *Clinical Pharmacology.* 9th ed. New York: Churchill Livingstone; 2003:37-40.

22. Miller RD, Katzung BG. Local anesthetics. In: Katzung BG, ed. *Basic & Clinical Pharmacology.* Philadelphia: McGraw-Hill; 2001:436-445.

23. Price DD, Stephen L, Wilsey B, Rafii A. Analysis of peak magnitude and duration of analgesia produced by local anesthetics injected into sympathetic ganglia of complex regional pain syndrome. *Clin J Pain.* 1998; 14(3):216-226.

24. Schneider LH, Berger-Feldscher S. Tenolysis: dynamic approach to surgery and therapy. In: Hunter JM, Mackin EJ, Callahan AD, eds. *Rehabilitation of the Hand: Surgery and Therapy.* Philadelphia: Mosby; 1995:463-476.

25. Klein SM, Nielsen KC, Martin A, et al. Interscalene brachial plexus block with continuous intraarticular infusion of ropivacaine. *Anesth Analg.* 2001;93(3):601-605.

26. Corda DM, Enneking FK. A unique approach to postoperative analgesia for ambulatory surgery. *J Clin Anesthesiol.* 2000;12(8):595-599.

27. Byl NN. The use of ultrasound as an enhancer for transcutaneous drug delivery: phonophoresis. *Phys Ther.* 1995;75(6):539-553.

28. Nunez M, Miralles ES, Boixeda P, et al. Iontophoresis for anesthesia during pulsed dye laser treatment of port-wine stains. *Pediatr Dermatol.* 1997;14(5):397-400.

29. Tachibana K, Tachibana S. Use of ultrasound to enhance the local anesthetic effect of topically applied aqueous lidocaine. *Anesthesiology.* 1993;78(6):1091-1096.

30. Mandabach MG. Perspectives in pain management: intrathecal and epidural analgesia. *Crit Care Clin.* 1999; 15(1):105-123.

31. Salerno E. *Pharmacology for Health Professionals.* New York: Mosby; 1999.

32. Linchitz RM, Raheb JC. Subcutaneous infusion of lidocaine provides effective pain relief for CRPS patients. *Clin J Pain.* 1999;15(1):67-72.

CHAPTER 12

DRUGS FOR THE TREATMENT OF PAIN AND INFLAMMATION

PHYSIOLOGY OF PAIN

Pain is usually a direct response to some event that produces tissue damage. The cause may be injury, inflammation, or cancer. However, it also may arise from an unrecognized event or cause (e.g., trigeminal neuralgia) and continue long after the precipitating injury has healed (e.g., phantom limb pain). Pain is also a subjective experience, difficult to see, difficult to quantify, and difficult to treat—especially if there is no known physical or anatomical reason for discomfort. Studying pain is complex because it is often related to an affective component that cannot be easily reproduced in an animal model. Commonly used procedures to test analgesic drugs involve applying a noxious stimulus to an animal and then watching the animal's response. Measuring the time it takes for a rodent to withdraw its tail when exposed to heat and measuring the threshold force that results in withdrawal of an inflamed paw when it is pinched repetitively with greater strength are two research methods commonly used. Similar tests are also conducted on human subjects, but they still lack the affective component that is intertwined with patients' pain.

Neural Mechanisms of Pain and Their Modulation

Two mechanisms may be involved with pain production, nociceptive afferent neurons and abnormal central control over the afferent input. One or both may be present with a pain syndrome. The nociceptive afferent neurons are unmyelinated C fibers and finely myelinated A delta fibers that have sensory endings in the peripheral tissue, which activate in response to noxious input from mechanical, thermal, or chemical stimuli. Stimulation of the A delta fibers produces sharp, intense, and well-localized discomfort; whereas stimulation of the unmyelinated C fibers produces a dull, burning, diffuse type of pain.[1]

Tissue injury results in the local release of several chemicals that stimulate the afferent receptors and neurons.[2,3] The cell bodies of these neurons lie in the dorsal root ganglia. The fibers enter the spinal cord via the dorsal root and terminate in the laminae. The A delta nociceptor fibers synapse in laminae I and V (Figure 12-1). C fibers synapse in laminae I and II (the substantia gelatinosa). They synapse with neurons containing excitatory amino acids and neuropeptides that act as neurotransmitters between the primary afferents and spinal cord nociresponsive neurons.

In the dorsal horn, nociceptive block is attained by N-methyl-D-aspartate (NMDA) blockers, by antagonists of substance P, and by inhibitors of nitric oxide synthesis.[4] Substance P is an excitatory transmitter released by the nociceptive afferent neurons, which produces a slow depolarizing response in the postsynaptic cell that increases in amplitude with repetitive stimulation. Substance P also enhances

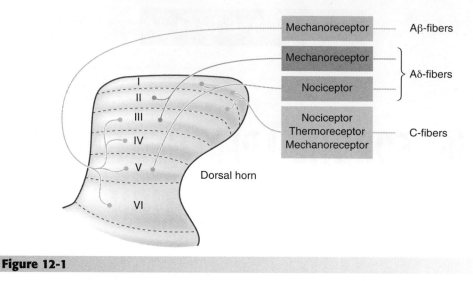

Figure 12-1

The termination of afferent fibers in the six laminae of the dorsal horn of the spinal cord. (From Rang HP, Dale MM, Ritter JM, Moore JL. *Pharmacology.* 5th ed. New York: Churchill Livingstone; 2003.)

NMDA receptor transmission resulting in calcium (Ca^{2+}) influx and activation of nitric oxide synthesis. The released nitric oxide enhances pain perception and transmission in ways that have not yet been fully explained. Substance P also acts in the periphery to produce inflammation, as does calcitonin gene-related peptide released along with substance P.

The cells of the substantia gelatinosa are mainly short inhibitory interneurons that project to laminae I and V.[1] These interneurons regulate transmission at the first synapse in this pain pathway, between the primary afferents and the spinothalamic tract. It is often given the gatekeeper function allowing impulses from one group of afferent fibers to regulate the transmission of nociceptive fibers. The substantia gelatinosa has plentiful opioid peptides and opioid receptors and is viewed as an important site for morphine-like drugs. From laminae I and V, sensory information is then projected upward to the thalamus.

Some descending pathways make up another gating mechanism that controls pain transmission in the dorsal horn.[2] This descending portion originates in the periaqueductal gray area of the midbrain. These fibers project downward first to the nucleus raphe magnus and then back down to lamina I where they synapse on enkephalinergic and serotoninergic interneurons. These neurotransmitters then diminish pain by blocking the release of substance P and inhibiting the spinothalamic neurons (Figure 12-2).

There is also a similar pathway from the locus ceruleus; this pathway inhibits transmission in the dorsal horn, which contains norepinephrine.

Chemical Mediators of Pain

Stimulation of nociceptive endings in the periphery is often chemical in nature. These chemicals are released as a result of inflammatory or ischemic changes in tissues. Further understanding of these chemicals and receptors may provide strategies for treatment.

The vanilloid receptor was recognized after it was observed that capsaicin, the chemical in chili peppers, caused intense pain when injected into the skin or applied on sensitive tissues.[5] It binds to the receptor, opening up an ion channel permeable to several cations that initiates a depolarization and an action potential. Other substances including hydrogen (H^+) and even heat produce a similar response on these receptors. Essentially, a large influx of Ca^{2+} occurs in the nerve terminal, producing release of substance P and calcitonin gene-related peptide. This Ca^{2+} may even be enough to produce nerve terminal degeneration. This has been the premise behind use of topical capsaicin, but the initial painful response has discouraged researchers from pursuing this treatment.

Bradykinin is another pain-producing substance that becomes more potent in the presence of

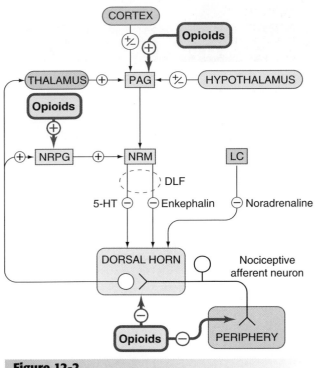

Figure 12-2

The descending control system, showing the main sites of action of opioids on pain transmission. Opioids excite neurons in the periaqueductal gray matter *(PAG)* and in the nucleus reticularis paragigantocellularis *(NRPG),* which in turn project to the rostroventral medulla, which includes the nucleus raphe magnus *(NRM).* From the NRM, 5-HT- and enkephalin-containing neurons run to the substantia gelatinosa of the dorsal horn, and exert an inhibitory influence on transmission. Opioids also act directly on the dorsal horn, as well as on the peripheral terminals of nociceptive afferent neurons. The *locus ceruleus (LC)* sends noradrenergic neurons to the dorsal horn, which also inhibit transmission. The pathways shown in this diagram represent a considerable oversimplification but depict the general organization of the supraspinal control mechanisms. *Shaded boxes* represent areas rich in opioid peptides. *DLF,* Dorsolateral funiculus; *5-HT,* 5-hydroxytryptamine. (From Rang HP, Dale MM, Ritter JM, Moore JL. *Pharmacology.* 5th ed. New York: Churchill Livingstone; 2003.)

prostaglandins.[5] Bradykinin receptors are coupled in some ways to the activation of the vanilloid receptor channel. Pain research is directed toward finding safe bradykinin antagonists that have analgesic and antiinflammatory properties.

Prostaglandins of the E and F series are released during inflammatory states and also during ischemia.[2] They do not produce pain in and of themselves but they enhance the pain-producing effects of other chemicals such as serotonin and bradykinin. The aspirin-type drugs inhibit prostaglandin synthesis and in turn reduce pain.

Other peripheral chemical mediators that initiate a painful response include serotonin, histamine, lactic acid, adenosine triphosphate, and potassium.[5] Antagonists to some of these mediators have been experimentally studied but produce only limited pain reduction.

Neurotransmitters Involved in the Nociceptive Pathway

Substance P and neurokinin (NK) A are members of the tachykinin family, which are characterized by a specific amino acid terminal sequence. They are dispersed widely throughout the central nervous system (CNS), especially in the nociceptive primary afferent neurons and in the dorsal horn. They are released from central and peripheral nerve terminals and trigger an inflammatory response known as *neurogenic inflammation.* The response of smooth muscle to tachykinins, including that in the gastrointestinal (GI) tract and bronchial airways, tends to be constriction. On blood vessels, there is a mix of constriction and dilation along with increased permeability, leading to edema. Substance P and NKA act on NK1 and NK2 receptors, respectively, creating a slow excitatory synaptic potential in dorsal horn neurons. This synaptic potential builds to become a burst of action potentials that continues after the stimulus stops called *wind-up.* Several tachykinin antagonists have been developed; unfortunately, they have not been very effective in decreasing pain in humans but have been somewhat useful in the treatment of depression.[6]

Other neurotransmitters acting centrally involved in pain production include glutamate, γ-aminobutyric acid (GABA), serotonin, norepinephrine, and adenosine.[7] Glutamate is an excitatory amino acid that is involved in fast synaptic transmission at the first synapse in the dorsal horn by acting on α-amino-3-hydroxy-5-methylisoxazole-4-propionate (AMPA) receptors. Glutamate also acts on NMDA receptors, facilitating the wind-up phenomenon. GABA is released by interneurons in the spinal cord and inhibits some of the excitatory impulses in the dorsal horn. Serotonin is involved in the descending pathway from the nucleus raphe magnus to the dorsal horn, acting to interrupt pain impulses in the ascending pathway. Norepinephrine is the neurotransmitter from the locus ceruleus to the dorsal horn, acting as an antinociceptive pathway. Adenosine also plays a role in regulating the pain pathways by producing analgesia when acting on A_1 receptors but causes the reverse when acting on A_2 receptors.

Theoretically, any compound that acts on the neurotransmitters and chemical mediators listed previously should have an impact on the pain pathways. However, in practice, coming up with an effective drug for pain has been a bit more challenging.

Opiate Peptides and Their Receptors

The term *opioid* refers to any substance, whether endogenous or synthetic, that produces morphine-like effects that are blocked by the morphine antagonist, naloxone.

The naturally occurring opioids in plants are called *opiates*, and those found in humans are called *opioid peptides*. They originate from three protein precursors: proopiomelanocortin, prodynorphin, and proenkephalin, producing β-endorphin, met-enkephalin, leu-enkephalin, and dynorphin.[8] A fifth opioid peptide has been discovered: it is called *nociceptin* and appears to have the opposite effect of the endorphins and enkephalins, producing pain. These peptides are widespread in the brain but also found in more localized areas of the spinal cord. Dynorphin is found mainly in the interneurons of the spinal cord; the enkephalins are detected in the long descending pathways from the midbrain to the dorsal horn and are involved in modulating ascending pain impulses.

There are three main types of opioid receptors, μ, δ, and κ, which mediate the pharmacological actions of opiates.[2,9] Each has distinctive subtypes, and all are located in central regions involved with nociception, as well as in the periphery.[10,11] In addition, peripheral inflammation or chronic arthritis has been shown to increase the expression of the opioid receptor genes, resulting in receptor manifestation in inflamed synovia.[8] Interaction with the μ receptor produces analgesia and euphoria but is also associated with respiratory depression, bradycardia, emesis, a slowing of GI motility, and a high abuse potential. The δ receptors produce spinal analgesia and respiratory depression and have a low abuse potential. The κ receptor produces spinal

Table 12-1

Functional Effects Associated with the Main Types of Opioid Receptors			
	μ	**δ**	**κ**
Analgesia			
Supraspinal	+++	−	−
Spinal	++	++	+
Peripheral	++	−	++
Respiratory depression	+++	++	−
Pupil constriction	++	−	+
Reduced GI motility	++	++	+
Euphoria	+++	−	−
Dysphoria	−	−	+++
Sedation	++	−	++
Physical dependence	+++	−	+

From Rang HP, Dale MM, Ritter JM, Moore JL. *Pharmacology*. 5th ed. New York: Churchill Livingstone; 2003.
GI, Gastrointestinal.

analgesia, miosis, constipation, and sedation and is associated with a low abuse potential. A fourth receptor, σ, was thought to be responsible for some of the dysphoric effects of the opiates, namely anxiety, hallucinations, and bad dreams; but at present, it is unclear whether these are true opioid receptors.[2] See Table 12-1 for the main pharmacological effects produced by an interaction with the opiate receptors. All of the opioid receptors are G-protein linked and facilitate the opening of potassium channels, producing hyperpolarization. The result is inhibition Ca^{2+} influx and blocking of neurotransmitter release.[11]

MORPHINE AND SIMILAR OPIOID ANALGESICS

Opium is derived from the juice of the seedpod of the poppy (*Papaver somniferum*) plant. It has been used for centuries to reduce pain and produce analgesia and sleep and also as an anti-diarrheal agent.[12] It was primarily used in the Middle East by citizens of all means but was used only by the elite in Europe and the United States. In the 1800s use of morphine-containing tinctures became more common, and it became widely available from doctors and pharmacists. However, with the invention of the hypodermic syringe in the 1900s, street use of opioids in the form of heroin escalated. By the end of the 1940s when the nature of opiate addiction became known, opioid use became tightly restricted by government regulation. Legal use of opioids is now controlled solely by health care providers (e.g., physicians, dentists, nurses). However, this presents certain problems because a health care provider could face criminal charges if he or she prescribes these drugs inappropriately. This has led to reluctance on the part of physicians to prescribe opioids, often leaving chronic pain that is not related to a terminal illness untreated. Consensus statements put out by the American Academy of Pain Medicine and American Pain Society support the use of opioids after nonopioid therapy has failed and after a comprehensive medical exam has been conducted, along with mutually agreed on goals for treatment and specific follow-up.[13]

Opioid drugs are the first choice for treatment of severe pain. On a basic science level, these drugs decrease the influx of Ca^{2+} in the presynaptic terminal, preventing the release of substance P and glutamate.[11] They also increase potassium influx, resulting in hyperpolarization and a decrease in nerve transmission. A third area of action is the inhibition of GABAergic transmission in the brainstem where GABA inhibits a pain inhibitory neuron. There is also evidence that these drugs are involved with the mesolimbic dopamine system to produce euphoria, which is separate from their action on the pain pathways.

Analgesics That Are Strong μ-Agonists

Opiates may be divided according to how strongly they interact with their receptors. Those drugs that fall within the "strong agonist" category include morphine, fentanyl, hydromorphone, methadone, and meperidine. They have a strong affinity for the μ receptor and less affinity for the δ and κ receptors. They have similar pharmacodynamic effects, but they differ in terms of analgesic potency and elimination half-life. Some of the strong agonists metabolize into active metabolites, which extend the duration of action. Morphine in particular metabolizes into morphine-6-glucuronide, extending its analgesic activity. Morphine-6-glucuronide is 20 to 40 times more potent than morphine.[14] It is eliminated by the kidneys, so it will quickly accumulate in patients with renal failure. Accumulating metabolites also present problems even in patients with healthy kidneys when therapy is continued for more than 1 to 2 days.

Most opioids, including the strong agonists, are available in a variety of different dose forms and modes of administration, including oral, transdermal, intramuscular, intravenous (bolus, continuous infusion, patient controlled), subcutaneous infusion, rectal, epidural, intrathecal, intranasal, and transmucosal (lollipop). Proper dosing can be complicated, especially during a switch from one mode of administration to another, and therefore should be conducted by a skilled, experienced clinician. For example, the relative potency of intramuscular to oral morphine is 1:6, but this ratio changes with repeated administration or when patients receive the drug on a regular schedule. In these circumstances, the intramuscular to oral ratio is reduced to 1:2 or 1:3.[11] Delayed-release preparations are also available for some opioids. MS-Contin is oral morphine that provides pain relief for 8 to 12 hours. This provides for better compliance and longer-lasting pain relief before repeated dosing. For management of "breakthrough" pain, immediate-release morphine, IR-Contin, can be used. Transdermal fentanyl is also a useful drug for improving compliance and for providing longer pain relief. It is indicated for patients who could benefit from continuous infusion of an opioid and also for those patients who are unable to swallow or have GI problems. The half-life is long, and patches need only be replaced every 72 hours.[15] However, care must be taken when patients are switched from immediate-release formulations to other modes of administration because adverse drug events can become exaggerated.[16]

Switching from one opioid to another also presents certain challenges. Even though fentanyl and sufentanil are in the same category as morphine, potency vastly differs.[14] Sufentanil is 625 times more potent than morphine and 12 times more potent than fentanyl. When sufentanil is injected intravenously, analgesia is achieved just about instantly, but with morphine, minutes are required before pain relief occurs. Methadone has potency equal to that of morphine but a much longer duration of action. However, because methadone is converted to two inactive metabolites, in terms of pain control, its analgesic effects often wear off before the signs of physical withdrawal develop. Patients with opioid addiction may be given methadone to assist with the withdrawal process.[17,18] It is given in two to three daily doses and then tapered over time, producing a much gentler withdrawal. In addition, when injected in the presence of methadone, morphine injection does not cause the same euphoria as it does alone.[2]

Diamorphine (heroin) is rapidly converted to morphine, so its effects should be similar.[2] However, it has greater lipid solubility, so it crosses the blood-brain barrier more rapidly than morphine, giving the patient a greater "rush." It also has a shorter duration of action than morphine.

When pain relief with the strong opioids is inadequate, a common quandary for the physician is whether to change the drug or keep the drug but change its mode of administration.[19] When the physician desires to change the drug and not the mode of administration, comparisons regarding equianalgesic doses must be made. When changing the mode of administration, the dose must be adjusted. This is especially true when switching from an oral route to a parenteral route. Debate regarding the best course of action continues.

Weak Opioids

Drugs that fall within the mild to moderate agonist category include codeine, oxycodone, tramadol, and propoxyphene. These are considered to be the "weak opioids," although they are effective in treating pain of moderate intensity. However, withdrawal from these drugs may not be any easier than withdrawal from the stronger opioids. They are often prescribed in combination with nonsteroidal antiinflammatory drugs (NSAIDs). The rationale behind combining drugs in pain management is based on the fact that one drug is not always capable of controlling pain.[20] If only one drug were administered, a higher dose might be required to control the pain than if two different drugs were used at lower doses. Therefore combining drugs may be a useful way to reduce side effects.

Codeine is 20% less potent than morphine, but it is absorbed well when given orally, which makes it the preferred opioid in some cases.[2] It has almost no pain-relieving action on its own, but it converts to morphine and then to morphine-6-glucuronide. It also has a marked antitussive effect, so it is often formulated as a cough medicine.

Oxycodone is often marketed with either aspirin (Percodan) or acetaminophen (Percocet) for an additive effect. However, since 1996, the manufacturer has released this drug as a single entity and in the controlled-release tablet form (OxyContin) in doses ranging from 10 to 160 mg.[21] The tablets are intended for use every 12 hours, but they have become a popular drug for abuse. OxyContin tablets are being crushed to make the entire dose immediately available and are then snorted or dissolved in water and injected intravenously. When taken in this manner by people who have not built up tolerance to the drug, a single 80-mg dose can be fatal. For this reason, the 160-mg tablets were withdrawn from the market shortly after their introduction.

Tramadol is another weak μ and κ receptor agonist. It is an oral opioid that also blocks reuptake of norepinephrine and serotonin and is marketed for moderate pain relief. It is about one tenth as potent as morphine but is available in combination with acetaminophen for better efficacy.[14,22] It is not widely known as an opioid, and some physicians have actually used it as an antiinflammatory agent. The assumption has been that it does not produce dependence, but some opioid-type dependence has been reported.

Opioid Agonist-Antagonists (Partial Mixed Agonists)

The opiate agonist-antagonist drugs are agonists at the κ and δ receptors but show partial and weak agonist activity at the μ receptor.[11] Included in this category are pentazocine, butorphanol, and nalbuphine. They produce an analgesic effect in patients who cannot tolerate morphine but precipitate a withdrawal reaction in those patients who had previously been receiving the strong agonist drugs. The reason for this is that the strong agonist is displaced off the receptor by the partial mixed agonist drug, thereby triggering withdrawal.

The mixed agonist drugs play a limited role in clinical pain relief. They are useful for decreasing mild to moderate pain but can exacerbate psychiatric conditions.[2] They can produce dysphoria, nightmares, and hallucinations. The real advantage of these drugs over some of the other opioids is that there is less potential for abuse.

Partial Agonist Opioids

Buprenorphine is a new opioid that shows high affinity for the μ receptor but has lower efficacy than the other opioids. The maximal effect (Emax) on the dose-response curve is less than the maximal effect produced by a full agonist, so it cannot control pain as well as the strong agonists.[14] However, it appears to be quite effective as an alternative to methadone for preventing withdrawal symptoms in patients who are physically dependent on morphine or heroin.[23] A systematic review revealed that sublingual buprenorphine given three times a week was just as effective as methadone for maintenance. Buprenorphine is available in tablet forms for sublingual and oral administration. The major limitation of this drug is that the maximum effective dose of buprenorphine is equivalent to only 70 mg of oral methadone, lower than what is needed to combat heroin addiction.

Adverse Effects of Opioids

The adverse effects of opioids can be divided into CNS effects and peripheral effects. The major CNS effects include sedation, respiratory depression, cough suppression, miosis, truncal rigidity, and vomiting. The sedative effect is one of drowsiness with some depressed mentation and impaired reasoning.[24] Cognitive impairment appears to be worse during the first few days of use and in the first few hours after a dose is given. Patients also score poorly on timed performance tests in psychomotor function when taking these drugs. The respiratory depression is produced by a depressed response to carbon dioxide at the respiratory centers in the pons and medulla and occurs at usual doses. Thus opiates should be avoided in patients with respiratory diseases because rate and depth of respiration will be reduced. Cough suppression, which might be considered a positive effect of opioids for a patient with a chronic cough, may cause harm in the elderly patient recovering from surgery who is at risk for pneumonia. Pupillary constriction is caused by stimulation of the oculomotor center. The patient may also have reddened eyes from cerebral vessel dilation. This dilation is a result of the respiratory depression and hypoxia. It is an important diagnostic finding because most other causes of coma and respiratory depression produce papillary dilation. Lastly, nausea and vomiting result from stimulation of the chemoreceptor trigger zone located in the medulla. Most of these adverse effects, with the exception of miosis, diminish after prolonged administration.

The peripheral side effects include constipation, urinary retention, and bronchospasm. These effects occur as a result of activation of opiate receptors in the perspective areas. Delayed gastric emptying can retard the absorption of other drugs. Biliary tract irritability may also occur because opioids produce contraction of the gall bladder but at the same time cause constriction of the sphincter. Therefore opioids should be avoided in patients with gall bladder disease. Some opiates also cause histamine release from mast cells, which is responsible for pruritus or frictopathia, as well as bronchoconstriction.

Opioids have the potential to produce complex immunosuppressant and hormonal effects. Animal studies and in vitro assays show that opioids can depress immune function.[12,25] They have been shown to increase immunosuppression in patients with AIDS and may actually increase viral load.[26] Other than the obvious danger of sharing needles, this fact helps explain the prevalence of AIDS in opioid-addicted individuals. In terms of hormonal effects, opioids influence the hypothalamic-pituitary-adrenal axis and the hypothalamic-pituitary-gonadal axis. Morphine reduces plasma cortisol levels and also results in a decrease in luteinizing hormone, follicle-stimulating hormone, testosterone, and estrogen.[12] In combination, these effects lead to decreased libido, aggression, and amenorrhea. However, prolactin levels are noticeably increased and may result in galactorrhea.

Tolerance and Dependence

There is no doubt that opioids have helped many people who have severe pain. However, more people could be helped by these drugs than those who actually receive them. Patients may fear addiction and refuse to take these medications. Physicians are also reluctant to prescribe opioids. Many stories of celebrity drug addictions reinforce the notion that addiction is a real concern. However, according to the American Geriatrics Society, addiction problems related to these drugs are unusual in older patients.[27] In addition, rarely do patients with cancer pain become addicted. Proponents of opioid therapy for relief of pain believe that it is unlikely that a patient who does not have a history of addiction or alcoholism will experience problems with these drugs.[28]

The CNS-mediated effects of opioids are the most likely to lead to misuse after long-term administration and include psychological and physical dependence.[11] The development of physical dependence and tolerance is predictable, but these are separate entities from psychological dependence (addiction). Unfortunately, tolerance to opioids develops quickly, and the patient must continually administer a higher dose to get the same effect. Tolerance begins after the first administration, and often, an increase in dose is needed in just 2 to 3 weeks. When given regularly over time, withdrawal symptoms begin within 6 to 10 hours after a dose is missed. This onset of withdrawal is usually accompanied by feelings of anxiety, irritability, and alternating chills and hot flashes. Other signs include body aches, runny nose, diarrhea, shivering, gooseflesh, stomach cramps, insomnia, sweating, tachycardia, yawning, nausea, and vomiting.[29] Symptoms reach their peak at 24 to 72 hours. These are physical impairments indicating that the patient was physically dependent, but not necessarily psychologically dependent, on the drug.

Addiction refers to deliberately seeking out a drug for its mood-altering abilities.[29] This tends to occur when opioids are used in excessive doses after the need for pain relief has passed. Opioids mediate this effect by increasing synaptic dopamine levels in the limbic system in susceptible patients. It is believed that the drug triggers biological changes that lead to a compulsive craving. Addiction can be treated with pharmaceuticals, but treatment is not always successful. The usual daily morphine dose that prevents withdrawal symptoms is equal to about one fourth of the previous day's dose.[11] This dose is labeled *the detoxification dose* and is divided into four daily doses. After a few more days, the dose is cut in half and again administered in four daily doses. This continues until the total dose per day is down to 10 to 15 mg of morphine. In another 2 days, the morphine can be discontinued. The alternative is to switch the patient to methadone by using one quarter of this dose as the initial detoxification dose and proceeding as described previously. This produces a much gentler withdrawal. In comparison with morphine withdrawal, signs of withdrawal from methadone do not begin until a dose has been missed for 36 to 48 hours.

Opioid Antagonists

Naloxone in repeated doses is used to reverse respiratory depression and coma in opioid overdose.[2] It is a competitive antagonist at the μ, κ, and δ receptors but has the highest affinity for the μ receptor. This explains why it rapidly reverses the respiratory insufficiency but has little effect on analgesia. It is given intravenously, and its actions are almost immediate. It also precipitates withdrawal in physically dependent patients but produces no effect in healthy subjects. It is also used during labor to reverse the effect of an opioid on a newborn baby. Naltrexone is similar to naloxone but has a longer duration of action.

Patient-Controlled Analgesia

Patient-controlled analgesia (PCA), allows the patient to self-administer the analgesic medication on an as-needed basis, usually on top of a preprogrammed continuous infusion.[30] This method consists of an infusion pump that is electronically controlled and connected to a timing device. PCA devices may be small pumps that are worn by the patient, implantable delivery devices, or larger pumps that are attached to a pole or rest on a bedside table. The catheter delivering the medication may be placed intrathecally, intravenously, or in the epidural space.[31] The patient presses on a thumb button whenever he or she feels pain. The pump then releases a preset amount of drug through the indwelling intravenous catheter. The timer is programmed to lock out additional doses until the first dose has had a chance to reach peak effect. The "lock out" interval can be changed as necessary.

PCA has grown in popularity since the development of the infusion pumps.[30,32] Patients seem to like the fact that they can give themselves medication without having to rely on a nurse. A background of continuous analgesia prevents the peaks and troughs associated with drug administration every 4 hours. Supporters of PCA also report that recovery from surgery is accelerated because factors such as muscle guarding, poor chest expansion, and immobility caused by pain are avoided. However, this mode of administration is not without problems.

Programming errors, mechanical problems, adverse reactions associated with the medication, and infections such as epidural abscesses and meningitis can occur.[33] Simple kinking of the tube may cause changes in the dose the patient receives, although there is a pump occlusion alarm to alert the patient if it occurs. The catheter can move from the epidural space into the subarachnoid space or from the subarachnoid space into the vascular system.[34] In addition, the catheter may press on neural tissue, nerve roots, or the spinal cord. Signs of catheter migration include aspiration of cerebrospinal fluid as indicated by a wet catheter dressing and the patient complaining of a throbbing, continuous occipital headache. If the catheter has migrated into the vascular system, blood will be apparent in the catheter. The therapist should also be on the alert for any sudden nausea and vomiting, hypotension, and respiratory depression. Compression of nerve tissue is indicated by motor weakness and bowel and bladder dysfunction. There has also been a case report of a delayed diagnosis of a myocardial infarction in a patient who received PCA after a radical cystoprostatectomy.[35]

The Medical Device Reporting Regulations require that manufacturers, distributors, and facilities that use the devices report deaths or serious injuries associated with these pumps to the Food and Drug Administration.[36] In addition, health care providers are encouraged to voluntarily report adverse events to the Food and Drug Administration through MedWatch. Errors that have been reported include those related to product packaging, drug concentration programming errors, and improper installation of tubing.[36] In several cases, patients experienced respiratory depression related to overdose of morphine when part of the shipping package was left in place, allowing a free flow of drug into the patient. Narcotic overdose can also result when the pump is programmed with a lower concentration of drug than what is actually filled in the drug reservoir. The pump's calculation of the rate of infusion is based on the drug concentration in the reservoir. A higher infusion rate occurs if the concentration is underestimated.[33] Another problem is faulty installation of tubing, resulting in continuous drug infusion. Ideally, the pumps should be designed so that parts fit together only in one way.

Some new types of infusion pumps are undergoing extensive testing and are expected to cut down on drug programming errors.[37] To program these devices a health care provider can scan a barcoded label on a drug package or intravenous fluid container. This will automatically program the pump to the correct infusion rate. A patient-controlled transdermal fentanyl patch that uses iontophoresis to deliver the drug is currently under investigation for postsurgical pain control.[38] However, until these devices are widely accepted, apnea monitoring and arterial blood gas analysis should continue to be performed to minimize the risk of respiratory depression.

Therapeutic Concerns with Opioids

Physical therapists working with patients who have recently started using opioids need to be prepared for side effects. The patient may experience drowsiness or dizziness, and dulled cognitive function may be apparent. In many cases, the patient will develop tolerance for the side effects with the exception of miosis and constipation. Until these symptoms disappear, patients should take commonsense precautions such as not driving, avoiding hazards (such as throw rugs), holding onto the stair railings, and not making any important decisions.[27]

Physical therapy should be scheduled when the opioid has nearly reached its peak action so that the patient can fully cooperate with the program. However, this also means that the patient will not be able to accurately report when a technique is painful. In addition the therapist must consider the respiratory depression when planning an exercise program.

ANTIINFLAMMATORY AGENTS

NSAIDs are quite possibly the most widely used group of drugs in the world.[2] They are often self-administered or prescribed by a physician for musculoskeletal pain and injury or to treat an inflammatory condition such as rheumatoid arthritis. At least 20 different NSAIDs are available in the United States, but none are perfect in eliminating symptoms or benign in terms of side effects. Many of them work by primarily blocking prostaglandin synthesis.

Prostaglandins and Their Role in Inflammation

Prostaglandins have been detected in almost every tissue of the body in response to cell damage. They are not stored but rather released when an injury, inflammation, or tumor is present. There are several types of prostaglandins delineated by letter (A, B, C, D, E, F, H, I) and nonprostaglandins (thromboxanes).[39] Subscript numbers are added to indicate that a prostaglandin exists in a series (e.g., PGH_2). PGI_2 is also known as *prostacyclin*. All prostaglandins are derived from arachidonic acid, which is a fatty acid that is ingested through diet and stored as phospholipids in the cell membrane. Arachidonic acid is cleaved by the enzyme phospholipase A_2 and is then acted on by two enzyme systems, cyclooxygenase (COX) and lipoxygenase. Prostaglandins, prostacyclins, and thromboxanes come from the cyclooxygenase pathway, and leukotrienes come from the lipoxygenase pathway (Figure 12-3).

Prostaglandins have many diverse actions: PGAs, PGEs, and prostacyclin produce vasodilation; PGF_2 and thromboxanes produce vasoconstriction and make platelets sticky; other actions include increased cardiac output, increased capillary permeability, stimulation of uterine contractions, either vasodilation or constriction of bronchioles (PGE_1 and PGE_2 dilate; PGF_2 constricts), pain production, platelet aggregation, inhibition of gastric acid secretion and stabilization of the gastric mucosa, elevation of body temperature, and vascular dilation in the kidneys to help regulate renal vascular resistance. Some of these effects, particularly those on the kidneys and GI mucosa, are quite helpful; whereas other effects produce pain and dis-

comfort.[40,41] Along with prostaglandins, kinins also play a role in inflammation. Kinins, including bradykinin, are formed as a result of injury and are strong vasodilators. Vasodilation is accompanied by increased permeability of capillaries, resulting in redness, edema, and pain. Leukotrienes, histamines, and serotonin have similar roles.

Cyclooxygenase Enzyme

There are two different isoforms of the COX enzyme, but they are incompletely understood.[39,42] COX-1 is found in the platelets, kidneys, and stomach. COX-2 is induced and found in synoviocytes, endothelial cells, and macrophages and catalyzes the conversion of arachidonic acid to PGF_2. Both forms are found in synovial fluid of patients with rheumatoid arthritis. Drugs that act solely on the COX-2 form of the enzyme have been developed and are called *COX-2 inhibitors.*

Both COX-1 and COX-2 are long channels associated with the cell membrane, with COX-2 being wider than COX-1. Each has a bend toward the terminal end of the channel. Arachidonic acid enters the channel and becomes twisted around the bend.[2] At this point two oxygen molecules are inserted and a free radical is extracted. The result is the five-carbon ring recognized as a prostaglandin.

A third form of the enzyme, COX-3, has recently been identified in the human brain, spinal cord, and heart and in canine and murine species.[43] This enzyme is inhibited by acetaminophen but is relatively insensitive to aspirin and shows reduced sensitivity to diclofenac and indomethacin (nonselective NSAIDs).[44-46] This may explain acetaminophen's role in fever reduction.

Aspirin

Aspirin (acetylsalicylic acid) is one of the most widely used analgesic, antipyretic, and antiinflammatory drugs.[47] A national survey conducted in US households between 1998 and 1999 showed that 17% of subjects reported taking an aspirin in the preceding week, 23% reported using acetaminophen, and another 17% reported using ibuprofen. Given the prevalence of use of these agents, it is prudent to thoroughly review the pros and cons of these drugs. Aspirin blocks prostaglandin synthesis by blocking the action of both forms of COX. It binds irreversibly to a specific serine molecule (serine 530 for

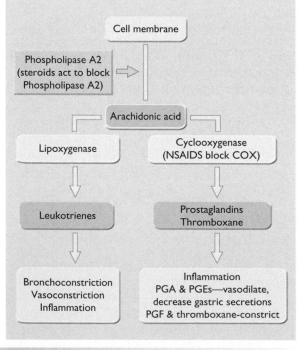

Figure 12-3

The cyclooxygenase *(COX)* and lipoxygenase pathway. *NSAIDs,* Nonsteroidal antiinflammatory drugs; *PG,* prostaglandin.

COX-1 and serine 516 for COX-2) toward the end of the tubular channel, inactivating the enzyme.[39]

Beneficial Effects of Aspirin

Aspirin has major beneficial effects including an antipyretic effect, an analgesic effect, an anti-inflammatory effect, and an antithrombotic effect.[2] The antipyretic action results from blockade of prostaglandins in the hypothalamus. Bacterial endotoxins produce the release of pyrogens from macrophages, which stimulate PGEs. These PGEs raise the set point for body temperature. COX-2 and COX-3 have a role in inducing pyrogen release, causing fever. The analgesic effect of aspirin results from decreased production of prostaglandins that sensitize nociceptors and the antiinflammatory response comes from blockade of prostaglandin-induced increased vascular permeability. As previously described, aspirin is also used in vascular disorders to inhibit platelet-induced thrombus formation by irreversibly inhibiting thromboxane production (80 mg/day). However, this positive effect of aspirin can cause serious bleeding. Bleeding time is increased and bruising is more common. The inhibition of platelet aggregation is a desirable effect for some patients, but the therapist must always be alert to excessive bleeding and bruising, especially if it occurs with a minor injury.

Higher doses are needed for analgesic activity (two 300-mg tablets administered four times per day) and even higher doses (12 to 20 tablets) are needed for antiinflammatory effects. Other beneficial effects include reducing the incidence of colon and rectal cancers.[40,48] There is also early evidence that aspirin delays the onset of Alzheimer's disease by inhibiting aggregation of amyloid-beta and by scavenging for radicals.[49-51] However, other studies indicate that aspirin and NSAIDs fail to produce changes in cognitive function in these patients.[52]

Adverse Effects of Aspirin

Regular aspirin use produces GI problems ranging from minor stomach discomfort to hemorrhage and ulceration. Even at normal doses, between 3 and 8 mL of blood may be lost in the feces per day and may cause anemia. Normally, PGI_2 inhibits gastric acid secretion, and PGE_2 stimulates mucus production in both the stomach and small intestine. Both of these prostaglandins are the result of COX-1 action. If these functions are blocked by aspirin, the epithelial membrane of the stomach will be

damaged.[40] Common GI side effects include dyspepsia, diarrhea, nausea, vomiting, and gastric bleeding and ulceration. It is estimated that one in five aspirin and NSAID users will experience some gastric injury. This damage may grow silently for years until hemorrhage and/or perforation results. Therefore it is suggested that aspirin be taken with food and a large volume of fluid to diminish the GI problems. Misoprostol, a PGE_1 analog, or omeprazole, a proton pump inhibitor, is sometimes given along with aspirin or NSAIDs to decrease the incidence of GI problems.[53,54]

One of the other major adverse effects of aspirin is renal dysfunction.[41] PGE_2 and PGI_2 are important for maintaining renal blood flow by helping to dilate the renal artery, particularly in individuals who have angiotensin-mediated vasoconstriction. Loss of this mechanism results in decreased sodium, potassium, and water excretion and facilitates hypertension. High doses can also produce acute renal failure.

Another problem with aspirin is that it readily binds to plasma proteins, producing several drug-drug interactions. Examples include raising unbound methotrexate levels, enhancing the hypoglycemic affect of sulfonylurea drugs used for diabetes, and increasing the anticoagulant effect of warfarin.

Salicylates produce metabolic changes that increase with the dose.[2] Large but normal doses can alter the acid-base balance. The increase in acidity leads to higher levels of carbon dioxide production, which stimulates respiration. Hyperventilation produces a respiratory alkalosis, which in turn is compensated for by renal excretion of bicarbonate. However, as the plasma aspirin level increases, respiration is suppressed, leading to retention of carbon dioxide on an already low bicarbonate level and metabolic acidosis. Fever is likely to be present because of an increased metabolic rate, and dehydration caused by vomiting may follow. Salicylate poisoning is also associated with headache, nausea, tinnitus, and confusion. It is more serious in children in whom the primary disturbance tends to be metabolic acidosis, whereas in adults, it results primarily in respiratory alkalosis.

Less common side effects of aspirin include skin rashes and photosensitivity, bronchospasm in patients with aspirin-sensitive asthma, liver dysfunction, and bone marrow depression. Aspirin has also been epidemiologically linked with an encephalitis (Reye's syndrome) when given to children with viral infections.

Nonsteroidal Antiinflammatory Drugs (Nonselective Cyclooxygenase Inhibitors)

NSAIDs act by reversibly inhibiting the COX enzyme, with varying effects on COX-1 versus COX-2 (Figure 12-4). In contrast, aspirin displays irreversible binding to the COX enzyme. NSAIDs are also more potent than aspirin at equal doses, and they have just about identical beneficial and adverse effects with the exception that they are not used for cardiac protection as will be explained later. Among the elderly, they are responsible for 10 to 20 of 1000 hospitalizations per year for peptic ulcer disease and for a fourfold increased risk of death from GI bleeding.[55]

The individual NSAIDs have differences in potency, toxicity, patient tolerance, and relative selectivity for COX-1 and COX-2. For example, diclofenac is said to be more GI sparing and sulindac is safer on the kidneys (Figure 12-5). NSAIDs associated with a shorter half-life produce less injury to the GI system than those with longer half-lives as measured by the degree of fecal blood loss. The theory is that the gastric mucosa has a chance to repair itself between doses of short-acting drugs but not with a longer-acting agent.[56] Indomethacin and ketoprofen produce greater degrees of GI toxicity and have longer half-lives.[57] Sulindac is somewhat renal sparing because it is converted to an inactive drug in the kidneys and thus may inhibit renal COX to a lesser extent than the other NSAIDs.[57] However, both of these drugs have the tendency to produce liver damage. Effects on the CNS also vary among the NSAIDs. Indomethacin, naproxen, and ibuprofen have been reported to pro-

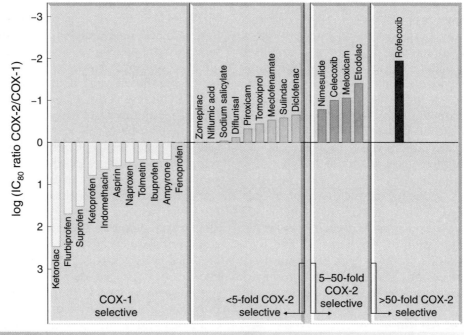

Figure 12-4

A comparison of cyclooxygenase *(COX)* isozyme selectivity of nonsteroidal antiinflammatory drugs *(NSAIDs)*. The graph shows the effect of various NSAIDs on COX-1 at a dose that gives an 80% inhibition of COX-2. The zero line indicates equal potency. Those below the line have selectivity for COX-1. Some above the line have a less than fivefold selectivity for COX-2. The next group (containing meloxicam, etodolac, celecoxib, and nimuselide) has a 50-fold selectivity for COX-2; but note that all can produce full inhibition of COX-1. Only rofecoxib has a greater than 50-fold selectivity for COX-2. Activity measured in whole blood assay. (From Rang HP, Dale MM, Ritter JM, Moore JL. *Pharmacology.* 5th ed. New York: Churchill Livingstone; 2003. Modified from Warner et al. *Proc Natl Acad USA.* 1999;96:7563-7568 as adapted by Vane SJ. Aspirin and other antiinflammatory drugs. *Thorax.* 2000;55 Suppl:S3-S9.)

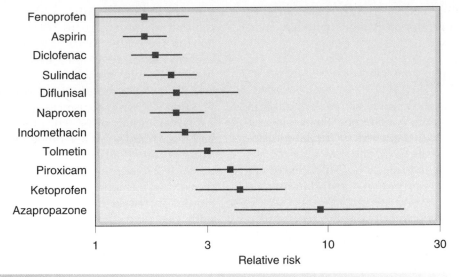

Figure 12-5

The risk of gastrointestinal complications with various nonsteroidal antiinflammatory drugs *(NSAIDs)*, relative to the risk with ibuprofen (relative risk = 1). Ibuprofen, given in a dose of 1200 mg daily, itself carries a risk of double that of placebo. The lines represent 95% confidence intervals. (From Hawkey CJ. Gastrointestinal toxicity of non-steroid anti-inflammatory drugs. In: Vane JR, Botting RH [eds]. Therapeutic Roles of Selective COX-2 Inhibitors. London: William Harvey Press; 2001.)

duce occasional cognitive dysfunction, confusion, behavioral disturbances, and dizziness.[58] In general, if a patient has a negative reaction to one NSAID, it does not automatically imply that he or she will react in the same manner to other agents in this class.

Cyclooxygenase-2 Inhibitors

As mentioned previously, two different isoforms of the COX enzyme are well known. COX-1 is found in various locations in the body, whereas COX-2 is more prevalent when induced by inflammation or surgery. The development of COX-2 inhibitors is a fairly new approach to preventing some of the traditional aspirin and NSAID renal and GI complications while exploiting their antiinflammatory action.[59] Celecoxib and rofecoxib are the oldest and most studied of the group. They have been found to produce less GI toxicity than the nonselective NSAIDs.[53] However, the hypertensive effects and nephrotoxic potential may remain.[41,60,61] Animal studies have revealed that the COX-2 isoform is important for renal PGE_2 synthesis, and in human studies in which celecoxib was compared with naproxen, both drugs showed similar decreases in

sodium excretion. However, in another study in which rofecoxib was compared with indomethacin, only indomethacin caused a decrease in glomerular filtration rate.[62] The authors hypothesized that the COX-1 enzyme is important in maintaining renal perfusion and the COX-2 enzyme is important in sodium regulation.

Several single-dose, randomized, double-blind studies have shown that COX-2 inhibitors are as effective as ibuprofen or naproxen in reducing postsurgical pain.[63] Rofecoxib has also been found to be as effective as ibuprofen in the treatment of osteoarthritis, but valdecoxib was found to be less effective than naproxen when studied in patients with rheumatoid arthritis.[64]

Besides their effects on the GI and renal systems, the nonselective COX inhibitors and the COX-2 inhibitors have a few other differences.[59] These selective inhibitors do not inhibit platelet aggregation or increase bleeding time, so they are of no value in decreasing thrombotic effects. However, the fact that they do not influence bleeding time makes them useful as pain medication after surgery. NSAID use after surgery has been previously limited because of concerns about blood loss. In addition, postoperative use of these drugs has been shown to reduce opioid use, pain, vomiting, and sleep disturbances and to improve range of motion in patients who have had orthopedic surgery.[65]

Acetaminophen

Acetaminophen (also known as paracetamol in Europe) is a common nonnarcotic analgesic and antipyretic agent. It is believed to inhibit prostaglandin synthesis in the CNS, and new research has demonstrated its ability to block the COX-3 enzyme.[44] It has only weak peripheral antiinflammatory properties.

Acetaminophen is primarily used to reduce pain and fever. Although not quite as effective as NSAIDs, it has become standard treatment for osteoarthritis when NSAIDs can no longer be tolerated.[66,67] Trends in medication use show a decline in NSAID use replaced by an increase in acetaminophen use for osteoarthritis.[68] Acetaminophen is also used in combination with NSAIDs to reduce the NSAID dose needed for symptom relief. This in turn will reduce the adverse effects associated with the antiinflammatory agents.

The advantage of acetaminophen over aspirin is that at a normal therapeutic dose it is free of adverse effects and can also be used for prolonged periods without problems.[69] However, at high doses (two to three times the maximum therapeutic dose), especially when combined with alcohol, acetaminophen may produce significant liver and kidney damage. The initial signs of acetaminophen toxicity are nausea and vomiting. The hepatotoxicity may be delayed for 24 to 48 hours. Antidotes given within 12 hours of acute ingestion can be used to reduce liver damage.

Nonsteroidal Antiinflammatory Drugs and Heart Disease

Some short- and long-term studies indicate that NSAIDs can produce elevations in blood pressure, leading to a diagnosis of hypertension.[47,70] This includes aspirin, but at antiinflammatory doses, not at the lower doses used to prevent thrombotic events. In 1990 questions were added to the Nurses' Health Study survey regarding the frequency of use of aspirin, acetaminophen, and other NSAIDs and the onset of hypertension. Follow-up questions were mailed every 2 years for 8 years. The study was completed in 51,630 women between the ages of 44 and 69 years who had no history of high blood pressure at the beginning of the study. However, by the end of the study, 10,579 new cases of hypertension were identified. The women who had the highest risk of developing elevated blood pressure were those who consumed these drugs between 15 and 22 days per month. What was really surprising was that women who used aspirin or acetaminophen 1 day per month or NSAIDs for 5 days per month had significantly higher blood pressure than nonusers. Another surprise was that hypertension was linked to acetaminophen, which at the time was not thought to influence renal function at usual doses. Similar increases in blood pressure are also seen with celecoxib and rofecoxib.[71] In another study among Medicaid beneficiaries in New Jersey, the odds of filling a first antihypertensive prescription were two times greater for subjects who had filled a prescription for an NSAID in the previous year than for those who had not.[70] In addition, the Joint National Committees Sixth Report on Hypertension states that NSAIDs adversely affect blood pressure.[72]

The mechanism of action for this link is probably interference with the synthesis of the renal vasodilator prostaglandins and sodium excretion from the kidney tubules. However, it was surprising that acetaminophen was associated with hypertension because this drug is supposed to block prostaglandin synthesis in the CNS and not in the peripheral tissue.[72] Perhaps the COX-3 isoform exists in the kidneys, or acetaminophen acts on a CNS site for blood pressure regulation.

Another observation regarding NSAIDs and high blood pressure is that these drugs actually make antihypertensive medication less effective.[72-74] Elderly patients who were taking hydrochlorothiazide to lower blood pressure found that their supine systolic and standing systolic pressures were significantly increased when they were taking ibuprofen compared with placebo.[73] Other studies that examined the combination of aspirin and angiotensin-converting enzyme (ACE) inhibitors in patients with heart failure also showed a dose-mediated conflict between the two drugs.[75,76] Aspirin alters arterial properties by blocking the synthesis of certain vasodilating prostaglandins. Therefore the vasodilating goal of an ACE inhibitor is attenuated by the use of aspirin in a dose-dependent manner. A significant effect on arterial properties is evident at an aspirin dose of 325 mg/day, but not at 100 mg/day. In fact, this dose of aspirin may be responsible for inhibiting half of the effectiveness of an ACE inhibitor in patients with difficult-to-treat heart failure.[77]

The second issue regarding the use of NSAIDs in patients with cardiac disease has to do with the increased risk of cardiovascular events associated with COX-2 inhibitors. By targeting only the COX-2 enzyme, they lose the cardioprotection afforded by blocking the COX-1 enzyme. As mentioned earlier, activation of the COX-1 enzyme induces the synthesis of thromboxane A_2 in the platelet, enhancing its clotting function. Blocking this enzyme is the principle behind using low-dose aspirin for cardiac protection. Four major studies, in which 16,000 subjects were enrolled, compared the number of cardiac events among patients who took a COX-2 inhibitor with those among patients who received a traditional NSAID. COX-2 inhibitors, specifically rofecoxib, increased the absolute risk of cardiovascular events by 1% compared with an increase in risk of 0.47% with naproxen [78-80] Those patients who took 50 mg of rofecoxib (higher than the recommended 25-mg dose) were five times more likely to have a myocardial infarction than those who were given 1000 mg of naproxen. At the time of this finding, it was not known whether this result was due to a reduction in cardiovascular events with the nonselective agent, an increase in cardiovascular events with the COX-2 inhibitor, or coincidence.[81] Continued study revealed that patients taking rofecoxib at a dose of 50 mg were almost two times more likely to have a coronary event than patients taking nonselective NSAIDs, but there was no increased risk associated with a dose of 25 mg or lower.[82] Some confounding factors in this study were that 17% of the rofecoxib users were taking 50 mg for 30 days but only 5 days is recommended at this dose, and the study included some subjects with the diagnosis of rheumatoid arthritis, which is also associated with an increased cardiovascular risk.[83,84] Comparisons of COX-2 inhibitors also demonstrated that rofecoxib was associated with an increased risk of cardiac events, whereas an increased risk was not seen with celecoxib.[85] Finally, on September 30, 2004, Merck & Company announced a worldwide withdrawal of rofecoxib.[86] This decision was based on a 4-year study designed to assess the drug's effectiveness in treating colon polyps. Analysis of data from 2600 patients revealed that in the group of patients taking rofecoxib, there were twice as many cardiovascular events, including strokes, compared with the placebo group. Further analysis of the data to determine the cause of these

events is likely to continue. Current speculation is that the drug's increased risk of cardiovascular disease is due to its inhibition of prostacyclin formation and lack of a positive effect on platelet aggregation.[87]

The last issue to discuss regarding the use of NSAIDs and heart disease is the fact that NSAIDs reduce the cardioprotective effects of low-dose aspirin.[88,89] The original study that sounded the alarm regarding this issue included 80 healthy volunteers. These subjects were given low-dose aspirin (81 mg) each morning, followed by 400 mg of ibuprofen 2 hours later, for 6 days. Another group of subjects followed the same procedure with the aspirin, but 2 hours later they were given acetaminophen, rofecoxib, or diclofenac. The next week the order of drug administration was reversed so that the NSAID was given first, followed 2 hours later by the low-dose aspirin. The investigators found that taking the aspirin a few hours before ibuprofen irreversibly inhibited platelet aggregation. However, when ibuprofen was taken before the aspirin, platelet aggregation was reversibly inhibited, eliminating the cardioprotective effects. The reason for this is that aspirin binds to the COX enzyme in the platelet for the life of the platelet. If it is taken first, the aspirin will block access to the binding site for the NSAID. However, if the NSAID binds to the COX first, it will keep the aspirin from entering its binding site, but only temporarily. Reversible binding implies that the NSAID disengages from the platelet so that its antithrombotic action does not persist throughout the dosing interval. The other drugs examined did not influence the beneficial effect of aspirin, regardless of timing of administration. In another study, 7000 men with heart disease who took low-dose aspirin were followed up for an 8-year period and tracked regarding their NSAID use. Those who took ibuprofen and aspirin together were almost twice as likely to have died from a cardiovascular problem than those who took only aspirin.[88] However, naproxen and diclofenac appeared to preserve aspirin's ability to prevent blood clots.

Therapeutic Concerns with Nonsteroidal Antiinflammatory Drugs

The main therapeutic concerns with NSAIDs have to do with bruising and increased risk of bleeding.

If GI side effects are present, the therapist should be on the alert for any diarrhea or vomiting that may interfere with physical therapy services. Last, because so many patients are taking aspirin for its cardioprotective effects and also taking NSAIDs for their musculoskeletal aches and pains, patients should be questioned regarding the timing of these medications and referred to their physicians for counseling if the drugs are not being administered properly. Because many patients take over-the-counter NSAIDs, the drugs are often viewed as being insignificant and thus never discussed with the physician. Also, some patients may be taking a prescription NSAID as well as an over-the-counter NSAID without the physician's knowledge.

NEUROPATHIC PAIN

Neuropathic pain is pain that is associated with disease or injury to the peripheral or central nervous system.[90] Diabetes, immune deficiencies, shingles, trauma, multiple sclerosis, ischemic issues, and cancer can all produce neuropathic pain. It is thought that sustained noxious input leads to altered processing of noxious information and that this plasticity can occur at several neural levels from the spinal cord on up to the cortex.

Mediators of inflammation that may be involved in neuropathic pain syndromes include the neuropeptides (bradykinin, calcitonin gene-related peptide, substance P, vasoactive intestinal peptide), cytokines (interleukins 1β, 6 and 8 and tumor necrosis factor-α), and eicosanoids ($PGF_2\alpha$ and PGE_2 and leukotriene B_4).[91,92]

Clinical signs of neuropathic pain include a variety of stimulus-independent and stimulus-dependent pains. Stimulus-independent pain can be shooting, shock-like, aching, crushing, burning, or electric shock-like. These types of pain may be related to nerve compression or entrapment syndromes. The underlying mechanism may be increased sensitization of C and A delta fibers. Stimulus-dependent pains result from mechanical, thermal, or chemical stimuli. Patients may experience hyperalgesia (including cold or heat hyperalgesia), mechanical allodynia, dysesthesias, paresthesias, and paroxysms. Paroxysms involve shooting, electric- or shock-like pain that results from a benign tactile stimulus. Referred pain, sympathetic hyperactivity, and a loss of some afferent sensory function are also common in neuropathic pain conditions.

Single types of drugs are usually insufficient to treat neuropathic pain. In fact, even though neuropathic pain can be diminished with the traditional analgesics, this syndrome is unfairly represented among patients who respond poorly to opioids.[93] The reason for combining drugs in pain management is that one drug does not always eliminate pain and use of two or more drugs with different mechanisms of action enhances pain relief.[20] Antidepressants and anticonvulsants are frequently used as adjuncts in the treatment of these pain syndromes.[94] Antidepressants such as amitriptyline and imipramine have been used to treat pain associated with diabetic neuropathy, postherpetic neuralgia, polyneuropathy, and nerve injury associated with cancer. The mechanism of action for decreasing pain has not been identified, but it appears to be separate from their antidepressive effect. The assistance with analgesia occurs at lower doses than those used to treat depression. In addition, these medications can relieve symptoms commonly seen in patients with chronic pain such as sleeping problems.[95] The older tricyclic antidepressants have a sedating effect that helps to ease the patient into a more restful sleep. The newer serotonin reuptake inhibitors are less sedating but have also been effective in decreasing chronic pain.

Anticonvulsants such as carbamazepine, phenytoin, lamotrigine, and gabapentin are also effective in the treatment of neuropathic pain.[96-98] Although the pathogenesis of neuropathy is not directly known, and in many cases the exact mechanism of action of the antiseizure drugs is not known, there is speculation that relief of pain with these drugs is due to blockade of sodium channels.

Other medications for neuropathic pain include clonidine and oral cannabinoids.[99-101] Epidural clonidine is indicated for neuropathic pain and is effective in approximately 50% of patients who do not respond to epidural opioids. Clonidine may decrease pain by its action on α_2-adrenergic receptors. Oral cannabinoids (dronabinol) have demonstrated pain-relieving effects in animal models of nerve injury but may not offer significant relief in refractory neuropathic pain. Investigations on the use of these drugs in pain syndromes are ongoing and may provide some new forms of pain relief for difficult cases.

In an effort to improve pharmacological effectiveness in the treatment of neuropathic pain, there has been a push toward pairing individual symptoms to treatment with specific drugs.[90] For patients whose primary complaints are static hyperalgesia (pain in response to gentle pressure caused by sensitized C-fiber nociceptors), the drugs of choice are systemic and topical lidocaine and opioids. When there is hyperalgesia in response to light stroking of the skin, NMDA antagonists such as ketamine and dextromethorphan (a low-affinity NMDA channel blocker) may be indicated. The pain-producing mechanism in this case may be "central sensitization" from increased input. In cases in which the symptoms are related to sympathetic hyperactivity, norepinephrine blockade is recommended with either clonidine or a stellate ganglion block with lidocaine. In summary, the recommended protocols are as follows: opioids or lidocaine for sensitized C-nociceptors, adrenergic blockers for sympathetic maintained pain, lidocaine for pain and itching associated with vasodilation, and NMDA antagonists for centrally mediated pain produced by excess activity at these receptors.

PAIN RELATED TO CANCER

Cancer-related pain is pain that may result from primary tumor growth, metastatic disease, or the toxic effects of chemotherapy and radiation.[93] Invasion of bone, joint, or muscle can cause continuous pain. Bone pain appears to be common, but not all bone metastases become painful. The spine is the most common site for bone metastases. Extension of the tumor from the vertebra may produce spinal cord or cauda equina compression and result in neurological compromise. The pain complaints tend to be variable; patients may complain of aching pains or dysesthesias anywhere in the dermatomal area innervated by the compressed neural tissue.

Treatment-related pain syndromes are also common and can result from chemotherapy, radiation, or surgery. Necrosis of bone may result from treatment with steroids or radiation. Visceral pain may result from intraperitoneal chemotherapy, scar tissue from surgery, or radiation-induced fibrosis.

Regular administration of NSAIDs is the usual starting point for mild pain associated with cancer. However, the beneficial response of pain control needs to be balanced with the risks (GI problems, bleeding tendencies, and masking of fever that indicates infection). When these drugs are no longer effective, a weak opioid may be added to or substituted for the NSAID. Codeine and hydrocodone preparations are recommended. When combinations of codeine-like drugs and NSAIDs are not sufficient and pain is severe, strong opioids are recommended. Morphine, hydromorphone, transdermal fentanyl, and oxycodone are appropriate. Sequential opioid trials (opioid rotations) are used to identify the drug that strikes the best balance between pain relief and side effects. During a switch to a stronger opioid, the dose of the new drug is reduced by approximately 30% to 50%.[93] Fixed schedule dosing appears to be preferred over dosing on an as-needed basis. Patients with limited opioid exposure are started out with a low dose, equivalent to 5 to 10 mg of parenteral morphine every 4 hours. Rescue medication is supplied for breakthrough pain. Patients with bone cancer pain generally require significantly higher doses of morphine than those with postoperative pain.[102]

When the opioid regimen fails to control pain, the adjuvant pain medications discussed earlier (antidepressants, NMDA antagonists, antiseizure medications, and local anesthetics) can be added, or the mode of administration (e.g., PCA or patches) can be changed.[93] The oral mode of administration is preferred but may need to be avoided if the patient has dysphagia or is vomiting. Corticosteroids can be administered after full opioid effectiveness has been exploited. Steroids are considered multipurpose drugs to relieve pain, anorexia, and nausea. They can also reduce tumor size in certain types of cancers (lymphomas). Drugs for bone pain include the bisphosphonates (see Chapter 15) and calcitonin, which can be added to the opioid regimen.[103] Even the Ca^{2+} channel blocker nifedipine has been used to decrease bone pain. Aggressive management of opioid and chemotherapy side effects also reduces discomfort. Anticholinergics can be used to reduce vomiting, and laxatives can be used for relief of opioid-induced constipation.

ACTIVITIES 12

■ 1. You are treating a 62-year-old woman with metastatic breast cancer in her home. This patient is currently receiving intravenous morphine through a PCA device. When you arrive at the patient's house, you find the front door open and a note from the patient's caregiver that she had a family emergency and had to leave. You suspect that the caregiver had left several hours ago, which means that the patient had not been checked or repositioned during that time. When you arrive at the patient's bedside, she is difficult to awake. She responds to stimuli but falls back to sleep. Blood pressure is 120/70 mm Hg, pulse is 86 beats/min, and respirations are 6 breaths/min. On your last visit, the patient was weak but fully responsive and cooperative with therapy.

Questions

a. What is your immediate course of action?
b. What factors could have contributed to the patient's change in condition?
c. What drug might be prescribed for this patient?
d. What did this case teach you about working with patients who are receiving opiates?
e. If this patient were receiving morphine through an epidural catheter, what signs would indicate catheter malposition?

■ 2. A 63-year-old man presents with severe, unrelenting midthoracic pain. The patient reports an insidious increase in pain over the past 2 months. He denies any falls or injuries to his back. He also reports a loss of 15 lb in the same period and constipation. Medical history includes squamous cell carcinoma of the lung 2 years ago, treated with chemo until remission 6 months

ago; hypertension, benign prostatic hypertrophy, and hyperlipidemia. Current medications include finasteride, simvastatin, and enalapril.

Labs
Alanine aminotransferase level, 40 IU/L; aspartate aminotransferase level, 45 IU/L; γ-glutamyl transferase level, 100 IU/L; alkaline phosphatase level, 350 IU/L; blood urea nitrogen level, 20 mg/dL; total calcium concentration, 30 mEq/L; total cholesterol level, 260 mg/dL; sodium concentration, 140 mEq/L; chloride concentration, 105 mEq/L; potassium concentration, 3.0 mEq/L; serum creatinine level, 1.0 mg/dL, red blood cell count, 5.0×10^6/mm^3, white blood cell count, 7000/mm^3; platelets, 80,000/mm^3

X-Ray
Compression fracture of T9-T12

Bone Scan
Metastatic disease localized in areas of ribs and spine

Questions

a. Analyze the patient's lab values and physical findings and list his medical problems.
b. How would you manage the patient's pain, both from a pharmacological perspective and a physical therapy perspective?
c. Discuss the issue of psychological dependence and addiction associated with opiate use in patients with cancer.
d. How should the patient be monitored in terms of efficacy, tolerance, and adverse effects?

References

1. Holtzman SG, Sung YF. Pain control with opioid analgesics. In: Brody MJ, Larner J, Minneman KP, eds. *Human Pharmacology: Molecular to Clinical.* 3rd ed. Philadelphia: Mosby; 1998:395-408.
2. Rang HP, Dale MM, Ritter JM, Moore JL. *Pharmacology.* 5th ed. New York: Churchill Livingstone; 2003.
3. Carr DB, Goudas LC. Acute pain. *Lancet.* 1999; 353:2051-2058.
4. Parsons CG. NMDA receptors as targets for drug action in neuropathic pain. *Eur J Pharmacol.* 2001;429:71-78.

5. Julius D, Basbaum AI. Molecular mechanisms of nociception. *Nature*. 2001;413:203-210.

6. Longmore J, Hill RG, Hargreaves RJ. Neurokinin-receptor antagonists: pharmacological tool and therapeutic drugs. *Can J Physiol Pharmacol*. 1997;75:612-621.

7. Yaksh TL. Spinal systems and pain processing: development of novel analgesic drugs with mechanistically defined models. *Trends Pharmacol Sci*. 1999;20(8):329-337.

8. Przewlocki R, Przewlocki B. Opioids in chronic pain. *Eur J Pharmacol*. 2001;429:79-91.

9. Dhawan BN, Cesselin F, Raghubir R, Reisine T, Bradley PB, Portoghese PS. International Union of Pharmacology. XII. Classification of opioid receptors. *Pharmacol Rev*. 1996;48(4):567-592.

10. Stein C, Yassouridis A. Peripheral morphine analgesia. *Pain*. 1997;71:119-121.

11. Inturrisi CE. Clinical pharmacology of opioids for pain. *Clin J Pain*. 2002;18(suppl 4):S3-S13.

12. Ballantyne CM, Mao J. Opioid therapy for chronic pain. *N Engl J Med*. 2003;349(20):1943-1953.

13. Portenoy RK. Opioid therapy for chronic nonmalignant pain: a review of the critical issues. *J Pain Symptom Manage*. 1996;11(4):203-217.

14. Camu F, Vanlersberghe C. Pharmacology of systemic analgesics. *Best Pract Res Clin Anaesthesiol*. 2002; 16(4):475-488.

15. Vallerand AH. The use of long-acting opioids in chronic pain management. *Nurs Clin North Am*. 2003; 38(3):435-445.

16. Kornick CA, Santiago-Palma J, Moryl N, Payne R, Obbens EA. Benefit-risk assessment of transdermal fentanyl for the treatment of chronic pain. *Drug Saf*. 2003;26(13):951-973.

17. Amato L, Davoli M, Ferri M, Ali R. Methadone at tapered doses for the management of opioid withdrawal. *Cochrane Database Syst Rev*. 2003;(3):CD003409.

18. Layson-Wolf C, Goode JV, Small RE. Clinical use of methadone. *J Pain Palliat Care Pharmacother*. 2002; 16(1):29-59.

19. McQuay H. Opioids in pain management. *Lancet*. 1999;353:2229-2232.

20. Curatolo M, Sveticic G. Drug combinations in pain treatment: a review of the published evidence and a method for finding the optimal combination. *Best Pract Res Clin Anaesthesiol*. 2002;16(4):507-519.

21. Oxycodone and OxyContin. *Med Lett Drugs Ther*. 2001; 43(1113):80-81.

22. Schnitzer T. The new analgesic combination tramadol/acetaminophen. *Eur J Anaesthesiol*. 2003;20(suppl 28): 13-17.

23. Buprenorphine: an alternative to methadone. *Med Lett Drugs Ther*. 2003; 45(1150):13-15.

24. Chapman SL, Byas-Smith MG, Reed BA. Effects of intermediate- and long-term use of opioids on cognition in patients with chronic pain. *Clin J Pain*. 2002; 18(4):S83-S90.

25. Sacerdote P, Manfredi B, Mantegazza P, Panerai AE. Antinociceptive and immunosuppressive effects of opiate drugs: a structure-related activity study. *Br J Pharmacol*. 1997;121:834-840.

26. Peterson PK, Sharp BM, Gekker G, Portoghese PS, Sannerud K, Balfour HH. Morphine promotes the growth of HIV-1 in human peripheral blood mononuclear cell cocultures. *AIDS*. 1990;4(9):869-873.

27. Potent painkillers: addictive? *Johns Hopkins Med Lett Health After 50*. 2004;16(1):1-2, 7.

28. Strain EC. Assessment and treatment of comorbid psychiatric disorders in opioid-dependent patients. *Clin J Pain*. 2002;18(4):S14-S27.

29. Savage SR, Joranson DE, Covington EC, Schnoll SH, Heit HA, Gilson AM. Definitions related to the medical use of opioids: evolution towards universal agreement. *J Pain Symptom Manage*. 2003;26(1):655-667.

30. Ballantyne JC, Carr DB, Chalmers TC, Dear KB, Angelillo IF, Mosteller F. Postoperative patient-controlled analgesia: meta-analyses of initial randomized control trials. *J Clin Anesthesiol*. 1993;5:182-193.

31. Jones TF, Feler CA, Simmons BP, et al. Neurologic complications including paralysis after a medication error involving implanted intrathecal catheters. *Am J Med*. 2002;112(1):31-36.

32. Shang AB, Gan TJ. Optimising postoperative pain management in the ambulatory patient. *Drugs*. 2003; 63(9):855-867.

33. Vicente KJ, Kada-Bekhaled K, Hillel G, Cassano A, Orser BA. Programming errors contribute to death from patient-controlled analgesia: case report and estimate of probability. *Can J Anaesthesiol*. 2003;50(4): 328-332.

34. Kuhn M. *Pharmacotherapeutics: A Nursing Process Approach*. 4th ed. Philadelphia: FA Davis; 1998.

35. Finger MJ, McLeod DG. Postoperative myocardial infarction after radical cystoprostatectomy masked by patient-controlled analgesia. *Urology*. 1995;45(1): 155-157.

36. Brown LS, Bogner MS, Parmentier CM, Taylor JB. Human error and patient-controlled analgesia pumps. *J Intraven Nurs*. 1997;20(6):311-316.

37. authors N. General-purpose infusion pumps. evaluating the B. Braun Outlook Safety Infusion System. *Health Devices*. 2003;32(10):382-395.

38. Viscusi ER, Reynolds L, Chung F, Atkinson LE, Khanna S. Patient controlled transdermal fentanyl hydrochloride vs intravenous morphine pump for postoperative pain. *JAMA*. 2004;291(11):1333-1341.

39. Bjorkman DJ. The effect of aspirin and nonsteroidal anti-inflammatory drugs on prostaglandins. *Am J Med*. 1998;105(1, suppl 2):8S-12S.

40. Eberhart CE, Du Bois RN. Eicosanoids and the gastrointestinal tract. *Gastroenterology*. 1995;109:285-301.

41. Brater DC. Effects of nonsteroidal antiinflammatory drug on renal function: focus on cyclooxygenase-2 selective inhibition. *Am J Med*. 1999;107:65S-71S.

42. Vane J. Towards a better aspirin. *Nature*. 1994;367:215-216.

43. Chandrasekharan NV, Dai H, Roos LT, et al. COX-3, a cyclooxygenase-1 variant inhibited by acetaminophen and other analgesic/antipyretic drugs: cloning, structure, and expression. *Proc Natl Acad Sci USA*. 2002; 99(21):13926-13931.

44. Warner TD, Mitchell JA. Cyclooxygenase-3 (COX-3): filling in the gaps toward COX continuum? *Proc Natl Acad Sci USA*. 2002;99(21):13371-13373.

45. Schwab JM, Schluesener HJ, Laufer S. COX-3: just another COX or the solitary elusive target of paracetamol. *Lancet*. 2003;361:981-982.

46. Schwab JM, Beiter T, Linder JU, Laufer S, Schulz JE, Meyermann R. COX-3—a virtual pain target in humans? *FASEB J*. 2003;17(15):2174-2175.

47. Dedier J, Stampfer M, Hankinson S, Willett W, Speizer F, Curhan G. Nonnarcotic analgesic use and the risk of hypertension in US women. *Hypertension.* 2002; 40:604-608.

48. Hulley SB, Furberg CD, Barrett-Connor E, et al. Non-cardiovascular disease outcomes during 6.8 years of hormone therapy: Heart and Estrogen/Progestin Replacement Study follow up. *JAMA.* 2002;288(1):58-66.

49. Asanuma M, Nishibayashi-Asanuma S, Miyazaki I, Kohno M, Ogawa N. Neuroprotective effects of non-steroidal anti-inflammatory drugs by direct scavenging of nitric oxide radicals. *J Neurochem.* 2001;76(6):1895-1904.

50. Thomas T, Nadackal TG, Thomas K. Aspirin and non-steroidal anti-inflammatory drugs inhibit amyloid-beta aggregation. *Neuroreport.* 2001;12(15):3261-3267.

51. Etminan M, Gill S, Samii A. Effect of non-steroidal anti-inflammatory drugs on risk of Alzheimer's disease: systematic review and meta-analysis of observational studies. *BMJ.* 2003;327(7407):128-138.

52. Aisen PS, Schafer KA, Grundman M, et al. Effects of rofecoxib or naproxen vs placebo on Alzheimer disease progression: a randomized controlled trial. *JAMA.* 2003;289(21):2819-2826.

53. Chan F, Hung L, Suen B, et al. Celecoxib versus diclofenac and omeprazole in reducing the risk of recurrent ulcer bleeding in patients with arthritis. *N Engl J Med.* 2002;347(26):2104-2110.

54. Scheiman J, Arbor A, Isenberg J. Agents used in the prevention and treatment of nonsteroidal anti-inflammatory drug-associated symptoms and ulcers. *Am J Med.* 1998;105(5A):32S-38S.

55. Way RA, Stein MC, Byrd V, et al. Educational program for physicians to reduce use of non-steroidal anti-inflammatory drugs among community-dwelling elderly persons: a randomized controlled trial. *Med Care.* 2001;39(5):425-435.

56. Scharf S, Kwiatek R, Ugoni A, Christophidis N. NSAIDs and faecal blood loss in elderly patients with osteoarthritis: is plasma half-life relevant? *Aust N Z J Med.* 1998;28:436-439.

57. Furst DE, Munster T. Nonsteroidal anti-inflammatory drugs, disease-modifying antirheumatic drugs, nonopioid analgesics, & drugs used in gout. In: Katzung BG, ed. *Basic & Clinical Pharmacology.* 8th ed. New York: McGraw-Hill; 2002:596-623.

58. St Lawrence KS, Ye FQ, Lewis BK, Weinberger DR, Frank JA, McLaughlin AC. Effects of indomethacin on cerebral blood flow at rest and during hypercapnia: an arterial spin tagging study in humans. *J Magn Reson Imaging.* 2002;15(6):628-635.

59. Drugs for pain. *Med Lett Drugs Ther.* 2000;42(1085): 73-78.

60. Perazella MA. COX-2 selective inhibitors: analysis of the renal effects. *Expert Opin Drug Saf.* 2002;1(1):53-64.

61. Gambaro G, Perazella MA. Adverse renal effects of anti-inflammatory agents: evaluation of selective and non-selective cyclooxygenase inhibitors. *J Intern Med.* 2003; 253(6):643-652.

62. Catella-Lawson F, McAdam B, Morrison BW, et al. Effects of specific inhibition of cyclooxygenase-2 on sodium balance, hemodynamics, and vasoactive eicosanoids. *J Pharmacol Exp Ther.* 1999;289:735-741.

63. Rofecoxib for osteoarthritis and pain. *Med Lett Drugs Ther.* 1999;41(1056):59-61.

64. Valdecoxib (Bextra): a new cox-2 inhibitor. *Med Lett Drugs Ther.* 2002;44(1129):39-40.

65. Buvanendran A, Kroin JS, Tuman KJ, et al. Effects of perioperative administration of a selective cyclo-oxygenase 2 inhibitor on pain management and recovery of function after knee replacement. *JAMA.* 2003;290(18):2411-2418.

66. Acetaminophen for osteoarthritis. *Cochrane Database Syst Rev.* 2003;2(CD004257).

67. Case JP, Baliunas AJ, Block JA. Lack of efficacy of acetaminophen in treating symptomatic knee osteoarthritis: a randomized, double-blind, placebo-controlled comparison trial with diclofenac sodium. *Arch Intern Med.* 2003;163(2):169-178.

68. Ausiello JC, Staffore RS. Trends in medication use for osteoarthritis treatment. *J Rheumatol.* 2002;29(5):999-1005.

69. Acetaminophen safety. *Med Lett Drugs Ther.* 2002; 44(1142):91-93.

70. Gurwitz JH, Avorn J, Bohn RL, Glynn RJ, Monane M, Mogun H. Initiation of antihypertensive treatment during nonsteroidal anti-inflammatory drug therapy. *JAMA.* 1994;272(10):781-786.

71. Whelton A, White W, Bello A, Puma J, Fort J, Investigators S-V. Effects of celecoxib and rofecoxib on blood pressure and edema in patients >65 years of age with systemic hypertension and osteoarthritis. *Am J Cardiol.* 2002;90:959-963.

72. Egan BM. Nonnarcotic analgesic use and the risk of hypertension in US women. *Hypertension.* 2002;40(5): 601-603.

73. Gurwitz JH, Everitt DE, Monane M, et al. The impact of ibuprofen on the efficacy of antihypertensive treatment with hydrochlorothiazide in elderly persons. *J Gerontol A Biol Sci Med Sci.* 1996;51(2):M74-M79.

74. Meune C, Mourad JJ, Bergmann JF, Spaulding C. Interaction between cyclooxygenase and the renin-angiotensin-aldosterone system: rationale and clinical relevance. *J Renin Angiotensin Aldosterone Syst.* 2003; 4(3):149-154.

75. Meune C, Mahe I, Mourad JJ, et al. Aspirin alters arterial function in patients with chronic heart failure treated with ACE inhibitors: a dose-mediated deleterious effect. *Eur J Heart Fail.* 2003;5(3):271-279.

76. Park MH. Should aspirin be used with angiotensin-converting enzyme inhibitors in patients with chronic heart failure? *Congest Heart Fail.* 2003;9:206-213.

77. Hall D. The aspirin-angiotensin-converting enzyme inhibitor tradeoff: to halve and halve not. *J Am Coll Cardiol.* 2000;35:1808-1812.

78. Mukherjee D, Nissen SE, Topol EJ. Risk of cardiovascular events associated with selective COX-2 inhibitors. *JAMA.* 2001;286(8):954-959.

79. Fowles RE. Potential cardiovascular effects of COX-2 selective nonsteroidal antiinflammatory drugs. *J Pain Palliat Care Pharmacother.* 2003;17(2):27-50.

80. Cardiovascular safety of COX-2 inhibitors. *Med Lett Drugs Ther.* 2001;43(1118):99-100.

81. Cleland JGF. No reduction in cardiovascular risk with NSAIDs-including aspirin? *Lancet.* 2002;359(9301): 92-93.

82. Ray WA, Stein MC, Daugherty JR, Hall K, Arbogast PG, Griffin MR. COX-2 selective non-steroidal anti-inflammatory drugs and risk of serious coronary heart disease. *Lancet.* 2002;360(9339):1071-1073.

83. DeMaria AN. Relative risk of cardiovascular events in patients with rheumatoid arthritis. *Am J Cardiol*. 2002; 89(suppl):33D-38D.

84. Griffin MR, Stein CM, Graham DJ, Daugherty JR, Arobogast PG, Ray WA. High frequency of use of rofecoxib at greater than recommended doses: cause for concern. *Pharmacoepidemiol Drug Saf*. 2004;13(6):339-343.

85. Solomon DH, Schneeweiss S, Glynn RJ, et al. Relationship between selective cyclooxygenase-2 inhibitors and acute myocardial infarction in older adults. *Circulation*. 2004;109(17):2068-2073.

86. Cohen R, Silverman E. FDA blasted for how it handled Vioxx after studies raised flags. *The Sunday Star-Ledger*. October 3, 2004;sect 3(1).

87. Ray WA, Stein CM, Hall K, Daugherty JR, Griffin MR. Non-steroidal anti-inflammatory drugs and risk of serious coronary heart disease: an observational cohort study. *Lancet*. 2002;359(9301):118-123.

88. MacDonald T, Wei L. Effect of ibuprofen on cardioprotective effect of aspirin. *Lancet*. 2003;361:573-574.

89. Catella-Lawson F, Reilly MP, Kapoor SC, et al. Cyclooxygenase inhibitors and the antiplatelet effects of aspirin. *N Engl J Med*. 2001;345(25):1809-1817.

90. Jensen TS, Gottrup H, Sindrup SH, Bach FW. The clinical picture of neuropathic pain. *Eur J Pharmacol*. 2001;429:1-11.

91. Huygen F, de Bruijn A, Klein J, Zijlstra FJ. Neuroimmune alterations in the complex regional pain syndrome. *Eur J Pharmacol*. 2001;429:101-113.

92. Boddeke E. Involvement of chemokines in pain. *Eur J Pharmacol*. 2001;429:115-119.

93. Portenoy RK, Lesage P. Management of cancer pain. *Lancet*. 1999;353:1695-1700.

94. Sindrup SH, Jensen TS. Efficacy of pharmacological treatments of neuropathic pain: an update and effect related to mechanism of drug action. *Pain*. 1999; 83:389-400.

95. Asburn MA, Staats PS. Management of chronic pain. *Lancet*. 1999;353:1865-1869.

96. Eisenberg E, Damunni G, Hoffer E, Baum Y, Krivoy N. Lamotrigine for intractable sciatica: correlation between dose, plasma concentration and analgesia. *Eur J Pain*. 2003;7(6):485-491.

97. Serpell MG. Gabapentin in neuropathic pain syndromes: a randomised, double-blind, placebo-controlled trial. *Pain*. 2002;99(3):557-566.

98. Simpson DM, Olney R, McArthur JC, Khan A, Godbold J, Ebel-Frommer K. A placebo-controlled trial of lamotrigine for painful HIV-associated neuropathy. *Neurology*. 2000;54(11):2115-2119.

99. Attal N, Brasseur L, Guirimand D, Clermond-Gnamien S, Atlami S, Bouhassira D. Are oral cannabinoids safe and effective in refractory neuropathic pain? *Eur J Pain*. 2004;8(2):173-177.

100. Ackerman LL, Follett KA, Rosenquist RW. Long-term outcomes during treatment of chronic pain with intrathecal clonidine or clonidine/opioid combinations. *J Pain Symptom Manage*. 2003;26(1):668-677.

101. Martin TJ, Eisenach JC. Pharmacology of opioid and nonopioid analgesics in chronic pain states. *J Pharmacol Exp Ther*. 2001;299(3):811-817.

102. Luger NM, Sabino MA, Schwei MJ, et al. Efficacy of systemic morphine suggests a fundamental difference in the mechanisms that generate bone cancer vs inflammatory pain. *Pain*. 2002;99(3):397-406.

103. Fine PG. Analgesia issues in palliative care: bone pain, controlled release opioids, managing opioid-induced constipation and nifedipine as an analgesic. *J Pain Palliative Care Pharmacother*. 2002;16(1):93-97.

CHAPTER 13

DRUG TREATMENT FOR ARTHRITIS-RELATED CONDITIONS

DRUG TREATMENT OF RHEUMATOID ARTHRITIS

Rheumatoid arthritis (RA) is a chronic and progressive inflammatory disorder, primarily affecting the synovium of the joints and leading to pain, stiffness, joint damage, and disability. The progression and general virulence of the disease may vary, but the course of disease is generally downward, with 50% of individuals becoming unable to work within 10 years of diagnosis.[1,2] Despite years of study, the cause and the mechanisms of disease in RA remain unknown.[3] Even the diagnostic process of using a set of clinical criteria is unrefined by today's standards of biological markers for disease. Treatment of RA has not been sensibly based on a thorough understanding of the pathogenesis but has instead been borrowed from other diseases. Treatment has consisted of an array of antiinflammatory and immunosuppressive drugs with their weak justification following some clinical efficacy. However, certain strides in treatment have been made and consist of extensive use of methotrexate (a chemotherapy agent), aggressive early treatment, and the development of effective combination treatments with methotrexate.[4]

Clinical Presentation

RA typically develops slowly over weeks to months, and symptoms include fatigue, weakness, low-grade fevers, and joint pain.[2] Stiffness, particularly of the hands, and myalgias precede the onset of inflammation. Joint involvement is commonly symmetrical and tends to affect the small joints of the hands, wrist, and feet; but some larger joints such as the elbows, shoulders, hips, knees, and ankles may also be involved. Symptoms of inflammation and joint swelling may be visible or palpable. The soft tissue around the joints feels soft, spongy, and warm and appears erythematous. Over time, slow destruction of the ligaments and tendons leads to joint deformities including metacarpophalangeal subluxations and other deformities involving the proximal interphalangeal joints such as swan-neck deformity, boutonniere deformity, and ulnar deviation. Extraarticular systemic involvement is also prevalent including vasculitis, pleural effusion, pericarditis, and lymphadenopathy.

Diagnosis is based on the American Rheumatism Association's criteria for classification of RA.[5] The criteria include the presence of morning stiffness, symmetrical arthritis, rheumatoid nodules, radiographic changes, and some laboratory values. Laboratory tests may show anemia, depressed bone marrow, elevated erythrocyte sedimentation rate, positive rheumatoid factor (60% to 70% of patients), and a positive antinuclear antibody (ANA) titer (25% of patients).

Pathogenesis of Rheumatoid Arthritis

RA has typically been considered an autoimmune disease; however, none of the laboratory markers strictly support this notion. In addition, a "unique autoantigen" has not been found, proving that this is strictly an autoimmune disorder.[3] At present, much of the attention regarding the pathogenesis of RA centers on the role of the T lymphocytes in the inflamed joint and proinflammatory cytokines.

RA is genetically linked to the histocompatibility antigens HLA DR 1 and 4.[6] This genetic connection is related to the presentation of antigen to the T lymphocytes that signal inflammation with synovial lining cell hyperplasia, T-lymphocyte infiltration, and the secretion of toxic proteases into the joint (collagenases, stromelysin, and free radicals). Activation of the cellular and humoral immune responses (B cell and cell mediated) begins with involvement of chemokines, cell adhesion molecules, and cytokines, resulting in loss of cartilage and bony erosions.

Because T lymphocytes are abundant in inflamed synovial tissue, researchers have spent time developing T-cell–depleting agents (novel monoclonal antibodies), but this approach has been largely ineffective.[3] Researchers' disappointment with this approach has led to a new focus on the other cellular components of the inflamed synovium, macrophage-like synoviocytes and fibroblastic synoviocytes, and a new model of RA as a "chronic tissue specific inflammatory process" with a variety of immune mediators playing a role.

Analysis of the inflamed synovium has shown that it contains principally two types of synoviocytes in abundance, type A and type B. Type A synoviocytes are members of the monocyte-macrophage family, which secretes large amounts of proinflammatory cytokines. This family is also known for its phagocytic ability. Type B synoviocytes are the specialized fibroblasts that produce hyaluronic acid and collagen, but under inflammatory conditions, these cells may also secrete cytokines and proteases into the joints. Neutrophils in the synovial fluid and chondrocytes in the cartilage also contribute inflammatory mediators.

The focus of research has become even more narrowed as new information about cytokines has been discovered. Cytokines are proteins that work as intercellular messengers for the immune system. Some cytokines have been classified as interleukins, but others have been named according to their function, such as tumor necrosis factor-α (TNF-α). Cytokines are produced in response to other cytokines (sort of a chain reaction) and also activated in response to specific stimuli such as microbial

products. Specifically, they bind to specific cell receptors that ultimately signal transduction systems that regulate transcription of specific genes. They tend to act locally but can have significant systemic effects. Cytokines have been shown to induce metabolic effects, including alterations in lipids and peripheral insulin resistance that promote atherogenesis, and they may be responsible for early death caused by coronary heart disease in patients with RA.[7,8]

In RA, cytokines are involved extensively in all aspects of inflammation and joint destruction. Table 13-1 lists the cytokines seen in inflamed synovial tissue, with TNF and interleukin-1 (IL-1) being the most abundant.[3,9] TNF was originally discovered as a factor that can induce regression and cell death in some tumors, but it may also be responsible for cachexia in cancer. Its level in RA coincides with the extent of inflammation and bone erosion, as well as with the expression of adhesion molecules, synthesis and release of proteases, and synovial neoangiogenesis (production of blood vessels in the synovium). IL-1 has many of the same properties as TNF.

With all this new understanding of RA, research has been directed toward neutralizing or blocking TNF.[3] Monoclonal antibodies to TNF are being used clinically. These drugs block TNF expression and also produce decreases in IL-1, IL-6, and some other adhesion molecules, reducing inflammatory infiltration. Another new approach is the administration of soluble TNF receptors that bind TNF, reducing its biological activity. The TNF blockers and soluble receptors show great promise for patients with RA. However, research on these agents is new, and it is still unknown whether they are more effective than the traditional drugs used for treatment of RA. Many of the initial studies have been placebo-controlled trials, and only recently have these drugs been compared with the gold standard treatment, methotrexate. Another concern is that these new drugs have still not elucidated a clear cause of RA, but the research has helped explain why some of the older agents such as antimalarials, gold, sulfasalazine, and steroids have been useful because all of them inhibit cytokine production to some extent.

Antirheumatoid Drugs

Three primary categories of drugs are used to treat RA: nonsteroidal antiinflammatory drugs (NSAIDs)

Table 13-1

Cytokines Detected in Rheumatoid Arthritis Synovial Tissue or Fluid				
Cytokine	Source	Target	Abundance	Effect on Inflammation or Tissue Damage
TNF	M	Multiple	+++	+++
IL-1β	M	Multiple	+++	+++
IL-6	M, F	Multiple	++	++
IL-8	Multiple	Neutrophils	++	++
IL-10	M, T	T	++	−
IL-12	M	T	+	++
IL-15	F, M	T	+	++
IL-2	T	T	+/−	+
IL-17	T	F	+	++
IFN-γ	T	Multiple	+	++
TGF-β	Multiple	T	++	−
GM-CSF	M, T	Multiple	++	++

From Fox DA. Cytokine blockade as a new strategy to treat rheumatoid arthritis: inhibition of tumor necrosis factor. *Arch Intern Med.* 2000;160:437-444.

TNF, Tumor necrosis factor; *IL,* interleukin; *IFN,* interferon; *TGF,* transforming growth factor; *GM-CSF,* granulocyte-macrophage colony-stimulating factor; *M,* monocyte/macrophage; *F,* fibroblast; *T,* T lymphocyte; −, inhibitory effect; +, low abundance/mild effect; ++, moderate abundance/moderate effect; +++, high abundance/high effect.

including aspirin and other salicylates for their antiinflammatory actions, disease-modifying antirheumatic drugs (DMARDs) for their attempt to alter the disease, and corticosteroids, which bridge the gap between the two. NSAIDs and the cyclooxygenase 2 (COX-2) inhibitors are used early in the course of the disease but only provide symptomatic relief rather than prevent joint destruction. Because these drugs have been extensively reviewed in Chapter 12, they will not be discussed in this section, but they are very important for the patient with RA.

Corticosteroids

The corticosteroid drug prednisone can produce quick and significant symptomatic improvement in inflammation. Prednisone is the synthetic version of our natural endogenous corticosteroid, cortisol. Cortisol is secreted from the adrenal cortex in response to adrenocorticotropic hormone (ACTH) coming from the anterior pituitary gland. The major physiological effects of cortisol include increasing gluconeogenesis and lipolysis to provide fuel for activity and for brain function. Cortisol also enhances epinephrine synthesis and sensitizes tissues to the effect of catecholamines. It is considered to be the

"stress hormone," meaning that physical, emotional, or chemical stress triggers its release.

Prednisone is used in the treatment of RA because it reduces inflammation and suppresses the immune system. When given exogenously, prednisone interferes with inflammatory cell adhesion and migration through vascular endothelium, impairs leukotriene and prostaglandin synthesis by blocking phospholipase A_2, impairs transport of immune complexes, makes antigens susceptible to phagocytosis, and inhibits release of immune cytokines through inhibition of their transcription factors.[10] Additionally, steroids have a direct effect on depressing bone marrow cells, resulting in neutropenia, leukopenia, and eosinopenia. The result is immune system depression.

Excess glucocorticosteroids, given for extended periods, are associated with a variety of negative side effects, leading to reluctance to prescribe them on a long-term basis. Steroids have a catabolic effect on all types of supportive joint tissue, producing osteoporosis, increased incidence of fracture, tendon rupture, thinned skin, and muscle wasting. Exogenous steroid use leads to Cushing's syndrome, which is characterized by muscle weakness, truncal obesity, "moon facies," fragile skin and capillaries, easy bruising, hypertension, diabetes, and neuro-psychiatric disorders.[11] Poor wound healing, increased risk of infection, stomach ulcers, acne, and cataracts can also occur.

Because osteoporosis occurs in about 50% of patients with RA, the American College of Rheumatology has developed some guidelines to prevent loss of bone density. The recommendations include administering the lowest effective dose. In addition, patients should adhere to certain lifestyle principles that have been shown to slow bone resorption. Avoidance of smoking, limiting alcohol intake, and maintaining a healthy weight are suggested. A baseline bone scan should be performed before steroid treatment is started, and follow-up scans should be done every 6 months to 1 year. Patients must also take 1500 mg of calcium and 400 to 800 IU of vitamin D daily. Administration of growth hormone is useful for children receiving steroids to prevent slowing of linear bone growth.[12] Treatment with the anti-osteoporosis drugs, alendronate, risedronate, and calcitonin, is also recommended (see Chapter 15).

Side effects of steroids may be minimized by alternate-day dosing or by using an alternative route of administration such as inhalation or topical application. Alternate-day dosing only works with prednisone and only if it is given at precisely the correct time. Another problem with using prednisone for chronic conditions is that patients must be convinced to withdraw the drug when the time is appropriate. Steroids produce a therapeutic effect but also create some euphoria and energizing effects, and patients may be reluctant to discontinue using them.

Because the adrenal glands stop producing steroids during exogenous administration (negative feedback), discontinuation of these drugs is performed slowly over time. The purpose of the weaning process is to give the adrenal glands time to resume production of steroids and also to help prevent a recurrence of the arthritis, which often occurs.

There has been renewed interest in the use of low doses of prednisone as a treatment for RA, given the belief that many of the side effects are dose related. A dose of prednisone may range anywhere from 5 to 150 mg/day. A low dose of prednisone is considered to be around 10 mg/day and is usually given in divided doses (5 mg twice a day). Several studies have shown this level of prednisone to be effective in limiting the number of tender and swollen joints, improving grip strength, and retarding the progression of bony erosions as compared with placebo when used as monotherapy in patients with a recent diagnosis of RA.[13-15] Prednisone can slow the course of RA, but this effect is limited. Therefore it is not recommended as monotherapy but should be combined with some other DMARDs for added benefit. Low-dose prednisone is well tolerated, although some side effects including high blood sugar levels, weight gain, bruising, and osteopenia are still documented.[16] Tapering is usually started at 6 months and is performed slowly with 1-mg decreases every couple of weeks to a month.[17]

Antimalarials

The antimalarial drug most commonly used in practice is hydroxychloroquine.[6] Approximately 30% of patients with RA respond to this drug, but improvement usually does not occur for 3 to 6 months. It has an extremely long half-life of around 40 days, so reaching a steady-state plasma concentration may take months. Its mechanism of action is to inhibit the response of lymphocytes to antigens. It is considered less effective than some of the other DMARDs but can be used as an adjunct. Side effects are not common but may include diarrhea, loss of appetite, gastrointestinal (GI) cramping, itching, and dizziness. Patients receiving long-term therapy may experience a rare retinopathy characterized by a progressive decrease in visual fields and irreversible blindness, so vision monitoring is recommended twice a year. These drugs are considered the least effective of the DMARDs, but they may also have the fewest toxic effects.

Azathioprine and Cyclosporine

Azathioprine is considered to be an antimetabolite, meaning that it blocks a normal metabolic process.[6] However, it is generally used as an immunosuppressant to prevent rejection of transplanted organs. It impairs the synthesis of DNA and RNA precursors and is also cytotoxic to inflammatory cells. It takes 2 to 3 months to be effective. Azathioprine is very toxic, producing fever, chills, fatigue, nausea, bone marrow suppression, and liver and renal failure. It is associated with an increased susceptibility to infection and abnormal bleeding. Because of these adverse events azathioprine is only used when the severe symptoms of RA fail to respond to the safer drugs. In addition, it is less effective than methotrexate.[18]

Cyclosporine is another anti-rejection drug used in the treatment of RA. It has a low therapeutic index and produces nephrotoxicity. It may be used alone or in combination with other DMARDs in patients with RA that is refractory to treatment.[19]

Gold

Gold is available in an oral preparation and also for parenteral intramuscular administration; injectable gold is believed to be more effective.[19] Gold salts inhibit maturation of phagocytes. Gold selectively accumulates in synovial cells but also in bone marrow, lymph nodes, liver, and spleen. It suppresses synovial inflammation during active RA. It is rarely used today except for patients who cannot tolerate NSAIDs or methotrexate. Effectiveness is not recognized for about 3 to 6 months.

Gold injections begin at 10 mg a week, and then the dose is increased in increments of up to 50 mg. One injection is given per week. The oral formula is given twice a day. Adverse reactions include rashes, sweating, syncope, thrombocytopenia, hepatitis, and inflammation of the skin and mucous membranes of the mouth. In addition to these side effects, diarrhea is common with the oral formulation. After 3 to 6 years, many patients experience toxic effects or can no longer tolerate the drug.

Penicillamine

Penicillamine is a chelator of heavy metals that also slows T-cell function. It appears to reduce symptoms of RA (within 2 to 3 months) but has not been successful in slowing joint destruction.[6] Penicillamine produces challenging side effects similar to those of the drugs already reviewed. It may cause diarrhea, nausea and vomiting, mouth ulcers, fever, rash, and bone marrow depression. In addition, iron-containing supplements must *not* be taken within 2 hours of penicillamine administration.

Sulfasalazine

Sulfasalazine is used more commonly today than the previously mentioned DMARDs. It suppresses the immune system in 1 to 3 months. The mechanism of action is unclear, but it may reduce natural killer cell activity and alter lymphocyte function. It also has some antimicrobial action and has been used for the treatment of ulcerative colitis.

Nausea and rash are fairly common adverse effects, but serious reactions such as hepatitis and bone marrow suppression are rare. A lupus-like reaction has been reported in some patients. The efficacy of sulfasalazine may be equal to that of hydroxychloroquine, but it may act more quickly.[20]

Methotrexate

Methotrexate is a folic acid antagonist that impairs DNA synthesis by inhibiting purine biosynthesis.[6] It is known to decrease levels of IL-1 and inhibit proliferation of rapidly replicating monocytes and lymphocytes. It basically acts as an immunosuppressant but was originally and is still used as a chemotherapy agent at a higher dose. It is now the drug of choice for patients with RA and often produces improvement within 1 month, more quickly than many of the other DMARDs.

Methotrexate administration is started at a dose of 7.5 to 10 mg once a week, which can be taken as a single dose or over a 24-hour period.[19] Intramuscular or subcutaneous injections are also available. Methotrexate is generally well tolerated at this low dose. However, it is most frequently associated with stomatitis, anorexia, and abdominal cramping and rarely with alopecia. Administration of folic acid is an effective way to reduce methotrexate's side effects. The more severe side effects include bone marrow suppression and pulmonary and hepatic toxic effects. Measurements of the liver transaminases must be performed regularly. Also, infections such as herpes zoster and pneumocystis carinii are more common among patients taking this drug. There is even a link to lymphoma, which spontaneously resolves when the drug is discontinued. Methotrexate is teratogenic and therefore has found use as an abortifacient in ectopic pregnancy. Concurrent use with NSAIDs increases the toxic effects of methotrexate, especially in elderly patients with diminished renal function.

Research on methotrexate has led to some major changes in rheumatology practice. Several clinical trials have indicated that aggressive pharmacological treatment of RA should occur early in the disease.[20] The beneficial effect of methotrexate is greater for patients during the first 2 years of the disease than for those who have had RA for 2 to 5 years.[21] Longitudinal studies show that the drug can retard radiographic progression of the disease. Additionally, methotrexate has been found to lower mortality risk in RA by protecting against cardiovascular events.[22] It is the standard against which all new DMARDs are evaluated. Additional studies have shown that methotrexate is even more effective when combined with some of the other DMARDs.[23]

Leflunomide

Leflunomide is a prodrug whose active metabolite inhibits the enzyme required for the pyrimidine nucleotide synthesis, ribonucleotide uridine monophosphate.[24] In regard to RA, this drug interferes with the synthesis of activated lymphocytes by interfering with their cell cycle progression because of inadequate stores of uridine monophosphate (see Chapter 23). Cells undergoing division need an adequate supply of pyrimidine nucleotides, but in the presence of leflunomide, this supply is dramatically reduced.

Patients begin a leflunomide regimen with 100 mg a day for 3 days and then switch over to a maintenance dose of 10 to 20 mg/day.[25] The reason for the loading dose is that the drug is almost completely protein bound. It has a long half-life, 15 days, which indicates that the effectiveness of the drug lasts for a while after its discontinuation. However, in the case of pregnancy or adverse reactions, there are ways to remove the drug. Leflunomide undergoes repeated enterohepatic recirculation, so patients can take the resin cholestyramine, which will bind the drug in the GI tract with final elimination in the stool.

In a clinical trial that included 482 patients with active disease, there was more than 20% improvement in swollen joints, and in general, more than 40% of subjects experienced a reduction in symptoms.[26] This was compared with 35% improvement in the methotrexate-treated group and 19% improvement in the placebo group. In addition, the Sharp x-ray score (a measure of disease progression) showed the least progression in subjects taking leflunomide. In another year-long study of 402 patients, researchers found that this drug was as effective as methotrexate (50% success rate in both groups).[27] Side effects reported included diarrhea, alopecia, rash, and increases in aminotransferase activity, indicating some liver damage. Leflunomide is also carcinogenic and teratogenic in animals.

Tumor Necrosis Factor Inhibitors

TNF represents a new target for inhibition in patients with RA. Etanercept and infliximab are two new drugs that can bind and inactivate TNF. Etanercept is an artificial bioengineered molecule that consists of two TNF receptors attached to a human immuno-globulin molecule.[28] This drug is administered subcutaneously two times per week, and long-term self-administration is required. This is significant in terms of patient compliance because some patients with RA will not have the dexterity to administer the injections.

Etanercept has been shown to be effective when compared with placebo and in some cases has been shown to be more effective than methotrexate.[29,30] Adverse effects reported have been mainly injection-site reactions, which do not necessitate removal of the drug. Repeated dosing is associated with the development of antinuclear antibodies, and a few patients have experienced a lupus syndrome. Demyelinating disorders including multiple sclerosis and myelitis have rarely been associated with etanercept.[31]

Infliximab is an antibody that targets TNF. It is administered intravenously every 8 weeks. Repeated administration has been associated with the development of antibodies to the drug. For this reason infliximab has only been studied with simultaneous administration of methotrexate. The combination of infliximab plus methotrexate has been shown to be as effective as etanercept plus methotrexate and more effective than methotrexate plus placebo.[32] Side effects have included headache, infusion reactions (fever, urticaria, dyspnea, and hypotension), aseptic meningitis, and worsening congestive heart failure.[19] In some patients, anti-infliximab antibodies have developed, but combining use of this drug with methotrexate may decrease the development of these antibodies.

Serious infections, including reactivation of tuberculosis and sepsis, have been reported with both etanercept and infliximab.[19] These usually occur within the first 2 to 7 months of treatment. Lupus-like symptoms have also been reported. Skin testing for *Mycobacterium tuberculosis* and a chest x-ray are now recommended before therapy with these drugs is started. These drugs should not be given to patients with a recent malignancy.

Adalimumab is a new TNF inhibitor that is administered by weekly subcutaneous injection.[33] This drug may be effective in the treatment of severe RA that is refractory to other drugs such as methotrexate when given either as a single agent or in combination with methotrexate. Side effects are similar to those of the other two drugs in this category. No comparison studies of the TNF inhibitors have been released.

Anakinra

Anakinra is another new drug that is a genetically engineered IL-1 receptor antagonist.[19] Compared with placebo, this drug has produced only modest improvements in signs and symptoms of RA, and therefore it will probably be used in combination with methotrexate. Side effects include injection-site reactions and infections similar to those caused by the TNF inhibitors, but there has been no report of reactivation of tuberculosis. Complications appear to occur more often when anakinra is combined with the TNF inhibitors.

Rehabilitation Concerns with Disease-Modifying Antirheumatic Drugs

The DMARDs have not been studied with respect to how they affect exercise performance or how exercise affects their efficacy or pharmacokinetics. Most can be toxic, producing renal and liver toxic effects, and are immunosuppressive. Most also produce fatigue. Frequent laboratory tests are necessary to evaluate liver function and to monitor for bone marrow suppression as indicated by anemia, thrombocytopenia, and neutropenia. The therapist should also watch for clinical signs of bone marrow suppression, such as easy bruising and lowered exercise tolerance; and patients must be monitored for any infections, particularly if they are taking TNF inhibitors. Many of these drugs also produce skin rashes, which are often a sign of drug toxicity. Skin inspection should be a regular part of the therapy appointment. In addition, patients should remain hydrated to protect renal function. Some of these drugs produce toxic metabolites that undergo renal elimination; keeping fluids moving through the kidneys can help decrease accumulation of these metabolites. Last, for patients also receiving steroids, the catabolic effects of DMARDs should be considered, especially when strengthening, stretching, or deep tissue work is performed so that tissue injury and rupture may be avoided.

Rational Dosing and Combination Therapy for Rheumatoid Arthritis

Combination therapy for RA has definitely been shown to be more effective than the use of individual drugs because individual agents are active at different stages of joint inflammation (Figure 13-1).[20,25,34] Most rheumatologists begin treatment with an NSAID and a DMARD. Because the selective COX-2 inhibitors are less likely to cause GI problems, they are typically the ones chosen for treatment.

Hydroxychloroquine is the DMARD of choice for mild RA, but sulfasalazine may act as a substitute. The triple combination of sulfasalazine, hydroxychloroquine, and methotrexate may also be used early because treatment with this triad has shown some marked clinical responses with toxic effects similar to those of methotrexate monotherapy. In fact, this combination of drugs shows such promise that some rheumatologists argue for further studies on the older drugs because there is more long-term experience with these drugs. Others argue that methotrexate should always be started first, followed by the addition of the newer TNF-inhibiting agents. What is clear in this argument is that it is too early in the data-gathering process to make adamant statements regarding which drug is better than the others or which combination is superior. More long-term data on safety and efficacy are needed, especially for the TNF inhibitors.

DRUG TREATMENT OF GOUT

Gout is a metabolic disorder in which the plasma urate concentration is elevated because of overproduction (hyperuricemia), deficient elimination, or a combination of the two.[35] Uric acid is produced by the degradation of purines, and the level tends to increase with age. Hyperuricemia is defined as a plasma level of more than 7.0 mg/dL in men and more than 6.0 mg/dL in women.[36] Hyperuricemia by itself does not always lead to gout; however, hyperuricemia is a necessary factor in the development of gout.

Gout tends to be more common in men in their thirties and forties and also in postmenopausal women. It is associated with cardiovascular disease, alcoholism, obesity, hypertriglyceridemia, and insulin resistance; and it is also seen in patients with renal insufficiency. Elevated uric acid production is responsible for approximately 10% of cases of gout, which can be associated with an inherited enzyme deficiency or a myeloproliferative disorder. In the remaining 90% of cases, patients appear to have diminished urinary excretion of uric acid. Treatment with some drugs—including the thiazide diuretics,

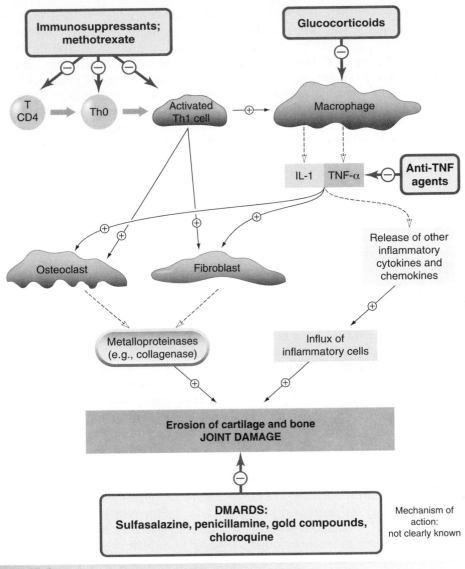

Figure 13-1

A schematic drawing of the cells and mediators involved in the pathogenesis of rheumatoid joint damage indicating the action of antirheumatoid drugs. The anti–tumor necrosis factor agents are etanercept and infliximab. *IL-1*, Interleukin-1, *TNF-α*, tumor necrosis factor-α; *DMARDs*, disease-modifying antirheumatoid drugs. (From Rang HP, Dale MM, Ritter JM, Moore JL. *Pharmacology.* 5th ed. New York: Churchill Livingstone; 2003.)

angiotensin receptor blockers, and cyclosporine (used to prevent transplant rejection)—is also associated with a greater risk of developing gout because these drugs are thought to interfere with the kidneys' ability to excrete urate.[37,38] High doses of aspirin appear to be uricosuric, but low doses cause uric acid retention. In fact, low-dose aspirin produces significant changes in renal function in patients with no known renal disease. Given the

widespread use of low-dose aspirin for cardiac protection, it is recommended that health care providers become alert to the signs and symptoms of gout.

The clinical manifestations of gout include intermittent bouts of acute monoarthritis produced by the deposition of crystals of sodium urate in the joint synovial fluid or a tophus (a nodular or needle-shaped bundle of urate crystals in the soft tissue).[36]

The classic presentation is arthritis of the first metatarsophalangeal joint, but it can occur at the knee and even inside the carpal canal, producing carpal tunnel syndrome.[39] The onset of the arthritis is often rapid; and the affected joint becomes warm, erythematous, painful, and swollen. Monoarthritis is the most common form, but a patient, especially an elderly person, may present with involvement of several of the proximal interphalangeal and distal interphalangeal joints of the hand. An inflammatory response results, involving synthesis and activation of lipoxygenase products and kinins and neutrophil migration to the area. The crystals become engulfed by phagocytosis, producing tissue damage and release of proteolytic enzymes. Patients may also have systemic involvement such as symptoms associated with uric acid kidney stones (urolithiasis).

Management of gout involves treating the arthritic inflammation and urolithiasis, if present, and also lowering uric acid levels to prevent exacerbations.[36,40] Drugs used are those that inhibit uric acid synthesis, increase uric acid excretion, inhibit migration of white cells into the joints, and reduce inflammation.

Treatment of Acute Gout

NSAIDs can be very effective in reducing the symptoms of acute gout. Indomethacin is the most common drug used, but there is little evidence that one NSAID is better than another.[36] Because gout is related to worsening renal function, caution should be used when these drugs are prescribed, particularly for the elderly. COX-2 inhibitors might be quite effective in this disorder because COX-2 has also been implicated in crystal formation.[40,41] Opioids are frequently prescribed for pain relief.

Colchicine is an old drug but one that is still quite effective in reducing the symptoms of gout. In a placebo-controlled trial, two thirds of patients in the colchicine group experienced improvement within 48 hours compared with only one third in the placebo group.[42] The drug prevents migration of neutrophils by binding to tubulin (a major protein that helps form the intracellular skeleton of the mitotic spindle), impairing the cells' ability to achieve chemotaxis and thus decrease phagocytosis.[3,5] Colchicine may also inhibit crystal-induced COX-2 expression. It is administered by the oral route every 1 to 2 hours until pain subsides or a specific maximal dose is reached. Its use is primarily limited by GI side

effects, which begin before the acute gouty symptoms are relieved. Adverse effects include severe diarrhea, nausea, and vomiting. Large doses may also produce GI hemorrhage and kidney damage. After an acute bout of gout, colchicine may be used at low doses along with some of the other preventive agents to prevent flare-ups. However, long-term use has been associated with bone marrow depression, renal failure, and even rhabdomyolysis and polyneuropathy.[43] In cases in which patients do not respond to NSAIDs or colchicine or the side effects of this therapy cannot be tolerated, good alternatives include oral prednisone and intravenous or intraarticular steroids.[44]

Long-Term Treatment of Gout

Drugs used to treat chronic gout or to prevent recurrence include medications that lower blood uric acid levels. The uricosuric agents (probenecid and sulfinpyrazone) increase excretion of uric acid by the kidneys. They block the reabsorption of filtered uric acid in the renal tubules, leading to increased clearance. They are most effective in patients whose urine contains only small amounts of uric acid and those who have good renal function. They are not helpful for the treatment of acute gout attacks and should not be administered until the acute attack subsides. The most common adverse effects of these drugs are rash and GI discomfort. Another limitation of these drugs is that they should not be given concurrently with doses of aspirin greater than 325 mg/day because salicylates interfere with their uricosuric effects. However, low-dose aspirin is acceptable as long as patients are counseled to stay away from other aspirin-containing products.[45] Lastly, sufficient hydration is imperative, particularly during intensive exercise sessions.

Allopurinol represents another approach to the long-term management of gout.[35] This drug inhibits uric acid synthesis by blocking the enzyme xanthine oxidase, which controls the last two steps in purine metabolism (conversion of adenine or guanine to uric acid). This drug tends to be more effective for patients whose urine contains large amounts of uric acid, indicating excessive production.[46] Like the uricosuric agents, allopurinol is not helpful during acute attacks, and if administration is started during this time, it may actually prolong the attack. However, allopurinol is quite helpful in preventing future attacks and kidney stones. Adverse effects are usually minor and include headaches, heartburn, and diarrhea. However, it can produce a number of drug interactions, most significantly inactivation of oral anticoagulants. Patients taking allopurinol must undergo frequent monitoring of their blood clotting ability with an international normalized ratio.

Rasburicase is a new uricolytic agent that is currently in clinical trials.[47] It has been used successfully in patients with elevated uric acid levels associated with use of chemotherapy agents. It was found to be more effective than allopurinol and was well tolerated. Future study is necessary to determine whether it will be effective in preventing gouty arthritis in patients with hyperuricemia.

Although the choice of drugs for the treatment of gout is clear, when to start administration of urate-lowering drugs is controversial.[37] Some physicians recommend starting therapy only in patients who experience more than four flare-ups per year. Others recommend treatment earlier, believing that it is more cost-effective to treat patients who have only had two attacks per year. Complicating the decision is the fact that gout is not always a progressive problem and patients with hyperuricemia do not always have gout. A trial of nonpharmacological management (diet, reduction in alcohol consumption, and weight reduction) may be a useful alternative. Many unanswered questions regarding the treatment of this disease remain, for example, how low plasma urate levels should be, how long patients should be treated with urate-lowering drugs, and whether intermittent use of the drugs is equal in effectiveness to continuous use.

DRUG TREATMENT OF SYSTEMIC LUPUS ERYTHEMATOSUS

Systemic lupus erythematosus (SLE) is an autoimmune disease affecting a variety of organs.[48] Constitutional symptoms such as fever, weight loss, and fatigue are common, as are a number of other clinical manifestations affecting the skin, joints, kidneys, heart, and vascular and nervous systems (Table 13-2).

The immunological dysfunction includes the development of antinuclear antibodies to components of the cell nucleus, particularly to double-stranded DNA.[49,50] This disorder promotes B-cell activity to both self-antigens and foreign antigens. Normally, the B lymphocytes provide help for T cells, produce cytokines, trigger antigen-induced

Table 13-2

Clinical Presentation of Lupus by System	
System	**Presentation**
Musculoskeletal	Arthritis of small joint of the hand and wrist but without joint erosions
Skin and mucosal surfaces	Photosensitivity
	Malar or butterfly rash (30%)
	Discoid lesions (raised, erythematous plaques on face, scalp, & neck)
	Papulosquamous rash on trunk
	Diffuse alopecia
	Oral ulcers (40%)
	Raynaud's phenomenon
Neuropsychiatric	Cognitive dysfunction
	Mood disorder
	Headaches
	Cerebrovascular accident
	Autonomic neuropathy
	Peripheral neuropathy
Renal	Glomerulonephritis
	Interstitial nephritis
Cardiovascular	Valvular heart disease
	Coronary artery disease
	Vasculitis
	Pericarditis
Pulmonary	Pleuritis
	Acute pneumonitis
Gastrointestinal	Peritonitis
	Hepatitis
	Pancreatitis
Hematological	Anemia
	Leukopenia
	Thrombocytopenia

production of immunoglobulin antibodies, and act as memory cells awaiting antigen re-exposure.[51] However, in SLE the B lymphocytes provide help to the autoreactive T cells; induce production of autoantibodies, creating destructive immune complexes; and undergo clonal proliferation. The direct infiltration of these immune complexes into the kidneys, joints, liver, and other organs leads to the destruction of tissue and the development of clinical symptoms.

Treatment of SLE involves a combination of anti-inflammatory and immunosuppressive drugs, and even some chemotherapy agents. The appropriate medication depends on the particular array of symptoms, organ involvement, and severity of disease.

Treatment of Mild to Moderate Systemic Lupus Erythematosus

In patients with mild to moderate SLE without major organ involvement, treatment tends to be a combination of NSAIDs, corticosteroids, and the antimalarial agent hydroxychloroquine.[48] NSAIDS are quite helpful in reducing the pain and inflammation associated with arthritis and arthralgias, and they are useful in combating SLE-induced fevers.

Acute inflammation in the skin and joints may be treated with steroids. Options include topical creams for inflammatory rashes and low-dose oral steroids for immune modulation. Prednisone is the preferred oral agent, because it is available in small doses that allow for convenient titration if symptoms progress.

Hydroxychloroquine has also been shown to be effective for the skin lesions and arthritis.[52] This drug can also reduce fatigue and prevent more serious flare-ups of the disease. A placebo-controlled trial that examined the effect of discontinuing hydroxychloroquine in stable SLE demonstrated that flares were 2.5 times more frequent in the group that discontinued the drug.[53] Methotrexate and leflunomide are two other drugs that can be used to treat moderate SLE.

Treatment of Severe Systemic Lupus Erythematosus

Patients with major organ involvement such as glomerulonephritis, pneumonitis, or neurological disease are considered to have severe disease. Prompt treatment is necessary to prevent death or long-term organ damage. Initial therapy involves high-dose corticosteroids, usually administered intravenously. Other immunosuppressive medications—including cyclophosphamide, methotrexate, azathioprine, and mycophenolate mofetil—can be added.

Cyclophosphamide might be the most effective agent at this time for treating severe SLE.[54] It is a chemotherapy agent that covalently binds to nucleic acids with an alkyl group (saturated carbon atoms). The drug may bind to one or both strands of DNA, producing cross-linkages between the strands. Essentially, this inhibits the activation of inflam-

matory cell division. High-dose cyclophosphamide induces maximal immunosuppression. In a small study of 14 patients with refractory SLE, high-dose cyclophosphamide was shown to achieve a complete response in five patients and a partial response in six patients.[55] Outcomes were defined by using the Responder Index for Lupus Erythematosus (RIFLE). At follow-up 32 months later, the five complete responders continued to be free of disease, and the partial responders had their symptoms controlled with drugs that were previously ineffective for them. Although the authors of this study report that the treatment was well tolerated, cyclophosphamide has some very serious side effects. In addition to alopecia, nausea, vomiting, diarrhea, and bone marrow depression, it produces hemorrhagic cystitis, leading to bladder fibrosis. Toxic metabolites (acrolein) are eliminated in the urine, but not before they have done damage. In this study the patients were well hydrated, and they also received an intravenous (IV) injection of MESNA (sodium 2-mercaptoethane sulfonate) to help inactivate these toxic compounds. MESNA binds to the irritant metabolites in the bladder to prevent cystitis. It was given intravenously 30 minutes before cyclophosphamide and again at 3, 6, and 8 hours after the alkylating agent was administered. In addition, patients received IV ondansetron for nausea and antibiotics, antivirals, and antifungal agents to prevent infection until their white blood cell counts returned to safe levels, aided by granulocyte cell-stimulating factors (see Chapter 23). Treatment with this agent is quite involved and requires tremendous cooperation from the patient. In another study in which high-dose treatment with cyclophosphamide was compared with a low-dose regimen, little difference in the percentage of responders was found, but the high-dose group experienced a significantly greater number of severe infections.[56]

Other immunosuppressive agents are currently available for the treatment of lupus. Mycophenolate mofetil was found to be as effective for SLE nephritis as prednisone combined with cyclophosphamide.[57] Cyclosporine, an anti-rejection drug, continues to be under study but so far has only shown modest improvement in arthralgias and myalgias.[54] A hope for the future may lie with the newly synthesized biological agents. These agents include rituximab and another drug, which is still in clinical trials, called *LJP 394*. Rituximab is engineered to target activated mature B lymphocytes.[51] Because these

B cells are implicated in the pathogenesis of SLE, anti-B-cell therapy may hold some promise for this disease.

Therapeutic Concerns with Drugs for Systemic Lupus Erythematosus

Because disease-modifying therapy for SLE consists largely of immunosuppressive agents, treatment carries significant risks of infection.[58] Patients with SLE appear to have a propensity for infection, and when this is combined with treatment with cyclophosphamide and high-dose steroids, special concern is warranted. Bacterial infections account for the majority of infections in SLE, greater than 80%. The most common infections are *Staphylococcus aureus, S. pyogenes, S. pneumoniae,* and *Escherichia coli.* Clinical presentations vary from full-blown sepsis to soft-tissue infection. Tissues most affected include lung, sinus, skin, and bone. The most common viral infection is herpes zoster, and fungal infections are most commonly caused by *Candida* species.

Therapists should regularly monitor the skin and soft tissue for their patients who are receiving immunosuppressive therapy and should look for reddened and warm areas. In addition, patients should be instructed to report any low-grade fever that occurs. Equipment should be kept clean, and patients should be isolated from anyone who might be infectious.

Another concern for patients with lupus is exposure to UV-A and UV-B sun rays.[54,59] It has been determined that both forms of light are harmful to patients with lupus because they induce inflammatory events in which local lymphocyte activation occurs. Other drugs such as the thiazide diuretics, neuroleptics, and tetracyclines also cause photosensitivity that may compound this problem for patients with lupus. Patients should wear sun-protective clothing and use broad-spectrum sunscreens frequently. The optimal sunscreen should contain titanium dioxide or zinc oxide and UV-A absorbers such as Parsol 1789 or Mexoryl-SX. Common sense dictates that UV light therapy is contraindicated for these patients. However, studies have indicated that phototherapy has some benefit for both cutaneous and systemic lupus.[60] The underlying mechanism of action is unknown, but studies to determine it are ongoing. For now, UV therapy should be avoided in patients with lupus.

Drug-Induced Rheumatic Syndromes

Many new and older drugs have resulted in a drug-induced rheumatic syndrome.[61] To qualify for a diagnosis of a drug-related syndrome, a patient must be exposed to the drug, exhibit clinical and laboratory evidence of the syndrome without having a history of the syndrome, and demonstrate rapid improvement in symptoms and laboratory values after discontinuation of the drug. Specifically, drug-induced rheumatic syndromes include SLE, vasculitis, scleroderma, and myositis.

Currently, more than 80 drugs are associated with SLE.[61] One of the more recently implicated drugs is minocycline, a tetracycline antibiotic used to treat acne. A recent prospective study included 20 patients with minocycline-induced SLE with arthritis, a positive ANA titer, and at least one other symptom of lupus.[62] By the sixteenth week after drug discontinuation, all symptoms were resolved. Similar situations have occurred with etanercept and sulfasalazine, both used in the treatment of RA.[63]

Other commonly used drugs implicated in SLE include lisinopril, an angiotensin-converting enzyme inhibitor, and simvastatin, a cholesterol-lowering drug.[61] Fosinopril, another angiotensin-converting enzyme inhibitor, has also been implicated in drug-induced scleroderma, and the statin drugs are associated with drug-induced myositis.

DRUG TREATMENT OF OSTEOARTHRITIS

Osteoarthritis is the most frequently diagnosed chronic medical condition.[64,65] It is responsible for 40% to 60% of degenerative states of the musculoskeletal system. It is characterized by cartilage degeneration, subchondral bone thickening, osteophytes, and bone cysts. Usually, the weight-bearing joints of the legs are affected, but osteoarthritis can also occur in the smaller joints of the hands and in the spine. These anatomical changes result in gradual development of joint pain, stiffness, and loss of range of motion.

Pathophysiology of Osteoarthritis

The common prevailing theory on osteoarthritis is that this disease reflects the aging process, meaning that repetitive use of joints results in cartilage

...ver, recent studies have introduced ...ation for this condition, describing ... as a complex interaction of genetic, ...and biological factors.[67]

...rticular cartilage can absorb shock and reduce ...tion at the joint surfaces.[65] Collagen fibers provide the strength to counter the shear forces during movement. Within this network of fibers are proteoglycans made of glycosaminoglycans attached to protein chains. These give the cartilage its elasticity and ability to resist compression through their fluid-absorbing abilities. Under pressure, the fluid is squeezed out, providing hydrostatic lubrication. As the cartilage ages, it loses fluid; the proteins become fragmented; and the levels of chondroitin sulfate, keratin sulfate, and hyaluronic acid change, but the cartilage retains most of its functions.

In contrast, in osteoarthritis, the cartilage has an increase in fluid content and normal proteins; but the levels of glycosaminoglycans, hyaluronic acid, and keratin sulfate decrease. The balance between cartilage synthesis and degradation is disrupted, and the structural properties of the collagen change. The chondrocytes, which are initially stimulated to repair the damage, also produce cytokines such as IL-1β and TNF-α, which are proinflammatory. The chondrocytes themselves produce abnormal types of collagen and increase their synthesis of proteinases, specifically matrix metalloproteinases (MMPs), causing the breakdown of proteoglycans.

Another area of study is the role of bone, especially subchondral bone in the development of osteoarthritis.[68] The progression of cartilage degeneration is associated with intensive remodeling of the subchondral bone. New bone synthesis, as evidenced by higher osteopontin (a bone-specific matrix protein) levels and elevated alkaline phosphatase levels, occurs. Both osteopontin and alkaline phosphatase are produced by the osteoblast. Proinflammatory cytokines (IL-1β, IL-6, prostaglandin E_2, and leukotriene B_4) are also products of the dysfunctional osteoblast.[69] IL-1β and IL-6 promote matrix degradation as a result of their activation of the MMPs. Prostaglandin E_2 stimulates bone formation at low concentrations but inhibits it as the concentration increases. Leukotrienes activate the osteoclasts. It is theorized that these cytokines run through the bone-cartilage interface to activate cartilage breakdown through channels and fissures. Thus the subchondral bone

changes and cartilage destruction mirror each other, with the cytokines being the go-between.

Therapeutics for Osteoarthritis

Aspirin, NSAIDs, and acetaminophen are the main treatments offered to reduce pain in osteoarthritis. However, given the fact that these drugs do not actually alter pathogenesis or repair damage already present, there is new interest in viscosupplementation, as well as in drugs that may repair damaged cartilage.

Aspirin and Acetaminophen

The primary treatments for osteoarthritic pain are acetaminophen and NSAIDs. Acetaminophen has been the drug preferred by physicians, as evidenced by a decline in NSAID use from 1989 to 1998.[70] The reason for this decline has been the recognition by physicians of the adverse cardiac and renal effects of the NSAIDs, particularly in the elderly. This decline has been met with an increase in acetaminophen use, although to reach the same level of effective pain relief as the NSAIDs, regular dosing of up to 4 g/day may be necessary.[65] However, several studies have shown that acetaminophen is not as effective in reducing pain as the NSAIDs, even at a dosage of 4 g/day.[71,72] In a small study of seven patients with osteoarthritis in which a crossover design was used, NSAIDs and acetaminophen were each favored by one patient, whereas five patients reported experiencing no difference between the two treatments. These five subjects went on to take acetaminophen, but 3 months later, they had all switched to use of an NSAID for greater effectiveness.

Hyaluronan

Viscosupplementation is a relatively new treatment option for patients with osteoarthritis of the knee. This procedure involves injecting a derivative of hyaluronan, a component of synovial fluid responsible for its lubrication properties, into the knee joint. The Food and Drug Administration has approved three hyaluronan derivatives: two containing sodium hyaluronate (Hyalgan and Supartz), which are injected once a week for 5 weeks, and Hylan G-F 20 (Synvisc), which is injected three times with 1 week between injections. This is a costly treatment resulting in only modest improvements.[73,74] Some patients experience only a slight reduction in pain compared with placebo injections or use of oral naproxen. In addition, there is no overall effect on joint space width.[75,76] Side effects include pain at the injection site, swelling, and a rash that dissipates in time.

Glucosamine and Chondroitin Sulfates

More than 250 years ago, a British naval surgeon designed the first controlled, prospective, clinical experiment in which lemons and oranges were used to cure scurvy.[77] This led to the recognition that dietary deficiencies can cause disease. Out of this research was born the belief that eating cartilage or its component molecules rebuilds joints and prevents arthritis. However, for years, knowledgeable scientists have refuted claims made by the dietary food industry that glucosamine and chondroitin can relieve the pain of osteoarthritis, stimulate proteoglycan synthesis in articular cartilage and hyaluronan synthesis in synovial tissue, and also decrease cartilage degradation. Neither glucosamine nor chondroitin is approved by the Food and Drug Administration; rather, both are considered dietary supplements. This has led to widespread use by the public without rigorous scientific documentation of their effectiveness. However, recently, several well-conducted studies have demonstrated that glucosamine and chondroitin might be effective not just in terms of reducing pain but also in preventing the progression of the disease.[78]

Glucosamine is an aminosaccharide that acts as a basic constituent and building block for the synthesis of the glycosaminoglycans and proteoglycans in the cartilage matrix and synovial fluid, particularly the proteoglycan aggrecans, a matrix structural protein.[79,80] Aggrecans plays an essential role in maintaining the health of cartilage by regulating its fluid content.[81] In vitro studies show that glucosamine appears to stimulate cartilage cells to synthesize aggrecans and to reduce MMPs.[81,82] In animals, oral glucosamine has a beneficial effect on immune-mediated arthritis. Chondroitin is a glycosaminoglycan that is found in articular cartilage, bone, skin, ligaments, and tendons. Along with aggrecans, it plays a role in creating an osmotic pressure that expands the cartilage matrix. In animal studies, chondroitin has been reported to maintain joint viscosity, stimulate cartilage repair,

and inhibit the enzymes involved in cartilage degradation. However, some sources indicate that the chondroitin molecule is too large to enter the synovium.

Human studies of lengths varying from 4 weeks to 3 years in which glucosamine was primarily used, with chondroitin added for some of the trials, demonstrated beneficial effects for patients with mild to moderate osteoarthritis, primarily of the knee.[80,83] Outcome measures used in many of the studies included measures of pain (visual analog scale during walking), joint space narrowing shown on plain radiographs, and the Western Ontario and McMaster Universities (WOMAC) Osteoarthritis Index Pain Subscale. One study in particular was a double-blind trial in which 212 patients were treated with either 1500 mg of glucosamine or placebo, once daily for 3 years.[84] The treated group demonstrated a 20% to 25% reduction in symptoms on the WOMAC Osteoarthritis Index Pain Subscale, whereas the placebo group showed a slight worsening of symptoms. Careful measurements of joint space narrowing with fluoroscopy to correct lower limb positioning and x-ray beam alignment showed no average loss of joint space in the patients receiving glucosamine, but those receiving placebo had significant changes detected on x-ray films. Similar numbers of patients in the two groups took at least one dose of a "rescue drug," either acetaminophen or an NSAID. Consumption of these drugs was inconsistent between the groups and also within each group. Adverse effects were similar in both groups and were no more serious than GI complaints of abdominal pain and diarrhea. Routine laboratory tests did not show any abnormalities in either group, and there was no change in glucose tolerance.

Even though significant positive outcomes were reported in these studies, the therapist should not recommend these drugs to patients with osteoarthritis. Because glucosamine and chondroitin are classified as dietary supplements and the active ingredients are not regulated, the purity of such products may be questionable. Further studies are needed to evaluate for possible drug-drug interactions. The National Institutes of Health is currently sponsoring a randomized controlled trial of glucosamine alone, chondroitin alone, and the two together to determine how they compare with celecoxib and placebo.[85] This study is expected to be completed in November 2005. In *The Medical Letter on Drugs and Therapeutics* the investigators reported that they could not locate a supplement with a consistent amount of the active ingredients for their study, so they had to manufacture these agents themselves.[78]

Future Agents to Control the Osteoarthritic Process

As discussed previously, the pharmacological management of osteoarthritis has been mainly symptomatic, with little emphasis placed on the biological factors leading to joint degradation. In part, this has been due to inadequate outcome measures that make documenting efficacy difficult. Pain and functional assessment have been used for the symptom-modifying drugs, but joint space narrowing assessed by plain radiographs has been used for structure-modifying agents. This standard measurement for joint space does not give us any information on the cartilage itself because it is not imaged. Newer techniques in magnetic resonance imaging now allow adequate visualization of the joint structures, particularly the cartilage and its pathological progress.[64] Some new quantitative measurements (assessment of cartilage volume) may be obtained, allowing specific, sensitive, and valid assessment of the progression of the disease. Incorporation of these outcome measurements into the research is the key to identifying possible structure-modifying agents for osteoarthritis.

Other advances in pharmacotherapy for osteoarthritis include the discovery of an IL-1β receptor antagonist and an IL-1β–converting enzyme blocker, both of which can be used to reduce several different cartilage breakdown processes.[64] The IL-1β–converting enzyme inhibitor is in clinical trials and is responsible for blocking the conversion of IL-1β into its mature form. Research is also being conducted on finding agents to block the activity of MMPs. Efforts are directed toward inhibiting their synthesis or blocking the conversion of the proMMPs into active MMPs. In addition, inhibition of the intracellular signaling pathways that signal the cell to produce MMPs is another attractive target. Another interesting route under study in osteoarthritis has to do with the activation of inflammation by nitric oxide (NO).[86,87] NO and its byproducts are capable of inducing tissue damage and may cause chondrocyte death. NO is also capable of increasing the activity of COX-2. In fact, a selective inhibitor of NO synthase showed a significant reduction in the severity of cartilage lesions in dogs. The mechanism of action appears to be the ability of the inhibitor to reduce IL-1β and MMP levels and also to reduce chondrocyte death. Lastly, licofelone, a new COX and lipoxygenase inhibitor, has been found to block the production of leukotriene B_4 and prostaglandin E_2, as well as several biomarkers seen in osteoarthritis.[88,89]

ACTIVITIES 13

■ 1. Review some of the literature presented in this chapter for outcome measures that are used to determine drug efficacy in RA. Indicate which ones might be useful in determining the effectiveness of a physical therapy intervention.

■ 2. Interview a patient with RA regarding drugs he or she has taken since the diagnosis was made. List the drugs and indicate the length of time they were administered, adverse effects, and the impact the drugs had on disease progression. In addition, indicate the reason for discontinuing the drugs.

■ 3. A 62-year-old woman fell on her right knee 2 years ago. She treated her injury with ice, elevation, and compression. The acute pain and swelling resolved within 2 weeks. However, over the past year, she has experienced increasing pain and stiffness in this knee. She reports morning stiffness and additional discomfort with activity. She is a retired elementary school teacher. She lives alone in a second-floor walk-up. Medical history includes: hypertension for 5 years.

Meds
Ibuprofen, hydrochlorothiazide

Physical Exam
Range of motion (ROM)
Knee: right 20°-70°/20°-75° left 0°-100°/
    0°-110° Hips: slight limitations in flexion and
    extension bilaterally
Strength
Quads: right 3+/5 due to pain; left 4/5
Hamstrings: right 4/5; left 4/5
Hip flexors: right 4/5; left 4/5
Hip extensors: right 4/5; left 4/5

X-Ray
Knee: narrowed joint spaces bilaterally, right
    more than left, consistent with osteoarthritis

Questions

a. What information do you need to know about this patient before prescribing meds?
b. Would you change her existing medications? If yes what would you prescribe?
c. How would you monitor this patient for adverse effects and efficacy of the meds?
d. What nonpharmacological therapies are indicated?

References

1. Pincus T, Callahan LF, Sale WG, Brooks AL, Payne LE, Vaugh WK. Severe functional declines, work disability, and increased mortality in seventy-five rheumatoid arthritis patients studied over nine years. *Arthritis Rheum*. 1984;27:864-872.
2. Pincus T, Callahan LF. The 'side effects' of rheumatoid arthritis: joint destruction, disability and early mortality. *Br J Rheumatol*. 1993;32(suppl 1):28-37.
3. Fox DA. Cytokine blockade as a new strategy to treat rheumatoid arthritis: inhibition of tumor necrosis factor. *Arch Intern Med*. 2000;160:437-444.
4. Quinn MA, Emery P. Window of opportunity in early rheumatoid arthritis: possibility of altering the disease process with early intervention. *Clin Exp Rheumatol*. 2003;5(suppl 31):S154-S157.
5. Wells BG, Dipiro JT, Schwinghammer TL, Hamilton CW. *Pharmacotherapy Handbook*. 5th ed. New York: McGraw Hill; 2003.
6. Day R, Quinn D, Williams K, Handel M, Brooks B. Connective tissue and bone disorders. In: Carruthers SG, Hoffman BB, Melmon KL, Nierenberg DW, eds. *Melmon and Morrelli's Clinical Pharmacology*. 4th ed. New York: McGraw Hill; 2000:645-702.
7. Sattar N, McCarey DW, Capell H, McInnes IB. Explaining how "high-grade" systemic inflammation accelerates vascular risk in rheumatoid arthritis. *Circulation*. 2003; 108(24):2957-2963.
8. del Rincon I, Escalante A. Atherosclerotic cardiovascular disease in rheumatoid arthritis. *Curr Rheumatol Rep*. 2003; 5(4):278-286.
9. Redlich K, Schett G, Steiner G, Hayer S, Wagner EF, Smolen JS. Rheumatoid arthritis therapy after tumor necrosis factor and interleukin-1 blockade. *Arthritis Rheum*. 2003;48(12):3308-3319.
10. Rang HP, Dale MM, Ritter JM, Moore JL. *Pharmacology*. 5th ed. New York: Churchill Livingstone; 2003.
11. Buckbinder L, Robinson RP. The glucocorticoid receptor: molecular mechanism and new therapeutic opportunities. *Curr Drug Targets Inflamm Allergy*. 2002;1(2):127-136.
12. Mauras N. Growth hormone therapy in the glucocorticosteroid-dependent child: metabolic and linear growth effects. *Horm Res*. 2001;56(suppl 1):13-18.
13. van Everdingen AA, Jacobs J, Siewertsz van Reesema DR, Bijlsma J. Low-dose prednisone therapy for patients with early active rheumatoid arthritis: clinical efficacy, disease-modifying properties, and side effects: a randomized, double-blind, placebo-controlled clinical trial. *Ann Intern Med*. 2002;136(1):1-12.
14. Bijlsma J, van Everdingen AA, Huisman M, De Nijs RN, Jacobs JW. Glucocorticoids in rheumatoid arthritis: effects on erosions and bone. *Ann N Y Acad Sci*. 2002; 966:82-90.
15. Gotzsche PC, Johansen HK. Short-term low-dose corticosteroids vs placebo and nonsteroidal antiinflammatory drugs in rheumatoid arthritis. *Cochrane Database Syst Rev*. 2001;2(CD000189).
16. Conn DL, Lim SS. New role for an old friend: prednisone is a disease-modifying agent in early rheumatoid arthritis. *Curr Opin Rheumatol*. 2003;15(3):193-196.
17. Lim SS, Conn DL. The use of low-dose prednisone in the management of rheumatoid arthritis. *Bull Rheum Dis*. 2001;50(12):1-4.
18. Willkens RF, Sharp JT, Stablein D, Marks C, Wortmann R. Comparison of azathioprine, methotrexate, and the combination of the two in the treatment of rheumatoid arthritis. A forty-eight-week controlled clinical trial with radiologic outcome assessment. *Arthritis Rheum*. 1995; 38(12):1799-1806.
19. Drugs for rheumatoid arthritis. *Treat Guidel Med Lett*. 2003;1(5):25-32.
20. Kwoh CK, Anderson LG, Greene JM, et al. Guidelines for the management of rheumatoid arthritis: 2002 update. *Arthritis Rheum*. 2002;46(2):328-346.
21. Weinblatt ME. Rheumatoid arthritis: treat now, not later. *Ann Intern Med*. 1996;124:773-774.
22. Choi HK, Hernan MA, Seeger JD, Robins JM, Wolfe F. Methotrexate and mortality in patients with rheumatoid arthritis: a prospective study. *Lancet*. 2002; 359(9313):1173-1177.

23. Landewe RB, Boers M, Verhoeven AC, et al. COBRA combination therapy in patients with early rheumatoid arthritis: long-term structural benefits of a brief intervention. *Arthritis Rheum.* 2002;46(2):347-356.

24. Fox RI, Herrmann ML, Frangou CG, et al. Mechanism of action for leflunomide in rheumatoid arthritis. *Clin Immunol.* 1999;93(3):198-208.

25. Kremer JM. Rational use of new and existing disease-modifying agents in rheumatoid arthritis. *Ann Intern Med.* 2001;134(8):695-706.

26. New drugs for rheumatoid arthritis. *Med Lett Drugs Ther.* 1998;40(1040):110-112.

27. Strand V, Cohen S, Schiff M, et al. Treatment of active rheumatoid arthritis with leflunomide compared with placebo and methotrexate. *Arch Intern Med.* 1999; 159:2542-2550.

28. Moreland L, Baumgartner SW, Schiff M, et al. Treatment of rheumatoid arthritis with a recombinant human tumor necrosis factor receptor (p75)-Fc fusion protein. *N Engl J Med.* 1997;337(3):141-147.

29. Genovese MC, Bathon JM, Martin RW, et al. Etanercept versus methotrexate in patients with early rheumatoid arthritis: two-year radiographic and clinical outcomes. *Arthritis Rheum.* 2002;46(6):1443-1450.

30. Bathon JM, Martin A, Fleischmann R, et al. A comparison of etanercept and methotrexate in patients with early rheumatoid arthritis. *N Engl J Med.* 2000; 343(22):1586-1593.

31. Robinson WH, Genovese MC, Moreland LW. Demyelinating and neurologic events reported in association with tumor necrosis factor alpha antagonism: by what mechanisms could tumor necrosis factor alpha antagonists improve rheumatoid arthritis but exacerbate multiple sclerosis? *Arthritis Rheum.* 2001; 44(9):1977-1983.

32. Maini R, St Clair EW, Breedveld F, et al. Infliximab (chimeric anti-tumour necrosis factor alpha monoclonal antibody) versus placebo in rheumatoid arthritis patients receiving concomitant methotrexate: a randomised phase III trial. ATTRACT Study Group. *Lancet.* 1999; 354(9194):1932-1939.

33. Adalimumab (humira) for rheumatoid arthritis. *Med Lett Drugs Ther.* 2003;45(1153):25-27.

34. Pincus T, O'Dell JR, Kremer JM. Combination therapy with multiple disease modifying antirheumatic drugs in rheumatoid arthritis: a preventative strategy. *Ann Intern Med.* 1999;131(10):768-774.

35. Wortmann R. Gout and hyperuricemia. *Curr Opin Rheumatol.* 2002;14(3):281-286.

36. Rott KT, Agudelo CA. Gout. *JAMA.* 2003;289(21): 2857-2860.

37. Schlesinger N, Schumacher HR. Gout: can management be improved? Curr Opin Rheumatol. 2001;13(3): 240-244.

38. Schlesinger N, Schumacher HR. Update on gout. *Arthritis Care Res.* 2002;47(5):563-565.

39. Mockford BJ, Kincaid RJ, Mackay I. Carpal tunnel syndrome secondary to intratendinous infiltration by tophaceous gout. *Scand J Plast Reconstr Surg Hand Surg.* 2003;37(3):186-187.

40. Terkeltaub RA. Gout. *N Engl J Med.* 2003;349(17): 1647-1655.

41. Agudelo CA, Wise C. Gout: diagnosis, pathogenesis, and clinical manifestations. *Curr Opin Rheumatol.* 2001; 13(3):234-239.

42. Ahern MJ, Reid C, Gordon TP, McCredie M, Brooks PM, Jones M. Does colchicine work? The results of the first controlled study in acute gout. *Aust N Z J Med.* 1987; 17(3):301-304.

43. Hsu WC, Chen WH, Chang MT, Chiu HC. Colchicine-induced acute myopathy in a patient with concomitant use of simvastatin. *Clin Neuropharmacol.* 2002;25(5):266-268.

44. Groff GD, Franck WA, Raddatz DA. Systemic steroid therapy for acute gout: a clinical trial and review of the literature. *Semin Arthritis Rheum.* 1990;19(6):329-336.

45. Harris M, Bryant LR, Danaher P, Alloway J. Effect of low dose daily aspirin on serum urate levels and urinary excretion in patients receiving probenecid for gouty arthritis. *J Rheumatol.* 2000;27:2873-2876.

46. Perez-Ruiz F, Calabozo M, Pijoan JI, Herrero-Beites AM, Ruibal A. Effect of urate-lowering therapy on the velocity of size reduction of tophi in chronic gout. *Arthritis Care Res.* 2002;47(4):356-360.

47. Pui CH. Rasburicase: a potent uricolytic agent. *Expert Opin Pharmacother.* 2002;3(4):433-442.

48. Dall'Era M, Davis JC. Systemic lupus erythematosus. *Postgrad Med.* 2003;114(5):31-40.

49. Rekvig OP, Nossent JC. Anti-double-stranded DNA antibodies, nucleosomes, and systemic lupus erythematosus: a time for new paradigms? *Arthritis Rheum.* 2003; 48(2):300-312.

50. Criscione LG, Pisetsky DS. B lymphocytes and systemic lupus erythematosus. *Curr Rheumatol Rep.* 2003;5(4): 264-269.

51. Silverman GJ, Weisman S. Rituximab therapy and autoimmune disorders: prospects for anti-B cell therapy. *Arthritis Rheum.* 2003;48(6):1484-1492.

52. Fabbri P, Cardinali C, Giomi B, Caproni M. Cutaneous lupus erythematosus: diagnosis and management. *Am J Clin Dermatol.* 2003;4(7):449-465.

53. The Canadian Hydroxychloroquine Study Group. A randomized study of the effect of withdrawing hydroxychloroquine sulfate in systemic lupus erythematosus. *N Engl J Med.* 1991;324(3):150-154.

54. Wallace DJ. Management of lupus erythematosus: recent insights. *Curr Opin Rheumatol.* 2002;14(3):212-219.

55. Petri M, Jones RJ, Brodsky RA. High-dose cyclophosphamide without stem cell transplantation in systemic lupus erythematosus. *Arthritis Rheum.* 2003; 48(1):166-173.

56. Houssaiau FA, Vasconcelos C, D'Cruz D, et al. Immunosuppressive therapy in lupus nephritis: The Euro-Lupus Nephritis Trial, a randomized trial of low-dose versus high-dose intravenous cyclophosphamide. *Arthritis Rheum.* 2002;46(8):2121-2131.

57. Chan TM, Li FK, Tang CS, et al. Efficacy of mycophenolate mofetil in patients with diffuse proliferative lupus nephritis. *N Engl J Med.* 2000;343(16):1156-1162.

58. Kang I, Park SH. Infectious complications in SLE after immunosuppressive therapies. *Curr Opin Rheumatol.* 2003;15(5):528-534.

59. Millard TP, Hawk JL, McGregor JM. Photosensitivity in lupus. *Lupus.* 2000;9(1):3-10.

60. Millard TP, Hawk JL. Ultraviolet therapy in lupus. *Lupus.* 2001;10(3):185-187.

61. Brogan BL, Olsen N. Drug-induced rheumatic syndromes. *Curr Opin Rheumatol.* 2003;15(1):76-80.

62. Gordon MM, Porter D. Minocycline induced lupus: case series in the West of Scotland. *J Rheumatol.* 2001; 28(5):1004-1006.

63. Shakoor N, Michalska M, Harris CA, Block JA. Drug-induced systemic lupus erythematosus associated with etanercept therapy. *Lancet*. 2002;359(9306):579-580.

64. Martel-Pelletier J, Pelletier JP. Osteoarthritis: recent developments. *Curr Opin Rheumatol*. 2003;15(5):613-615.

65. Morehead K, Sack KE. Osteoarthritis. *Postgrad Med*. 2003;114(5):11-17.

66. Verzijl N, Bank RA, TeKoppele HM, DeGroot J. AGEing and osteoarthritis: a different perspective. *Curr Opin Rheumatol*. 2003;15(5):616-622.

67. Aigner T, Dudhia J. Genomics of osteoarthritis. *Curr Opin Rheumatol*. 2003;15(5):634-640.

68. Laufer S. Role of eicosanoids in structural degradation in osteoarthritis. *Curr Opin Rheumatol*. 2003;15(5):623-627.

69. Lajeunesse D, Reboul P. Subchondral bone in osteoarthritis: a biologic link with articular cartilage leading to abnormal remodeling. *Curr Opin Rheumatol*. 2003;15(5):628-633.

70. Ausiello JC, Stafford RS. Trends in medication use for osteoarthritis treatment. *J Rheumatol*. 2002;29(5):999-1005.

71. Case JP, Baliunas AJ, Block JA. Lack of efficacy of acetaminophen in treating symptomatic knee osteoarthritis: a randomized, double-blind, placebo-controlled comparison trial with diclofenac sodium. *Arch Intern Med*. 2003;163(2):169-178.

72. Towheed TE, Judd MJ, Hochberg MC, Wells BG. Acetaminophen for osteoarthritis. *Cochrane Database Syst Rev*. 2003;2(CD004257).

73. Lo GH, LaValley M, McAlindon T, Felson DT. Intra-articular hyaluronic acid in treatment of knee osteoarthritis: a meta-analysis. *JAMA*. 2003;290(23):3115-3121.

74. Felson DT, Anderson J. Hyaluronate sodium injections for osteoarthritis: hope, hype, and hard truths. *Arch Intern Med*. 2002;162:245-247.

75. Jubb RW, Piva S, Beinat L, Dacre J, Gishen P. A one-year, randomised, placebo (saline) controlled clinical trial of 500-730 kDa sodium hyaluronate (Hyalgan) on the radiological change in osteoarthritis of the knee. *Int J Clin Pract*. 2003;57(6):467-474.

76. Cubbage K. Does intra-articular hyaluronate decrease symptoms of osteoarthritis of the knee? *J Fam Pract*. 2002;51(5):411.

77. Buckwalter JA, Callaghan JJ, Rosier RN. From oranges and lemons to glucosamine and chondroitin sulfate: clinical observations stimulate basic research. *J Bone Joint Surg*. 2001;83(A-8):1266-1268.

78. Update on glucosamine for osteoarthritis. *Med Lett Drugs Ther*. 2001;43(1120):111-112.

79. Towheed TE, Anastassiades TP. Glucosamine and chondroitin for treating symptoms of osteoarthritis. *JAMA*. 2000;283(11):1483-1485.

80. Richy F, Bruyere O, Ethgen O, Cucherat M, Henrotin Y, Reginster JY. Structural and symptomatic efficacy of glucosamine and chondroitin in knee osteoarthritis. *Arch Intern Med*. 2003;163:1514-1522.

81. Reginster JY, Bruyere O, Lecart MP, Henrotin Y. Naturocetic (glucosamine and chondroitin sulfate) compounds as structure-modifying drugs in the treatment of osteoarthritis. *Curr Opin Rheumatol*. 2003; 15(5):651-655.

82. Deal CL, Moskowitz RW. Nutraceuticals as therapeutic agents in osteoarthritis. *Rheum Dis Clin North Am*. 1999;25:778-799.

83. McAlindon T, LaValley M, Gulin JP, Felson DT. Glucosamine and chondroitin for treatment of osteoarthritis: a systematic quality assessment and meta-analysis. *JAMA*. 2000;283(11):1469-1475.

84. Reginster JY, Deroisy R, Rovati LC, et al. Long-term effects of glucosamine sulphate on osteoarthritis progression: a randomised, placebo-controlled clinical trial. *Lancet*. 2001;357:251-256.

85. Glucosamine/Chondroitin Arthritis Intervention Trial (GAIT). Available at: http://www.clinicaltrials.gov. Accessed April 4, 2004.

86. Pelletier JP, Martel-Pelletier J. Therapeutic targets in osteoarthritis: from today to tomorrow with new imaging technology. *Ann Rheum Dis*. 2003;62(suppl II):ii79-ii82.

87. Pelletier JP, Jovanovic DV, Lascau-Coman V, et al. Selective inhibition of inducible nitric oxide synthase reduces progression of experimental osteoarthritis in vivo. *Arthritis Rheum*. 2000;43(6):1290-1299.

88. Paredes Y, Massicotte F, Pelletier JP, Martel-Pelletier J, Laufer S, Lajeunesse D. Study of the role of leukotriene B4 in abnormal function of human subchondral osteoarthritis osteoblasts: effects of cyclooxygenase and/or 5-lipoxygenase inhibition. *Arthritis Rheum*. 2002; 46(7):1804-1812.

89. Jovanovic DV, Fernandes JC, Martel-Pelletier J, et al. In vivo dual inhibition of cyclooxygenase and lipoxygenase by ML-3000 reduces the progression of experimental osteoarthritis: suppression of collagenase 1 and interleukin-1b synthesis. *Arthritis Rheum*. 2001; 44(10):2320-2330.

5

Endocrine Pharmacology

CHAPTER 14

SELECTIVE TOPICS IN ENDOCRINE PHARMACOLOGY

OVERVIEW OF THE ENDOCRINE SYSTEM

The endocrine system consists of a group of duct-less glands that release hormones into the circulation for transport to their target organs.[1] In most instances the release of hormones is controlled through a negative feedback mechanism in which the stimulus initiates a response that reduces the original stimulus; or more simply stated, hormones inhibit their own release. The glands involved in this system include the hypothalamus, pituitary gland, thyroid gland, adrenal glands, gonads, pancreatic islets, and the parathyroid glands. See Table 14-1 for a review of the functional anatomy of the endocrine system.

Hypothalamic-Pituitary Axis

The hypothalamus and pituitary glands integrate physiological signals to produce the release of hormones that regulate the function of other glands. The hypothalamus produces releasing or inhibiting hormones that travel to the anterior pituitary gland via a portal venous system in the pituitary stalk (Figure 14-1).[1] These include growth hormone–releasing hormone, growth hormone–inhibitory hormone (also known as somatostatin), prolactin-releasing factor, thyrotropin-releasing hormone, corticotrophin-releasing hormone, gonadotropin-releasing hormone (GnRH), melanocyte-stimulating

hormone, and prolactin-inhibiting factor (Table 14-2). This portal venous system provides a delivery route for the hypothalamic hormones that regulate anterior pituitary function. The hypothalamus also synthesizes antidiuretic hormone (ADH) and oxytocin, which undergoes neurosecretory release into the posterior pituitary gland for storage and future systemic secretion.

In response to the hypothalamic releasing hormones, the anterior pituitary gland secretes GH, thyroid-stimulating hormone (TSH), adreno-corticotropic hormone (ACTH), follicle-stimulating hormone (FSH), luteinizing hormone (LH), and prolactin, which then bind to specific receptors in a variety of target tissues.[1]

An example of how the hypothalamic-pituitary axis integrates with a target tissue, such as the adrenal glands, is as follows. If a low concentration of circulating cortisol is sensed by the hypothalamic receptors sensitive to this hormone, there is a resultant release of corticotrophin-releasing hormone from the hypothalamus. This hormone is then released into the portal veins to act on receptors in the anterior pituitary gland. Stimulation of receptors in the anterior pituitary gland leads to the release of ACTH into the systemic venous system. The adrenal glands are then directed to synthesize and release cortisol into the general circulation. As the level of cortisol is increased, the hypothalamus reduces the amount of corticotrophin-releasing hormone released, forming a negative feedback loop. Similar

Table 14-1

Functional Anatomy of the Endocrine and Metabolic Systems			
Endocrine Function	**Regulatory Factors**	**Endocrine Organ/Hormone**	**Target Tissues**
Availability of fuel	Serum glucose, amino acids, enteric hormones (somatostatin, cholecystokinin, gastrin, secretin), vagal reflex, sympathetic nervous system	Pancreatic islets of Langerhans/insulin, glucagon	All tissues, especially liver, skeletal muscle, adipose tissue, indirect effects on brain and red blood cells
Metabolic rate	Hypothalamic thyrotropin-releasing hormone (TRH), pituitary thyrotropin (TSH)	Thyroid gland/ triiodothyronine (T_3)	All tissues
Circulatory volume	Renin, angiotensin II, hypothalamic osmoreceptor	Adrenals/aldosterone Pituitary/vasopressin	Kidney, blood vessels, CNS
Somatic growth	Hypothalamic growth hormone–releasing hormone (GHRH), somatostatin, sleep, exercise, stress, hypoglycemia	Pituitary/growth hormone Liver/insulin-like growth factors (IGFs)	All tissues
Calcium homeostasis	Serum Ca^{2+} and Mg^{2+} concentration	Parathyroid glands/ parathyroid hormone, calcitonin, vitamin D	Kidneys, intestines, bone
Reproductive function	Hypothalamic gonadotropin-releasing hormone (GnRH), pituitary follicle-stimulating hormone (FSH), and luteinizing hormone (LH), inhibins	Gonads/sex steroids Adrenals/androgens	Reproductive organs, CNS, various tissues
Adaptation to stress	Hypothalamic corticotrophin-releasing hormone (CRH), pituitary adrenocorticotropic hormone (ACTH), hypoglycemia, stress	Adrenals/glucocortico-steroids, epinephrine	Many tissues: CNS, liver, skeletal muscle, adipose tissue, lymphocytes, fibroblasts, cardiovascular system

From Page C, Curtis AB, Sutter MC, Walker L, Hoffman BB, eds. *Integrated Pharmacology*. Philadelphia: Mosby; 2002.
The endocrine and metabolic systems regulate seven major bodily functions. For each target tissue effect, endocrine glands release hormones in response to regulating factors, which include physiological (e.g., sleep and stress), biochemical (e.g., glucose and calcium), and hormonal (e.g., hypothalamic and enteric hormones) stimuli.

types of feedback loops exist for thyroid and sex hormone release.

There are many clinical uses for drugs in endocrinology.[2] One of the most common uses is replacement therapy. In diabetes, exogenous insulin is given if the body can no longer produce its own.

GH is also administered when there is a deficiency. Another use of endocrine drugs is to help make a diagnosis of an endocrine disorder. The dexamethasone suppression test will suppress cortisol release when the dysfunction is at the pituitary gland but will not in the presence of a cortisol-secreting

Table 14-2

Hormones Secreted by the Hypothalamus and the Anterior Pituitary

Hypothalamic Factor/Hormone (and Related Drugs)	Hormone Affected in Anterior Pituitary (and Related Drugs)	Main Effects of Anterior Pituitary Hormone
Corticotropin-releasing factor (CRF)	Adrenocorticotropic hormone (ACTH; corticotropin, tetracosactide)	Stimulates secretion of adrenal cortical hormones (mainly glucocorticoids); maintains integrity of adrenal cortex
Thyrotropin-releasing hormone (TRH; protirelin)	Thyroid-stimulating hormone (TSH; thyrotropin)	Stimulates synthesis and secretion of thyroid hormones, thyroxine and triiodothyronine; maintains integrity of thyroid gland
Growth hormone–releasing factor (GHRF)	Growth hormone (GH; somatotropin)	Regulates growth, partly directly, partly through evoking the release of somatomedins from the liver and elsewhere. Increases blood glucose, stimulates lipolysis
Growth hormone–releasing inhibiting factor (GHRIF; somatostatin, octreotide)	Growth hormone	As above
Gonadotropin-releasing hormone (GnRH; somatorelin, sermorelin)	Follicle-stimulating hormone (FSH)	Stimulates the growth of the ovum and the Graafian follicle in the female and gametogenesis in the male; with LH, stimulates the secretion of estrogen throughout the menstrual cycle and progesterone in the second half
	Luteinizing hormone (LH) or interstitial-cell-stimulating hormone (ICSH)	Stimulates ovulation and the development of the corpus luteum; with FSH, stimulates secretion of estrogen and progesterone in menstrual cycle. In males, regulates testosterone secretion
Prolactin release-inhibiting factor (PRIF, probably dopamine)	Prolactin	Together with other hormones, prolactin promotes development of mammary tissue during pregnancy; stimulates milk production in the postpartum period
Prolactin-releasing factor (PRF)	Prolactin	As above
Melanocyte-stimulating hormone (MSH) releasing factor (MSH-RF)	α-, β-, and γ-MSH	Promotes formation of melanin, which causes darkening of skin; MSH is antiinflammatory and helps to regulate feeding
MSH release-inhibiting factor (MSH-RIF)	α-, β-, and γ-MSH	As above

From Rang HP, Dale MM, Ritter JM, Moore JL. *Pharmacology.* 5th ed. New York: Churchill Livingstone; 2003.

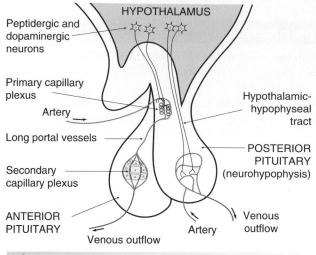

Figure 14-1

Schematic diagram of vascular and neural relationships between the hypothalamus, the posterior pituitary, and the anterior pituitary. The main portal vessels to the anterior pituitary lie in the pituitary stalks and arise from the primary plexus in the hypothalamus, but some (the short portal vessels) arise from the vascular bed in the posterior pituitary (not shown). (From Rang HP, Dale MM, Ritter JM, Moore JL. *Pharmacology.* 5th ed. New York: Churchill Livingstone; 2003.)

tumor in the adrenal gland. Birth control pills alter normal endocrine function by providing low doses of estrogen and progestin to suppress ovulation because the estrogen causes a negative feedback effect on the release of LH and FSH.

PATHOPHYSIOLOGY AND PHARMACOLOGY RELATED TO THE PITUITARY GLAND

Hypothalamic and pituitary disease may affect either single or multiple hormonal systems, leading to symptoms that appear similar to deficiencies of the target organs. Given the critical role of the hypothalamic and pituitary glands in regulation of the endocrine system, dysfunction at this level affects many organ functions.

Pituitary Hypofunction (Hypopituitarism)

Pituitary hypofunction may be caused by neoplasms, trauma, infection, or vascular infarction.[3]

There might be hypofunction of several hormones or diminished levels of a single hormone. Multiple endocrine deficits such as hypogonadism (decreased FSH and LH levels), secondary adrenal insufficiency (decreased ACTH), altered fluid regulation (decreased ADH), hypothyroidism (decreased TSH), and diminished growth (decreased GH) may all occur. The treatment is to replace the hormones that are deficient.

Adrenocorticotropic Hormone

The primary use of ACTH is diagnostic for differentiating between primary adrenal insufficiency (Addison's disease) and secondary adrenal insufficiency caused by poor secretion of ACTH by the pituitary gland.[4] In Addison's disease, the addition of ACTH will have no effect on cortisol production, but in secondary adrenal insufficiency, the added ACTH will cause the adrenals to produce the glucocorticosteroid. ACTH stimulates the adrenocorticosteroid pathway, converting cholesterol to cortisol in the adrenal cortex (Figure 14-2). Cortisol is then responsible for providing the necessary glucose for brain function and fuel.

Antidiuretic Hormone

ADH has a critical role in maintaining proper fluid balance in the body. An increase in plasma osmolality is one of the main stimuli for ADH release. A decrease in blood volume is also responsible for hormone release. Baroreceptors in the cardiovascular system sense a decrease in blood pressure, resulting in release from the posterior pituitary gland. ADH has two main target tissues: vascular smooth muscle via stimulating V1 and V3 receptors, leading to an influx of calcium into the cell, and the kidney distal tubule and collecting duct via a V2 receptor.[5] Renal actions include increasing the number and rate of water channels in the luminal membrane, thus increasing water reabsorption, which results in concentrated urine. Nonrenal effects include contraction of smooth muscle, particularly in the cardiovascular system, although this is only seen when the levels of ADH are elevated.

Various analogs of ADH are offered for replacement therapy. Vasopressin, which is actually ADH itself, has a short duration of action and must be given by subcutaneous or intramuscular injection. It is not highly selective for the V2 receptors, so its use will result in nonrenal effects. Desmopressin is more selective for V2 and also has a longer duration

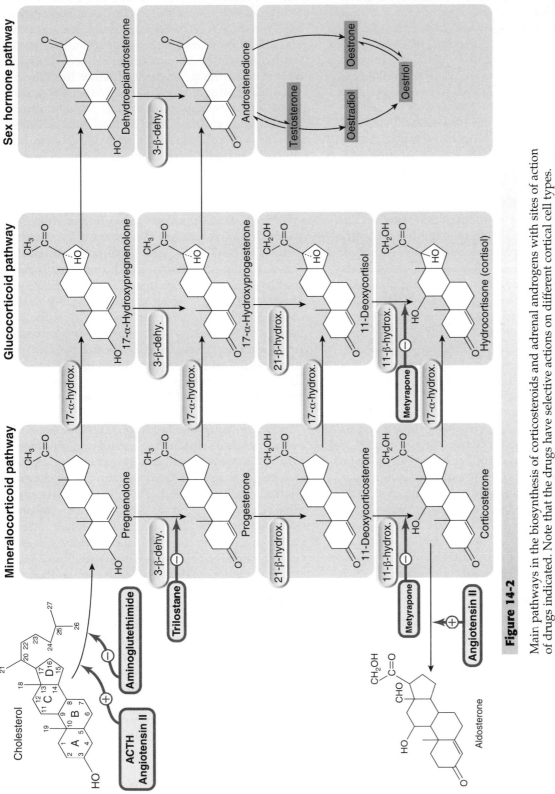

Figure 14-2

Main pathways in the biosynthesis of corticosteroids and adrenal androgens with sites of action of drugs indicated. Note that the drugs have selective actions on different cortical cell types. Glucocorticoids are produced by cells of the zona fasciculate, and their synthesis is stimulated by ACTH; aldosterone is produced by cells of the zona glomerulosa, and its synthesis is stimulated by angiotensin II. Metyrapone inhibits glucocorticoid synthesis; aminoglutethimide inhibits both glucocorticoid and sex hormone synthesis, and trilostane blocks synthesis of all three types of adrenal steroids. *ACTH*, Adrenocorticotropic hormone; *3-β-dhy, 3-β-dehydrogenase; 17-β-hydrox, 17-β-hydroxylase; 21-β-hydrox, 21-β-hydroxylase; 11-β-hydrox, 11-β-hydroxylase.* (From Rang HP, Dale MM, Ritter JM, Moore JL. *Pharmacology.* 5th ed. New York: Churchill Livingstone; 2003.)

of action. It is usually administered in the form of a metered nasal spray.

ADH and its analogs are used to treat diabetes insipidus and also to stop bleeding of esophageal varices through their action on smooth muscle. In addition, desmopressin is used for nocturnal enuresis in older children and adults and in patients with mild to moderate hemophilia to prevent bleeding. Parenteral desmopressin increases the concentration of factor VIII in blood. Adverse effects of these drugs are related to water intoxication and hyponatremia and include headache and tremors.

Growth Hormone Deficiency

GH originates in the somatotroph cells in the anterior pituitary. This gland contains more GH than any of the other pituitary hormones. Secretion is high in the newborn, decreasing to an intermediate level by the age of 4 years, and declining further after puberty. Secretion is pulsatile, varying throughout the day, with higher levels during deep sleep and in the early morning hours. The plasma concentration may fluctuate from 10-fold to 100-fold during the day.

GH has anabolic effects on several tissues, including skeletal muscle and epiphyseal cartilage.[6] It stimulates protein synthesis and the uptake of amino acids into cells. It stimulates production of insulin-like growth factor 1 (IGF-1) from the liver, which mediates the anabolic effect of GH. IGFs are also called *somatomedins.* Somatomedin receptors exist on many cell types, including liver and fat cells. The result of IGF production is stimulation of bone and muscle growth.

A deficiency in GH results in pituitary dwarfism. This condition may be produced by a lack of GH–releasing hormone or a diminished production of IGF. The pharmacological treatment is replacement with recombinant human GH, somatropin, or an analog called *somatrem*. Both of these are marketed for pediatric GH deficiency, short stature related to Turner's syndrome, and idiopathic, non-GH-deficient short stature in children more than 2.25 standard deviations below the mean height for their age.[7,8] Administration of the hormone results in linear skeletal growth and anabolic effects on organs and soft tissue. Children, ages 9 to 15 years who received somatropin three times per week over a 4-year period, had a final height measurement of 3.3 cm taller than children who received placebo. In another study in which a high dose and a low

dose of somatropin were compared, children who received the higher dose were 3.3 cm taller than those who had received the lower dose. Eighty-two percent of the subjects in the higher dose group who were followed up into adulthood were found to have achieved an adult height greater than the 5th percentile compared with 47% in the lower dose group. A meta-analysis of 10 controlled studies of children with short stature showed that GH injections for 5 years resulted in a gain of 4 to 6 cm.[9]

GH is usually administered as intramuscular injections three times per week until epiphyseal closure occurs. The total dose per week is determined by the weight of the child, but GH may be given in divided doses as often as six times per week.[8] This resembles the pulsatile release of endogenous GH. Side effects are minimal, with no effect on pubertal development, but may include insulin resistance or glucose intolerance. Some cases of intracranial hypertension, probably related to increased sodium retention, have been reported. There have also been some reports of gynecomastia, pancreatitis, and increased growth of preexisting nevi. Children should be monitored for these effects if they have an appropriate risk profile. For example, obese children should be screened periodically for diabetes.

In 1989 two placebo-controlled studies of GH replacement in GH-deficient adults were published. GH administered to individuals in these studies was found to be beneficial in terms of body composition and lipid levels.[10] Since then, more published evidence has indicated beneficial but inconsistent effects of GH for adults with hypopituitarism, patients with HIV disease, patients with fibromyalgia, children with cystic fibrosis, and even frail elderly patients.[11-13] In general, GH given to adults reduces central obesity, improves lipid levels, and increases bone density and lean body mass. When given along with resistive training to healthy elderly men for 12 weeks, GH was found to increase isokinetic muscle strength compared with exercise alone, exercise with placebo injection, or placebo alone.[14] Exercise alone produced a significant increase in muscle strength, but the GH-only group did not show any improvement. The investigators concluded that in healthy elderly men, GH can augment the strengthening effect of exercise, but not when it is the only therapy. Subjects who took GH did, however, show positive changes in body composition consisting of decreased fat mass.

A similar study performed with frail elderly patients for 6 months demonstrated that GH combined with exercise and exercise alone did increase muscle strength significantly.[12] Treatment with GH alone resulted in a nonsignificant trend toward increased quadriceps strength. Musculoskeletal side effects reported among the adults included carpal tunnel syndrome, arthralgias, and lower extremity edema. Although further study is needed to determine the benefits of GH administration in adults, the current guidelines indicate that if a patient perceives no benefit after 6 months of treatment, withdrawal should begin.[3]

Another indication for GH administration is to offset some of the negative side effects associated with long-term use of steroids for certain disease processes.[15] Steroids suppress linear growth and become GH antagonists, particularly when given to children. However, because both therapies are associated with insulin resistance and hyperglycemia, children receiving this regimen must be monitored frequently for type 2 diabetes.

Therapeutic Concerns with Hypopituitarism

As reviewed previously, hypopituitarism can entail the partial or complete loss of anterior pituitary hormone secretion. Once it occurs, it is generally permanent and requires multiple hormone replacement therapies. In patients who have panhypopituitarism (multiple deficiencies), cortisol should be replaced first, followed by thyroxine (T_4) (see discussion of thyroid deficiency and corticosteroid deficiency).[3] Sex steroids may be replaced when the patient's medical condition has stabilized. The last to be replaced is GH.

Hypopituitarism requires complicated treatment regimens that are often imprecise, with levels sometimes exceeding the normal range.[3] Achieving the optimum dose is a trial-and-error process. The therapist treating patients who are receiving hormone replacement must be alert to the side effects of excessive hormone levels. Unexpected interactions between hormones may also occur; therefore any ailment not usually seen should be reported to the patient's endocrinologist. Children and adults who have low GH levels have decreased bone mineral density and therefore are at increased risk for fractures. Slipped capital femoral epiphyses have been associated with GH deficiency.[8] It might be prudent to suggest that these children have GH levels determined, especially if they have any other

metabolic bone disease or renal insufficiency. Likewise, children with known GH deficiency who have hip pain should be thoroughly evaluated.

Acromegaly

Acromegaly results from excessive production of GH caused by a pituitary adenoma in adults.[6] The clinical features include excessive growth of bone and soft tissue with their resultant musculoskeletal problems, as well as some complex metabolic abnormalities (hyperglycemia, insulin resistance, elevated IGF-1 levels). Patients with this disorder display skin thickening; thyroid enlargement; excessive sweating; enlarged hearts; and enlargement of the hands, feet, and facial features (Figure 14-3). Severe arthritis, carpal tunnel syndrome, sleep apnea, and impaired cardiovascular function with hypertension are also seen. When this disorder occurs in children, it is labeled *gigantism* and results in linear bone growth because the growth plates are still active.

Treatment of GH-secreting tumors usually involves surgery and radiation.[16] However, if the patient is

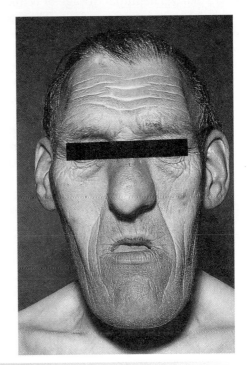

Figure 14-3

Characteristic facial features of acromegaly. (Courtesy Dr. C. D. Forbes and Dr. W. F. Jackson. From Rang HP, Dale MM, Ritter JM, Moore JL. *Pharmacology*. 5th ed. New York: Churchill Livingstone; 2003.)

not a candidate for surgery, drug intervention can be used. The dopamine agonist bromocriptine can block GH release in a certain percentage of patients. In healthy individuals, bromocriptine will increase secretion of GH; however, in patients with acromegaly, the drug appears to have a paradoxical effect. Because bromocriptine is not always effective, somatostatin analogs have become the drugs of choice.

Somatostatin diminishes GH concentration in both healthy subjects and patients with acromegaly. Somatostatin has multiple functions, acting as a neurotransmitter, regulating the release of GH—and when secreted by the pancreatic delta cells—acting to inhibit both insulin and glucagon release.[17] During the initial studies, this hormone showed promise in the treatment of diabetes. However, its benefit is limited by its extremely short half-life (1 to 3 minutes).

Octreotide is a longer-acting synthetic somatostatin analog. Its half-life is 80 to 100 minutes, and it is effective in reducing GH levels in 94% of patients and can help lower IGF-1 to normal levels in about 70% of patients.[18] The initial dosage of octreotide is three subcutaneous injections daily. The dose and number of injections may be increased if needed. Some newer depot preparations of octreotide have improved compliance by reducing the need for injections to only once or twice a month. Side effects of octreotide include nausea, abdominal cramps, diarrhea, flatulence, and gallbladder dysfunction. Tolerance for these adverse effects develops quickly.

The Food and Drug Administration has recently approved a GH receptor antagonist, pegvisomant, as parenteral treatment for acromegaly.[19] This treatment is reserved for patients who are not candidates for surgery or in cases in which surgery has failed. This drug binds to the GH receptors and blocks attachment by endogenous GH.

The patient is initially given a 40-mg subcutaneous loading dose, followed by daily doses starting at 10 mg. In a 12-week trial, reported side effects included injection-site reactions, nausea, diarrhea, chest pain, and flu-like symptoms. Increased hepatic enzyme levels have also been seen in a few patients.

THYROID DISEASES

Thyroid hormone (TH) controls the basal metabolic activity of all tissues by regulating genes that increase cell metabolism and protein synthesis.[20] In addition, these hormones stimulate tissue oxygen consumption, complement the sympathetic nervous system, and enhance gluconeogenesis, but at the expense of wasting tissue in order to supply glycogen. TH increases the metabolism of carbohydrates, fats, and proteins by influencing insulin, glucagon, glucocorticoids, and the catecholamines—either directly or indirectly—by regulating the activity of some enzymes involved in carbohydrate metabolism. Other important physiological effects of TH include regulating body temperature, increasing cardiac rate and contractility, and enhancing red blood cell mass and circulatory volume. An adequate TH level is critical for normal bone growth, and there is evidence that TH stimulates both osteoblasts and osteoclasts, but in patients with hyperthyroidism, the net effect on bone cells is bone resorption, leading to osteoporosis and increased risk of fracture.[21]

The thyroid gland secretes three main hormones: T_4, triiodothyronine (T_3), and calcitonin.[5] Calcitonin is involved in regulating the plasma calcium level and will be discussed in Chapter 15. T_3 and T_4 are formed by the iodination of tyrosine residues on a large peptide (thyroglobulin), which is synthesized and secreted into the lumen of the follicle (the functional unit of the thyroid gland). The follicles are surrounded by a rich capillary network, which produces a high rate of blood flow into the gland.

The first step in producing TH is the uptake of iodide by the follicle cells (Figure 14-4).[5] Iodide is taken up by a sodium/iodine (Na^+/I^-) cotransporter, which receives energy from the Na^+/K^+-ATPase pump. Next, the iodide is oxidized by the enzyme, thyroperoxidase, and attaches to the tyrosine residue on thyroglobulin. The coupling of two iodinated tyrosines forms diiodotyrosine. When two diiodotyrosines are coupled they form T_4 (Figure 14-5). Hormone secretion occurs when endocytotic vesicles fuse with the wall of the follicle cell. Thyroglobulin is resorbed into the follicle cells, and T_4 and T_3 are secreted into the circulation. Most of T_3 is formed by the deiodination of T_4 in extrathyroidal tissues, generating about 80% of the circulating T_3.[22] T_3 is the more active hormone with a higher affinity for thyroid receptors.

The regulation of thyroid function comes from the hypothalamus releasing TSH and subsequent release of thyrotropin-releasing hormone from the

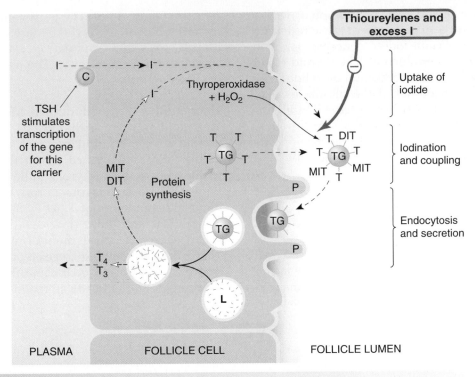

Figure 14-4

Diagram of thyroid hormone synthesis and secretion with the sites of action of drugs that modify it. The carrier *(C)* is a symport that transports sodium and iodine (I⁻) into the cell. See text for details. *TSH*, Thyroid-stimulating hormone (thyrotropin); *TG*, thyroglobulin; *T*, tyrosine; *MIT*, monoiodotyrosine; *DIT*, diiodotyrosine; T_4, thyroxine; T_3, triiodothyronine; *L*, lysosome; *P*, pseudopod. (From Rang HP, Dale MM, Ritter JM, Moore JL. *Pharmacology*. 5th ed. New York: Churchill Livingstone; 2003.)

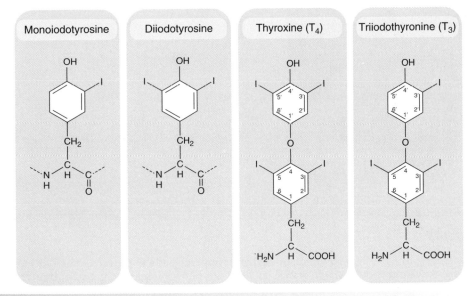

Figure 14-5

Iodinated tyrosine residues. Monoiodotyrosine and diiodotyrosine are shown in peptide linkage, as in thyroglobulin. When thyroxine (T_4) is used as a drug, it is given as the salt of the amino acid. (From Rang HP, Dale MM, Ritter JM, Moore JL. *Pharmacology*. 5th ed. New York: Churchill Livingstone; 2003.)

anterior pituitary gland.[5] The production of TSH is also regulated by a negative feedback effect from T_3 and T_4. The plasma iodide concentration also influences hormone production. The thyroid gland requires uptake of at least 500 nmol of iodide daily (equal to 70 mg of iodine). If the plasma level of iodide is reduced, there will be a reduction in hormone production and an increase in TSH secretion. An elevated level of plasma iodide has the opposite effect, a reduction in hormone production.

Hyperthyroidism (Thyrotoxicosis)

Hyperthyroidism is due to an overproduction of the endogenous hormone or excessive ingestion of exogenous hormone.[23] Symptoms include nervousness, weight loss, heat intolerance, tremor, tachycardia, hyperhidrosis, exophthalmos, and enhanced reflexes (Figure 14-6). The most common cause for hyperthyroidism is Graves' disease, an autoimmune disease in which circulating immunoglobulins stimulate the TSH receptor. The result is sustained overproduction of TH.

Thionamides (Propylthiouracil, Methimazole)

Treatment for hyperthyroidism includes antithyroid drugs, surgical removal, and radioactive iodine.[23] Propylthiouracil and methimazole inhibit iodine coupling to thyroglobulin by binding to the peroxidase enzyme. Propylthiouracil also inhibits deiodination of T_4 to T_3. Skin rashes, fever, arthralgias, and bone marrow depression may occur; therefore close monitoring is important. These drugs require 6 weeks of administration before success is realized because they do not affect the thyroglobulin already stored in the gland.

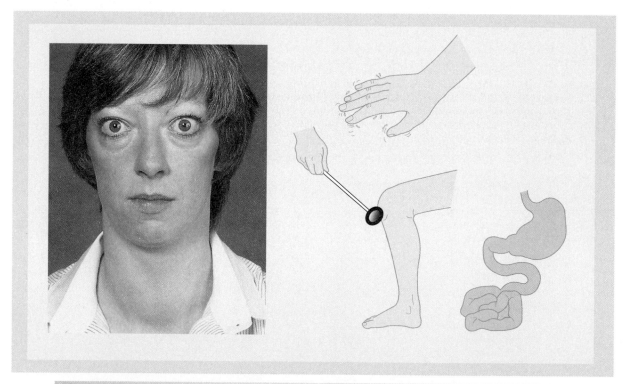

Figure 14-6

Signs and symptoms of hyperthyroidism. Hyperthyroidism leads to characteristic symptoms of nervousness, weight loss, heat intolerance, and fatigue. Signs such as tachycardia, tremor, accelerated reflexes, smooth skin, hyperhidrosis, and ocular stare are common to hyperthyroidism of any cause. Proptosis, diplopia, and corneal inflammation are specific findings in Graves' disease. (Photograph courtesy Dr. C. D. Forbes and Dr. W. F. Jackson. From Page C, Curtis AB, Sutter MC, Walker L, Hoffman BB, eds. *Integrated Pharmacology*. Philadelphia: Mosby; 2002.)

Iodide and Radioactive Iodine

Another treatment for hyperthyroidism is the administration of iodide, which in excess will inhibit the iodination of tyrosines. It is often used during a "thyroid storm" or to reduce TH levels until surgery can be performed. It is called *Lugol's solution* and consists of liquid drops added to fruit juice taken three times a day. Side effects include diarrhea, nausea, burning of the mouth, and a metallic taste.

Destruction of the thyroid gland can be achieved with radioactive iodine (^{131}I).[23] The radioisotope is taken up into the thyroid follicular cells and slowly destroys the gland. Onset of action is within 2 to 4 weeks and peaks between 2 and 4 months. Treatment with the thionamides should precede this treatment because administering radioiodine to an overactive thyroid gland can precipitate a thyroid crisis. Once the thyroid gland is destroyed, supplemental TH is required.

β-Adrenoceptor Antagonists

β-Blockers are considered adjuncts in the treatment of hyperthyroidism.[23] They are usually given to help reduce some of the symptoms of excess TH levels until the radioisotope treatment is effective. These drugs are effective in reducing symptoms related to adrenergic hyperstimulation such as tachycardia and tremor. Use of a β-blocker continues until the patient becomes euthyroid.

Treatment of Thyroid Storm

Thyroid storm represents a severe form of thyrotoxicosis and is considered a medical emergency.[23] Symptoms include fever, delirium, excessive tachycardia, hypotension, vomiting, and diarrhea. Supportive treatments such as intravenous hydration, cortisol, and large doses of propylthiouracil are needed. Oral potassium iodide to block TH release and β-blockers to lower heart rate are also needed.

Hypothyroidism

TH deficiency is usually caused by autoimmune destruction of the gland or directed destruction as a result of treatment for hyperthyroidism.[24] Symptoms include bradycardia, lethargy, weight gain, cold intolerance, and myxedema. Hypothyroidism is also associated with altered lipoprotein metabolism, resulting in elevated low-density lipoprotein (LDL) cholesterol levels and cardiovascular disease.[25] A goiter may form as a result of constant stimulation by TSH because there is no negative feedback.

Levothyroxine

Treatment of hypothyroidism is replacement therapy with synthetic oral levothyroxine. This drug is actually a T_4 look-alike that requires metabolic activation to form active T_3. Levothyroxine has a long elimination half-life of about 6 days because of extensive binding to plasma thyroid-binding globulin and to albumin. In chronic diseases, however, this is preferred because the effects of a missed dose would be minimized. The disadvantage is its slow rate of achieving a steady state, which means that dose adjustments can only be made after several weeks (4 to 8) of therapy. An overdose of levothyroxine might result in arrhythmias, angina, and symptoms of hyperthyroidism. For this reason, elderly patients with hypothyroidism are initially given low doses of levothyroxine with small increases at 4-week intervals. Doses are adjusted to keep TSH levels within normal limits.

Therapeutic Concerns for Patients Receiving Therapy for Hypothyroidism

It is well known that hyperthyroidism increases bone resorption, leading to osteoporosis and increased risk of fractures.[26] Some studies have demonstrated a similar risk for patients receiving long-term levothyroxine therapy. In a recent large study of 23,183 subjects receiving TH, fracture of the femur was significantly associated with levothyroxine therapy in male subjects. The suggested mechanism for this risk is subclinical hyperthyroidism. Therefore it is prudent for therapists to take this fracture risk into consideration, particularly when treating elderly male subjects receiving TH replacement. Therapists should also watch for any signs of hyperthyroidism, especially in their older clients, so that adjustment in dose can be made as quickly as possible to avoid adverse effects.

DRUG THERAPY FOR ADRENAL DYSFUNCTION

The adrenal cortex is responsible for the secretion of three types of steroid hormones: glucocorticoids, mineralocorticoids, and sex steroids. The endogenous glucocorticoids include hydrocortisone (cortisol) and corticosterone and primarily affect carbohydrate and protein metabolism. Aldosterone is the endogenous mineralocorticoid and is responsible for water and electrolyte balance. The primary sex steroids that are released are mainly in the form of androgens.

Glucocorticoids

The glucocorticoids are secreted from the adrenal cortex in response to ACTH from the anterior pituitary gland.[27] The initial step in cortisol synthesis is the conversion of cholesterol to pregnenolone (Figure 14-2). Basal release follows a diurnal variation with a marked elevation in the pre-dawn hours of the morning and a marked reduction during the late evening hours.[2] Replacement therapy attempts to mimic this normal cycle (Figure 14-7). Psychological factors and physical stimuli such as excessive heat or cold, injury, surgery, illness, or infection will increase secretion, which is why cortisol is called *the stress response hormone*.[28]

Cortisol activates the GRα and GRβ receptors located in the cell cytoplasm in almost every tissue of the body.[5,29] This steroid-receptor complex then moves to the nucleus of the cell and binds to steroid-response elements in the DNA. The net effect is to turn off transcription of genes for the cyclooxygenase-2 enzyme, various cytokines and adhesion factors, the vitamin D_3 induction of the osteocalcin gene in osteoblasts, and nitric oxide synthase. Another effect of this steroid-receptor complex is to induce the formation of annexin-1 (previously known as lipocortin-1).[30] Annexin-1 has strong antiinflammatory actions, as well as negative feedback action, on the hypothalamus and anterior pituitary gland.

The major metabolic effects of cortisol include increasing gluconeogenesis and lipolysis to provide fuel for physical activity and brain function.[4] Cortisol also produces a decrease in the uptake of glucose, resulting in a trend toward hyperglycemia. The effect on proteins is an increase in catabolism, and the effect on fat is redistribution to the trunk. Cortisol also decreases calcium absorption from the gastrointestinal tract and increases its excretion in the kidney tubules.

The antiinflammatory and immune suppressive actions of cortisol are the pharmacological reasons for its use.[5] In the area of inflammation, influx and activity of leukocytes, eicosanoids, and fibroblasts are decreased. In chronic inflammation, prolifer-

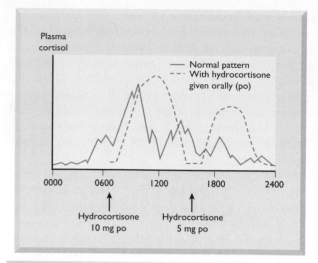

Figure 14-7

Glucocorticosteroid replacement therapy. An average adult produces approximately 10 mg of cortisol per day. Cortisol production shows marked diurnal variation, with an initial elevation in the pre-waking hours. Physiological replacement with oral hydrocortisone attempts to mimic this endogenous pattern. (From Page C, Curtis AB, Sutter MC, Walker L, Hoffman BB, eds. *Integrated Pharmacology.* Philadelphia: Mosby; 2002.)

ation of blood vessels is decreased. In the lymphoid areas production of T and B cells, cytokines, tumor necrosis factor, and immunoglobulin G is decreased.

Excess Glucocorticoids (Cushing's Syndrome)

Excess glucocorticoids lead to Cushing's syndrome, characterized by muscle weakness, osteoporosis, central obesity, moon faces, fragile skin and capillaries, hypertension, diabetes, and neuropsychiatric disorders (Figure 14-8). This syndrome resembles the unwanted effects of cortisol and the adverse drug effects of exogenous steroid administration. Cushing's syndrome may result from a ACTH-secreting adenoma, a cortisol-secreting adrenal tumor, or ectopic ACTH production from certain tumors in the lungs or gastrointestinal tract. Treatment for Cushing's syndrome is usually surgical, but drug treatment, with metyrapone, is advocated for several weeks before surgery to reverse some of the catabolic and metabolic effects.[5] This drug blocks the enzyme 11β-hydroxylase, inhibiting the terminal step in cortisol synthesis (Figure 14-2). The precursors of these pathways, such as 17-hydroxyprogesterone, are funneled into the

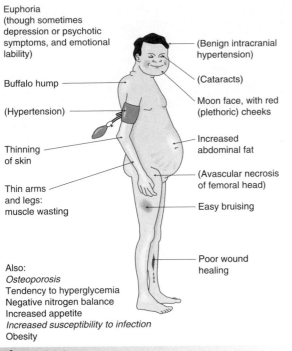

Euphoria
(though sometimes depression or psychotic symptoms, and emotional lability)

Buffalo hump

(Hypertension)

Thinning of skin

Thin arms and legs: muscle wasting

(Benign intracranial hypertension)

(Cataracts)

Moon face, with red (plethoric) cheeks

Increased abdominal fat

(Avascular necrosis of femoral head)

Easy bruising

Poor wound healing

Also:
Osteoporosis
Tendency to hyperglycemia
Negative nitrogen balance
Increased appetite
Increased susceptibility to infection
Obesity

Figure 14-8

Effects of prolonged glucocorticoid excess: iatrogenic Cushing's syndrome. Italicized effects are particularly common. Less frequent effects, related to dose and duration of therapy, are shown in parentheses. (From Rang HP, Dale MM, Ritter JM, Moore JL. *Pharmacology.* 5th ed. New York: Churchill Livingstone; 2003. Adapted from Baxter & Rousseau, 1979.)

mineralocorticoid and sex hormone pathways, leading to adrenal androgen formation and hirsutism, salt formation, and hypertension. An alternate drug is trilostane, which inhibits an earlier enzymatic step in cortisol formation.

Glucocorticoid Deficiency

Diminished levels of cortisol lead to devastating effects, even in nonstressful situations.[5] This deficiency can result from hypothalamic-pituitary disease, autoimmune destruction of the adrenal cortex (Addison's disease), or suppression of the hypothalamic-pituitary-adrenal axis after steroid withdrawal. Symptoms include weight loss, fatigue, arthralgias, and reduced cardiovascular function. If the insult is at the adrenal gland, additional symptoms such as low blood pressure and hyperkalemia are present as a result of the loss of aldosterone. Treatment for deficiency is replacement therapy. An attempt is made to simulate physiological secretion

by giving 10 mg of steroid in the morning and 5 mg in the evening. Hydrocortisone is the drug of choice for replacement, whereas the more potent steroids such as prednisone, are reserved for inflammatory and immune disorders. Side effects of treatment include symptoms resembling Cushing's syndrome. Therapeutic concerns with steroids have been reviewed previously.

Mineralocorticoids

Aldosterone is the primary mineralocorticoid as described previously.[4] Its secretion is regulated by a variety of factors, with angiotensin II, hyponatremia, and hyperkalemia being primary. The actions of aldosterone include increasing the permeability of the kidney distal tubules (luminal side) to sodium by increasing the number of sodium channels. Water is then passively reabsorbed following the osmotic pressure gradient. Aldosterone also stimulates the Na^+/K^+-ATPase pump in the basolateral membrane, leading to sodium reabsorption and excretion of potassium and hydrogen.

Mineralocorticoid Deficiency

Mineralocorticoid deficiency is characterized by reduced extracellular volume, resulting in orthostatic hypotension, dehydration, oliguria, and poor skin turgor. Fludrocortisone is the synthetic version of aldosterone used for replacement therapy. Adverse effects include sodium retention, hypokalemia, and hypertension.

Mineralocorticoid Excess

Excess aldosterone is usually produced by an adenoma in the zona glomerulosa of the adrenal cortex (Conn's syndrome).[4] The primary treatment for this tumor is surgical resection, but drug therapy is recommended for patients who are not candidates for surgery. The drug of choice for this problem is the potassium-sparing diuretic, spironolactone.

DRUG TREATMENT FOR THE REPRODUCTIVE SYSTEM

The hypothalamic-pituitary-gonadal axis regulates short-term control over events such as spermatogenesis, follicular development, and the menstrual cycle but is also involved in long-term control to maintain the secondary sex characteristics and initiate puberty and then menopause.[2] Hypothalamic

GnRH is the master hormone that interacts in a complex way with the anterior pituitary gland to release LH and FSH. LH stimulates sex steroid production in the gonads and also converts the adrenal androgens to testosterone and estrogens. Estrogens are also produced by the aromatase enzyme in the gonads and adipocytes, which then become the sole source of estrogen in post-menopausal woman after ovarian failure. FSH is the major regulator of gamete production.

Androgens and the Male Reproductive System

Dihydrotestosterone (DHT) and its precursor testosterone are androgens that produce anabolic and masculinizing effects in both sexes.[2] They are produced by the androgenic precursors coming from the adrenal glands, dehydroepiandrosterone and androstenedione, in the testes, and in small amounts by the ovaries in response to LH. Testosterone is an active ligand in muscle and liver, but in other tissues (prostate, seminal vesicles, epididymis, and skin), it is converted to the more powerful DHT by the enzyme 5α-reductase (Figure 14-9). The aromatase enzyme in the gonads and adipose tissue converts the testosterone precursors to estrogens.

Actions of testosterone and DHT include development of the male testes, penis, epididymis, seminal vesicles, and prostate at puberty, along with growth of axillary, pubic, facial, and chest hair and maintenance of these tissues throughout adulthood. These hormones are also responsible for the stimulation of sexual function and behavior and, of course, spermatogenesis in the adult. In terms of their metabolic actions, they are anabolic agents, increasing the size of muscles and bone. Testosterone stimulates the synthesis of clotting factors in the liver and also stimulates the production of erythropoietin by the kidneys, giving men a higher hemoglobin concentration than women.

Androgen Deficiency

Diminished androgen levels in prepubertal boys will cause a delay in puberty, especially in the development of secondary sex characteristics. Failure of the testes to produce enough testosterone in adults leads to low energy, decreased libido, erectile dysfunction, decreased growth of axillary and pubic hair, anemia, osteoporosis, and atrophy

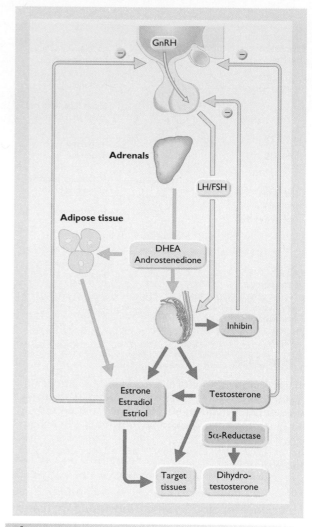

Figure 14-9

Regulation of sex steroids. Hypothalamic gonadotropin-releasing hormone *(GnRH)* stimulates the release of luteinizing hormone *(LH)* and follicle-stimulating hormone *(FSH)* from the gonadotrophs of the anterior pituitary. LH and FSH stimulate sex steroid production in the gonads. Adrenal androgens are further metabolized to more potent androgens in the gonads. The aromatase enzyme in both the gonads and adipose tissue converts androgens to estrogens. In certain target tissues, the enzyme 5α-reductase converts testosterone to the more potent androgen dihydrotestosterone. In postpubertal males, sex steroid production is constant. In females, gonadotropins and sex steroids are released in a complex pattern during the menstrual cycle. *ACTH,* Adrenocorticotropic hormone; *DHEA,* dehydroepiandrosterone. (From Page C, Curtis AB, Sutter MC, Walker L, Hoffman BB, eds. *Integrated Pharmacology.* Philadelphia: Mosby; 2002.)

of muscle. Testosterone serum levels normally decrease with age, 1% to 2% per year after the age of 30 years.[31] Hypogonadism can be primary from testicular failure or secondary from decreased GnRH secretion. Other causes of hypogonadism include Klinefelter's syndrome, mumps, orchiectomy, alcoholism, chemotherapy, and radiation therapy for pituitary or hypothalamic tumors. Treatment with testosterone will stimulate spermatogenesis and cause male sex characteristics to appear, regardless of whether the condition is due to primary testicular failure with elevated FSH and LH levels or secondary failure caused by decreased gonadotropin secretion.

Because testosterone has poor bioavailability, oral synthetic analogs, transdermal applications, intramuscular injections, and topical gels have been developed.[32] Some commonly used intramuscular preparations (testosterone enanthate, testosterone cypionate) have an oil-based solution to slow absorption from the site of injection. This allows dosing intervals of 2 to 4 weeks compared with an aqueous solution that only lasts 3 days. However, this mode of administration produces great peaks and troughs in concentrations.[33] The oral synthetic agents (methyltestosterone, oxandrolone) can produce a more evenly controlled serum level but have been associated with hepatic tumors. Testosterone patches are applied once daily and are also capable of producing a stable concentration; however, a patch worn on the scrotum has a tendency to fall off with exercise and sweating and requires that the scrotum be shaved frequently. A patch formulated to be worn on the upper arm, thigh, back, or abdomen is available, but it frequently produces skin reactions. It is estimated that 10% of the testosterone dose is absorbed through the skin from the patch. This then serves as a reservoir, slowly releasing the hormone into the body over a 24-hour period. A new buccal tablet is also available; it is placed inside the cheek or just above the incisor tooth and held there for 30 seconds.[34] The tablet remains in place by forming a gel that slowly releases the hormone across the oral mucosa. Twice-a-day dosing is necessary, and each tablet stays in place for 12 hours. Adverse effects have included gum and mouth irritation, as well as a bitter taste, but apparently, oral activities, such as eating and brushing the teeth, are not affected. Testosterone can also be rubbed onto the skin, but topical application requires 30 minutes to 4 hours to reach a normal concentration, and vigorous skin-to-skin contact 2 to 12 hours after application did result in a doubling of testosterone levels in female partners.[35]

Testosterone replacement therapy is associated with some potential risks and adverse events.[36] Lipid levels in patients taking testosterone are inconsistent but suggest a neutral effect when the hormone is administered as replacement; however, a significant reduction in high-density lipoprotein (HDL) levels is seen at supraphysiological doses. Other areas of concern are the potential for developing benign prostatic hyperplasia and prostate cancer. However, multiple studies have not demonstrated a worsening of voiding symptoms, an indication of increased prostate size, with replacement therapy. In addition, there is only a low frequency of prostate cancer associated with replacement therapy, despite the fact that lowering testosterone levels has treatment effects in both the benign disease and cancer. Monitoring prostate-specific antigen levels and performing digital rectal examinations are recommended. Other potential adverse events include hepatic neoplasms, seen only with the oral preparations, and sleep apnea. Some rather benign side effects include breast tenderness and reduced testicular size (from down-regulation of gonadal receptors).

Supraphysiological Use of Testosterone

Studies assessing muscle size and strength in healthy eugonadal men given high doses of testosterone have shown significant increases in bench-press and squat exercise capacity, as well as increases in fat-free mass, particularly when treatment was combined with exercise.[37] However, physiological doses of testosterone given to older men, not all of whom had hypogonadism, have shown inconsistent gains in strength and physical function. This explains why athletes abusing androgens not only use supraphysiological doses but also use several different androgen preparations simultaneously. The typical physiological dose is 100 mg of testosterone enanthate, given intramuscularly in weekly injections. The typical supraphysiological dose may be 1 g or more.[38] Therapists should be aware that although many people associate the term *steroid* with androgens, the term actually describes the basic chemical structure of many endogenous substances including cholesterol, estrogen, progesterone, and cortisol.

Two examples of anabolic steroids are nandrolone and stanozolol. Nandrolone is given by intramuscular injections, and stanozolol is taken orally. There are few medical indications for their use, although nandrolone has been used to promote erythropoiesis in aplastic anemia. Adverse effects that might be expected with these drugs include aggressive mood disorder, priapism, oligospermia, increased LDL levels, weight gain from muscle hypertrophy and fluid retention, and hepatotoxicity.[39] In addition, gynecomastia may occur as a result of the transformation of androgens to estrogens. Further investigations are needed to assess the risk for prostate or testicular cancer with these elevated levels of hormones.

The testosterone precursors, androstenedione and androstenediol, are considered dietary supplements, believed to enhance muscle strength.[40,41] However, when they were given according to the manufacturer's directions to men ages 35 to 65 years with normal testosterone levels, no greater strength was detected with the drugs compared with resistance training alone. This supplementation does result in increases in estrogen and abnormally affects the lipid profile.[42] However, it is important to recognize that many athletes who take these supplements consume much greater doses than recommended and that the adverse effects cannot always be anticipated.

Additional Uses for Testosterone

From the previous discussion, it is clear that testosterone is useful in physiological doses for men with hypogonadism; however, when administered in large amounts to eugonadal men, the adverse effects may outweigh the benefits. Despite this risk/benefit ratio, research is being conducted on the use of testosterone and its precursors in various states of illness. Synthetic testosterone analogs have been studied in men with AIDS wasting.[43,44] Wasting is defined as a loss of more than 10% of body weight. In several placebo-controlled studies, the testosterone group gained a significant amount of weight and lean body mass compared with the placebo group. Studies of women with AIDS wasting syndrome have also demonstrated weight gain with the hormone.[45] However, in both these populations, testosterone levels were below normal when matched to age-appropriate norms.

Another area in which testosterone and its analogs are used is treatment of androgen insuffi-ciency in women.[46] Low levels of androgens in women produce depression, fatigue, and decreased libido. Androgen replacement in these women improves the sex drive, increases bone density, reduces menopausal symptoms, and in general creates a feeling of well-being.[47,48] Side effects in this population may include acne, hoarse voice, virilization, and hirsutism, although these signs are much more prevalent at supraphysiological doses than the doses used for loss of libido.

Androgen Excess

Androgen excess in women is expressed by hirsutism and acne, which are common symptoms of polycystic ovary syndrome.[49] This syndrome presents as a hormone imbalance, high LH and low FSH (the reverse of normal) levels, and is associated with infertility, obesity, diabetes, and high estrogen and androgen levels. Danazol is an androgen analog used for the treatment of androgen excess and polycystic ovary syndrome.[50] It has few androgenic effects on peripheral tissues and is not converted to estrogen. However, it is able to provide feedback inhibition to the hypothalamus, reducing the release of GnRH. It is also used to reduce gonadal activity in endometriosis, precocious puberty, and fibrocystic breast disease. Adverse effects include nausea, fluid retention, mild hirsutism, reduction in breast size, hepatic dysfunction, and symptoms associated with menopause. Other agents that can be used for excess testosterone in women include spironolactone, which has potent antiandrogen properties, and some insulin-sensitizing agents such as metformin, which is used in diabetes.[2,51] Metformin was originally used in polycystic ovary syndrome to help obese women lose weight. It was later discovered that these patients had lowered androgen levels and improved menstrual cycle regularity when receiving the drug. The mechanism of action is not clear, but there seems to be a connection between insulin resistance and a high androgen level, so that if one is reduced, the other could be expected to follow.

Androgen excess in men may also be treated with spironolactone, but when androgen excess is combined with prostatic growth and male pattern baldness, the drug of choice is finasteride. Finasteride is a 5α-reductase inhibitor that is used for benign prostatic hypertrophy.[52] This results in a decrease in formation of DHT by the prostate, a subsequent decrease in prostate size, and improvement in urinary flow. It is mildly effective, reducing prostate size by about 20%. Side effects include decreased libido and impotence. This drug and the newer dutasteride must not be handled by pregnant women because they can be absorbed through the skin and may cause birth defects.[53]

Estrogen, Progesterone, and the Female Reproductive System

Each ovary contains about 7 million ova (eggs) at birth, but most die during childhood, leaving about 400,000 at puberty; of these, about 400 are actually ovulated.[2] GnRH, FSH, and LH maintain an intimate balance to ensure that one egg matures and undergoes ovulation each month from puberty to menopause. The menstrual cycle begins with shedding of the uterine endometrium, which lasts approximately 5 days. This is followed by the follicular or proliferative phase in which GnRH induces release of FSH and LH, which in turn stimulate follicles to develop. The prolonged low-level release of the gonadotrophic hormones results in continued maturation of one Graafian follicle. The remaining follicles undergo regression, but the developing follicle continues to mature and converts the androgens produced by the thecal cells of the follicle into estradiol (Figure 14-10). Estradiol in turn causes the uterine endometrium to proliferate. In the late follicular phase, the granulosa cells of the maturing follicle start to express LH receptors. These granulosa cells are then stimulated by LH to secrete progesterone. A higher estradiol concentration at mid cycle then promotes LH secretion and the LH surge, a reverse from the usual negative feedback mechanism. The LH surge begins to stop androgen and estrogen synthesis and induces the release of ovarian cytokines, prostaglandins, and histamine, causing a rupture of the ovary wall and ovulation. Ovulation starts the luteal phase when the ruptured follicle becomes a corpus luteum, producing progesterone. The progesterone readies the uterine endometrium for implantation. Plasma LH levels fall and remain low for the remainder of the cycle. The progesterone produced by the corpus luteum suppresses LH and FSH production by negative feedback on the hypothalamus and pituitary. If fertilization does not occur, the corpus luteum decreases its progesterone secretion and the endometrium starts to shed. When fertilization does occur, progesterone secretion is maintained by

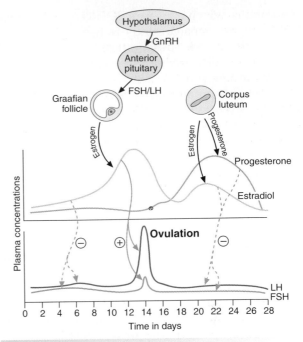

Figure 14-10

Endocrine control of the menstrual cycle. −, Negative feedback; +, positive feedback. (From Waller DG, Renwick AG, Hillier K. *Medical Pharmacology and Therapeutics.* New York: WB Saunders; 2001.)

human chorionic gonadotropin secreted from the fertilized egg until the placental hormones take over in about 6 to 8 weeks.

Contraceptive Agents

Oral contraceptives contain either a combination of a synthetic estrogen and a progestogen (synthetic progesterone) or progestogen alone.[4] The estrogen component is usually ethinyl estradiol, but occasionally, it is mestranol. These synthetic estrogens closely resemble the natural estradiol produced in the body. Ethinyl estradiol differs by only one substitution, making it more resistant to metabolism. Over the years, the dose of estrogen has been reduced, and the so-called second-generation pills produced now have only 20 to 30 µg of ethinyl estradiol compared with the 50 µg in the older preparations. Several different progesterones have also been used throughout the years. The first-generation progestogens had significant androgenic activity, causing acne and reduced HDL cholesterol levels. The newer third-generation progestogens lack androgenic effects and allow for greater expression of estrogen on lipoproteins, which increases HDL levels. Examples of the progestogens currently in use in the combination pill include desogestrel, gestodene, and norgestimate. A combined oral contraceptive that contains a new progestogen, drospirenone, is also available. This progestogen has some antimineralocorticoid activity that has been shown to decrease water retention; however, it is associated with a tendency to retain potassium. Other progestogens include the 17-hydroxyprogesterone acetate derivatives, which are also devoid of androgenic activity and are mainly used in intramuscular preparations for dysfunctional bleeding or for depot forms of contraception. Medroxyprogesterone (MPA) is also a derivative of the 17-hydroxyprogesterone acetate but is mainly used in hormone replacement therapy (HRT).

The mechanism of action of oral contraceptives is mainly the disruption of the precise hormonal balance that controls the menstrual cycle. The estrogen component suppresses LH and FSH secretion and follicular development by providing negative feedback to the hypothalamus and pituitary. The progestogen component also inhibits production of gonadotropins and makes the cervical mucus thick and unfriendly to sperm. Both components affect fallopian tube motility in opposite ways, thus altering the rate of ovum transport.

Oral combined contraceptives are available in three different combinations. The monophasic pill contains fixed amounts of estrogen and progestogen that are taken together for 21 days before drug administration is stopped to allow 1 week of withdrawal bleeding. There are also multiphasic combinations (biphasic and triphasic) that have a stepwise increase in both hormones and some that just provide increases in the progesterone concentration.

The progestogen-only pill is useful for women who should not take estrogen (especially those women who have a history of thromboembolic disorders). It is considered to be just a little less effective than the combined pills but must be taken within 3 hours of the usual time every day without any breaks. In addition, more irregular bleeding and breakthrough bleeding are associated with this type of pill. The intramuscular injection of progestogen can provide contraception for up to 8 to 12 weeks. Ovulation is more reliably inhibited than with the oral progestogen pill.

The oral contraceptive pills have several benefits in addition to preventing pregnancy. These pills reduce premenstrual tension, dysmenorrhea, and irregular bleeding and thus reduce anemia, ovarian cysts, and endometriosis. There is also strong evidence that they reduce the risk of ovarian cancer by simply limiting the explosive effect of ovulation on the ovary.[54]

Because noncompliance can be a problem with daily contraceptive regimens, there has been new emphasis on development of drugs for women who have trouble remembering to take a daily pill.[55,56] The norelgestromin–ethinyl estradiol patch and the etonogestrel–ethinyl estradiol vaginal ring are now available. The patch inhibits ovulation in the same manner as the daily pill, but the patch is applied once a week for 3 weeks, followed by a patch-free week for withdrawal bleeding. Application sites include the upper arm, buttocks, lower abdomen, and upper torso. The vaginal ring requires even less patient compliance. It releases ethinyl estradiol and etonogestrel; it is placed in the vagina for 3 weeks and then removed for 1 week. Menstrual bleeding occurs during the ring-free week. A new combined hormonal injection of MPA acetate and estradiol cypionate can be given monthly. Lastly, a long-acting progestin-only contraceptive consisting of six Silastic capsules containing 36 mg of levonorgestrel is available; it is implanted under the skin and remains in place for 5 years. The progestin is released at a constant rate. Because a surgical incision is required for insertion of the implants, complications such as pain, edema, and bruising may occur. There have also been reports of nerve injury with placement or removal, cellulitis, ulceration, and excessive scarring at the insertion site.

Some annoying side effects associated with birth control pills include breakthrough bleeding, nausea, headaches, and breast tenderness; but in time, most women are able to tolerate these.[57] The adverse drug reactions, which are more worrisome, include increased risk of deep vein thrombosis, ischemic stroke, myocardial infarction, and pulmonary embolism. However, since the doses of estrogen and progestin were reduced in the 1970s, the safety profile has improved. In addition, estrogens alone are associated with an increase in plasma HDL cholesterol levels, although this factor may be negated by the tendency to increase clotting factors, retain fluid, and produce more renin. Another problem is that some of the newer progestogens, especially norethisterone and MPA, oppose some of the beneficial effects of estrogens on lipid profiles, and gestodene and desogestrel may be associated with a slightly higher risk of deep venous thrombosis.[58] Critics speculate that the newer oral contraceptives pose no risk at all, if patients with other cardiovascular risk factors such as smoking, advanced age, and diabetes are excluded.

Despite years of study, the effect of oral contraceptive use on breast cancer continues to be controversial. Data from a pooled analysis of 54 studies published in 1996 showed a small increase in the risk of breast cancer with current use, but a more recent study, published in 2002, showed no increased risk among women who were currently using oral contraceptives.[59] The study also demonstrated no added risk for women who had ever used the pill or for those who had used the pill on a long-term basis. However, for those women who have a *BRCA1* or *BRCA2* gene mutation and for those with a strong family history of breast cancer, the increased risk has not been ruled out.

Postcoital Pill

High-dose estrogen and progestogen combinations have traditionally been administered within 72 hours of insemination to prevent pregnancy.[4] Although this approach is 75% successful, it is associated with a high degree of nausea and vomiting. Mifepristone (RU 486) is an antiprogestin that has been approved for the termination of a pregnancy of 49 days or less.[60] This drug has a high affinity for progesterone receptors. Removal of progesterone's influence on the pregnancy produces uterine contractions. In addition, the drug increases prostaglandins, which also stimulate uterine contractility. The recommended dose is three 200-µg mifepristone tablets taken as a single dose. If abortion does not occur within 3 days, then two more 200-µg misoprostol tablets (also given as a single dose) may be administered. Misoprostol also acts to stimulate uterine contractions. This drug combination terminates early pregnancy in approximately 95% of women. Side effects include vaginal bleeding and cramping abdominal pain. Recently, a dose as low as 10 mg has been shown to be effective.[61]

Treatment for Infertility

Infertility may be due to problems with ovulation, an anatomical abnormality of the fallopian tubes such as scarring or endometriosis, or male factors; or it may be unexplained.[62] Unexplained infertility is probably caused by poor quality or quantity of eggs. Ovulation induction or controlled ovarian hyperstimulation is the hallmark of assisted reproduction techniques and is used to treat most cases of infertility. Stimulating the maturation of multiple follicles improves the odds of becoming pregnant in combination with intrauterine insemination or in vitro fertilization. For these procedures to be successful, a complex protocol with several different drugs is needed.

Women undergoing these techniques begin with injections of GnRH agonists. Three are currently available in the United States: leuprolide acetate, nafarelin acetate, and goserelin.[63] Administration of any of these agents initially increases the pituitary release of FSH and LH, but after 7 to 10 days, gonadal secretions are diminished. The goal of this part of the protocol is to prevent premature ovulation. Side effects include those associated with menopause such as hot flashes. These drugs may also be used to treat precocious puberty, endometriosis, uterine fibroids, breast and uterine neoplasms, prostate cancer, and other hormone-sensitive cancers.

Once the reproductive system is turned off, patients are given injectable FSH and LH agonists in an attempt to stimulate growth of multiple follicles.[62] Daily injections over a period of 8 to 12 days will cause the maturation of many follicles in preparation for egg retrieval. The patient is monitored by means of ultrasonography and measurement of serum estradiol levels to determine when the follicles are ready to be harvested. When the follicles reach 18 to 20 mm in diameter, the patient will receive an injection of human chorionic gonadotropin to induce final egg maturation and ovulation by simulating an LH surge. The eggs are then subsequently retrieved and mixed with sperm to achieve fertilization.

During the time that the egg and sperm are mixing, the mother-to-be receives supplemental progesterone.[62] Most commonly, this entails daily intramuscular injections of progesterone in oil to prepare the uterine lining for implantation. Any time between day 3 and day 6 of fertilization, the embryos are transferred to the mother for implantation. Progesterone injections continue until the placenta begins its own progesterone support at around 8 weeks. If pregnancy is not achieved, administration of progesterone is discontinued, and shedding of the uterine lining begins.

Clomiphene is another drug for infertility to promote follicular maturation, although at much lower numbers than the FSH/LH combinations. Clomiphene is not a gonadotropin but rather an antiestrogen. It antagonizes the normal negative feedback of estrogen on the hypothalamus and pituitary and results in an increased FSH level. Ovarian enlargement is a necessary side effect.

Two major side effects are associated with induced ovulation.[62] Ovarian hyperstimulation syndrome is a serious complication in which fluid collects in the abdomen, leading to weight gain, severe pelvic pain, vomiting, and dyspnea. Fatalities are rare but have been reported. The other adverse effect of these drugs is enlargement of the ovaries in all women. This occurs because multiple eggs are maturing, which causes the ovaries to expand. Aerobic activity and activities that include jumping and running are contraindicated. Overheating may affect egg maturity, and jumping activities are contraindicated because an ovary may twist on itself, cutting off its blood supply.

Hormone Replacement Therapy

HRT has been used extensively by postmenopausal women experiencing the symptoms of decreasing estrogen levels. Estrogen therapy is useful in reducing vasomotor symptoms (hot flashes), atrophic vaginitis, osteoporosis, mood swings, and insomnia associated with menopause.[4] In addition, for years, physicians were convinced that HRT was cardioprotective because it produces a decrease in LDL and an increase in HDL cholesterol levels. However, in some recent well-conducted and large-scale studies, investigators have expressed major doubt as to the cardioprotection offered by HRT. These studies have given women more reason to worry about the risk of breast cancer as well.

HRT has been supplied most commonly in tablet form. Estrogen is taken daily with the addition of a progestin tablet for 10 to 14 days a month. This regimen leads to predictable monthly vaginal bleeding at least in the initial years of use. Another alternative has been to take an estrogen tablet daily and a progestin tablet for 10 to 14 days every 3 months. However, the most popular form of HRT has been a pill containing 0.625 mg of conjugated equine estrogen and 2.5 mg of MPA acetate, known by the trade name *Prempro* and manufactured by Wyeth-Ayerst. The typical regimen for women who have undergone a hysterectomy is use of estrogen alone (unopposed estrogen). The reason for this is that estrogen stimulates growth of the endometrial lining, which if left unchecked, can develop into endometrial cancer. However, women who no longer have a uterus do not need to be concerned about endometrial carcinoma.

The first study questioning the benefit versus risk of HRT appeared in the *Journal of the American Medical Association* in August 1998.[64] In this study, known as the HERS trial (Heart and Estrogen-Progestin Replacement Study), 2700 women between the ages of 44 and 79 years with known heart disease were examined. These women were randomly assigned to take conjugated estrogen plus progestin or placebo. The study showed that adding HRT did not reduce the incidence of heart attack. There was actually an increase in the number of deaths caused by coronary heart disease (CHD) in the first year of the study, followed by a decrease over the next 3 years, but without an overall reduction in events. A later report in which the same subjects were examined revealed no reduction in the risk of stroke.[65] The next study, released in August 2000 and called the Estrogen Replacement and Atherosclerosis (ERA) trial, indicated that the use of HRT did not slow the progression of coronary artery blockages.[66] The follow-up to the HERS trial, the HERS II trial, which extended observation of the original subjects, showed that after 6.8 years, HRT did not reduce the risk of CHD.[67] The most disturbing study, released in July 2002 and called the Women's Health Initiative Randomized Controlled Trial (WHI), indicated that the risks of HRT exceeded the benefits in healthy postmenopausal women.[68] In this study 16,608 women between the ages of 50 and 79 years were followed up for 5.2 years. They received either placebo or the same estrogen and progesterone combination used in the previous studies. The trial was stopped early because of an increased risk of coronary events, stroke, deep venous thrombosis, gall bladder disease, and invasive breast cancers. The incidence of breast cancer, which appeared to be greater for women who took HRT for more than 5 years, was also greater for women receiving the combination of estrogen and progesterone when compared with other studies of women taking estrogen alone. Absolute risks of taking the hormone combination per 1000 women per year were as follows: for breast cancer, 3.8 with HRT versus 3.0 with placebo; for strokes, 2.9 with HRT versus 2.1 with placebo; for myocardial infarction, 3.0 with HRT versus 2.3 with placebo; and for blood clots, 3.4 with HRT versus 1.6 with placebo. Positive outcomes included a reduction in hip fractures (33%) and colorectal cancers (37%).[69]

The important point is that these studies were performed with a specific type of HRT, conjugated equine estrogen plus MPA acetate, so that these results cannot be generalized to all kinds of HRT (e.g., estrogen ring or estrogen patch). In addition, the type of breast cancer exhibited in the WHI study was more invasive than the tumor that has been typically associated with estrogen. This has led to speculation that the culprit for the breast cancer is the MPA, and not the estrogen.

To determine which hormone is responsible for the increases seen in breast cancer and to more definitively determine the cardiovascular risk associated with estrogen, investigators allowed one arm of the WHI study to continue. The WHI investigators continued to study 10,739 healthy women who had previously had a hysterectomy in the WHI Estrogen-Alone Trial. These women were randomly assigned to receive unopposed estrogen or placebo. This study was also recently stopped prematurely, almost a year before its scheduled end.[70] This was a difficult decision made by the National Institutes of Health with the aid of extra advisors because the safety monitoring board could not reach a consensus. The hypothesis of this study was that hormone therapy would reduce the risk of CHD, which did not occur, although early CHD was reduced in the estrogen-alone group.[71] The risk of stroke was still present and was, in fact, a commonality for all three major studies—the HERS, WHI, and the WHI-Estrogen-Alone Trial. However, in the estrogen-alone trial, only 0.12% additional strokes were seen

per year. A pattern of increased pulmonary embolism was observed in all the studies, but it was not statistically significant in the estrogen-alone trial.

The major finding of the estrogen-alone trial was the effect of hormones on breast cancer. In the HERS and WHI studies, the risk of breast cancer was increased about 25%. In the WHI Estrogen-Alone Trial, the risk of breast cancer was reduced by 23%. Therefore combining the results of all three studies demonstrates that estrogen plus progestin, particularly MPA, is associated with a higher risk of breast cancer. In fact, some animal and human studies demonstrate that progestins are mitogenic on the human breast but that this risk varies among the different progestins.[72-74]

So who should be receiving HRT? It is clear that HRT has its benefits, such as reducing menopausal symptoms, osteoporosis, and colorectal cancers.[75] However, estrogen therapy is associated with stroke, venous thromboembolism, gall bladder disease, and breast cancer. MPA is associated with a different form of breast cancer and one that is more invasive. Women must carefully weigh the risks versus the benefits of this therapy. They must be adequately informed regarding the cardiovascular events that may occur within the first 1 to 2 years of therapy, and these should be balanced against the severity of menopausal symptoms. Perhaps HRT may be prescribed for a short time, 6 months, and only for women who do not have cardiovascular risk factors. Other forms of HRT such as skin patches, vaginal creams, and vaginal rings might not present the same risks; but further study of these products is warranted.[76]

ACTIVITIES 14

■ 1. Discuss some alternative drugs, dietary supplements, and lifestyle changes that are available to women who are experiencing menopause and who have cardiovascular risk factors.

■ 2. You are evaluating a 52-year-old woman for difficulty with fine motor skills caused by a fine tremor of her hands. As part of your evaluation, you attempt to take a detailed medical history. The patient does not remember when

the tremors started or what makes them better or worse. She only knows that skills such as buttoning and writing are becoming more difficult. The only other piece of information she offers is that she has felt very nervous and is hoping a massage could be part of her treatment program. You proceed with the evaluation.

This patient is a thin active woman who states she has trouble keeping weight on. She has prominent eyes and presents with hot, moist skin, despite the fact that she has been sitting in your waiting area for at least 45 minutes. Upper extremity range of motion is within normal limits, and strength is normal, although the patient reports some proximal weakness in her legs when she goes from sitting to standing. Likewise, cervical range is normal; however, you palpated a lump on the neck, which probably represents an enlarged thyroid gland.

Questions:

a. Discuss the most likely diagnosis for this patient and list some other symptoms associated with this condition. Which sign or symptom might negatively affect physical therapy intervention?

b. You are alarmed by your findings and refer the patient to her doctor. The patient's physician prescribes propylthiouracil. Why was this drug chosen?

c. After surgical removal of the thyroid gland, the patient will receive thyroid replacement therapy. What signs or symptoms should you look for and what should the patient know about replacement therapy?

■ 3. You are treating a 13-year-old boy for impairments related to cerebral palsy. The child also has a growth hormone deficiency and is currently taking somatrem. He has recently demonstrated more limitations in function, and you have noticed additional tightness in the hamstrings and heel cords bilaterally. You also notice that his clothes seem too short for his body. Review of the patient's chart reveals that he has grown at least 3 cm in the last 4 months. What are your recommendations?

REFERENCES

1. Guyton AC, Hall JE. *Textbook of Medical Physiology.* 10th ed. Philadelphia: W.B. Saunders Company; 2000.
2. Miller JW. Drugs and the endocrine and metabolic systems. In: Page C, Curtis AB, Sutter MC, Walker L, Hoffman BB, eds. *Integrated Pharmacology.* Philadelphia: Mosby; 2002:281-326.
3. Lamberts SW, de Herder WW, van der Lely AJ. Pituitary insufficiency. *Lancet.* 1998;352:127-134.
4. Waller DG, Renwick AG, Hillier K. *Medical Pharmacology and Therapeutics.* New York: WB Saunders; 2001.
5. Rang HP, Dale MM, Ritter JM, Moore JL. *Pharmacology.* 5th ed. New York: Churchill Livingstone; 2003.
6. Okada S, Kopchick JJ. Biological effects of growth hormone and its antagonist. *Trends Mol Med.* 2001; 7(3):126-132.
7. Growth hormone for normal short children. *Med Lett Drugs Ther.* 2003; 45(1169):89-90.
8. Vance ML, Mauras N. Growth hormone therapy in adults and children. *N Engl J Med.* 1999;341(16):1206-1216.
9. Finkelstein BS, Imperiale TF, Speroff T, Marrero U, Radcliffe DJ, Cuttler L. Effect of growth hormone therapy on height in children with idiopathic short stature. *Arch Pediatr Adolesc Med.* 2002;156(3):230-240.
10. Murray RD, Shalet SM. Adult growth hormone replacement: lessons learned and future direction. *J Clin Endocrinol Metab.* 2002;87(10):4427-4428.
11. Hutler M, Schnabel D, Staab D, et al. Effect of growth hormone on exercise tolerance in children with cystic fibrosis. *Med Sci Sports Exerc.* 2002;34(4):567-572.
12. Hennessey JV, Chromiak JA, DellaVentura S, et al. Growth hormone administration and exercise effects on muscle fiber type and diameter in moderately frail older people. *J Am Geriatr Soc.* 2001;49(7):852-858.
13. Paiva ES, Deodhar A, Jones KD, Bennett R. Impaired growth secretion in fibromyalgia patients: evidence for augmented hypothalamic somatostatin tone. *Arthritis Rheum.* 2002;46(5):1344-1350.
14. Lange KHW, Andersen JL, Beyer N, Isaksson F. GH administration changes myosin heavy chain isoforms in skeletal muscle but does not augment muscle strength or hypertrophy, either alone or combined with resistance exercise training in healthy elderly men. *J Clin Endocrinol Metab.* 2002;87(2):513-523.
15. Mauras N. Growth hormone therapy in the glucocorticosteroid-dependent child: metabolic and linear growth effects. *Horm Res.* 2001;56(suppl 1):13-18.
16. Colao A, Lombardi G. Growth-hormone and prolactin excess. *Lancet.* 1998;352(9138):1455-1461.
17. Lamberts SW, van der Lely AJ, de Herder WW, Hofland LJ. Octreotide. *N Engl J Med.* 1996;334:246-254.
18. Colao A, Merola B, Ferone D, Lombardi G. Extensive personal experience: acromegaly. *J Clin Endocrinol Metabol.* 1997;82:3395-3402.
19. Pegvisomant (Somavert) for acromegaly. *Med Lett Drugs Ther.* 2003;45(1160):55-56.
20. Zhang J, Lazar MA. The mechanism of action of thyroid hormones. *Ann Rev Physiol.* 2000;62:439-466.
21. Yen PM. Physiological and molecular basis of thyroid hormone action. *Physiol Rev.* 2001;81(3):1097-1142.
22. Wood AJ. Drugs and thyroid function. *N Engl J Med.* 1995;333(25):1688-1694.
23. Gittoes N, Franklyn JA. Hyperthyroidism. *Drugs.* 1998; 55(4):543-553.
24. Lindsay RS, Toft AD. Hypothyroidism. *Lancet.* 1997; 349:413-417.
25. Brent GA. The molecular basis of thyroid hormone action. *N Engl J Med.* 1994;331(13):847-853.
26. Sheppard MC, Holder R, Franklyn JA. Levothyroxine treatment and occurrence of fracture of the hip. *Arch Intern Med.* 2002;162:338-343.

27. Bakheit AMO, Thilmann AF, Ward AB, et al. A randomized, double-blind, placebo-controlled, dose-ranging study to compare the efficacy and safety of three doses of botulinum toxin type a (Dysport) with placebo in upper limb spasticity after stroke. *Stroke*. 2000; 31:2402-2406.

28. Lamberts SW, Bruining H, De Jong FH. Corticosteroid therapy in severe illness. *N Engl J Med*. 1997;337(18): 1285-1292.

29. Funder JW. Glucocorticoid and mineralocorticoid receptors: biology and clinical relevance. *Ann Rev Med*. 1997;48:231-240.

30. Buckingham JC, Flower RJ. Lipocortin 1: a second messenger of glucocorticoid action in the hypothalamo-pituitary-adrenocortical axis. *Mol Med Today*. 1997; 3(7):296-302.

31. Basaria S, Dobs AS. Hypogonadism and androgen replacement therapy in elderly men. *Am J Med*. 2001; 110(7):563-572.

32. Testim and Striant—two new testosterone products. *Med Lett Drugs Ther*. 2003;45(1164):70-72.

33. Dobs AS, Meikle AW, Arver S, Sanders SW, Caramelli KE, Mazer NA. Pharmacokinetics, efficacy, and safety of permeation-enhanced testosterone transdermal system in comparison with bi-weekly injections of testosterone enanthate for the treatment of hypogonadal men. *J Clin Endocrinol Metab*. 1999;84(10):3469-3478.

34. Dobs AS, Hoover DR, Chen MC, Allen R. Pharmacokinetic characteristics, efficacy, and safety of buccal testosterone in hypogonadal males: a pilot study. *J Clin Endocrinol Metab*. 1998;83(1):33-39.

35. Androgel. *Med Lett Drugs Ther*. 2000;42(1080):49-51.

36. Rhoden EL, Morgentaler A. Risks of testosterone-replacement therapy and recommendations for monitoring. *N Engl J Med*. 2004;350(5):482-492.

37. Bhasin S, Storer TW, Berman N, et al. The effects of supraphysiologic doses of testosterone on muscle size and strength in men. *N Engl J Med*. 1996;335:1-7.

38. Bhasin S, Woodhouse L, Storer TW. Proof of the effect of testosterone on skeletal muscle. *J Endocrinol*. 2001; 170:27-38.

39. Christiansen K. Behavioural effects of androgen in men and women. *J Endocrinol*. 2001;170:39-48.

40. Broeder CE, Quindry J, Brittingham K, Panton L. The Andro Project: physiological and hormonal influences of androstenedione supplementation in men 35 to 65 years old participating in a high-intensity resistance training program. *Arch Intern Med*. 2000;160:3093-3104.

41. Brown GA, Vukovich MD, Sharp RL, Reifenrath TA, Parsone KA, King DS. Effect of oral DHEA on serum testosterone and adaptations to resistance training in young men. *J Appl Physiol*. 1999;87(6):2274-2283.

42. King DS, Sharp RL, Vukovich MD, et al. Effect of oral androstenedione on serum testosterone and adaptations to resistance training in young men: a randomized controlled trial. *JAMA*. 1999;281(21):2020-2028.

43. Corcoran C, Grinspoon S. Drug therapy: treatments for wasting in patients with the acquired immunodeficiency syndrome. *N Engl J Med*. 1999;340(22):1740-1750.

44. Bhasin S, Storer TW, Javanbakht M, et al. Testosterone replacement and resistance exercise in HIV-infected men with weight loss and low testosterone levels. *JAMA*. 2000;283(6):763-770.

45. Miller KW, Corcoran C, Armstrong C, et al. Transdermal testosterone administration in women with acquired immunodeficiency wasting: a pilot study. *J Clin Endocrinol Metab*. 1998;83:2717-2725.

46. Chi MC, Lobo RA. Formulations and use of androgens in women. *Mayo Clin Proc*. 2004;79(4):S3-S7.

47. Shifren JL. The role of androgens in female sexual dysfunction. *Mayo Clin Proc*. 2004;79(4):S19-S24.

48. Kearns AE, Khosla S. Potential anabolic effects of androgens on bone. *Mayo Clin Proc*. 2004;79(4):S14-S8.

49. Guzick DS. Polycystic ovary syndrome. *Obstet Gynecol*. 2004;103(1):181-193.

50. Nissen D, ed. *Mosby's Drug Consult*. St Louis: Mosby, Inc; 2004.

51. Tsilchorozidou T, Prelevic GM. The role of metformin in the management of polycystic ovary syndrome. *Curr Opin Obstet Gynecol*. 2003;15(6):483-488.

52. McConnell JD, Bruskewitz R, Walsh P, et al. The effect of finasteride on the risk of acute urinary retention and the need for surgical treatment among men with benign prostatic hyperplasia. *N Engl J Med*. 1998;338(9):557-563.

53. Dutasteride (Avodart) for benign prostatic hyperplasia. *Med Lett Drugs Ther*. 2002;44(1146):109-110.

54. Ness RB, Grisso JA, Klapper J, et al. Risk of ovarian cancer in relation to estrogen and progestin dose and use characteristics of oral contraceptives. *Am J Epidemiol*. 2000;152(3):233-241.

55. Herndon E. New contraceptive options. *Am Fam Physician*. 2004;69:853-860.

56. Forinash AB, Evans SL. New hormonal contraceptives: a comprehensive review of the literature. *Pharmacotherapy*. 2003;23(12):1573-1591.

57. Petitti DB. Clinical practice. Combination estrogen-progestin oral contraceptives. *N Engl J Med*. 2003; 349(15):1443-1450.

58. Rosing J, Tans G, Nicolaes GA, et al. Oral contraceptives and venous thrombosis: different sensitivities to activated protein C in women using second- and third-generation oral contraceptives. *Br J Haematol*. 1997;97(1):233-238.

59. Marchbanks PA, McDonald JA, Wilson HG, et al. Oral contraceptives and the risk of breast cancer. *N Engl J Med*. 2002;346(26):2025-2032.

60. Mifepristone (RU 486). *Med Lett Drugs Ther*. 2000; 42(1091)101-102.

61. Gemzell-Danielsson K, Mandl I, Marions L. Mechanisms of action of mifepristone when used for emergency contraception. *Contraception*. 2003;68(6):471-476.

62. Drugs for assisted reproduction. *Treat Guidel Med Lett*. 2003;1(14):89-92.

63. Huirne JA, Lambalk CB. Gonadotropin-releasing-hormone-receptor antagonists. *Lancet*. 2001;358:1793-1803.

64. Hulley S, Grady D, Bush T, et al. Randomized trial of estrogen plus progestin for secondary prevention of coronary heart disease in postmenopausal women. *JAMA*. 1998;280(7):605-613.

65. Simon JA, Hsia J, Cauley JA, et al. Postmenopausal hormone therapy and risk of stroke: The Heart and Estrogen-progestin Replacement Study. *Circulation*. 2001; 103(5):638-642.

66. Herrington DM, Reboussin DM, Brosnihan KB, et al. Effects of estrogen replacement on the progressions of coronary-artery atherosclerosis. *N Engl J Med*. 2000; 343(8):522-529.

67. Grady D, Herrington DM, Bittner V, et al. Cardiovascular disease outcomes during 6.8 years of hormone therapy:

Heart and Estrogen/Progestin Replacement Study Follow Up. *JAMA.* 2002;288(1):49-57.

68. Investigators: Writing Group for the Women's Health Initiative. Principal results from the Women's Health Initiative Randomized Controlled Trial. *JAMA.* 2002;288(3):321-333.

69. Chlebowski RT, Wactawski-Wende J, Ritenbaugh C, et al. Estrogen plus progestin and colorectal cancer in postmenopausal women. *N Engl J Med.* 2004;350(10):991-1004.

70. Hulley S, Grady D. The WHI estrogen-alone trial—do things look any better? *JAMA.* 2004;291(14):1769-1771.

71. Anderson GL, Limacher M, Assaf AR, et al. Effects of conjugated equine estrogen in postmenopausal women with hysterectomy. *JAMA.* 2004;291(14):1701-1712.

72. Santen RJ. Risk of breast cancer with progestins: critical assessment of current data. *Steroids.* 2003;68(10-13):953-964.

73. Nilsen J, Brinton RD. Divergent impact of progesterone and medroxyprogesterone acetate (Provera) on nuclear mitogen-activated protein kinase signaling. *Proc Natl Acad Sci USA.* 2003;100(18):10506-10511.

74. Brinton LA, Schairer C. Postmenopausal hormone-replacement therapy—time for a reappraisal? *N Engl J Med.* 1997;336(25):1821-1822.

75. Kocjan T, Gordana M. Hormone replacement therapy update: who should we be prescribing this to now? *Curr Opin Obstet Gynecol.* 2003;15(6):459-464.

76. Stevenson JC, Oladipo A, Manassiev N, Whitehead MI, Guilford S. Randomized trial of effect of transdermal continuous combined hormone replacement therapy on cardiovascular risk markers. *Br J Haematol.* 2004;124(6):802-808.

CHAPTER 15

DRUG TREATMENT FOR OSTEOPOROSIS AND DIABETES

DRUG TREATMENT FOR OSTEOPOROSIS

Osteoporosis is the loss of bone mass caused by a loss of mineral content, which reduces the strength of bone. All individuals lose bone mass as they age, but for women, there is a marked increase in bone loss after menopause that corresponds to the loss of estrogen. Other factors that influence the loss of bone include smoking, significant alcohol use, immobility, and age.[1] Age-related bone loss results from increased bone resorption and increased apoptosis of osteocytes, decreasing the repair response. In addition, fracture risk is increased because of comorbid conditions, cognitive impairment, medications, deconditioning, and inadequate calcium and vitamin D intake. There is a lower incidence of osteoporosis among men, probably resulting from higher peak bone mass to begin with, shorter life expectancy, and a more gradual cessation of hormone production. Bone loss in the young elderly individual is associated with trabecular loss and may predispose the individual to spontaneous vertebral fractures. Osteoporosis in older patients is associated with loss of cortical bone, increasing the risk of traumatic fracture, particularly at the neck of the femur. Many drugs are marketed for the prevention and treatment of osteoporosis, particularly postmenopausal osteoporosis. However, drug intervention for this disorder has become much more complicated by the news that hormone replacement therapy increases the incidence of cardiovascular diseases and breast cancer.

Bone Remodeling

Bone is specialized connective tissue designed as a load-bearing structure. It is formed by a combination of dense compact (cortical) bone and cancellous (trabecular) bone. Trabecular bone is a honeycomb of vertical and horizontal bars filled with marrow and fat. Trabecular bone is located in the vertebral bodies, pelvis, and proximal femur.[2] The mineral components of bone are calcium and phosphorus, and the organic matrix is type I collagen. Two major cell types that are found in bone include the osteoclast, responsible for removing the mineralized matrix, and the osteoblast, responsible for producing the matrix. These cell types are the commanders of the bone remodeling process.

Bone is constantly undergoing remodeling with a delicate balance between resorption by osteoclasts and bone formation by osteoblasts.[3] Bone remodeling occurs in small packets of cells called *basic multicellular units* (BMUs). The BMU is approximately 1 to 2 mm long and 0.2 to 0.4 mm wide and is composed of a group of osteoclasts in the front, osteoblasts in the back, a central vascular capillary, and a nerve supply. Each BMU begins at a particular place and advances toward a target, which is the area that needs replacement. The BMU travels through bone across a surface, excavating and then replacing.

Osteoclasts adhere to bone and remove it by proteolytic digestion and acidification. Osteoblasts move to cover the excavated area and begin forming new bone. The lifespan of the BMU is 6 to 9 months, and at any one time there are 1 million active BMUs.

The precursors of osteoblasts are mesenchymal stem cells, which also give rise to bone marrow stromal cells, chondrocytes, muscle cells, and adipocytes; whereas the precursors of osteoclasts are hematopoietic cells of the monocytes/macrophage lineage.[4] The development and differentiation of these cells are controlled by growth factors and cytokines produced in the bone marrow environment. Several cytokines are involved in the early stages of hematopoiesis and in osteoclastogenesis. Interleukin 6, in particular, is involved in both pathways but alone is able to stimulate osteoclastogenesis and promotes bone resorption.

The regulation of cell numbers and alterations in the functional activity of the osteoclasts and osteoblasts, termed *cell vigor*, contributes to changes in rate of resorption and formation. Several molecules have been proposed to coordinate this function. Three proteins that are involved in this signaling pathway have been identified.[5] Two of these proteins are membrane-bound cytokine-like molecules called *receptor activator of nuclear factor* (RANK) and the RANK ligand (RANKL). RANK is present on osteoclast precursor cells, and when activated, promotes osteoclast maturation by increasing the expression of specific genes. RANKL is produced by and exists on the surface of osteoblasts. So if an osteoclast precursor encounters an osteoblast, the resulting interaction between RANK and RANKL stimulates the osteoclast precursor to mature into the bone-resorbing osteoclast. Activation of RANK by RANKL induces the expression of interferon-β in osteoclast precursor cells, which ultimately leads to a decrease in osteoclast differentiation by means of negative feedback.[6] Osteoblasts also produce osteoprotegerin, which binds to RANKL and prevents it from binding to RANK. This inhibits RANKL-mediated osteoclast maturation. It is believed that these chemical factors are involved in modulating the strength of the osteoclast response and in stimulating more frequent cycles of resorption.

The mature osteoblast secretes the bone matrix whose major product is type I collagen.[4] Extracellular processing of this collagen results in three-chained type I collagen molecules, which then form a collagen fibril. The osteoblasts also synthesize other proteins that are incorporated into the bone matrix, including osteocalcin and osteonectin (non-collagenous proteins), as well as glycosaminoglycans, biglycan, and decorin; osteoblasts also help regulate the local concentrations of calcium and phosphate in a way that promotes the formation of hydroxyapatite. Osteoblasts also express large amounts of alkaline phosphatase, which is thought to also play a role in mineralization of bone. Bone mineralization lags behind matrix production, and matrix synthesis determines the volume of bone, but mineralization of the matrix increases the density of bone by displacing water. Osteoblasts become osteocytes as they are buried within mineralized matrix. They are regularly spaced throughout the matrix and communicate with each other and with other cells on the bone surface via multiple extensions of their plasma membrane. Osteoblasts communicate with the cells of the bone marrow stroma. Communication actually extends from the osteocytes to the osteoblasts to bone marrow and finally to the endothelial cells of the vascular supply. So the location of the osteocytes can indicate the need for repair and transmit this need to the bone marrow to stimulate differentiation of additional osteoblasts. Osteocytes can also detect changes in the levels of hormones that circulate through the blood vessel, such as estrogen and glucocorticoids, which influence their function.

Osteoclasts are large multinucleated cells that have a ruffled border, described as a complex system of finger-shaped projections of membrane.[4] This structure is surrounded by a specialized area called *the clear zone*, which is what attaches the osteoclast to bone and seals off the area to be excavated. Here the osteoclast secretes the matrix metalloproteinases to degrade the matrix.

Systemic hormones, primarily parathyroid hormone (PTH) and 1,25-dihydroxyvitamin D_3, are strong stimulators of osteoclast formation and regulate calcium absorption and excretion from the intestine and kidneys, maintaining calcium homeostasis.[7] Specifically, PTH increases calcium reabsorption from bone, increases calcium reabsorption from the kidneys, increases intestinal absorption of calcium, and promotes the formation of 1,25-dihydroxyvitamin D_3. At the same time, PTH decreases phosphate reabsorption from the kidneys. The result is an increase in the serum calcium level and a decrease in the serum phosphate level.

Vitamin D is produced in the skin by UV light (D_3) or ingested in the diet (D_3 and D_2).[7] Because vitamins D_2 and D_3 have identical biological actions, they are referred to as vitamin D. However, vitamin D must undergo successive hydroxylations to act as a hormone. In the liver it is hydroxylated to 25-hydroxyvitamin D_3, and then in the kidneys, it is further activated to 1,25-dihydroxyvitamin D_3.[8] At physiological levels vitamin D increases bone formation. It stimulates absorption of calcium, phosphate, and magnesium from the intestines and plays a significant role in bone formation. Vitamin D is responsible for mineralization of newly formed osteoid along the calcification front. The mechanism of action may be the synthesis of osteocalcin and fibronectin. In addition, it increases calcium and phosphorus reabsorption from the kidneys. At high levels, however, the action of vitamin D mimics the action of PTH.

Calcitonin inhibits osteoclast development and promotes osteoclast apoptosis.[7] It decreases resorption and enhances bone formation. Other hormones including estrogen, androgen, glucocorticoids, and thyroid hormone have strong influences over the development of osteoblasts and osteoclasts by producing different cytokines.

Pathogenesis of Osteoporosis

The rate of differentiation of osteoblasts and osteoclasts, their relative vigor, and the timing of their death—all influence the bone repair process.[4] The life span of the osteoclast is about 2 weeks, whereas the osteoblast exists for 3 months. Normally, estrogen and androgens suppress interleukin 6, as well as directly act on osteoclasts to promote their cell death. The sex steroids also have an anti-apoptotic effect on osteoblasts. Therefore the loss of sex steroids, particularly after menopause, leads to a shortened lifespan for osteoblasts. In addition, a delay in the cell death of osteoclasts leads to the formation of deeper resorptive cavities and perforation of the trabeculae.

The amount of bone formed during each remodeling phase decreases with age, regardless of sex. Specifically, there is a decrease in wall thickness, and this has become a marker for reduced remodeling. Changes in the production of bone cells, that is, a reduction in progenitor cells, provide an explanation for osteoporosis caused by senescence independent from sex steroid loss. Decreased osteoblastogenesis

as a result of aging is associated with an increase in adipogenesis and myelopoiesis, suggesting a change in expression of the genes toward differentiation of multipotent mesenchymal stem cells to adipocytes instead of osteoblasts.[9,10] There is strong evidence for an association of dietary fat and lipoproteins with bone marrow differentiation, osteoporosis, and atherogenesis. In fact, mice fed a high-fat diet for 4 months showed decreases in osteogenic cell differentiation.[11,12]

The third major type of osteoporosis is drug-induced loss of bone mineral density (BMD). Glucocorticoids, in particular, have been shown to inhibit osteoblastogenesis and increase osteoblast cell death, making decreased bone formation the cardinal feature.[13] However, there is an early loss of BMD, suggesting that steroid use increases osteoclast numbers, despite decreasing osteoclast production, by decreasing osteoclast cell death. BMD can decrease by 2% to 4% after just 6 months of steroid use in healthy men, after which the rate of loss declines. In one short-term study, 10 days of steroid administration to mice increased osteoclast numbers. Therefore the adverse effect of steroids on bone occur in two phases, an early phase characterized excessive bone resorption and a slower, later phase in which the loss is due to decreased formation.[14] Another feature of glucocorticoid-induced osteoporosis is osteonecrosis, resulting in a collapse of the large joints.[15] This osteonecrosis is explained by still another mechanism, increasing osteocyte apoptosis.

Prevention and Treatment of Osteoporosis

For patients at risk for developing osteoporosis, the goals of treatment include obtaining optimal peak bone mass and minimizing further bone loss. Ideally, prevention begins in childhood with a healthy diet and adequate intake of calcium and vitamin D (see discussion of calcium and vitamin D). It is estimated that the highest rate of calcium accumulation occurs at a mean age of 12.5 years in girls and at 14 years in boys.[16] After this period of rapid accumulation, a period of bone consolidation occurs during which calcium levels change little but periosteal expansion occurs. The actual age of peak bone mass is unknown because of its variability but may be in the twenties at the proximal femur and near age 30 for the spine in healthy women. Multiple factors affect attainment of peak bone mass including nutrition, eating disorders, genetics, weight cycling, and conditions leading to hypoestrogenism such as heavy exercise, low body fat, and premature menopause. Although current data are insufficient to set specific recommendations for premenopausal women, it is clear that some interventions to prevent this disease must be instituted early. However, often women do not direct their attention toward preventing osteoporosis until later in life after fracture or loss of height has been noted.

Typically, the need for drug therapy is determined by bone densitometry.[1] Measurement of hip and spine BMD with dual-energy x-ray absorptiometry is the gold standard for an osteoporosis diagnosis. The test is based on the fact that calcium absorbs much more radiation than protein or soft tissue. The amount of energy that is absorbed by the calcium in a section of bone represents the bone mineral content. This is a noninvasive and painless test that is used to identify osteoporosis, determine the risk of fracture, and monitor the patient's response to treatment. This test measures the patient's BMD and compares it with "young normal" (30-year-old healthy adult) and age-matched norms. The comparisons with the young normal norms are listed as T-scores, and the aged-matched comparisons are listed as Z-scores.[17] The World Health Organization defines osteoporosis on the basis of bone density levels. Individuals with a T-score within 1 standard deviation (SD) of the norm (+1 or –1) are considered to have normal bone density. Scores below the norm are indicated by negative numbers. Low bone mass or osteopenia is bone density 1 to 2.5 SDs below the young adult mean (–1 to –2.5 SDs). Osteoporosis is 2.5 SDs or more below the young adult mean (<–2.5 SDs). For this test, –1 SD equals approximately a 10% to 12% decrease in bone density. The current guidelines by the National Osteoporosis Foundation recommend that all white women aged 65 years or older be offered a screening test.[18] In addition, patients who are younger than 65 years old but who have strong risk factors for a fracture or another condition linked to osteoporosis should also be tested. This list includes a smoking history, body weight less than 56.3 kg, history of fracture after age 50, long-term (>3 months) oral steroid therapy, and the need to use arms when rising from a chair. Because nonwhite women and men have a lower incidence of osteoporosis, the evidence for making recommendations about testing is less clear.

BMD is usually measured every 1 to 2 years during drug therapy to determine whether the patient is responding.[17] However, determining a response is not always easy. Patients may lose BMD even if they are responding to medication; they may just be losing bone at a slower rate. In addition, some women lose bone with treatment, only to regain it, even if therapy is unaltered. There is variability within the test, but this is less than 5%.

When to start therapy is also not always easy to determine. At initial screening many patients have BMD too high to require treatment, but BMD may decline rapidly, especially within 5 years of menopause.[17] After about 60 years of age, bone loss declines so that women tend to lose less than 1% of hip bone density a year, reducing the T-score 1 point over 10 years. The general recommendation is that therapy should be started when T-scores fall below –1.5 for the femoral neck. Treatment recommendations for women who do not have a fracture history and whose BMD is >–1.5 are uncertain. The Fracture Intervention Study, in which the effects of alendronate on the risk of hip and nonspine fractures were examined, demonstrated clear benefits of treatment for women with T-scores less than –2.5 but not for women with higher scores.[19]

Currently, several effective treatments for osteoporosis can slow the rate of bone resorption. The decision about which drug to administer and the duration of therapy is based on careful consideration of the risks versus the benefits and the patient's individual risk factors for fractures, coronary events, and breast cancer.

Estrogens

Until recently, estrogen had been the number one drug used to prevent osteoporosis in postmenopausal women. A recent study in the elderly indicated that 0.625 mg of estrogens per day with or without progesterone increased both spine and hip BMD, and even lower doses of estrogen (0.3 or 0.45 mg/day) also increased bone density.[20,21] In the Women's Health Initiative study discussed in the Chapter 14, there was a significant reduction in the number of hip and vertebral fractures in women receiving hormone replacement therapy (HRT) compared with placebo.[22] However, as discussed previously, estrogen therapy was found to produce an increased risk of coronary heart disease, and when combined with medroxyprogesterone, was associated with a virulent form of breast cancer. Because long-term estrogen use was what was recommended to prevent bone loss, the women who were taking it for this purpose must now consider their individual risk versus benefit ratio and decide either to continue with this approach or choose an alternate therapy.

Calcium and Vitamin D

Dietary and supplemental calcium are effective in reducing the rate of bone loss in elderly women and those with very low calcium intake.[23,24] It was initially thought that supplementation with calcium would have an early positive effect but that this effect would not last despite continued dosing. However, one study demonstrated that the positive effects of calcium were at least sustained over a 4-year period. At present, all regimens approved for the treatment and prevention of osteoporosis include supplemental calcium and vitamin D. Current recommendations include an elemental calcium intake of 1000 mg for all adults between the ages of 19 and 50 years and 1200 mg for everyone older than 50 years.[25] Calcium salts (calcium carbonate, calcium gluconate, calcium lactate, and calcium phosphate) are used for nutritional supplementation. One of the most commonly used calcium salts is calcium carbonate. However, it requires an acid medium to form a soluble compound; whereas calcium citrate, calcium gluconate, and calcium lactate are pH independent, thus resulting in greater absorption.

The minimum daily requirement for vitamin D in adults younger than 50 years is 200 IU, but this increases to 400 IU for those ages 51 to 70. For those older than 70 years old, a minimum of 600 IU is recommended. Vitamin D is recommended along with calcium because it improves calcium absorption from the gastrointestinal (GI) tract, decreases calcium renal excretion, and is responsible for bone mineralization. This combination has been especially recommended for nursing home residents who have low sunshine exposure.[26]

Supplementation with calcium and vitamin D is generally safe.[27] GI problems such as constipation and excess gas may occur. Some side effects may be lessened when supplements are taken with a meal; this also improves bioavailability because acid secretion is greatest at mealtime. Supplements should be used with caution by persons who are prone to kidney stones.

Bisphosphonates

Bisphosphonates inhibit bone resorption by reducing recruitment of osteoclasts and programming their cell death.[27] They have a strong affinity for calcium phosphate and therefore are absorbed directly into bone. The bisphosphonates have different antiresorptive potentials, with the potencies of etidronate, pamidronate, alendronate, and risedronate being 1, 100, 1000, and 5000 in order. Their oral bioavailability is very low, 1% to 3%, and is further impaired by food, calcium, iron, coffee, tea, and orange juice. They must be taken with a full glass of water, and patients must maintain an upright position for 30 minutes after intake to avoid heartburn. The safety profile is good, but clients report mild to moderate GI discomfort consisting of esophagitis, nausea, and abdominal pain.

Studies of alendronate in approximately 4000 postmenopausal women with either an existing vertebral fracture or osteoporosis, as defined by a T-score less than –2.5 at the femoral neck, but without vertebral fracture showed a significant reduction in fracture rate during a 3- to 4-year period when compared with placebo.[28,29] Other studies in which alendronate was used have also had positive outcomes. Alendronate given for 2 years to 1174 postmenopausal women younger than 60 years without osteoporosis increased BMD at the lumbar spine (3.5%) and at the hip (1.9%), and when the original study performed on patients with osteoporosis was extended, it was found that the drug was effective and well tolerated over a 10-year period.[30,31] Studies performed with risedronate have also shown positive outcomes. This drug demonstrated an increase in BMD in patients with normal and low BMD in the spine and hip.[25] Both alendronate and risedronate are available in a once-a-week formulation. This type of administration is just as effective as daily dosing but is associated with improved compliance.[32]

Selective Estrogen Receptor Modulators

Tamoxifen and raloxifene are estrogen agonists in some tissues and antagonists in other tissues. Tamoxifen has been used for the treatment of estrogen-sensitive breast cancer because it blocks estrogen receptors in breast tissue. It is a partial agonist in bone but also in the endometrium and may cause endometrial cancer. Raloxifene is a related drug that has been found to be an agonist in bone but an antagonist in both breast tissue and endometrium, which favors its use in the treatment of osteoporosis.[33]

In a double-blind, placebo-controlled, 2-year study of more than 600 postmenopausal women, raloxifene was shown to increase BMD in the lumbar spine, hip, and femoral neck.[34] Three different doses of raloxifene were administered, resulting in greater BMD with a greater dose. Concentrations of total cholesterol and low-density lipoprotein (LDL) cholesterol decreased in the treatment group, whereas these measures did not change in the placebo group. No change in endometrial thickness was detected. In terms of cardiovascular events, a 4-year study in which raloxifene was compared with placebo showed that the drug did not affect the overall risk of cardiac events but did significantly reduce the number of events in women who had cardiac risk factors at the beginning of the study.[35] In addition, raloxifene was associated with a reduction in breast cancer over a 4-year period.[36] Although these studies have positive outcomes, raloxifene is assumed to be less effective than estrogen or the bisphosphonates.[37]

Side effects of raloxifene are similar to those of estrogen and include hot flashes, leg cramps, and an increased risk of thromboembolic events.[25] Long-term studies are needed to more fully assess these side effects, as well as to look for endometrial hyperplasia.

Tibolone is an oral steroid derived from norethynodrel that is not exactly considered a selective estrogen receptor modulator. However, this drug has estrogenic, progestogenic, and weak androgenic activity. It has been used in Europe for prevention of osteoporosis but is not available in the United States.[38] Several studies show that tibolone has beneficial effects on the vasculature and cholesterol levels.[39,40] However, there is some indication that this drug may promote tumor cell growth in breast cells.[41,42]

Calcitonin

Calcitonin is a peptide produced by thyroid cells that binds to receptors on osteoclasts to inhibit their function.[25] It is approved for the treatment of but not the prevention of osteoporosis. It is available as a subcutaneous injection or a nasal spray. A tablet form is not available because when calcitonin is taken orally, much of the drug is broken down in the GI tract. A 5-year study with salmon calcitonin showed a reduction in vertebral fractures, but not in peripheral fractures.[27,43] Subcutaneous injection may produce nausea and flushing, and rhinitis is associated with the nasal preparation, but no other side effects have been reported.

Anabolic Therapies

All the osteoporotic treatments discussed previously are considered antiresorptive agents that generally work on osteoclasts to reduce bone loss. They do increase BMD, but by only a few percentage points. These treatments are not curative and if medication is stopped, bone loss resumes. However, a new class of drugs called *anabolic agents,* capable of stimulating significant increases in BMD, is under development.[44] The goal of these agents is to increase bone mass and mechanical strength over a short time to replace the bone lost. The agents currently under study include the statin drugs, PTH and related peptides, growth hormone, fluoride, and insulin-like growth factor-1. Of these agents, the statins and PTH-related peptides look most promising. Fluoride stimulates new bone formation but interferes with bone mineralization so that the new bone is not resistant to fractures. Studies of growth hormone demonstrate increases in bone mass; however, this effect is inconsistently sustained after treatment.[45-47] Insulin-like growth factor-1 stimulates the proliferation of osteoblasts, but this therapy has been associated with edema, hypotension, and tachycardia.[48,49] Further studies on all of these agents are continuing.

Native PTH (hPTH-[1-84]) is the principal regulator of serum calcium, and as discussed earlier, an increase in PTH leads to excessive bone resorption and bone loss.[48] However, there is evidence that intermittent PTH injections improve bone strength by stimulating new bone formation. The primary target with this type of administration is the osteoblast. Osteoblasts are stimulated to express genes for factors such as insulin-like growth factor-1, vascular endothelial growth factor, and transforming growth factor β, which stimulate the proliferation of osteoblast precursor cells. PTH works by increasing the number of osteoblasts and extending their lifespan. The results are an increase in size of remaining trabeculae and increased cortical thickness from bone added at the endocortical surfaces. PTH requires the first two amino acids plus parts of the remaining amino acids to activate a G-protein–linked receptor. The compounds under study resemble the native PTH in size, but smaller fragments, such as teriparatide (hPTH-[1-34]), may prove to be just as effective with minimal side effects.

Animal and human studies with hPTH-(1-84) and teriparatide have shown favorable outcomes. Many of the animal studies have used the sexually mature oophorectomized rat model required by the Food and Drug Administration (FDA) for evaluation of new therapies for osteoporosis. Oophorectomized rats experience tremendous loss of trabecular bone during the initial weeks after removal of the ovaries. Daily injections of small amounts of PTH simulate new cortical and trabecular bone in these animals.[50] PTH has also been noted to greatly increase callus volume of a fractured rat tibia by 175% over control values.[51] Similar to the animal studies, daily doses of 15 to 50 mg of PTH given to 1600 postmenopausal women significantly increased BMD at the spine and hip compared with placebo.[52] In fact, this was the study that convinced the FDA to approve teriparatide, despite some reservations regarding the development of osteosarcomas in PTH-treated rats.

Because PTH receptors are found throughout the body, it might be assumed that PTH and PTH analogs would have many side effects.[48] However, other than hypercalcemia, there have been no serious side effects. There are some reports of hypotension and tachycardia, but no fatalities; however, it should be kept in mind that patients have not been receiving PTH for more than 3 to 4 years.

Besides PTH, the other big news regarding anabolic agents for osteoporosis is the use of the statin drugs. This is an exciting development because these drugs have already been shown to offer many positive benefits. It was originally noted that the statins induced a bone protein involved in osteoblastogenesis, and when lovastatin or simvastatin was injected into the calvariae of mice, a significant increase in bone formation was seen.[44] Clinical studies support these animal studies by showing a reduction in fracture risk in postmenopausal women; however, the exact manner in which the statins get into bone remains unknown.[53,54]

Combination Therapy

Because there are several different types of drugs now available for the treatment of osteoporosis, combi-nation therapy may be an option for patients with severe osteoporosis.[55] Combinations of alendronate with HRT, and alendronate and raloxifene, have already been shown to increase BMD more than each agent independently.[56,57] Even sequential treatment with PTH and alendronate resulted in an increase in spinal bone density over each agent separately. This treatment regimen might offer the best hope for preserving the anabolic effects of PTH, particularly because the long-term effects of PTH injections are not known yet.

Therapeutic Concerns Regarding Anti-Osteoporosis Agents

In general, anti-osteoporosis agents do not have direct physical therapy concerns. The action of these drugs appears to have limited effects on physical therapy interventions. However, a few guidelines should be remembered when patients receiving these drugs are treated. First, many of these agents are administered by daily injections. Patients should be asked where their injection sites are located, and use of modalities or exercise in these areas should be avoided. For patients receiving the bisphosphonates, exercises that increase intraabdominal pressure and exercises performed in the supine position should be avoided. The reason for this is that many patients taking these drugs have esophagitis or esophageal reflux, and lying supine or increased abdominal pressure will exacerbate this condition.

DRUG TREATMENT FOR DIABETES

Diabetes is a chronic metabolic disorder characterized by hyperglycemia associated with either insulin insufficiency (type 1) or combined insulin insufficiency with insulin resistance (type 2). The incidence of diabetes in the United States alone has tripled since the late 1950s, making what was once considered only a minor disease a major threat worldwide.[58,59] The estimated number of persons with diabetes is expected to rise from the current figure of around 150 million worldwide to 220 million in 2010 and then to 300 million by 2025. Changes in the environment and lifestyle have resulted in escalating obesity, which is linked to diabetes.

Pathophysiology of Diabetes

Hyperglycemia occurs in both types of diabetes as a result of uncontrolled hepatic glucose production and reduced uptake by cells. Glycogen synthesis is also reduced. The normal response to eating a meal is that carbohydrates from food are converted to glucose, which enters the plasma. Glucose also enters the blood from the breakdown of stored glycogen in the liver, which is caused by the hormone glucagon and other hormones (Table 15-1). In response to the rise in blood sugar, the pancreas produces insulin from its beta cells, which is secreted into the bloodstream. The insulin then interacts with its receptors on cell surfaces enhancing glucose entry into the cell for fuel. Leftover glucose is converted to glycogen in the liver and muscles and stored for future use. As a result, the blood glucose level drops, reducing the need for insulin.

Type 1 diabetes is considered an autoimmune disease in which the body produces antibodies that attack the beta cells.[60] Patients with type 1 diabetes tend to be young (children or adolescents) and not obese. There is a strong inherited predisposition, and associations with some specific histocompatibility antigens exist, but it is believed that exposure to a virus is the precipitating event. Initially, the ability of the beta cells to produce insulin is just impaired, but as time goes on (usually less than a year), the pancreas ceases to produce the hormone. In response

to a meal, because little or no insulin is being produced, the blood sugar level rises. The pancreas tries to compensate by producing more insulin, but eventually it cannot keep up with demand.

In type 2 diabetes, insulin is plentiful, at least in the beginning of the illness, but resistance to the hormone is present. The liver and muscles become less sensitive to the action of insulin. Sensing an elevated blood glucose level, the pancreas attempts to increase production of insulin, but eventually the pancreas "burns out." At that point the patient with type 2 diabetes will need supplemental insulin. Unlike type 1 diabetes, this form of the disease is associated with obesity.[61] Obesity itself can cause some degree of insulin resistance. Patients who are not considered obese may have an increased percentage of body fat distributed in the abdominal area. Type 2 diabetes usually develops during adult life, although the growing number of children with this disease is emerging as a major public health problem.[58]

Heredity also plays a role in type 2 diabetes.[62] A polygenic basis for type 2 diabetes has been discussed because many patients with this disease have a relative with diabetes. It has also been shown that nondiabetic first-degree relatives of diabetic

Table 15-1

Effect of Hormones on Blood Glucose Levels			
Hormone	Main Actions	Main Stimulus for Secretion	Main Effect
MAIN REGULATORY HORMONE			
Insulin	↑ Glucose uptake ↑ Glycogen synthesis ↓ Glycogenolysis ↓ Gluconeogenesis	Acute rise in blood glucose	↓ Blood glucose
MAIN COUNTERREGULATORY HORMONES			
Glucagon	↑ Glycogenolysis ↑ Gluconeogenesis	Hypoglycemia (i.e., blood glucose <3 mmol/L), e.g., with exercise, stress, high-protein meals, etc.	↓ Blood glucose
Adrenaline	↑ Glycogenolysis ↓ Glucose uptake		
Glucocorticosteroids	↑ Gluconeogenesis ↓ Glucose uptake and utilization		
Growth hormone	↓ Glucose uptake		

From Rang HP, Dale MM, Ritter JM, Moore JL. *Pharmacology*. 5th ed. New York: Churchill Livingstone; 2003.

patients are insulin resistant. Parental history of hypertension and diabetes has also been associated with diabetic nephropathy in offspring with type 1 diabetes.[63]

Other specific types and causes of diabetes have been identified.[61] Genetic defects may be present in the beta cell. In fact, this is associated with the onset of hyperglycemia before the age of 25 years and is referred to as maturity-onset diabetes of the young. It is characterized by impaired insulin secretion but with minimal or no insulin resistance. Some genetic defects prevent the conversion of proinsulin to insulin, resulting in mild glucose intolerance, as well as defects that alter the structure of the insulin receptor. Acquired processes are also involved in the development of diabetes. Any injury to the pancreas caused by infection, carcinoma, or trauma and endocrinopathies such as acromegaly, Cushing's syndrome, pheochromocytoma, and glucagonomas can also produce diabetes. Several drugs, such as steroids, thiazide diuretics, and protease inhibitors (used for the treatment of AIDS), raise the blood glucose level and trigger diabetes in susceptible patients. Gestational diabetes mellitus is an acquired glucose intolerance seen during pregnancy. This may disappear after delivery but can also predict future problems of impaired glucose tolerance.

The terms *impaired glucose tolerance* and *impaired fasting glucose* refer to a metabolic state intermediate between normal carbohydrate metabolism and diabetes. These are not considered clinical entities by themselves but are risk factors for the development of diabetes and cardiac disease. Both are associated with insulin resistance syndrome (formerly known as syndrome X or the metabolic syndrome). Insulin resistance syndrome includes decreased sensitivity to insulin, compensatory hyperinsulinemia, abdominal obesity, dyslipidemia (high triglyceride and/or low high-density lipoprotein [HDL] cholesterol levels) and hypertension.[64] A body mass index greater than 25, family history of type 2 diabetes, gestational diabetes, and polycystic ovary syndrome are associated with this disorder.

Symptoms of Diabetes

The initial symptoms of diabetes are related to hyperglycemia.[59] Diabetic ketoacidosis may appear suddenly in type 1 disease when there is nearly a complete absence of insulin and the body is forced to utilize other sources for energy. In an effort to produce fuel, fatty acids are released from adipose tissue and broken down in the liver into ketone bodies. These strong acids accumulate in the blood, leading to metabolic acidosis. In addition, the excess blood glucose is filtered through the kidney glomerulus, taking with it large quantities of water, causing polyuria and severe dehydration. Other symptoms of ketoacidosis include a fruity breath, nausea, slowing respirations, changes in mental state, and finally a collapse of the cardiovascular system.

In contrast to type 1 diabetes, type 2 diabetes may develop very slowly, so that some patients may not notice symptoms for years. The classic symptoms include polyuria, polydipsia, weight loss despite increased food intake, and weakness. Other symptoms may occur including blurred vision caused by changing levels of glucose in the eye, recurrent vaginal yeast infections, and frequent skin infections.

Long-term complications are also common with this disease, especially if a patient has had difficulty controlling his or her glucose level. Several prospective studies have demonstrated greater degrees of microvascular and macrovascular disease with long-term poor control of glucose level.[65-67] Retinopathy, nephropathy, neuropathy, autonomic neuropathy, glaucoma, cataracts, skin infections, coronary heart disease, stroke, and peripheral vascular disease are more likely to occur when glycemic control is not maintained. Advanced glycation end products have been implicated in the development of dysfunction of the vascular endothelium. These are nonenzymatic products of glucose and albumin. Oxygen-derived free radicals and increased activation of the diacylglycerol–protein kinase C signal transduction pathway have also been identified in diabetic animals.[68] Protein kinase C activation leads to deposition of extracellular matrix, resulting in a thickening of the capillary basement membrane. This change is associated with increased vascular permeability, impaired regulation of vascular tone, endothelial cell proliferation, and microaneurysm formation, leading to many of the ischemic events seen in diabetes. Specific diacylglycerol–protein kinase C pathway inhibitors are being explored as adjunct treatments for diabetes.

Diagnostic Testing for Diabetes

In an effort to promote early detection, the American Diabetes Association recommends that persons age

45 and older be tested for diabetes every 3 years.[61] However, the presence of symptoms or risk factors for diabetes should prompt earlier testing. These risk factors include having a first-degree relative with diabetes, being in a high-risk ethnic group (black, Hispanic, or Native American), obesity, previous gestational diabetes, hypertension, a high triglyceride level, and a low HDL cholesterol level.[69]

A diagnosis of diabetes can be made in three ways, but any positive result needs to be followed up with another test on a subsequent day.[61] A diagnosis of diabetes can be made when the blood glucose level climbs above 200 mg/dL in a blood sample obtained at any time of the day and under any circumstances, along with the classic symptoms of thirst, frequent urination, and weight loss. A diagnosis can also be made with a fasting blood glucose (FBG) test or an oral glucose tolerance test. The FBG test requires that the patient abstain from eating or drinking for 12 hours before a blood sample is obtained. A normal FBG test result is less than 100 mg/dL. A positive result for the disease is an FBG value greater than or equal to 126 mg/dL. FBG values between 100 and 125 mg/dL indicate impaired glucose tolerance and identify patients who may need counseling regarding diet and exercise and also those who must be regularly screened in the future.[70,71] The oral glucose tolerance test is performed by having the patient drink a solution containing 75 g of glucose, followed by sampling the blood every half hour for 2 hours. Glucose levels of 140 mg/dL and lower obtained at 2 hours after glucose administration are considered normal. Impaired glucose tolerance is defined by a level between 140 and 200 mg/dL 2 hours after administration, and any value of 200 mg/dL or greater is considered positive for diabetes.

The normal and diagnostic values cited previously are the updated values recently adopted by the American Diabetes Association.[61] This diagnostic "cut point" for diabetes and impaired glucose tolerance results from collection of clinical and epidemiological data that correlate glucose levels with the onset of microvascular and macrovascular disease, indicating that measurements above these values are associated with a significant increase in morbidity.

Another test called *the hemoglobin A_{1c} (HbA$_{1c}$) test*, also known as the glycohemoglobin or the glycated hemoglobin test, is not used for diagnostic purposes but is used to assess blood glucose control over the previous 3 months in persons known to have the disease.[61] The test is based on the fact that some glucose absorbed from the intestine attaches to hemoglobin and remains there for the life of the red blood cell, which is approximately 120 days. This combination of glucose and hemoglobin is called *glycosylated hemoglobin*. When glucose levels are consistently high, the amount of glycosylated hemoglobin increases. A normal HbA$_{1c}$ value in persons without the disease is between 4% and 6%. The American Diabetes Association recommends an HbA$_{1c}$ value under 7% for people with diabetes. This test is given twice a year to people who successfully manage their glucose level and is recommended every 3 months for those patients who have inconsistent levels or for those who might not be as interested in managing their blood glucose level as they should be.

Other laboratory tests important to perform for patients with diabetes include tests of blood urea nitrogen, blood creatinine, and protein (albumin) in the urine, which provide useful data for evaluating kidney damage. Measurements of triglyceride, total, LDL, and HDL cholesterol levels are also needed on a regular basis to assess for cardiac risk factors.

Self-Monitoring of Blood Glucose Level

Self-monitoring of blood glucose level is essential for patients with diabetes. Regular measurement and keeping a log of the values, food intake, and activity level are recommended. Not only is monitoring useful for indicating when a patient needs to be more aggressive in management, it also allows the patient to make rapid changes in diet, medication, or activity level to keep glucose levels within an acceptable range. High or low levels at the same time of the day suggest the need for a medication change. Although unexpected alterations in glucose readings may simply be traced to eating an unusually large or small amount of food, they may also be caused by variation in activity level or even psychological stress that the patient might be experiencing on a particular day. The log is helpful for identifying these anomalies. Patients are encouraged to check glucose levels frequently; before meals, 2 hours after meals, and before bedtime. Optimal blood glucose control is a preprandial level and a bedtime glucose level between 70 and 90 mg/dL.[72] Glucose monitoring requires only a single drop of blood, which can be withdrawn by a lancet or by the meter itself from a fingertip. The blood is placed on a reagent strip containing an enzyme called *glucose oxidase*. The strip is inserted into a meter, which provides a digital readout of the blood glucose level.

Many different types of monitors with variable features are available. Factors to consider when choosing a monitor include how large the numbers are on the readout, how difficult the meter is to use, and whether it has memory features that could make record keeping easy. Some models can download meter results to a computer and print out summaries. The type of test strips required by the monitor should also be considered. These strips have a shelf life and therefore are packaged either in a vial or individually wrapped in foil. A patient with arthritis might have difficulty opening the individually wrapped strips. Some monitors have a roll of test strips inserted inside so the patient does not have to handle them directly. Elderly patients should be informed that Medicare pays for meters and testing supplies.

In the past few years, the FDA has approved several new methods for testing glucose levels.[73] The Freestyle blood glucose monitoring system (TheraSense, Alameda, Calif), the One Touch FastTake system (LifeScan, Milpitas, Calif), and the Sof-Tac Diabetes Management System (Abbott Laboratories, MediSense Products, Bedford, Mass) all allow blood to be drawn from the forearm, which is less sensitive than the fingertip. Studies have shown that blood glucose measurements obtained from the arm with the automated devices are just as accurate as those obtained from finger sticking. The Sof-Tac device, in particular, is easy to use as well, combining lancing the skin and transferring of blood to the test strip. The patient places the device on either the forearm or upper arm. When the device is engaged, it creates a vacuum seal against the skin, releasing the lancet and drawing blood onto the strip. Strips can be loaded up to 8 hours before testing. Blood glucose results are provided in 40 seconds from the time the device is engaged.

The GlucoWatch Biographer (Cygnus, Inc., Redwood City, Calif) represents another innovation in testing.[74] This is an automatic, noninvasive glucose monitoring device. It is worn on the wrist like a watch and consists of a disposable single-use electrochemical sensor that contains two glucose

oxidase–containing gel disks and two electrodes. A small electric current is emitted through the skin, which by means of reverse iontophoresis, measures glucose-containing interstitial fluid from adjacent cells. Glucose measurements may be obtained as often as once every 20 minutes within a 12-hour period. Each reading is the average of two 10-minute periods and lags behind blood glucose readings because of processing and the 5-minute delay between blood and tissue sugar levels. This device demonstrates good correlation with the glucose measurements obtained from fingerstick methods, but the manufacturer states that it is not meant to replace regular blood monitoring. However, it is not accurate in low ranges of blood glucose and may cause persisting edema and redness of the skin under the device. Another problem is that it must be recalibrated with the fingerstick readings every 12 hours before use. Nevertheless, this device represents a crucial step in improving blood glucose monitoring technology.

Insulin and the Other Pancreatic Islet Hormones

The pancreatic islets of Langerhans contain at least three main types of cells: beta cells that secrete insulin, alpha cells that secrete glucagon, and delta cells that secrete somatostatin.[75] Each islet contains mainly the beta cells surrounded by the alpha cells interspersed with delta cells.

The main action of insulin is to preserve energy stores by stimulating the uptake and storage of glucose, amino acids, and fats after a meal. It responds quickly to reduce the blood glucose level by acting on the liver, muscle, and fat. In the liver, insulin inhibits glycogenolysis (glycogen breakdown) and gluconeogenesis (synthesis of glucose from amino acids) while enhancing glycogen synthesis and increasing glucose utilization (Table 15-2). In addition, insulin stimulates carrier-mediated transport of glucose into several tissues. These carriers are called *glut carriers* and range in number from 1 to 5. Glut 4 carriers are responsible for glucose entry into muscle and adipose tissue (Figure 15-1). In adipose tissue, insulin enhances glucose metabolism, resulting in the formation of glycerol, a precursor to triglycerides, and also inhibits lipolysis. In terms of insulin's effect on protein metabolism, it stimulates the uptake of amino acids into muscle and increases protein synthesis.

Table 15-2

Summary of the Effects of Insulin on Carbohydrate, Fat, and Protein Metabolism in Liver, Muscle, and Adipose Tissue

Type of Metabolism	Liver Cells	Fat Cell	Muscle
Carbohydrate metabolism	↑↓ Gluconeogenesis ↓ Glycogenolysis ↑ Glycolysis ↑ Glycogenesis	↑ Glucose uptake ↑ Glycerol synthesis	↑ Glucose uptake ↑ Glycolysis ↑ Glycogenesis
Fat metabolism	↑ Lipogenesis ↓ Lipolysis	↑ Synthesis of triglycerides ↑ Fatty acid synthesis ↓ Lipolysis	—
Protein metabolism	↓ Protein breakdown	—	↑ Amino acid uptake ↑ Protein synthesis

From Rang HP, Dale MM, Ritter JM, Moore JL. *Pharmacology.* 5th ed. New York: Churchill Livingstone; 2003.

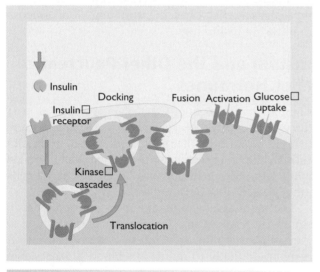

Figure 15-1

Intracellular kinase cascades cause translocation of glucose transporters from an endosomal compartment to the plasma membrane where they increase glucose uptake. (From Page C, Curtis AB, Sutter MC, Walker L, Hoffman BB, eds. *Integrated Pharmacology.* Philadelphia: Mosby; 2002.)

Insulin is initially synthesized as one long peptide chain called *preproinsulin* in the rough endoplasmic reticulum. Preproinsulin is then transported to the Golgi apparatus where it is cleaved into a smaller peptide called *proinsulin* and then finally to insulin and a fragment called *C-peptide*. The exact function of the C-peptide is unknown, but it is stored in granules in the beta cells along with insulin and released by exocytosis in equimolar amounts. Some proinsulin may be released as well.

Beta cells respond to an absolute glucose concentration in the blood and also to a change in concentration. Glucose enters the beta cell via a Glut 2 transporter. There it undergoes metabolism, producing intracellular adenosine triphosphate (ATP). This ATP blocks a specialized ion channel called *an ATP-sensitive potassium (K+) channel* (Figure 15-2). The channel closes, blocking the outflow of K+ ions from the cell and producing a membrane depolarization. The positive change in membrane potential opens the voltage-gated calcium channels, leading to calcium (Ca^{2+}) influx. Calcium entry triggers exocytosis and insulin release.

The beta cell responds to glucose in two phases, an initial rapid secretion of insulin, followed by a slower delayed release.[76] In addition, a low-level basal release of insulin occurs (Figure 15-3). Many factors other than just glucose control the release of insulin. The GI hormones (e.g., gastrin, secretin, cholecystokinin) trigger the release of insulin. These hormones are released by both the visual and physical activity of eating and explain why there is a greater release of insulin in response to food than when the same amount of glucose is given intravenously. Other stimuli for insulin release include amino acids, fatty acids, and the parasympathetic nervous system (Figure 15-4). The sympathetic system exerts an inhibitory effect on insulin release.

Once released, insulin binds to a specialized

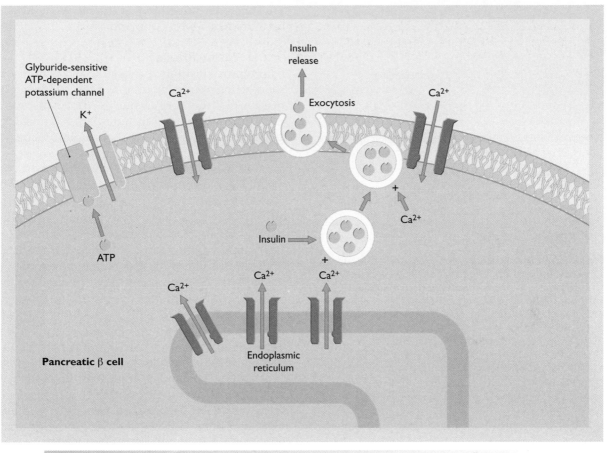

Figure 15-2

Insulin secretion. Insulin release from pancreatic beta cells is stimulated by the release of calcium (Ca^{2+}) from the endoplasmic compartment by voltage-sensitive channels and by influx of extracellular Ca^{2+}. The adenosine triphosphate (ATP)–dependent potassium (K^+) channel on the plasma membrane maintains the intracellular resting potential. Inhibition of this K^+ channel by sulfonylurea or meglitinide agents results in depolarization and activation of Ca^{2+} channels, resulting in enhanced insulin secretion. (From Page C, Curtis AB, Sutter MC, Walker L, Hoffman BB, eds. *Integrated Pharmacology.* Philadelphia: Mosby; 2002.)

membrane-bound receptor linked to a tyrosine kinase (Figure 15-5). This is a large receptor consisting of two α- and two β-subunits. The α-subunits are extracellular, and each contains an insulin-binding site. The β-subunits exist in both outside and inside cells and have tyrosine kinase activity. Tyrosine kinase activity allows autophosphorylation of the receptor, leading to a signal cascade that ultimately turns on several genes involved in cell growth and metabolism. The development of insulin resistance is thought to be related to the loss of this tyrosine kinase activity.

Glucagon acts as the opposite to insulin, increasing the blood glucose level and stimulating protein and fat breakdown.[76] Its secretion is stimulated by low levels of glucose and fatty acids in the plasma and a high-protein meal but is inhibited by high levels of glucose and fats. Sympathetic nerve activity and circulating epinephrine also stimulates glucagon release. Essentially, this hormone guarantees available plasma glucose to fuel the brain and muscles for activity. Glucagon stimulates glycogen breakdown and gluconeogenesis.

Somatostatin opposes the action of both insulin and glucagon because it inhibits their secretion.[76] It is widely found outside the pancreas, secreted by the hypothalamus, which then inhibits the release of growth hormone from the anterior pituitary.

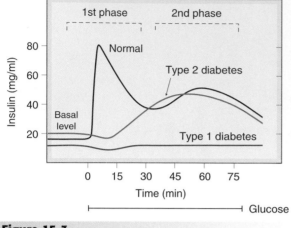

Figure 15-3

Schematic diagram of the two-phase release of insulin in response to constant glucose infusion. The first phase is missing in type 2 (non-insulin-dependent) diabetes mellitus, and both phases are missing in type 1 (insulin-dependent) diabetes mellitus. The first phase is also produced by amino acids, sulfonylureas, glucagons, and gastrointestinal tract. hormones. (Data from Pfeifer et al. *Am J Med.* 1981;70:579-588.) (From Rang HP, Dale MM, Ritter JM, Moore JL. *Pharmacology.* 5th ed. New York: Churchill Livingstone; 2003.)

Hence, this hormone lowers the blood glucose level by several mechanisms.

Insulin Treatment

All insulins were originally isolated from beef or pork pancreases until 1982 when genetically engineered human insulin became available.[77] This innovation has led to a number of insulin analogs that have improved pharmacokinetic properties; however, replacement of physiological insulin and return of glycemic control remain difficult goals to achieve.

The goal of insulin therapy is to match plasma insulin level to food intake and exercise.[77] In healthy individuals, the concentration of glucose in the plasma remains within a narrow range throughout the day, despite the amount of food consumed and activity level. After eating, the glucose level rises to a peak in 30 to 60 minutes and then returns to baseline concentrations within 2 to 3 hours. The lowest glucose level exists around 2:00 to 3:00 AM in the morning, but basal secretion rises again before breakfast, probably in response to growth hormone secretion. Insulin must be secreted or provided in appropriate amounts to match this level of glucose.

This includes meal-related secretion, a low-level basal release, and the morning rise.

Insulin Formulations

Four types of insulin are available: ultra-short-acting, short-acting or regular, intermediate, and long-acting insulin. Ultra-short-acting insulins (lispro and aspart) can be taken 5 minutes before a meal, peak at 1 hour, and have a duration of 3 to 5 hours.[78-80] An ultra-short-acting insulin acts more rapidly but for a shorter time than regular insulin. Regular insulin has an onset of action within 30 minutes, peaks in about 2 hours, and has a duration of action of 6 to 8 hours.[81] Regular insulin has no additives to delay absorption. The ultra-short-acting insulins offer slightly better control of the postprandial rise in the glucose level, but there may be a more rapid onset of hypoglycemia and less time for symptom recognition. In addition, the use of the ultra-short-acting agents alters the glucose monitoring schedule. It is customary for the patient to measure the pre-meal glucose levels to determine the amount of regular insulin needed.[72] However, if the patient uses lispro or aspart at noon with the anticipation that the next dose will be at 6:00 PM before dinner, the pre-dinner glucose measurement would be inaccurate. This is because the rapid-acting analogs might only be effective for 4 hours compared with the 6 hours for regular insulin. By dinner time, the pre-meal glucose levels will be quite high, and the patient will then have the tendency to increase the next insulin dose, possibly triggering a hypoglycemic event.

Intermediate-acting insulin has a more gradual onset. It begins working after about 1 to 4 hours, and peak action occurs after about 6 to 12 hours. Effects may continue for 14 to 24 hours. A cationic protein, protamine (neutral protamine Hagedorn or NPH, is added to regular insulin zinc suspensions to slow absorption. The intermediate-acting insulins have the advantage of longer duration but also slower onset than the short-acting agents.

Long-acting insulin (Ultralente) contains zinc and a buffer to delay absorption, postponing onset for 4 to 6 hours with duration lasting up to 36 hours. Ultralente peaks between 8 and 20 hours. Insulin glargine is a new long-acting insulin that has recently been approved.[82] The mean onset of action is within 1 hour of injection, but the duration of action is similar to that of Ultralente. It has no peak and instead mimics continuous infusion of rapid-acting

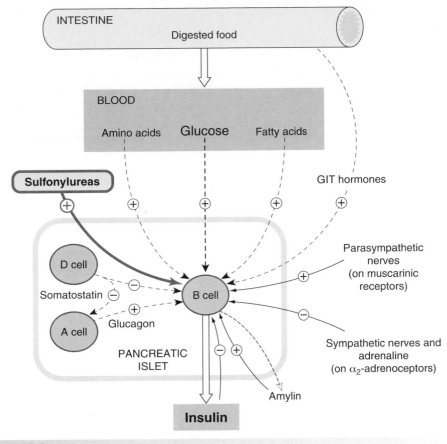

Figure 15-4

Factors regulating insulin secretion. Blood glucose is the most important factor. Drugs used to stimulate insulin secretion are shown in boxes. Glucagon potentiates insulin release but opposes some of its peripheral actions and increases blood glucose. *GIT*, Gastrointestinal tract. (From Rang HP, Dale MM, Ritter JM, Moore JL. *Pharmacology.* 5th ed. New York: Churchill Livingstone; 2003.)

regular insulin from a subcutaneous pump. Long-acting insulins are intended to provide adequate basal insulin concentrations in a single daily dose.[77]

All insulins are available in concentrations of 100 units/mL.[81] There is one regular insulin formulation available in a 20-mL vial containing 500 units/mL for patients who require more than 200 units/day. Regular and ultra-short-acting insulins can be combined in the same syringe with intermediate-acting insulin and Ultralente but not with glargine (another long-acting insulin) because glargine will delay the absorption of the shorter-acting agent.[83] Patients can check the appearance of an insulin to help identify it. Regular and ultra-short-acting insulins and glargine are clear; the other insulins appear cloudy. Premixed insulins are available containing 70% NPH and 30% regular,

70% insulin aspart protamine and 30% aspart, or 75% insulin lispro protamine and 25% lispro.

Unopened insulin products may be kept at room temperature, but once the stopper or seal has been punctured, the insulin is considered to be "in use."[81] In-use insulin vials can be kept at room temperature for up to 28 days. However, it has been recommended that in-use measured syringes containing mixtures of insulins be stored in the refrigerator. Any unused insulin must be discarded if it freezes. Insulin travel packs are also available.

Insulin Regimens for Type 1 Diabetes
Combinations of insulin types are used to control glucose.[76,84] This strategy of mixing types is known as the "basal/bolus regimen."[85] Low levels of insulin are required from bedtime until early morning, and

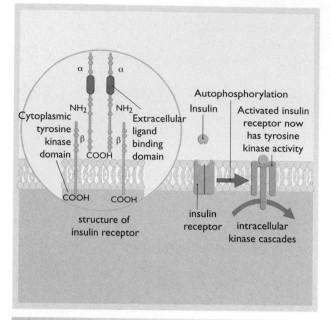

Figure 15-5

Insulin action. The insulin receptor is a heterodimeric transmembrane receptor consisting of two α and two β subunits. The intracellular portions of the β subunits contain tyrosine kinase activity. Insulin receptor stimulation leads to phosphorylation of multiple intracellular signaling molecules. Phosphorylation of tyrosine kinase residues on intracellular kinases leads to activation of serine/threonine kinase cascades. (From Page C, Curtis AB, Sutter MC, Walker L, Hoffman BB, eds. *Integrated Pharmacology*. Philadelphia: Mosby; 2002.)

higher levels are required during the daytime hours with significant increases at meal times. One regimen is called *split and mixed* and consists of a mixture of rapid-onset insulin (regular or ultra-short-acting) with intermediate or Ultralente insulin given before breakfast and a second injection given before supper (Figure 15-6). The supper dose of the NPH may be adjusted to achieve euglycemia before breakfast the next morning without producing hypoglycemia in the middle of the night. When the desired fasting morning level of glucose is achieved, the morning dose of the intermediate-acting insulin may be adjusted to attain euglycemia before supper. This regimen requires two injections per day. A disadvantage to this regimen is that there might not be enough active insulin available to cover lunch. Also, nocturnal hypoglycemia may occur around midnight, especially if the patient did not eat a snack after dinner. In addition, and perhaps more

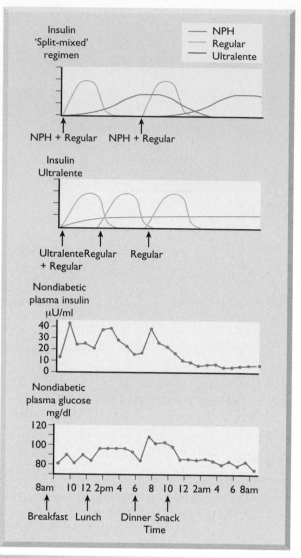

Figure 15-6

Insulin therapy. Exogenously administered insulin does not mirror the rapid meal-related increases of pancreatic insulin secretion as a result of delayed absorption from the site of injection. The goal of insulin dosing regimens is to coordinate peaks in insulin delivery with meal times. Systemic insulin levels are higher during insulin therapy of type 1 diabetes mellitus than with endogenous pancreatic regulation. Pancreatic insulin release into the portal venous system may suppress hepatic gluconeogenesis at lower doses than those needed with systemic insulin administration. (From Page C, Curtis AB, Sutter MC, Walker L, Hoffman BB, eds. *Integrated Pharmacology*. Philadelphia: Mosby; 2002.)

important, patients rarely achieve adequate control with this program.[85]

For the purpose of improving nighttime control, the second intermediate-acting insulin can be held until bedtime (9:00 PM). This regimen is called *split and mixed with bedtime intermediate*. Three injections are required: one at breakfast consisting of regular or ultra-short-acting insulin mixed with NPH, short-acting insulin at dinner, and an injection of intermediate-acting insulin before bed. Nocturnal hypoglycemia is delayed, instead corresponding to the early morning hyperglycemia.

The "multiple dosing" regimen includes preprandial regular insulin and bedtime intermediate insulin for a total of four injections. This system covers each meal, as well as the slow climb toward hyperglycemia in the 5:00 to 8:00 AM period. The longer-acting insulins (Ultralente and glargine) may be substituted for the intermediate-acting insulin at bedtime, depending on the patient's caloric intake and activity level.[86] This regimen offers the most flexibility in terms of meal size and timing in that each meal is covered with regular insulin and the longer-acting agents cover the basal insulin release during the night. However, any large depot of insulin can easily lead to hypoglycemia (see the following section).

Dosing Guidelines

Insulin doses are expressed in units instead of milliliters. The injection is standardized so each milliliter contains 100 *United States Pharmacopeia (USP)* units. For the initial insulin dose, most patients are started with an average dose of intermediate-acting insulin. This dose may range from 10 to 30 units per day. The obese patient may require a greater amount. The dose is then adjusted to meet the patient's diet and activity level. Patients are asked to coordinate increases in dose with their fasting plasma glucose test. A fasting plasma glucose value of 120 to 140 requires an increase of 4 U/day and 140 to 180 requires an increase of 6 U/day. If the fasting plasma glucose value is over 180, the dose is adjusted by 8 U/day. Insulin level is increased weekly as long as there are no severe hypoglycemic events (plasma glucose <72 mg/dL).

After dosing with the intermediate- or long-acting insulins, the meal-related dose must be configured. Short-acting insulins administered with each meal should achieve a peak postprandial blood glucose level of less than 160 mg/dL (Table 15-3).[72] Blood

Table 15-3

Ideal and Acceptable Blood Glucose Levels at Various Times of the Day		
	Ideal	Acceptable for Diabetics
Preprandial	70-90 mg/dL	91-120 mg/dL
Postprandial (peak)	70-135 mg/dL	136-160 mg/dL
Bedtime	70-90 mg/dL	110-135 mg/dL
2:00-4:00 AM	70-105 mg/dL	70-130 mg/dL

glucose at bedtime should be between 110 and 135 mg/dL. Patients are encouraged to check glucose levels frequently, especially after a change in regimen, and also around 2:00 AM to check for hypoglycemia. Nightmares may be a signal that the patient is hypoglycemic during sleep.

Insulin Regimens for Type 2 Diabetes

Insulin is also a very important adjunct in the treatment of type 2 disease when glycemic control can no longer be achieved with a combination of oral hypoglycemic agents, diet, and exercise. More than a third of all patients with type 2 diabetes will require treatment with insulin.[59] Therefore early insulin replacement in type 2 diabetes is becoming a new strategy for development of optimal metabolic control. It is believed that this strategy improves insulin sensitivity by reducing "glucotoxicity" and may reduce cardiovascular risk.[85]

In general, patients with type 2 diabetes begin therapy with an oral insulin sensitizer or insulin secretagogue (see discussion of oral hypoglycemic agents).[85] As insulin resistance develops, the patient begins receiving an evening basal insulin replacement in addition to the oral agents. This requires only one daily injection without the need to mix different preparations. Insulin-naïve patients start with an average dose of 15 U of glargine at night and then make adjustments according to the FBG test result the next morning. If patients are switching to glargine from once-daily NPH or Ultralente, the initial dose remains the same. However, if they are switching from twice-daily NPH, the initial dose of glargine must be reduced by 20%. Comparison studies of NPH insulin and glargine at bedtime showed equivalent glycemic control and similar weight gain. However, patients who took glargine had less symptomatic hypoglycemia and better control glycemic control in the late afternoon.[87]

Adverse Effects of Insulin

The main adverse effect of insulin is hypoglycemia, which may occur as a result of a delayed or missed meal, excess insulin, decreased carbohydrate content of a meal, increased insulin absorption rates, or exercising without first eating a snack.[83] Symptoms include sweating, tachycardia, nervousness, headache, faintness, weakness, and numbness in the fingers and around the mouth. These responses occur as a result of epinephrine release and are considered to provide a warning for the patient to eat something with sugar, usually fruit juice (4 to 6 oz) or hard candy (5 to 7 pieces).[59] Glucose tablets are also available. Other signs include double vision, confusion, and finally seizures, coma, and death. Once the confusion begins, the patient may not be able to seek either food or help.

Patients using insulin should carry at least 15 g of carbohydrate to be administered orally in the event of a hypoglycemic event.[83] The glucose level can be stabilized in about 15 minutes with 10 to 15 g of carbohydrate in cases of mild hypoglycemia. Family members and friends should receive instruction on how to use glucagon in cases in which the patient cannot be given sugar orally. Quick fixes that can be administered by the patient include 4 oz of orange juice, 6 oz of regular soda, 6 to 8 oz of 2% or skim milk, three graham crackers, six jelly beans, and 2 tablespoons of raisins.[88] Patients who take β-blockers or who have had nerve damage from their diabetes may not be able to recognize the signs of hypoglycemia and must be quite vigilant about measuring their glucose levels.

Other side effects of insulin include lipoatrophy, a benign condition in which a loss of subcutaneous fat occurs at the injection site; lipohypertrophy; local injection site reactions; and the Somogyi effect or rebound hyperglycemia.[59] The Somogyi effect can occur 6 to 12 hours after periods of hypoglycemia.

Delivery of Insulin

Insulin must be injected to be effective because it is destroyed by digestive enzymes if taken orally. It is usually injected subcutaneously in several different places: the abdomen (except for 2 inches around the navel), the front and outer side of the thigh, the upper part of the buttocks, and the outer side of the

upper arm.[59] Injection locations need to be varied to prevent inflammation and lipodystrophy. Injections of at least two finger widths apart are recommended, and no injection site should be used more than once in a month. Absorption is most rapid when insulin is injected into the abdomen; it occurs more slowly when injected in the arms and even more slowly when injected in the thigh or buttocks. The exception is when a patient is exercising or receiving a massage.[89] Absorption under these circumstances will be greatly increased. In fact, exercise and massage are contraindicated in the area of injection for the length of the time that the drug is expected to be active. Injections in the abdomen are frequently used during the day, and the thigh and buttock locations are used in the evening so that insulin will persist longer in the circulation during the night.

Insulin is usually injected with a syringe specially calibrated for insulin and ultrafine needles.[59] Insulin pens combine an insulin container and syringe in one device. The cartridges come prefilled, and the patient simply dials in the dose. Some are reusable and others are disposable. In a study in which patient preferences were compared, the prefilled, disposable pen was clearly preferred over the vial and syringe setup.[90] Jet injectors use a high-pressure jet of air to send a stream of insulin through the skin, eliminating the use of a needle. External insulin pumps that provide continuous insulin infusion and supplemental regular insulin for mealtime are also available. These pumps offer excellent control with programs that are easily adjusted.

Two new methods for delivery of insulin are currently being investigated and refined. These include inhaled insulin and continuous subcutaneous insulin infusion. Inhalation of insulin is performed in a manner similar to the method used by people with asthma.[91] The insulin comes in a dry powder form dispersed by aerosol into particles. The patient inhales the dry powder through the mouth into the lungs, which then enters the bloodstream. The current inhaler is about the size of a flashlight and dispenses regular insulin. Studies have been performed with patients who have type 2 disease who also take oral hypoglycemic agents. Specifically, two small studies (one with 26 patients and the other with 68 patients) demonstrated improved glycemic control when inhaled insulin was given at pre-meal times. These studies were performed with individuals whose diabetes could not be controlled with the oral hypoglycemic agents alone. When inhaled insulin was added to the regimen of oral drugs, patients experienced significant reductions in glycosylated hemoglobin values, fasting plasma glucose levels, and postprandial glucose increases compared with the patients receiving only the oral drugs.[92] In addition, there was a marked reduction in fasting triglyceride levels. Negative aspects of inhaled insulin included weight gain and a much greater incidence of hypoglycemia, although all events but one were classified as mild to moderate. Only one event resulted in severe hypoglycemia, when third-party assistance was needed to provide a glucose source.

Continuous subcutaneous insulin infusion with external pumps is another alternative to multiple daily injections. These pumps provide continuous insulin infusion with supplemental regular insulin for mealtime. Doses can be adjusted fairly easily, allowing total flexibility with meals and snacks. A study in which multiple injections with the pen injector (NovoPen) were compared with subcutaneous continued infusion in patients type 2 diabetes demonstrated similar glycemic control but significant improvement in satisfaction scores for the subjects who used the pump.[93] The safety profile was also similar between the groups in terms of hypoglycemic events, but a few users of the pump had to struggle with clogs and blockages. Similar results were seen in a study in which continuous insulin infusion was compared with multiple daily injections in children with type 1 diabetes.[94]

Oral Hypoglycemic Agents and Treatment of Type 2 Diabetes

Oral hypoglycemic drugs are used by patients with type 2 disease who do not require insulin to prevent ketoacidosis, although insulin is often added as resistance increases. These drugs act to increase insulin secretion or to improve the sensitivity of tissues to insulin. They are classified according to whether they increase insulin secretion, improve insulin sensitivity, or block glucose uptake.

Biguanides (Metformin)

Metformin is one of the most commonly used antidiabetic agents. It will reduce gluconeogenesis in the liver and improve glucose utilization in skeletal muscle, thereby reducing insulin resistance.[95,96] It does not stimulate insulin secretion, lowering the risk of hypoglycemia. It is often used as a first-line oral agent or in combination with a sulfonylurea (see discussion on sulfonylureas). In addition, this drug lowers cholesterol and triglyceride levels and may even help the patient lose weight.[97] Adverse effects include transient nausea and diarrhea. Lactic acidosis is a rare complication. This drug is usually administered twice daily, with breakfast and then again with dinner.

Sulfonylureas

These agents block the ATP-sensitive K^+ channel in the beta cells of the pancreas.[98] This action depolarizes the cell and ultimately produces release of insulin. Examples include tolbutamide, glipizide, glimepiride, and glyburide.[99,100] They all have similar chemical structures and modes of action, so if a patient loses responsiveness to one sulfonylurea, he or she should be switched to a drug in another classification. Tolbutamide was the first sulfonylurea available and thus has been given the relative potency number of 1. Glipizide is considered a second-generation sulfonylurea and has a relative potency number of 100 relative to tolbutamide.[60] The most common side effect is hypoglycemia, which is more likely to occur in elderly malnourished patients or those with liver abnormalities. Alcohol, skipped meals, and exercise might trigger hypoglycemia with these drugs.[101] However, there is a concern regarding cardiac protection with glyburide.[102,103] ATP-sensitive K^+ channels are also expressed in cardiac and vascular myocytes. Here they are thought to be involved in the adjustment of vascular tone and myocardial contractility. Blocking this channel provides less protection of contractility during hypoxia. In addition, clinical studies have shown greater ischemia and more electrophysiological abnormalities in patients taking glyburide compared with other sulfonylureas.

These drugs may be given once a day or in divided doses 15 to 30 minutes before a meal. Glipizide is now available as an extended release formulation called *Glucotrol XL*. In addition, glyburide is available in a fixed-dose combination with metformin. Used together, these drugs demonstrate better glycemic control than either drug alone.[104]

Repaglinide and Nateglinide are two other drugs that act like the sulfonylureas but lack the sulfonylurea moiety.[100,105] They are rapidly absorbed and eliminated so there is a lower risk of hypoglycemia than with the standard sulfonylureas. In addition, they are relatively selective for the ATP-sensitive K^+ channel in the beta cells and do not affect these channels in cardiac tissue, thus reducing the cardiac risk. They also produce less weight gain compared with the sulfonylureas. They are given before a meal to reduce the postprandial glucose rise.

Thiazolidinediones (Glitazones)

The thiazolidinediones were developed as a result of the surprising finding that a clofibrate analog, ciglitazone, which was being developed for its lipid-lowering abilities, was found to lower blood glucose levels. Rosiglitazone and pioglitazone, two other drugs in this category, have since been developed for treatment of type 2 diabetes. These agents improve glycemic control by increasing insulin sensitivity in muscle, liver, and adipose tissue.[100] Thiazolidinediones bind to peroxisome proliferator–activated receptor γ on intranuclear transcription factors. Genes that are involved in modulating lipid metabolism and insulin action are activated, particularly in adipose and muscle tissues. They have also been shown to influence the beta cell directly by reducing the proinsulin/insulin ratio seen in type 2 disease but do not produce hypoglycemia. They are particularly effective for patients who are obese with predominant central adiposity because of the association with insulin resistance. Plasma triglyceride levels are reduced, HDL cholesterol levels are increased, and small LDL particles are transformed into larger particles that are less atherogenic.[106] These agents also have favorable effects on coagulation and blood pressure. Side effects of these agents include fluid retention, so patients need to be monitored for worsening congestive heart failure. Because the first clinically available glitazone (troglitazone) produced some fatal liver toxicity and has been withdrawn, it is suggested that liver enzymes be regularly monitored with the remaining glitazones.[107]

Because insulin resistance precedes the development of type 2 disease and also leads to the decline in beta cell function, it is reasonable to suggest that either the thiazolidinediones or the biguanides be started very early at the first sign of disease.[100] Metformin exerts its effect primarily by decreasing glucose production, whereas the glitazones improve insulin-mediated uptake of glucose; therefore it would seem that the first choice in the treatment of insulin resistance should be the thiazolidinediones. However, metformin has a better safety profile and produces weight loss, so the first agent of choice really depends on individual patient factors.

α-Glucosidase Inhibitors

Acarbose and miglitol inhibit GI absorption of carbohydrates by inhibiting the α-glucosidase enzymes in the intestines.[100] The drugs are taken just before meals and therefore lower the peak glucose levels seen after a meal. These drugs may also be given in combination with metformin, a sulfonylurea, or a glitazone. Adverse drug reactions include flatulence, diarrhea, and abdominal discomfort. Hypoglycemia may be a problem when the drug is administered with other agents but does not occur when α-glucosidase inhibitors are administered as monotherapy.

Selection of Agents for Type 2 Diabetes

Diet and exercise are the first-line treatments for type 2 diabetes; however, they often do not control blood glucose levels, and many clinicians are forced to prescribe drugs. Popular initial choices for medications tend to be metformin or a sulfonylurea prescribed as monotherapy. However, only a small proportion of patients can achieve adequate glycemic control with one drug alone. As mentioned previously, there appears to be a good rationale for starting with an insulin sensitizer rather than an insulin secretagogue. Because the hallmark of type 2 disease is insulin resistance, it makes sense to begin therapy with a glitazone or metformin, which improves insulin sensitivity, does not cause hypoglycemia, and can normalize the HbA1c levels. Given that this disease is progressive and glycemic control worsens with time, patients who initially responded to monotherapy will likely require combination therapy. The addition of another oral agent or insulin to the existing maximum dose of the initial therapy is the next step. Choice of agent depends on several individual patient factors such as weight and lipid profile and the safety profile of the medications. Several clinical studies prove the efficacy of combination therapy: metformin and rosiglitazone; pioglitazone and a sulfonylurea; and triple therapy with troglitazone, glyburide, and metformin.[108-110] These studies demonstrate that combination therapy significantly improves fasting plasma glucose and lipid levels over those achieved with monotherapy.

However, combination therapy is also associated with a greater risk of hypoglycemia.

Management of the Nonglycemic Side Effects of Type 2 Diabetes

Complications associated with type 2 diabetes can be reduced with other medications. Management of cardiovascular disease with antihypertensive and lipid-lowering drugs has been shown to contribute significant clinical efficacy.[111] A subgroup analysis of 202 diabetic patients participating in the Scandinavian Simvastatin Survival Study who were given simvastatin demonstrated reduced major coronary heart disease events equal to the reductions seen in nondiabetic patients over a 5.5-year period.[112] The benefit of lowering cholesterol is viewed as being even more significant for diabetic patients who have coronary artery disease than for nondiabetic patients with the same disease process because diabetes magnifies the risk of atherosclerotic events. The Cholesterol and Recurrent Events (CARE) trial evaluated the effect of pravastatin compared with placebo for the prevention of recurrent cardiovascular events in 586 patients with diabetes and average cholesterol readings.[113] The patients with diabetes who received active drug experienced a significant reduction in cardiovascular events compared with those who received placebo. These studies are so convincing regarding the use of the statins in diabetes that the American College of Physicians recently developed guidelines on the management of hypercholesterolemia in persons with type 2 disease.[114] The recommendations call for the use of statins for the primary prevention of macrovascular complications for all patients with cardiovascular risk factors and diabetes. The Clinical Efficacy Assessment Subcommittee of the American College of Physicians cites many studies as evidence for this recommendation, several of which have been previously reviewed in this book: the Air Force Coronary Atherosclerosis Prevention Study/Texas Coronary Atherosclerosis Prevention Study (AFCAPS/TexCAPS), the Antihypertensive and Lipid-Lowering to Prevent Heart Attack Trial–Lipid-Lowering Trial (ALLHAT-LLT), the Cholesterol and Recurrent Events (CARE) trial, the Anglo-Scandinavian Cardiac Outcome Trial—Lipid Lowering Arm (ASCOT-LLA), and the Scandinavian Simvastatin Survival Study.

In addition to lowering cholesterol, reducing hypertension in patients with diabetes is paramount.

There is a significant amount of evidence that angiotensin-converting enzyme (ACE) inhibitors improve cardiovascular outcomes in these patients. The Heart Outcomes Prevention Evaluation (HOPE) trial examined the effect of ramipril on the number of cardiac events in 3577 patients with diabetes.[115] This study was stopped 6 months early (after 4 to 5 years) when the evidence was overwhelming in favor of this therapy for diabetes. Treatment with ramipril reduced the risk of cardiac death by 37%, the risk of stroke by 33%, and the risk of myocardial infarction by 22%. There was also a significant reduction in nephropathy with this treatment. In another study, losartan, an ACE receptor blocker, was credited with significantly reducing the development of end-stage renal disease in patients with diabetes.[116] This study was a double-blind, placebo-controlled trial that included 1513 patients with type 2 disease. All subjects received maintenance therapy consisting of conventional antihypertensive agents, with the experimental group additionally receiving losartan. It is now the assumption that ACE inhibitors and ACE receptor blockers have the potential to interfere with the development of more extensive coronary atherosclerosis, with alterations in the fibrinolytic system that impair reperfusion after myocardial infarction, and with diabetic neuropathy with sympathetic/parasympathetic imbalance, either directly by altering the renin-angiotensin system or indirectly through their hemodynamic effect such that the beneficial effects are experienced by a greater degree in the diabetic population.[117]

EXERCISE AND DIABETES TREATMENT: THERAPEUTIC CONCERNS

Physical activity plays a crucial role in attaining health and preventing disease. However, some critical principles need to be followed before exercising someone with diabetes. During physical activity the skeletal muscles utilize their stores of glycogen and triglycerides, as well as free fatty acids from adipose tissue and glucose released from the liver, to meet energy requirements. Glucose levels in healthy patients remain adequate during most physical activity to meet these energy requirements and also to preserve central nervous system function. However, it is difficult for a diabetic individual to maintain the metabolic adjustments necessary. When there is an insufficient amount of insulin, the excessive release of the counter-insulin hormones, glucagon and catecholamines, which normally occurs with exercise will increase the already high levels of glucose and ketone bodies and may precipitate diabetic ketoacidosis. On the other hand, when there is a high plasma insulin level because of exogenous insulin injections, mobilization of glucose and other substrates that are released with exercise will be attenuated and hypoglycemia will be induced.

Exercise acts similarly to insulin by stimulating glut 4 transporters in muscle and improves the pathways for glycogen storage.[118] In addition, regular exercise is associated with overall improved insulin sensitivity. However, exercise can be dangerous by inducing hypoglycemia. It is especially important for the patient with type 1 diabetes to be able to adjust his or her nutrition and insulin regimen for safe participation in recreation or sports. In particular, self-monitored blood glucose levels and the patient's response to activity need to be recorded, preferably at the same time every day. Hypoglycemia may occur during, immediately after, or several hours after exercise.

Some general guidelines that may help improve glycemic response to exercise and avoid hypoglycemia are as follows.

1. Attain good glycemic control before exercise.[119] If glucose is below 100 mg/dL, the patient should eat a snack. Exercise is contraindicated if fasting glucose levels are >300 mg/dL and should be done with caution if glucose levels are >250 mg/dL.
2. Monitor blood glucose before and after exercise to determine when food must be consumed. Monitoring during exercise may be necessary for long periods of activity. In addition, it is important to learn how the patient's glycemic response varies with different exercises and under different conditions.
3. Consume carbohydrates as needed to avoid hypoglycemia and have these foods available after exercise as well. A snack may be required for every 30 minutes of activity.
4. Continue measuring glucose levels frequently for up to 6 to 12 hours after exercise because exercise-induced hypoglycemia may occur hours after activity is stopped.

5. Reduce the pre-meal insulin dose for postprandial exercise. Because exercise acts as insulin does and can trigger hypoglycemia, patients should be counseled to lower their pre-exercise insulin dose. The goal should be to end the exercise session with a plasma glucose level similar to that measured before the preceding meal. This recommendation came from a study that evaluated pre-meal insulin dose reductions for postprandial exercises of varying intensities to prevent exercise-induced hypoglycemia in type 1 disease.[120] For this study, eight male patients receiving Ultralente as the basal injection and lispro as the pre-meal insulin exercised at 25% maximum oxygen consumption (VO_{2max}), 50% VO_{2max}, and 75% VO_{2max} on a cycle ergometer. Each subject acted as his own control in a crossover design, and each received a pre-meal insulin dose based on the number of carbohydrates expected to be consumed at the meal before exercise. Subjects performed the exercises after receiving a full dose of insulin, 100% lispro, after 50% lispro, and after 25% lispro for either 30 or 60 minutes. Venous blood samples were retrieved at 10- to 15-minute intervals for determination of plasma glucose, insulin, and glucagon levels. Glucose monitoring continued for 18 hours after the experiment but at a reduced frequency. Subjects were also studied during a period of rest instead of exercise at each of the designated insulin doses. The results demonstrated that the full pre-meal insulin dose was associated with increased hypoglycemia at all the exercise intensities and even at rest in some subjects. Reductions in the pre-meal insulin dose resulted in far fewer episodes of hypoglycemia. A similar concern regarding the reduction of medication has also surfaced when exercise is combined with the sulfonylureas.[101] A reduction in dose of the oral hypoglycemic agent may be needed.
6. Exercise after meals improves glycemic control. The high glycemic response that occurs after food intake is more important in terms of microvascular risk than the pre-meal levels.[72] Therefore it makes sense to exercise

after a meal when physical activity is working in conjunction with the pre-meal insulin dose to control glycemic levels. In a study in which the effects of walking before and after a meal on blood glucose levels were compared in patients type 1 diabetes receiving intensive insulin therapy (pre-meal regular insulin and NPH at bedtime), walking after a meal was found to have a better effect on glycemic control.[121] Walking before breakfast produced some hyperglycemia, probably resulting from secretion of catecholamines and glucagon and an already high glucose level. Walking an hour after a meal did not produce hypoglycemia, either because walking is a light aerobic exercise producing smaller effects on blood sugar levels than running or because the peak effect of regular insulin had not been reached when the subjects started walking. The peak effect of regular insulin does not occur until 2 hours after injection. However, this timing of exercise should not be generalized to all types of short-acting insulins because insulin lispro peaks at 1 hour, not at 2 hours. In a study in which the glycemic response of regular insulin was compared with that of insulin lispro during exercise 1 hour after a meal, insulin concentrations were higher and peaked earlier with a significantly higher drop in glucose level with lispro.[122] Therefore when timing exercise with food intake and insulin dose, the therapist must also consider the type of short-acting insulin the patient received and should not exercise the patient vigorously during the peak insulin times.

7. Do not perform massage or exercise and do not apply a modality to a body part that has recently received an injection of insulin.[89,123] These activities will hasten absorption and may cause hypoglycemia. Wait until the duration of action for that insulin injection is over.

In general, the principles cited in the list for handling exercise in adults with diabetes also apply to children. Children may be prone to greater variations in glycemic control, not only with exercise but also with play activities.[119] In the case of adolescents, monthly hormonal changes, particularly in girls, will also make control of blood glucose levels challenging.[124]

ACTIVITIES 15

■ 1. Discuss pharmaceutical and physical therapy options for the following patients. Include questions you would ask regarding medical history that would help you make good treatment choices. Patient A is a 52-year-old woman who has just passed through menopause. BMD is currently within normal limits. Patient B is an 82-year-old woman who has just completed rehab for a total hip replacement as a result of a fall. She lives in a nursing home. Patient C is a 22-year-old competitive runner. She is 5′10″ but weighs only 110 lb. She has not had a menstrual period in more than a year, and bone density testing shows that she has a T-score of −2.7 at the femoral neck.

■ 2. A teenage girl with type 1 diabetes has been having bouts of hypoglycemia during the last period of the school day. There have even been two episodes when she became unconscious but responded to glucagon. She takes regular insulin with intermediate insulin every morning and again before supper.

Questions

a. What are the possible causes of this patient's hypoglycemia?

b. The timing of the glucose testing is very important. Testing at the following times gives what information regarding this patient's insulin regimen?

fasting blood sugar taken in the morning before breakfast

blood samples taken before lunch

blood sugar samples taken in the evening between 8:00 and 9:00 PM

blood sugar samples taken during the night

c. If this patient needed physical therapy, when would you schedule it?

d. This patient had an elevated glucose level at around 11:00 AM. Which insulin dose should be adjusted?

e. List the symptoms of hypoglycemia.

f. Discuss some guidelines for exercising a diabetic patient.

3. A 62-year-old woman has had type 2 diabetes for more than 5 years. She has been taking glyburide twice daily but does not have good glycemic control. Her HbA_{1c} level is 8.8%. She has lost approximately 15 lb during the last 5 years, but her HbA_{1c} level continues to climb even after the glyburide has been increased to the maximum allowable daily dose. What options should be discussed with the patient?

References

1. Wells BG, Dipiro JT, Schwinghammer TL, Hamilton CW. *Pharmacotherapy Handbook.* 5th ed. New York: McGraw Hill; 2003.

2. Marcus R. Treatment of osteoporosis. In: Carruthers SG, Hoffman BB, Melmon KL, Nierenberg DW, eds. *Melmon and Morrelli's Clinical Pharmacology.* 4th ed. New York: McGraw-Hill; 2000:703-711.

3. Hill PA. Bone remodelling. *Br J Orthod.* 1998;25(2):101-107.

4. Manolagas SC. Birth and death of bone cells: basic regulatory mechanisms and implications for the pathogenesis and treatment of osteoporosis. *Endocr Rev.* 2000;21(2):115-137.

5. Alliston T, Derynck R. Interfering with bone remodelling. *Nature.* 2002;416:686-687.

6. Takayanagi H, Sunhwa K, Matsuo K, et al. RANKL maintains bone homeostasis through c-Fos-dependent induction of interferon-b. *Nature.* 2002;416:744-749.

7. Genuth SM. Endocrine regulation of calcium and phosphate metabolism. In: Berne RM, Levy MN, eds. *Physiology.* 4th ed. Philadelphia: Mosby; 1998:848-871.

8. Bushinsky DA, Monk RD. Calcium. *Lancet.* 1998;352:305-311.

9. D'ippolito G, Schiller PC, Ricordi C, Roos BA, Howard GA. Age-related osteogenic potential of mesenchymal stromal stem cells from human vertebral bone marrow. *J Bone Miner Res.* 1999;14(7):1115-1122.

10. Parhami F, Gharavi N, Ballard AJ, Tintut Y, Demer LL. Role of the cholesterol biosynthetic pathway in osteoblastic differentiation of marrow stromal cells. *J Bone Miner Res.* 2002;17(11):1997-2003.

11. Diascro DD, Vogel RL, Johnson TE, et al. High fatty acid content in rabbit serum is responsible for the differentiation of osteoblasts into adipocyte-like cells. *J Bone Miner Res.* 1998;13(1):96-106.

12. Parhami F, Tintut Y, Beamer WG, Gharavi N, Goodman W, Demer LL. Atherogenic high-fat diet reduces bone mineralization in mice. *J Bone Miner Res.* 2001;16(1):182-188.

13. Weinstein RS, Chen JR, Powers CC, et al. Promotion of osteoclast survival and antagonism of bisphosphonate-induced osteoclast apoptosis by glucocorticoids. *J Clin Invest.* 2002;109(8):1041-1048.

14. O'Brien CA, Jia D, Plotkin LI, et al. Glucocorticoids act directly on osteoblasts and osteocytes to induce their apoptosis and reduce bone formation and strength. *Endocrinology.* 2004;145(4):1835-1841.

15. Weinstein RS, Manolagas SC. Apoptosis and osteoporosis. *Am J Med.* 2000;108(2):153-164.

16. Gourlay ML, Brown SA. Clinical considerations in premenopausal osteoporosis. *Arch Intern Med.* 2004;164(6):603-614.

17. Cummings SR, Bates DW, Black DM. Clinical use of bone densitometry. *JAMA.* 2002;288(15):1889-1897.

18. Bates DW, Black DM, Cummings SR. Clinical use of bone densitometry. *JAMA.* 2002;288:1898-1900.

19. Black DM, Cummings SR, Thompson DE, et al. Effect of alendronate on risk of fracture in women with low bone density but without vertebral fractures: results from the Fracture Intervention Trial. *JAMA.* 1998;280(24):2077-2082.

20. Lindsay RS, Gallagher C, Kleerekoper M, Pickar JH. Effect of lower doses of conjugated equine estrogens with and without medroxyprogesterone acetate on bone in early postmenopausal women. *JAMA.* 2002;287(20):2668-2676.

21. Villareal DT, Binder EF, Williams DB, Schechtman KB, Yarasheski KE, Kohrt WM. Bone mineral density response to estrogen replacement in frail elderly women. *JAMA.* 2001;286(7):815-820.

22. Roussouw, JE, Anderson GL, Prentice RL, et al. Risks and benefits of estrogen plus progestin in healthy postmenopausal women: principal results from the Women's Health Initiative randomized controlled trial. *JAMA.* 2002;288(3):321-333.

23. Reid I, Ames RW, Evans MC, Gamble GD, Sharpe SJ. Long-term effects of calcium supplementation on bone loss and fractures in postmenopausal women: a randomized controlled trial. *Am J Med.* 1995;98:331-335.

24. Dawson-Hughes B, Harris SS, Krall EA, Dallal GE. Effect of calcium and vitamin D supplementation on bone density in men and women 65 years of age or older. *N Engl J Med.* 1997;337(10):670-676.

25. Drugs for prevention and treatment of postmenopausal osteoporosis. *Treat Guidel Med Lett.* 2002;1(3)13-18..

26. Prince RL. Diet and the prevention of osteoporotic fractures. *N Engl J Med.* 1997;337(10):700-702.

27. Delmas PD. Treatment of postmenopausal osteoporosis. *Lancet.* 2002;359:2018-2026.

28. Black DM, Thompson DE, Bauer DC, et al. Fracture risk with alendronate in women with osteoporosis: The Fracture Intervention Trial. *J Clin Endocrinol Metab.* 2000; 85(11):4118-4124.

29. Black DM, Cummings SR, Karpf DB, et al. Randomised trial of effect of alendronate on risk of fracture in women with existing vertebral fractures. *Lancet.* 1996; 348:1535-1541.

30. Bone HG, Hosking D, Devogelaer JP, et al. Ten years' experience with alendronate for osteoporosis in post-menopausal women. *N Engl J Med.* 2004;350(12): 1189-1199.

31. Hosking D, Chilvers C, Christiansen C, et al. Prevention of bone loss with alendronate in postmenopausal women under 60 years of age. *N Engl J Med.* 1998; 338(8):485-492.

32. Once-a-week alendronate (Fosamax). *Med Lett Drugs Ther.* 2001;43(1100):26.

33. Clemett D, Spencer CS. Raloxifene: a review of its use in postmenopausal osteoporosis. *Drugs.* 2000;60(2): 380-411.

34. Delmas PD, Bjarnason NH, Mitlak BH, et al. Effects of raloxifene on bone and mineral density, serum cholesterol concentrations, and uterine endometrium in post-menopausal women. *N Engl J Med.* 1997;337(23): 1641-1647.

35. Barrett-Connor E, Grady D, Sashegyi A, et al. Raloxifene and cardiovascular events in osteoporotic post-menopausal women. *JAMA.* 2002;287(7):847-857.

36. Cauley JA, Norton L, Lippman ME, et al. Continued breast cancer risk reduction in postmenopausal women treated with raloxifene: 4-year results from the MORE trial. Multiple outcomes of raloxifene evaluation. *Breast Cancer Res Treat.* 2001;65(2):125-134.

37. Raloxifene for postmenopausal osteoporosis. *Med Lett Drugs Ther.* 1998;40(1026):54.

38. Swegle JM, Kelly MW. Tibolone: a unique version of hormone replacement therapy. *Ann Pharmacother.* 2004; 38(5):874-881.

39. Anedda FM, Velati A, Lello S, et al. Observational study on the efficacy of tibolone in counteracting early carotid atherosclerotic lesions in postmenopausal women. *Horm Res.* 2004;61(1):47-52.

40. Bots ML, Evans GW, Riley W, et al. The Osteoporosis Prevention and Arterial Effects of Tibolone (OPAL) study: design and baseline characteristics. *Control Clin Trials.* 2003;24(6):752-775.

41. Mueck AO, Lippert C, Seeger H, Wallwiener D. Effects of tibolone on human breast cancer cells and human vascular coronary cells. *Arch Gynecol Obstet.* 2003; 267(3):139-144.

42. Beral V, Million Women Study Collaborators. Breast cancer and hormone-replacement therapy in the Million Women Study. *Lancet.* 2003;362(9382):419-427.

43. Chestnut CH, Silverman S, Andriano K, et al. A randomized trial of nasal spray salmon calcitonin in postmenopausal women with established osteoporosis: the Prevent Recurrence of Osteoporotic Fractures study. *Am J Med.* 2000;109:267-276.

44. Rosen CJ, Bilezikian JP. Anabolic therapy for osteoporosis. *J Clin Endocrinol Metab.* 2001;86(3):957-964.

45. Holloway L, Butterfield G, Hintz RL, Gesundheit N, Marcus R. Effects of recombinant human growth hormone on metabolic indices, body composition, and bone turnover in healthy elderly women. *J Clin Endocrinol Metabol.* 1994;79(2):470-479.

46. Whitehead HM, Boreham C, McIlrath M, et al. GH treatment of adults with GH deficiency; results of a 13 month placebo controlled cross-over study. *Clin Endocrinol (Oxf).* 1992;36:45-52.

47. Biller BM, Sesmilo G, Baum HB, Hayden D, Schoenfeld D, Klibanski A. Withdrawal of long-term physiological GH administration. *J Clin Endocrinol Metab.* 2000;85(3): 970-976.

48. Morley P, Whitfield JF, Willick GE. Parathyroid hormone: an anabolic treatment for osteoporosis. *Curr Pharm Des.* 2001;7:671-687.

49. Ghiron L, Thompson J, Halloway L, et al. Effects of rhGH and IGF-1 on bone turnover in elderly women. *J Bone Miner Res.* 1995;10(12):1844-1852.

50. Baumann BD, Wronski TJ. Response of cortical bone to anti-resorptive agents and PTH in aged ovariectomized rats. *Bone.* 1995;16(2):247-253.

51. Andreassen TT, Ejersted C, Oxlund H. Intermittent parathyroid hormone (1-34) treatment increases callus formation and mechanical strength of healing fractures. *J Bone Miner Res.* 1999;14(6):960-968.

52. Neer RM, Arnaud C, Zanchetta JR, et al. Effect of parathyroid hormone (1-34) on fracture and bone mineral density in postmenopausal women with osteoporosis. *N Engl J Med.* 2001;344(19):1434-1444.

53. Chan AK, Andrade SE, Boles M, et al. Inhibitors of hydroxymethylglutaryl-coenzyme A reductase and risk of fracture among older women. *Lancet.* 2000;355(9222): 2185-2188.

54. Pasco JA, Kotowicz MA, Henry MJ, Sanders KM, Nicholson GC. Statin use, bone mineral density, and fracture risk. *Arch Intern Med.* 2002;162(5): 537-540.

55. Ettinger B, Bilezikian JP. For osteoporosis, are two antiresorptive drugs better than one? *J Clin Endocrinol Metab.* 2002;87(3):983-984.

56. Johnell O, Scheele WH, Lu Y, Reginster J-Y, Need AG, Seeman E. Additive effects of raloxifene and alendronate on bone density and biochemical markers of bone remodeling in postmenopausal women with osteoporosis. *J Clin Endocrinol Metab.* 2002; 87(3):985-992.

57. Bone HG, Greenspan SL, McKeever C, et al. Alendronate and estrogen effects in postmenopausal women with low bone density. *J Clin Endocrinol Metab.* 2000;85(2):720-726.

58. Zimmet P, Alberti KG, Shaw J. Global and societal implications of the diabetes epidemic. *Nature.* 2001; 4141:782-787.

59. Margolis S, Saudek CD. *The Johns Hopkins White Papers on Diabetes.* Baltimore, MD: Johns Hopkins Medical Institutions; 2002.

60. Rang HP, Dale MM, Ritter JM, Moore JL. *Pharmacology.* 5th ed. New York: Churchill Livingstone; 2003.

61. The Expert Committee on the Diagnosis and Classification of Diabetes Mellitus. Report of the Expert Committee on the Diagnosis and Classification of Diabetes Mellitus. *Diabetes Care.* 1998;21(1S):5S-19S.

62. Sreekumar R, Halvatsiotis P, Schimke JC, Nair KS. Gene expression profile in skeletal muscle of type 2 diabetes and the effect of insulin treatment. *Diabetes.* 2002; 51(6):1913-1920.

63. Roglic G, Colhoun HM, Stevens LK, Lemkes HH, Manes C, Fuller JH. Parental history of hypertension and parental history of diabetes and microvascular complications in insulin-dependent diabetes mellitus: the EURODIAB IDDM Complications Study. *Diabet Med.* 1998;15(5):418-426.

64. Insulin resistance syndrome. Altered sugar processing leads to a multitude of medical problems. *Mayo Clin Womens Healthsource.* 2002;6(11)1-2.

65. Levin SR, Coburn JW, Abraira C, et al. Effect of intensive glycemic control on microalbuminuria in type 2 diabetes. Veterans Affairs Cooperative Study on Glycemic Control and Complications in Type 2 Diabetes Feasibility Trial Investigators. *Diabetes Care.* 2000;23(10):1478-1485.

66. The Diabetes Control and Complications Trial Research Group. The effect of intensive treatment of diabetes on the development and progression of long-term complications in insulin-dependent diabetes mellitus. *N Engl J Med.* 1993;329(14):977-986.

67. Stratton IM, Adler AI, Neil HA, et al. Association of glycaemia with macrovascular and microvascular complications of type 2 diabetes (UKPDS 35): prospective observational study. *BMJ.* 2000;321(7258):405-412.

68. Way KJ, Katai N, King GL. Protein kinase C and the development of diabetic vascular complications. *Diabet Med.* 2001;18:945-959.

69. American Diabetes Association. Screening for type 2 diabetes. *Diabetes Care.* 2004;27(S1):S11-S14.

70. The Expert Committee on the Diagnosis and Classification of Diabetes Mellitus. Follow-up report on the diagnosis of diabetes mellitus. *Diabetes Care.* 2003;26(11): 3160-3167.

71. American Diabetes Association. Diagnosis and classification of diabetes mellitus. *Diabetes Care.* 2004;27:S5-S10.

72. Home PD. Therapeutic targets in the management of type 1 diabetes. *Diabetes Care.* 2002;18(suppl 1):S7-S13.

73. Fineberg SE, Bergenstal RM, Bernstein RM, Laffel L, Schwartz SL. Use of an automated device for alternative site blood glucose monitoring. *Diabetes Care.* 2001; 24(7):1217-1220.

74. Garg SK, Potts RO, Ackerman NR, Fermi SJ, Tamada JA, Chase HP. Correlation of fingerstick blood glucose measurements with GlucoWatch Biographer glucose results in young subjects with type 1 diabetes. *Diabetes Care.* 1999;22(10):1708-1714.

75. Guyton AC, Hall JE. *Textbook of Medical Physiology.* 10th ed. Philadelphia: WB Saunders Company; 2000.

76. Miller JW. Drugs and the endocrine and metabolic systems. In: Page C, Curtis AB, Sutter MC, Walker L, Hoffman BB, eds. *Integrated Pharmacology.* Philadelphia: Mosby; 2002:281-326.

77. Owens DR, Zinman B, Bolli GB. Insulins today and beyond. *Lancet.* 2001;358:739-746.

78. Homko C, Deluzoio A, Jimenez C, Kolaczynski JW, Boden G. Comparison of insulin aspart and lispro: pharmacokinetic and metabolic effects. *Diabetes Care.* 2003;26(7):2027-2031.

79. Insulin aspart, a new rapid-acting insulin. *Med Lett Drugs Ther.* 2001;43(1115):89-90.

80. Home PD, Barriocanal L, Lindholm A. Comparative pharmacokinetics and pharmacodynamics of the novel rapid-acting insulin analogue, insulin aspart, in healthy volunteers. *Eur J Clin Pharmacol.* 1999;55(3):199-203.

81. Allen J. Insulins. In: *Prescriber's Letter.* Stockton, Calif: Therapeutic Research Center; 2002.

82. Wang F, Carabino JM, Vergara CM. Insulin glargine: a systematic review of a long-acting insulin analogue. *Clin Ther.* 2003;25(6):1539-1540.

83. American Diabetes Association. Insulin administration. *Diabetes Care.* 2004;27(suppl 1):S106-S107.

84. Havas S. Educational guidelines for achieving tight control and minimizing complications of type 1 diabetes. *Am Fam Physician.* 1999;60(7):1997-1998.

85. Rosenstock J. Insulin therapy: optimizing control in type 1 and type 2 diabetes. *Clin Cornerstone.* 2001; 4(2):50-64.

86. Rosenstock J, Park G, Zimmerman J. Basal insulin glargine (HOE 901) versus NPH insulin in patients with type 1 diabetes on multiple daily insulin regimens. U.S. Insulin Glargine (HOE 901) Type 1 Diabetes Investigator Group. *Diabetes Care.* 2000;23(8):1137-1142.

87. Riddle MC. Timely initiation of basal insulin. *Am J Med.* 2004;116(3, suppl 1):3-9.

88. McKenry LM, Salerno E. Drugs affecting the endocrine system. In: *Pharmacology in Nursing.* 21st ed. Philadelphia: Mosby; 2003:819-881.

89. Linde B. Dissociation of insulin absorption and blood flow during massage of a subcutaneous injection site. *Diabetes Care.* 1986;9(6):570-574.

90. Korytkowski M, Bell D, Jacobsen JD, Suwannasari R. A multicenter, randomized, open-label, comparative, two-period crossover trial of preference, efficacy, and safety profiles of a prefilled, disposable pen and conventional vial/syringe for insulin injection in patients with type 1 or 2 diabetes mellitus. *Clin Ther.* 2003;25(11):2836-2848.

91. Cefalu WT, Skyler JS, Kourides IA, et al. Treating type 2 diabetes with inhaled insulin. *Ann Intern Med.* 2001;134(3):203-207.

92. Weiss SR, Cheng SL, Kourides IA, Gelfand RA, Landschulz WH. Inhaled insulin provides improved glycemic control in patients with type 2 diabetes mellitus inadequately controlled with oral agents. *Arch Intern Med.* 2003;163(19):2277-2282.

93. Raskin P, Bode BW, Marks JB, et al. Continuous subcutaneous insulin infusion and multiple daily injection therapy are equally effective in type 2 diabetes: a randomized, parallel-group, 24 week study. *Diabetes Care.* 2003;26(9):2598-2603.

94. Weintrob N, Benzaquen CD, Galatzer A, et al. Comparison of continuous subcutaneous insulin infusion and multiple daily injection regimens in children with type 1 diabetes: a randomized open crossover trial. *Pediatrics.* 2003;112(3):559-564.

95. Bailey CJ. Biguanides and NIDDM. *Diabetes Care.* 1992; 15(6):755-772.

96. Stumvoll M, Nurjhan N, Perriello G, Dailey G, Gerich JE. Metabolic effects of metformin in non-insulin-dependent diabetes mellitus. *N Engl J Med.* 1995;333(9):550-554.

97. DeFronzo RA, Goodman AM. Efficacy of metformin in patients with non-insulin-dependent diabetes mellitus. *N Engl J Med.* 1995;333(9):541-549.

98. Akiyoshi M, Kakei M, Nakazaki M, Tanaka H. A new hypoglycemic agent, A-4166 inhibits ATP-sensitive potassium channels in rat pancreatic beta-cells. *Am J Physiol*. 1995;268:E185-E193.

99. Hu S, Wang S, Fanelli B, et al. Pancreatic b-cell KATP channel activity and membrane-binding studies with nateglinide: a comparison with sulfonylureas and Repaglinide. *J Pharmacol Exp Ther*. 2000;293(2): 444-452.

100. Weissman PN. Reappraisal of the pharmacologic approach to treatment of type 2 diabetes mellitus. *Am J Cardiol*. 2002;90(5):42-50.

101. Larsen JJ, Dela F, Madsbad S, Vibe-Peterson J, Galbo H. Interaction of sulfonylureas and exercise on glucose homeostasis in type 2 diabetic patients. *Diabetes Care*. 1999;22(10):1647-1654.

102. Riddle MC. Sulfonylureas differ in effects on ischemic preconditioning—is it time to retire glyburide? [editorial] *J Clin Endocrinol Metab*. 2003;88(2):528-530.

103. Wascher TC, Boes U. Ischemia in type 2 diabetes: tissue selectivity of sulfonylureas and clinical implications. *Metabolism*. 2003;52(8):3-5.

104. Glyburide/metformin (Glucovance) for type 2 diabetes. *Med Lett Drugs Ther*. 2000;42(1092):105-106.

105. Repaglinide for type 2 diabetes mellitus. *Med Lett Drugs Ther*. 1998;40(1027):55-56.

106. Lebovitz HE. Rationale for and role of thiazolidinediones in type 2 diabetes mellitus. *Am J Cardiol*. 2002;90 (5, suppl 1):34-41.

107. Gale EA. Lessons from the glitazones: a story of drug development. *Lancet*. 2001;357:1870-1875.

108. Fonseca V, Rosenstock J, Patwardhan R, Salzman A. Effect of metformin and rosiglitazone combination therapy in patients with type 2 diabetes mellitus: a randomized controlled trial. *JAMA*. 2000;283:1695-1702.

109. Kipnes MS, Krosnick A, Rendell JW, Egan JW, Mathisen AL, Schneider RL. Pioglitazone hydrochloride in combination with sulfonylurea therapy improves glycemic control in patients with type 2 diabetes mellitus: a randomized, placebo-controlled study. *Am J Med*. 2001;111(1):10-17.

110. Yale JF, Valiquett TR, Ghazzi MN, Owens-Grillo JK, Foyt HL. The effect of a thiazolidinedione drug, troglitazone, on glycemia in patients with type 2 diabetes mellitus poorly controlled with sulfonylurea and metformin: a multicenter, randomized, double-blind, placebo-controlled trial. *Ann Intern Med*. 2001; 134(9):737-745.

111. Estacio RO, Jeffers BW, Gifford N, Schrier RW. Effect of blood pressure control on diabetic microvascular complications in patients with hypertension and type 2 diabetes. *Diabetes Care*. 2000;23(suppl 2):B54-B64.

112. Pyorala K, Pedersen TR, Kjekshus J, Faergeman O, Olsson AG, Thorgeirsson G. Cholesterol lowering with simvastatin improves prognosis of diabetic patients with coronary heart disease: a subgroup analysis of the Scandinavian Simvastatin Survival Study (4S). *Diabetes Care*. 1997;20(4):614-620.

113. Goldberg RB, Mellies MJ, Sacks FM, et al. Cardiovascular events and their reduction with pravastatin in diabetic and glucose-intolerant myocardial infarction survivors with average cholesterol levels: subgroup analyses in the Cholesterol and Recurrent Events (CARE) Trial. *Circulation*. 1998;98(23):2513-2519.

114. Snow V, Aronson MDH, R., Mottur-Pilson C, Weiss KB. Lipid control in the management of type 2 diabetes mellitus: a clinical practice guideline from the American College of Physicians. *Ann Intern Med*. 2004;140(8): 644-649.

115. Heart Outcome Prevention (HOPE) Study Investigators. Effects of ramipril on cardiovascular and microvascular outcomes in people with diabetes mellitus: results of the HOPE study and MICRO-HOPE substudy. *Lancet*. 2000;355:253-259.

116. Brenner BM, Cooper ME, de Zeeuw D, et al. Effects of losartan on renal and cardiovascular outcomes in patients with type 2 diabetes and neuropathy. *N Engl J Med*. 2001;345(12):861-869.

117. Zuanetti G, Latini R, Maggioni AF, M., Santoro L, Tognoni G. Effect of the ACE inhibitor lisinopril on mortality in diabetic patients with acute myocardial infarction: data from the GISSI-3 study. *Circulation*. 1997; 96(12):4239-4245.

118. Rice B, Janssen I, Hudson R, Ross R. Effects of aerobic or resistance exercise and/or diet on glucose tolerance and plasma insulin levels in obese men. *Diabetes Care*. 1999; 22(5):684-691.

119. American Diabetes Association. Physical activity/ exercise and diabetes. *Diabetes Care*. 2004;27(suppl 1): S58-S62.

120. Rabasa-Lhoret R, Bourque J, Ducros F, Chaisson J-L. Guidelines for premeal insulin dose reduction for postprandial exercise of different intensities and durations in type 1 diabetic subjects treated intensively with a basal bolus insulin regimen (Ultralente-lispro). *Diabetes Care*. 2001;24(4):625-630.

121. Yamanouchi K, Abe R, Takeda A, Atsumi Y, Shirchiri M, Sato Y. The effect of walking before and after breakfast on blood glucose levels in patients with type 1 diabetes treated with intensive insulin therapy. *Diabetes Res Clin Pract*. 2002;58(1):11-18.

122. Yamakita T, Ishii T, Yamagami K, et al. Glycemic response during exercise after administration of insulin lispro compared with that after administration of regular human insulin. *Diabetes Res Clin Pract*. 2002; 57(1):17-22.

123. Koivisto VA, Felig P. Effects of leg exercise on insulin absorption in diabetic patients. *N Engl J Med*. 1978; 298(2):79-83.

124. DeWitt DE, Dugdale DC. Using new insulin strategies in the outpatient treatment of diabetes. *JAMA*. 2003; 289(17):2265-2269.

6

SECTION

Psychopharmacology

❦

DRUG TREATMENT FOR DEPRESSION AND ANXIETY

❦

DEPRESSION

Depression is an extremely common condition with a high prevalence worldwide and is associated with a fair amount of morbidity and mortality.[1] Community surveys on depression in Europe have shown 1-year prevalence rates from 1.4% in rural Germany to as high as 9.3% in Finland.[2] One survey from Japan indicated that 53.4% of first-year university students were depressed.[3] Chronic depression is frequently associated with dysfunction in interpersonal, marital, occupational, and family functioning, so that many more individuals are affected by this disorder than just those who are classified as depressed.[4]

Depression is a disorder of mood, as opposed to a disorder of thought or reality. Symptoms range from mild and hardly noticeable to severe with hallucinations and delusions. The majority of depressions include some of the following symptoms: low mood, loss of interest in pleasurable activities, loss of motivation, loss of libido, pessimism, fatigue, sleep disturbances, poor self-esteem, suicidal thoughts, and disturbances in food intake.[5] Two major categories of depression outlined in the fourth edition of the *Diagnostic and Statistical Manual of Mental Disorders (DSM-IV)* are dysthymic disorder and major depressive disorder, chronic type.[4] Dysthymic disorder is a mild chronic depression defined by the presence of more depressive moments than not for at least 2 years, the persistence of the

depression for longer than 2 months, and an insidious onset. Patients with dysthymic disorder can display several of the symptoms of depression, but dysthymic disorder is usually characterized by more of the cognitive (low self-esteem, hopelessness), affective (low mood), and social dysfunction (loss of motivation and social withdrawal) aspects than disturbances in sleep or appetite. In addition, *DSM-IV* recognizes the diagnostic importance of symptoms that begin with an early onset, before the age of 21 years. For an actual diagnosis, the *DSM-IV* requires the presence of two of the following symptoms: fatigue or decreased energy, insomnia or hypersomnia, increased or decreased appetite, low self-esteem, poor concentration, and difficulty with decision making.[4]

Individuals with dysthymic disorder may also experience exacerbations in mood disturbance that meet the criteria for a major depressive episode. In fact, 75% to 90% of patients with a dysthymic disorder report having had a major depressive episode previously.[4] Approximately 25% of patients given a diagnosis of a major depressive episode report having a pervasive dysthymic disorder. For some patients, this may represent different phases of a single disease that waxes and wanes, depending on environmental stressors, rather than two distinct conditions. Those patients who are actually given a diagnosis of a major depressive episode may display the full gamut of symptoms described in the *DSM-IV*. However, one of the difficulties with classifying any of the depressions is that there is no "biological feature" or laboratory value that separates one type from another. Psychological tests can help with the diagnosis, but few primary care doctors will take the time to administer them. Therefore the classification system is based on the subjective description of symptoms.

Distinctions have been made between other types of depressive syndromes; for example, unipolar affective disorder is when the mood is in the same direction (depression), as opposed to bipolar affective disorder, in which the primary mood may be either depression or mania but may include periods when the opposite affect is interspersed. Unipolar affective disorder is further divided into reactive depression, precipitated by a stressful life event, and endogenous depression, which is unrelated to external stress and has a familial component.

At least three aspects of depression underline the urgency for a rapid diagnosis and initiation of treatment. Suicide is a consequence of depression and is the eighth leading cause of death in the United States and the third leading cause of death among children between the ages of 5 and 14 years.[1] Depression can lead to significant medical morbidity. There is evidence that depression affects cardiovascular health, resulting in a greater mortality rate among patients who have sustained a myocardial infarction.[6] Depression has also been linked to osteoporosis, peptic ulcer disease, and diabetes.[7] Even subthreshold psychiatric symptoms are associated with significant medical impairment.[8] Although several of these physical developments might be linked to an elevated cortisol level, which is a trend seen in patients with depression, they nevertheless highlight the physical manifestations of this mental illness. The third aspect of depression that demands concern is the chronicity of the disease. Studies have shown that many patients who experience a major depressive episode eventually have chronic disease.[4] This is particularly true if the depression is not appropriately treated or if the patient is undertreated. In the majority of medical illnesses, good therapeutic agents are developed as an outcome of having a thorough understanding of the biology of the condition. Unfortunately, little is known about the underlying mechanisms of depression.

Pathophysiology of Depression

The original biological hypothesis of depression has been referred to as *the monoamine hypothesis*.[5] It was popularized in the early 1960s as a result of the observation that patients taking reserpine to lower blood pressure became depressed. Depression was also observed when reserpine was used in high doses for the treatment of schizophrenia. Reserpine inhibits storage and subsequent release of the amine neurotransmitters, serotonin and norepinephrine, from the presynaptic nerve endings in the brain. Reserpine is rarely used today, but it is credited with having helped establish a neurochemical basis for depression. According to this theory, depression is related to a deficiency or imbalance of norepinephrine or serotonin or a deficiency in transmission of these amines. In addition, catecholamine depletion caused by low levels of tryptophan, a precursor to serotonin, has been associated with depression. In two studies, limiting dietary intake of tryptophan was found to produce a relapse in patients being treated for depression.[9,10]

Evidence for the monoamine theory has been presented and accepted by many researchers in the field of psychiatry, mainly because pharmacological evidence exists; limiting reuptake of these neurotransmitters with antidepressants increases their concentration at the synaptic cleft and reduces symptoms. However, years of research have uncovered several inconsistencies with this theory. First, the biochemical effects of the antidepressant drugs occur quickly, but the antidepressant effects may take weeks to materialize. This suggests that relief of depression is related to a secondary adaptive change in the brain rather than a direct action of the drug. A change in receptor sensitivity concurrent with a down-regulation of the receptor is another theory that has been difficult to prove.

Current theories are focused on the neuroendocrine system, as well as signal transduction pathways and growth factors, to help narrow down a pathophysiology for depression. Persistent stress is known to activate the sympathetic nervous system and the hypothalamus-pituitary-adrenal axis. Elevated levels of corticotrophin-releasing hormone are implicated in the pathophysiology of depression, which is borne out by studies that show cortisol fails to reduce corticotrophin-releasing hormone levels in depressed patients. Some researchers have even proposed that depressive subtypes could be related to different levels of corticotrophin-releasing hormone. Further support is provided by the observations that a significant number of patients with Cushing's disease have depression and are also known to have hippocampal volume depletion correlated with cortisol hypersecretion, similar to that seen in patients with depression.[11-13] This has been described as stress-induced neuronal atrophy or impairment in neuroplasticity. Additionally, it has been shown that stress and glucocorticoids reduce cellular resilience, a process by which neuronal cells become more susceptible to certain abuse such as ischemia, hypoglycemia, and excitatory amino acid toxicity.[14] Some of the current antidepressants increase hippocampal neurogenesis and improve neuroplasticity. Dysfunctions in growth hormone, thyroid hormone release, opioid receptors, and substance P are also being explored. The addition of thyroid hormone to antidepressant treatment in refractory depression has been successful, and blockade of substance P receptors has also shown promise.[15-17]

Mechanism of Action of the Antidepressants

In the absence of a definitive theory for the pathogenesis of depression, it is useful to look at some of the commonalities that exist among the antidepressants to help explain at least some of the pathophysiology. In general, these drugs act by blocking reuptake of either serotonin or norepinephrine (Figure 16-1).[18] Normally, the major mechanism by which neurotransmission is terminated is by reuptake of the transmitter from the synaptic cleft back into the nerve terminal. From there, the neurotransmitter is either metabolized or stored in vesicles for future release. Reuptake is performed by a transmembrane transporter that carries sodium and chloride ions along with the neurotransmitter into the cell cytoplasm. By blocking the reuptake transporter with drugs, excess neurotransmitter is allowed to accumulate in the synaptic cleft. Excess amounts of serotonin or norepinephrine in the synaptic cleft lead to down-regulation of their postsynaptic receptors. It is theorized that this down-regulation of the receptors is what ultimately produces relief from depression.

Amphetamine and cocaine are similarly transported into the neuron by the transmembrane transporter.[18] However, this presents a problem because the transporters also allow reverse movement of serotonin and norepinephrine when the chemicals are displaced from the storage vesicles into the cytoplasm through the action of amphetamines. Therefore it is extremely dangerous to combine antidepressants with an amphetamine. The result

would be extremely high neurotransmitter concentrations in the synaptic cleft.

Another mechanism exerted by antidepressants is desensitization of autoreceptors.[18] Somatodendritic and terminal autoreceptors regulate transmitter release through feedback inhibition. If excess neurotransmitter is released, the chemical makes its way to the autoreceptor and shuts down the nerve. These receptors are viewed as the neuron's shut-off switch in response to excessive firing. Drug desensitization of these autoreceptors would block this turn-off switch, allowing the neuron to continue firing and releasing neurotransmitter. The result would be similar to blocking reuptake of the neurotransmitter in that higher concentrations of the chemical in the synaptic cleft would produce a down-regulation of the respective postsynaptic receptors.

Even though many of the older antidepressants focused on promoting higher neurotransmitter concentrations at the synaptic cleft, it has been determined that the availability of serotonin is critical for relief of depression. A third mechanism by which antidepressants may achieve their goal is through enhancing norepinephrine release, which in turn enhances serotonergic cell firing. Norepinephrine acts on the α_1 receptor of the serotonin neuron to stimulate firing and release of serotonin (Figure 16-2). The result is an elevated neurotransmitter concentration at the synaptic cleft and subsequent down-regulation of the postsynaptic receptors.

Given the fact that antidepressants are effective in reducing the symptoms of depression in many patients, it is reasonable to speculate from their mechanisms of action on the pathophysiology of this disorder. The action of these drugs suggests that relief from depression may have more to do with the number of active receptors than with the absolute neurotransmitter concentration. This explanation fills in some of the gaps in the original monoamine hypothesis because down-regulation of the receptors takes several weeks to occur; thus even though elevated neurotransmitter release is observed fairly soon, the relief of depression occurs at a later date.

Tricyclic Antidepressants

The tricyclic antidepressants (TCAs) are a group of drugs that share a common three-ring chemical structure.[5] They are similar in structure to the phenothiazines (antipsychotic agents) except they have an extra atom in the central ring (Figure 16-3).

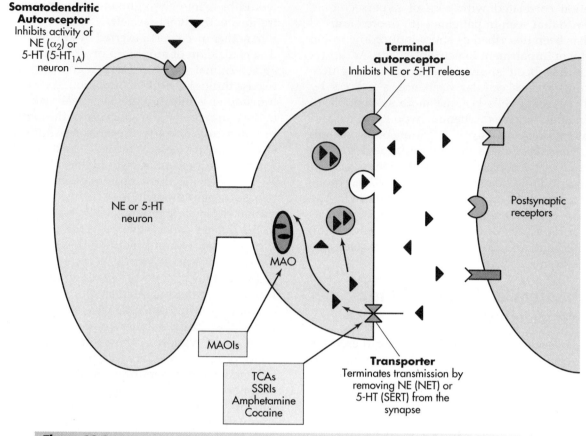

Somatodendritic Autoreceptor
Inhibits activity of NE (α_2) or 5-HT (5-HT_{1A}) neuron

Terminal autoreceptor
Inhibits NE or 5-HT release

NE or 5-HT neuron

MAO

MAOIs

TCAs
SSRIs
Amphetamine
Cocaine

Transporter
Terminates transmission by removing NE (NET) or 5-HT (SERT) from the synapse

Postsynaptic receptors

Figure 16-1

A noradrenergic or serotonergic synapse and sites at which some antidepressants may exert their actions. Tricyclic antidepressants, selective serotonin *(5-HT)* reuptake inhibitors, and some atypical antidepressants, as well as many other drugs such as amphetamine, act at the reuptake transporter *(NET* or *SERT* for norepinephrine *[NE]* or 5-HT, respectively). Monoamine oxidase *(MAO),* which is targeted by MAO inhibitors *(MAOIs),* is localized at the mitochondrial outer membrane. Somatodendritic and terminal autoreceptors regulate transmitter release through feedback inhibition of neuronal activity or inhibition of excitation-secretion coupling. The somatodendritic autoreceptors are innervated by recurrent collaterals from the same cell, by terminals from neighboring NE or 5-HT neurons, or by NE- or 5-HT–containing afferents from other brain regions. Dendritic release of transmitter may also activate somatodendritic autoreceptors. (From Brody MJ, Larner J, Minneman KP, eds. *Human Pharmacology: Molecular to Clinical.* 3rd ed. Philadelphia: Mosby; 1998.)

In fact, they were originally developed as antipsychotic drugs, but they were found to be useful only in reducing depression in schizophrenic individuals and not effective in reducing the psychosis.

Mechanism of Action of Tricyclic Antidepressants

As discussed previously, the main action of the TCAs is to block reuptake of serotonin and norepinephrine into the presynaptic terminal. Some are also effective at blocking dopamine uptake.[19] This is achieved by competitive inhibition of the binding site. However, synthesis of the neurotransmitters and their storage and release are not affected by these drugs.

Examples of TCAs include amitriptyline (also used to reduce pain in neurogenic pain syndromes), imipramine, nortriptyline, and clomipramine.[20] The choice of a TCA is based on the degree of sedation desired, or not desired, and the side effect profile (Table 16-1). For the most part, TCAs have equal effectiveness with a success rate of approximately

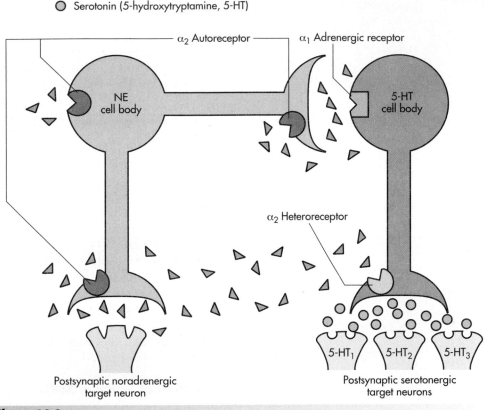

△ Norepinephrine
○ Serotonin (5-hydroxytryptamine, 5-HT)

Figure 16-2

Mechanisms for noradrenergic control of serotonin *(5-HT)* release. The mechanism whereby modulation of norepinephrine (NE) release may alter 5-HT release is shown. α_2-Adrenergic autoreceptors regulate NE release by a negative feedback process. Activation of somatodendritic autoreceptors decreases noradrenergic neuronal activity, and activation of terminal autoreceptors decreases release of the neurotransmitter. Noradrenergic terminals innervate 5-HT cell bodies, where stimulation of postsynaptic α_1-adrenergic receptors activates 5-HT cell activity, increasing 5-HT release. α_2-Adrenergic receptors also exist as heteroreceptors on serotonergic terminals, where their activation inhibits 5-HT release. Thus a drug that blocks α_2-adrenergic receptors, but not α_1-adrenergic receptors, increases NE release, and thereby increases 5-HT release. (From Brody MJ, Larner J, Minneman KP, eds. *Human Pharmacology: Molecular to Clinical.* 3rd ed. Philadelphia: Mosby; 1998.)

60%, which is similar to that of other antidepressant agents.[1]

Adverse Drug Reactions Associated with Tricyclic Antidepressants

TCAs have varying affinities for histamine, muscarinic, and α_1 adrenoceptors.[5] In fact, the action at these other neurochemical receptors is responsible for most of the side effects. TCAs act as antagonists at muscarinic receptors, producing dry mouth, constipation, urinary retention, blurred vision, and tachycardia. Blockade of histamine receptors produces sedation and weight gain, and the blockade at the adrenergic receptors produces orthostatic hypotension and dizziness. These side effects are especially problematic for the elderly patient because of an increased risk of falls. The TCAs also produce sexual dysfunction including decreased libido, abnormal ejaculation, and impotence. Prolongation of the QT interval on an electrocardiogram and its association with arrhythmia and sudden death pose another problem for the patient undergoing treatment.[21,22] This may be associated with the inhibition of a cardiac potassium channel

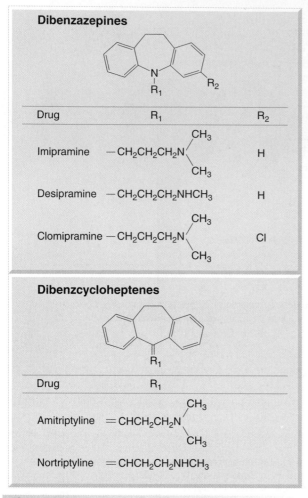

Figure 16-3

Chemical structures of tricyclic antidepressants. (From Rang HP, Dale MM, Ritter JM, Moore JL. *Pharmacology.* 5th ed. New York: Churchill Livingstone; 2003.)

in the ventricle known as the human ether-a-go-go related gene (HERG) channel. Because the TCAs bind to plasma proteins, their effects tend to be enhanced by aspirin, which competes with them for binding to albumin. In addition, these drugs potentiate the effect of alcohol and other sedatives.

TCAs have a narrow safety index; overdose occurs at about five times the daily dose.[23] Toxic effects include shock, metabolic acidosis, arrhythmias and conduction defects, tremors, delirium, and bowel and bladder paralysis. In addition, because most of the drugs have a long half-life, if a person survives the initial overdose, he or she is still at risk for cardiac events 3 to 4 days later.

Selective Serotonin Reuptake Inhibitors

The discovery of the selective serotonin reuptake inhibitors (SSRIs) represented a major advance in psychopharmacology. These were among the first drugs in psychiatry to have been developed through a process of rational drug development. Many of the other psychopharmaceuticals were developed serendipitously. The choice to selectively block the serotonin uptake pump was due to the presumed relationship between serotonin and depression, anxiety disorders, and pain syndromes, as well as the pharmacodynamics of the TCAs. In addition, they were developed to affect only the serotonin (5-hydroxytryptamine [5-HT) receptors (5-HT1A, 5-HT1D, 5-HT2A, 5-HT2C, and 5 HT3) and not the other neuroreceptors. Unlike the TCAs, SSRIs have no anticholinergic, histaminergic, or adrenergic properties. They also lack the cardiotoxic side effects commonly seen with the TCAs. Another important advantage to these drugs is that they have a higher safety index than the TCAs, but exactly how high has not been determined.[24]

Mechanism of Action of SSRIs

The leading hypothesis regarding the mechanism of action of these drugs is that they produce desensitization of the somatodendritic 5-HT1A autoreceptors in the midbrain raphe nucleus. Desensitization of these receptors increases serotonin levels in critical brain areas. In addition, studies on paroxetine show that in young depressed patients (20 to 30 years old), there is a down-regulation of the 5-HT2A, but this down-regulation is lessened in older subjects.[25,26]

Zimelidine, marketed by Astra, was the first SSRI to be developed.[24] It was approved for use in the early 1980s in Europe but was soon withdrawn because of reports of Guillain-Barré syndrome in some patients. Shortly after this withdrawal, fluoxetine and three other drugs in this category appeared on the market almost simultaneously: citalopram, sertraline, fluvoxamine, and paroxetine. The sixth and newest agent, escitalopram, has been released more recently. These are now among the most prescribed agents in medicine.

Although the five SSRIs listed previously have the same mechanism of action, there are some differences between them regarding their inhibition of the cytochrome P450 enzymes.[24,27] Paroxetine and fluoxetine are modest inhibitors of these enzymes,

Table 16-1

Side Effect Profiles of Selected Antidepressant Drugs

Drug	Side Effects						
	Anticholinergic	Drowsiness	Agitation	Orthostatic Hypotension	Arrhythmia	GI	Weight Gain
Amitriptyline	4^+	4^+	0	4^+	3^+	0	4^+
Desipramine	1^+	1^+	1^+	2^+	2^+	0	1^+
Imipramine	3^+	3^+	1^+	4^+	3^+	1^+	3^+
Trazodone	0	4^+	0	1^+	1^+	1^+	1^+
Bupropion	0	0	2^+	0	0	3^+	0
Fluoxetine	0	0	2^+	0	0	3^+	0
Paroxetine	0	0	2^+	0	0	3^+	0
Sertraline	0	0	2^+	0	0	3^+	0

Adapted from McKenry LM, Salerno E. *Mosby's Pharmacology in Nursing*. St Louis: Mosby; 2003.
0, Absent or seldom; *4*$^+$, very common; GI, gastrointestinal.
Data were obtained from the following: Depression Guideline Panel. (1993). Depression in Primary Care. Vol 2. Treatment of major depression. Clinical Practice Guideline #5. Rockville, MD: Department of Health and Human Services, Public Health Service, Agency for Health Care Policy and Research. DHCPR Pub. No. 93-0551.

whereas citalopram has little effect on them, indicating that it has fewer drug-drug interactions compared with the other four SSRIs. Paroxetine is viewed as having more side effects, particularly sexual dysfunction and weight gain.[28] Another difference between the SSRIs is in their half-lives. Fluoxetine has a half-life of 1 to 4 days, longer than the other drugs. This is helpful for the patient demonstrating poor compliance because omission of one daily dose will have virtually no effect on concentration. However, if it becomes necessary to switch to another drug (perhaps a TCA), the patient would have to endure a long washout period before the new drug could be administered.

Indications for Use of SSRIs

The number one indication for SSRIs is in the treatment of major depression. Studies have shown superiority of these agents compared with placebo, and several meta-analyses have indicated that the TCAs and SSRIs have equal efficacy.[29,30] In addition, TCAs and SSRIs have similar time lines with regard to onset of action. However, the major difference between the two drug categories in these studies was that fewer patients discontinued their SSRIs because of adverse drug reactions (ADRs).[31]

SSRIs have also been the focus of other large studies examining their effectiveness in the treatment of obsessive compulsive disorder (OCD), social phobia, generalized anxiety disorder (GAD), panic disorder, posttraumatic stress disorder, premenstrual syndrome, and eating disorders, as well as depression associated with medical illness. In fact, they have been shown to be superior to other drugs in the treatment of panic disorders, social phobia, and OCD; but for some of these disorders, a higher dose and longer duration of treatment may be necessary compared with the treatment for depression.[32-36] Treatment of these conditions also requires cognitive-behavioral therapy for improved efficacy. Expectations regarding the SSRIs for the treatment of eating disorders, anorexia nervosa, and bulimia nervosa have been lowered because clinical investigations with these drugs have resulted in mixed results. A lack of efficacy has been particularly observed in treatment of patients with anorexia who are typically malnourished and underweight. It is theorized that the lack of adequate nutrients affects serotonin synthesis, which lowers treatment efficacy because once a normalization of weight is achieved, the SSRIs reduce relapse rates.[37]

Side Effects of SSRIs

The SSRIs have relatively few side effects compared with the TCAs because they lack affinity for the adrenergic, muscarinic, and histaminergic receptors.

Minor ADRs include nausea, anorexia, and weight loss; but most patients develop tolerance to these effects with continued use. Gastrointestinal (GI) symptoms are exacerbated if these drugs are combined with a nonsteroidal antiinflammatory drug.[38] Lasting side effects include bleeding because SSRIs inhibit platelet aggregation and sexual dysfunction.[28,39] Sexual dysfunction (erectile dysfunction and delayed ejaculation in men and anorgasmia in women) is a leading reason for switching to another type of antidepressant.[24,40] However, the SSRIs, specifically fluoxetine, may be used in the treatment of premature ejaculation, exploiting the sexual dysfunction side effect.

Rarer ADRs include an association with the syndrome of inappropriate antidiuretic hormone secretion and serotonin syndrome.[24,41] The syndrome of inappropriate antidiuretic hormone secretion results in hyponatremia, which may manifest as nervousness, agitation, and worsening of depression. Serotonin syndrome usually occurs from the interaction of two or more drugs that potentiate the central effects of serotonin.[42] It is characterized by changes in mental state, restlessness, hyperreflexia, diaphoresis, shivering, and tremors. It has occurred with the combination of SSRIs and monoamine oxidase inhibitors (MAOIs) (see discussion of monoamine oxidase inhibitors) and the combination of SSRIs and the diet drug fenfluramine. In addition, some other drugs with MAOI activity, such as isoniazid, linezolid, dextromethorphan, tramadol, and St. John's Wort, can cause this syndrome when taken with an SSRI. On very rare occasions, it has occurred with SSRIs alone. Treatment is immediate withdrawal of the drugs and provision of supportive measures. Both of these syndromes can result in death.

More troublesome ADRs include neurological effects. Several movement disorders have been reported including akathisia, dystonia, dyskinesia, tardive dyskinesia, parkinsonism, and bruxism.[43] Most of these ADRs were observed in patients who had some predisposition, a history of antipsychotic use, or existing neurological diagnoses. Treatment strategies include lowering the dose, discontinuation of the drugs, and addition of a benzodiazepine, anticholinergic, or β-blocker to reduce tremors. Other neurological effects include the production or exacerbation of restlessness, agitation, anxiety, and headaches. Insomnia may also be a problem, but this can be treated by morning dosing.[44]

Abrupt discontinuation of many drugs produces some unpleasant withdrawal symptoms, and the SSRIs are not immune to this event.[45] The most common symptoms include GI problems, flu-like symptoms, disequilibrium, extrapyramidal symptoms, anxiety, crying spells, irritability, confusion, and sleep disturbances. Fluvoxamine and paroxetine have a greater risk of producing a withdrawal syndrome than the other drugs, possibly because paroxetine has some anticholinergic properties and sudden cessation of the drug could lead to a cholinergic rebound. Another explanation is that abrupt elimination of the drug would lead to a deficiency of serotonin, or at the very least, a neuronal dysregulation. In fact, sudden withdrawal of any of the antidepressants may create a stress response affecting many of the neuronal systems which could cause further dysfunction and compromise long-term outcome.[46] Patients with panic disorders are particularly susceptible to the withdrawal syndrome.

SSRIs and Suicide: Are They Safe for Children?

Whether SSRIs increase the risk of suicide and whether they are safe for children have emerged as two controversies stemming from some case reports that appeared in the literature in 1990, as well as a "Dear Colleague" letter from the United Kingdom's Committee on Safety of Medicine.[47] In this letter the committee advises physicians not to use paroxetine to treat childhood or adolescent depression.[48] The data (which were unpublished) leading to these recommendations came from three clinical trials presented to the Food and Drug Administration (FDA) by GlaxoSmithKline in a quest to gain approval for the use of paroxetine to treat OCD in children. According to the *Medical Letter,* which viewed the reports, in 1134 children, the effectiveness of paroxetine was no different from that of placebo. However, the treatment group did show significant emotional instability in the form of crying, mood alterations, suicidal thoughts, and attempted suicide. At present, only fluoxetine has been approved by the FDA for the treatment of depression in children, and only fluvoxamine and sertraline have been approved for the treatment of OCD in children. The FDA has followed the example of its counterpart in the United Kingdom by recommending that paroxetine not be prescribed for children.

To address the concerns over suicide rates with SSRIs, particularly in the lay press, the FDA recently reviewed suicide data for subjects who had participated in clinical trials of nine antidepressants including SSRIs and some newer atypical antidepressants (fluoxetine, sertraline, paroxetine, venlafaxine, nefazodone, mirtazapine, sustained-release bupropion, extended-release venlafaxine, and citalopram).[47,49] Rates of successful suicide were tabulated for each of the drugs investigated. A total of 48,277 depressed patients participated in the trials, and 77 committed suicide. The results demonstrated no difference in suicide rates between antidepressant- and placebo-treated individuals. In addition, there was no difference between the SSRIs and the other type of antidepressants. The FDA concluded that use of antidepressants from any of the classes of drugs had little effect on suicide rates in these clinical trials. However, there are a few problems with this report that indicate further studies on this subject are needed. First, with regard to children, the FDA study did not distinguish children from adults, so we do not know how many children committed suicide. Second, data were collected on successfully completed suicides but not on number of attempts. In addition, there was no information offered on the percentage of subjects who experienced an increase in suicidal ideation. Third, randomized controlled studies designed to prove clinical efficacy are typically brief compared with the length of time a patient would be expected to be taking an antidepressant. Some suicides may have been missed simply because they occurred after the study was terminated.[50]

Despite the FDA's current support of SSRIs, discussion on both sides of the argument continues. Physicians who argue that there is no increased risk of suicide with the SSRIs report that many studies show a marked reduction in suicidal ideation.[51] They also argue that although written prescriptions for these drugs are growing worldwide, this has coincided with a decrease in successful suicide attempts.[52] Others argue that if there were, in fact, an increase in suicides in some of the studies reviewed, it may have been a function of patient selection rather than a result of drug therapy.[53] Because patients who have a history of self-harm have an increased risk of suicide, if the studies did not include proper screening for this history, the review would represent a case of bias. In this case, what should be discussed are new therapeutic options for individuals who have resistant depression as opposed to the risk of suicide with

the SSRIs. Another point to consider is that many patients are undertreated and do not receive an adequate maintenance dose for a sufficient length of time. Perhaps the only conclusion that can be made from this ongoing debate is that further study on the safety of SSRIs is needed. The significant take-away message for physical therapists is to be alert for any increase in suicidal thoughts or behavior among their patients.

Returning to the issue of whether to give SSRIs to children, several studies have shown these drugs to be effective in the treatment of depression on at least a short-term basis.[48,54] Adverse effects have been similar to those reported in adults—nausea, nervousness, insomnia, and fatigue. However, increases in motor activity appear to be more prevalent in children than adults. Although these issues do not seem to be terribly significant, there are some concerns about dosing in children. The first is that in some children SSRI therapy appears to suppress growth hormone secretion enough that replacement therapy with somatropin is necessary.[55] Another concern is that the long-term effects of these drugs on the brain and personality development and behavior are unknown.

A New Look at SSRIs from a Neurologist's Perspective

It has been determined that drugs that increase brain amine concentrations increase the rate and level of motor recovery from brain lesions in animals. In addition, single doses of fluoxetine and paroxetine have been shown to improve motor performance through practice in healthy individuals.[56] As a result of these discoveries, plus the fact that depression in stroke is associated with a poor outcome, several researchers have examined the effects of fluoxetine on motor and functional performance in patients who sustained ischemic strokes.[57] In one study, subjects who were unable to walk after an ischemic stroke in the area of the middle cerebral artery received physical therapy with placebo, with the norepinephrine reuptake inhibitor maprotiline, or with fluoxetine. Activities of daily living were assessed by the Barthel Index; the degree of neurological impairment was assessed by a neurological scale for subjects with hemiplegia; and mood was assessed with a depression rating scale. After 3 months of treatment, the greatest improvement in motor performance was observed in the fluoxetine group, and the poorest performance was seen in the maprotiline group.[57] In another study, a single dose of fluoxetine was given to patients in the early phases of recovery (2 weeks) after lacunar stroke.[58] Data were collected during a finger-tapping activity and during a nine-hole peg test of finger dexterity. Improvements were noted in speed of execution. Fluoxetine also increased grip strength in the involved extremity compared with placebo. The very simplified explanation is that SSRIs, through the serotonin system, stimulate the pyramidal cells. Another explanation is that fluoxetine improves attention, resulting in improved motor performance. The coupling of motor activity with drug administration as therapy after a stroke is an exciting concept.

Serotonin and Norepinephrine Reuptake Inhibitors

In recent years, another controversy over selective versus multitransmitter antidepressants has erupted. TCAs have broad influence over many neurotransmitter systems and thus also produce many side effects. The SSRIs produce few side effects but technically just alter the serotonergic system. Now a drug that functions in between the two extremes of selectivity is available—venlafaxine.[59] Venlafaxine is very similar to the TCAs but lacks the cholinergic and histaminergic properties. It is a potent serotonin reuptake inhibitor at low doses, but at higher doses, it also acts to block norepinephrine reuptake. It is a weak inhibitor of dopamine uptake but has no affinity for the other neurotransmitter systems. Its potential for anticholinergic and orthostatic hypotensive effects is minimal.

Venlafaxine has shown efficacy in the treatment of GAD, depression, and at high doses, treatment-resistant depression. Traditionally, treatment of GAD has consisted of benzodiazepines, but the high comorbidity of GAD and depression has led to the use of antidepressants for this condition. In addition, results of recent studies suggest that GAD's pathophysiology relates to much more than just abnormalities of the γ-aminobutyric acid (GABA) system and gives credence to the use of drugs with a broader pharmacological spectrum.[60] Remission rates with extended-release venlafaxine for GAD have been consistently higher than those with placebo.[61,62] With regard to depression, venlafaxine has demonstrated superiority over SSRIs and placebo; remission rates are higher and remission is reached, on average, after 2 weeks of treatment as opposed to 4 weeks.[63-65] Most of the side effects associated with venlafaxine are similar to those of the SSRIs, except that venlafaxine can cause increases in blood pressure.

Mirtazapine is another antidepressant with broader activity than the SSRIs. It is actually labeled as a noradrenergic and specific serotonergic antidepressant.[5] This drug blocks α_2 autoreceptors on noradrenergic nerves and increases serotonergic neuronal firing by acting on the noradrenergic α_2 heteroreceptors sitting on the serotonin cell body. It is also a blocker at 5-HT$_{2A}$ and 5-HT$_3$ receptors. This drug produces less nausea and anxiety and fewer headaches than the SSRIs, but because it has some affinity for the muscarinic and histamine receptors, it produces an increase in appetite, weight gain, and sedation. This drug is being targeted for resistant depression and the prevention of relapses.[66] Comparative studies are needed to determine its effectiveness.

Atypical Antidepressants

Bupropion is a drug that resembles amphetamine in structure but is not clinically related. It appears to block reuptake of dopamine and norepinephrine. Because of its action on the dopaminergic system, it has been used to treat addictions (primarily smoking), as well as to relieve depression. Also because of its influence on the dopaminergic neurons, this drug is being investigated to determine its effect on periodic limb movement disorder brought on by the more traditional antidepressants.[67] ADRs include weight loss, nausea, increased sweating, tremor, and an increased risk of seizures, especially in persons with a prior diagnosis of bulimia.

Trazodone is another drug in this category. It blocks serotonin reuptake and also blocks the postsynaptic serotonin receptors. However, it does have α_1 antagonist and antihistaminergic properties.[68] It is considered an antidepressant but is currently used in the treatment of insomnia, having shown some benefit in depressed and nondepressed individuals.[69] The side effects include orthostatic hypotension, dizziness, and GI disturbances. Atrial and ventricular arrhythmias have also been reported with this drug.

Monoamine Oxidase Inhibitors

MAOIs directly increase the activity of noradrenergic synapses by inhibiting the enzymes MAO-A and

MAO-B, which are involved in the degradation of norepinephrine, dopamine, and serotonin.[5] These drugs were used with greater frequency years ago, but because of their adverse effects, they have largely been replaced by the SSRIs and other agents listed previously. Side effects include central nervous system (CNS) excitation, restlessness, irritability, sleep loss, tremor, confusion, dry mouth, and urinary retention—many of which result from central and peripheral anticholinergic actions. In addition, hypertensive reactions are likely if a patient consumes foods containing tyramine. Tyramine is normally degraded by MAO-A in the GI tract. However, if the enzyme is blocked, tyramine entering the circulation stimulates the release of norepinephrine. Foods rich in tyramine include cheese, beer, red wine, raisins, and avocados and must be avoided by patients taking these drugs. The exception is a new MAOI called *moclobemide*, which reversibly inhibits MAO-A, as opposed to the irreversible inhibition produced by the other drugs in this category. A risk of hypertension still exists, but higher levels of tyramine must be consumed before this occurs. Because of the risk of hypertension and several drug-drug interactions (cimetidine, meperidine, SSRIs, TCAs, and many over-the-counter-products), MAOIs are used only for drug-resistant or atypical depression.

Guidelines for the Use of Antidepressants/Therapeutic Concerns

The choice of antidepressant for a particular patient is usually made according to the drug's side effect profile and the relative risk posed by its drug-drug interactions. If a patient experiences a great deal of anxiety and insomnia, then an agent with a sedating effect is used. For patients who experience fatigue along with their depression, the SSRIs are chosen. However, young or middle aged men may reject these drugs because they diminish libido. In addition, if a drug has been used successfully in the past, it is usually tried again with subsequent bouts of depression. However, a risk of intermittent treatment is that the drug's effectiveness may diminish with each use. If one antidepressant is not effective after a reasonable trial period (6 to 8 weeks), then another agent with a different neurotransmitter action is administered. Loss of effectiveness with intermittent use is the reason that many psychiatrists

advocate continuous dosing even when symptoms improve.

The physical therapist treating patients taking antidepressants should always be aware of worsening symptoms. Patients should be assessed for appearance, behavior, speech, and level of interest. Negative changes in these areas should be reported to the physician, as well as any hypomania or manic behavior, because use of antidepressants may reveal undiagnosed bipolar illness. Blood pressure should be monitored for hypotension, and pulse should be checked for arrhythmias. Some of the TCAs and SSRIs may cause tremors so that success in performing fine motor tasks may be difficult to achieve. Success at strengthening activities may also be blunted because of sedation and a diminished level of alertness.

ANXIETY DISORDERS AND SEDATIVE AND ANXIOLYTIC DRUGS

The concept of anxiety has evolved to include a functional and normal mental state, as well as a pathological state or a symptom of a broader psychiatric disorder. Normal anxiety is useful in that it controls an animal's or human's response to a threat and assists in survival. Therefore anxiety is a normal response under appropriate conditions, but it becomes pathological when it is out of proportion to the situation.

The classification of anxiety disorders is based on the symptoms displayed by a patient. The *DSM-IV* divides anxiety disorders into the following categories: panic disorder without agoraphobia, panic disorder with agoraphobia (fearful avoidance), agoraphobia, specific phobia, social phobia (or social anxiety disorder), GAD, OCD, acute stress disorder, and posttraumatic stress disorder. Anxiety can also be divided according to whether it is a state (short-lived and dependent on stressors in the environment) or a trait that is a long-lasting feature of a person's personality. Although anxiety disorders present in a number of different forms, they probably all have some common neurological pathways.

There are several common somatic and psychological symptoms of anxiety.[60] Symptoms usually include a combination of somatic and psychological complaints. Patients might report restlessness, inability to relax, muscle aching or tension, fatigue, and some GI symptoms such as constipation or diarrhea or difficulty swallowing ("lump in the throat").

GAD usually occurs before the age of 40 years; this disorder is chronic, although symptoms may vary. During a panic attack, patients may describe other physical complaints including chest pain, palpitations, sweating, hyperventilation, hot flashes, nausea, tremor, or dizziness. Psychological issues reported include excessive worry, irritability, sleep disturbances, poor concentration, and fear.

Evidence regarding the neuroanatomy and neurochemistry of anxiety comes from animal studies including stimulation and ablation of neuroanatomical areas, human studies with magnetic resonance imaging and positron emission tomography, and information derived from pharmacological interventions.[70,71] The brainstem areas mediate the physiological manifestations of anxiety, fear, and panic. The periaqueductal gray matter (PAG) receives descending afferents from the paralimbic cortex and limbic systems and afferents from the deep sensory structures. Stimulation of the ventrolateral PAG produces hypotension, bradycardia, and analgesia; whereas stimulation of the lateral PAG produces tachycardia, increased blood flow, and other manifestations seen in anxiety and panic. Direct stimulation of the locus coeruleus (a noradrenergic nucleus located lateral to the PAG) also produces anxious behavior and panic. Anxiolytic drugs and antiadrenergic drugs block the locus coeruleus. The hypothalamus, which receives input from the limbic system and the locus coeruleus, is central to the neuroendocrine response to anxiety through the activation of the hypothalamus-pituitary-adrenal axis and secretion of hormones involved in stress reactions. Another neuroanatomical area associated with anxiety is the limbic system, which has a central role in producing emotions. Within the limbic system lies the amygdala, which has widespread connections to the other areas involved in anxiety and also has control over motor, neuroendocrine, autonomic, and respiratory responses seen during a panic attack. The amygdala has recently been recognized for its role in producing fear and therefore represents a target for anxiolytic agents.[72] Lastly, it has been shown that chronic stress and high levels of cortisol lead to a reduction in hippocampal volume, and the hippocampus also lies within the limbic system.

Most of the research into the neurochemistry of anxiety has centered on the monoamines: serotonin, norepinephrine, and the GABA-benzodiazepine receptor complex. The noradrenergic theory of anxiety states that increased noradrenergic release leads to arousal.[73] Supporting evidence based on the actions of amphetamines and cocaine, as well as β-agonists, in producing the peripheral symptoms of anxiety exists. Further support for the role of the sympathetic system in producing anxiety comes from the activation of the presynaptic α_2 adrenoceptors in the locus coeruleus. Blocking these α_2 receptors with yohimbine leads to anxiety, whereas administration of clonidine (an α_2 agonist) reduces sympathetic outflow and decreases anxiety.

A relationship between anxiety and the serotonergic system has been known to exist for a long time, but over the last decade, research into this area has dramatically increased. The impetus for this has come from the success of the SSRIs in reducing depression and the realization that depression and anxiety often exist together.[74,75] However, this relationship is very complex. Increases in serotonin at the PAG are thought to reduce panic, but increases at the amygdala are thought to be anxiogenic. This is further complicated by the fact that at least in depression, it is not the absolute concentration of the neurotransmitter that is important, but rather the activity at and sensitivity of the receptors. Some research suggests that activation of the $5-HT_{2C}$ receptor in the PAG exerts anti-panic effects.[76] Weeding out this complexity is clearly beyond the scope of this text.

The association of anxiety with the GABAergic system has been demonstrated clinically by the efficacy of the benzodiazepines in reducing acute anxiety. Alcohol, barbiturates, and benzodiazepines acting on the GABA-gated chloride channel produce a rapid anxiolytic action by inhibiting the release of many neurotransmitters.[77] Specifically, these agents facilitate the opening of the channel, allowing chloride ions to flow into the postsynaptic neuron and creating a more negative (inhibitory) membrane potential.[78] The benzodiazepines bind to the $GABA_A$ receptor, which is a pentameric complex containing 18 or more protein subunits.[79] A mutation in one of the α subunits of a single amino acid eliminates benzodiazepine sensitivity. This information has been transformed into a series of experiments on transgenic mice in which this mutation was induced in four different α subunits. Each of these mutations was responsible for eliminating one or two different effects of the benzodiazepines. For example, a mutation in the α_1-subunit (the most widely expressed variant in the wild) eliminated the sedative and amnesic actions but not the anxiolytic effects, and a mutation on the α_2-subunit eliminated the anxiolytic effects but did not alter the sedative effects. It is hoped that these experiments will lead to more information on the role of abnormal benzodiazepine receptors in psychiatric disorders and assist in the development of partial agonists at the benzodiazepine receptor site that can reduce anxiety without producing sedation.[80]

Because it is clear that anxiety states can be affected by either the serotoninergic or the GABAergic system, another area of study is the interconnections between the two systems. There is evidence that administration of a single dose of an SSRI (citalopram) to healthy volunteers increases GABA concentrations.[81] In addition, a clinical interaction has been demonstrated by a reduction in serotonin function with a benzodiazepine and the return of anxiety when the drug is withdrawn, coinciding with serotonin function.[75] In the future, efficacy may result from developing compounds that exert GABAergic control over serotonin neurons.[82]

Barbiturates

The barbiturates are CNS depressants capable of producing effects that range from mild sedation and a reduction in anxiety to unconsciousness and death by respiratory and cardiac failure in a dose-dependent manner.[5] They act at the $GABA_A$ receptor to enhance the action of GABA but at a different site than that targeted by the benzodiazepines. Because of the risk of overdose and dependence, only a few barbiturates, with very specific indications, are used today. The ultra-short-acting thiopental is used to induce anesthesia and the longer-acting phenobarbital is used to control seizures.

Barbiturates are, for the most part, rapidly absorbed and have a quick onset of action because of their high lipid solubility.[83] Initially, patients experience dizziness, followed by sedation. The adverse effects are extensions of the CNS depression and include confusion, ataxia, and impairment of mental and psychomotor functions. All of these effects are increased if the drug is combined with other CNS depressants. Because of their lipid solubility, barbiturates tend to collect in the adipose tissue, only to be released slowly back into the circulation to again pass into the brain. This is what produces the "hangover" effect the next day. Paradoxical

reactions consisting of excitement, confusion, and hostility may also occur and are more common in the elderly. Other side effects that are not neurologically related include joint and muscle pain, vomiting, sore throat, fever, and angioedema.

Barbiturates are inducers of the P450 enzyme system, which means they increase the activity of the enzymes that metabolize them.[84] Tolerance to the sedative-anxiolytic effect develops within 7 to 14 days, and use of these drugs for a period of only 1 month can lead to physical dependence. The drugs with the shorter half-life tend to be the more troublesome drugs because sudden discontinuation will produce a rapid and severe withdrawal syndrome. Sudden withdrawal produces anxiety, irritability, agitation, tremor, insomnia, and weakness.[85] Some patients may have generalized seizures or experience acute psychosis. Cessation of administration of the longer-duration agents will produce a withdrawal syndrome that is slower in onset and less severe but of longer duration. For the purpose of avoiding severe withdrawal symptoms, patients are switched to a drug with a longer half-life, and then the dose is reduced by one eighth every 2 weeks.

Benzodiazepines

The first benzodiazepine, chlordiazepoxide, was synthesized by accident in 1961 by Hoffman la Roche Laboratories.[5] As soon as its pharmacological action was noted, it quickly became one of the most popular drugs worldwide. The benzodiazepines continue to be commonly prescribed but because of tolerance and dependence issues, interest has begun to wane.[86] Expert panels have recommended a reduction in the use of benzodiazepines for anxiety disorders, with the exception of short-term use for acute anxiety and panic, but these drugs continue to be preferred by primary care physicians as first-line agents for all anxiety disorders except OCD.[87]

The benzodiazepines act like the barbiturates by binding to the $GABA_A$ receptor and facilitating the opening of the chloride channel. Therefore side effects are also similar to those of the barbiturates but are milder.[88,89] Sedation, vertigo, dizziness, dysarthria, and ataxia are common effects, as are alterations in judgment, memory, and concentration. Tasks requiring speed and accuracy can be markedly disrupted. The elderly, in particular, are sensitive to the psychomotor impairments associated with these drugs, leading to an increased risk of falls, and the memory loss may be mistaken for dementia. Driving or operating heavy machinery can be dangerous under the influence of these drugs. Epidemiological data indicate that benzodiazepines contribute to car accidents. Even though effects are strongly dose related, some benzodiazepines, such as diazepam, are more sedating than others. In addition, the longer-acting agents are more likely to produce excessive sedation, which can last for much of the day. Paradoxical arousal responses can also occur and present a major management problem. The patient may become panicky or anxious and may even become hostile or experience uncontrollable crying. Reduction in dose or total drug withdrawal may be needed to reverse the reaction.

Benzodiazepines have a few advantages over the barbiturates in that they have a lower potential for abuse and fewer drug interactions and are associated with fewer fatalities. Overdose rarely ends in death unless a benzodiazepine is combined with other CNS depressants such as alcohol, opioids, or barbiturates. Antegrade amnesia, the inability to remember events that occur after dosing, may be considered either an adverse or beneficial effect, depending on the patient and the desire to remember a medical procedure in which he or she has been sedated.

At least 13 benzodiazepines are available. They have basically identical mechanisms of action, but differences in their pharmacokinetics exist. In addition, a few show some selectivity of action; for example, clonazepam possesses good anticonvulsant activity with less sedation. The main differences between the drugs are related to duration of action. Diazepam, chlordiazepoxide, and flurazepam are long acting with duration of action lasting 1 to 3 days. These are long acting because they are broken down to active metabolites that have additional half lives. Lorazepam is considered an intermediate-acting drug with a half-life of 10 to 20 hours. Triazolam is a short-acting benzodiazepine with a half-life of only 2 to 4 hours.

Patients may develop tolerance to both the therapeutic effects and ADRs associated with benzodiazepines.[88,90] However, this tolerance issue is not as dramatic as that seen with narcotics. Patients receiving high doses or those who have taken the drugs for long periods can have severe or even fatal withdrawal reactions if the medication is stopped abruptly. Withdrawal symptoms begin

5 to 10 days after a long-acting drug is stopped (diazepam) and as soon as 48 hours after withdrawal of an intermediate-acting drug. Withdrawal symptoms are similar to those of barbiturate withdrawal but may also include perceptual dysfunction such as photophobia, hyperacusis, and the feeling of being in constant movement. For the purpose of avoiding withdrawal, patients who have taken the short-acting drugs should be switched to longer-acting ones, and then the dosage should be reduced slowly over time (6 to 8 weeks). Slow withdrawal will also minimize the rebound insomnia that may occur with these agents.

Clinical Considerations with Benzodiazepines

Many patients take benzodiazepines for long periods. However, benzodiazepines are designed to treat symptoms of anxiety for short periods (no more than 3 to 4 months) while the patient works on the causative factors of a disorder.[91] Many elderly patients take the long-acting agents over an extended period, which leads not only to dependence but also to daily fatigue, ataxia, increased risk of falls, and problems with judgment.[92] This presents a challenge for the treating therapist because these side effects are not compatible with many of our physical therapy goals, particularly strengthening interventions.

The benzodiazepines interfere with the sleep cycle, even though they are often prescribed for sleep disturbances.[68] The normal sleep cycle consists of non-rapid eye movement (non-REM) sleep and REM sleep. The non-REM portion is further divided into four stages, with the depth of sleep increasing from stage 1 to stage 4. Stages 3 and 4 together are known as deep sleep. Cycling between the stages occurs throughout the night, with each cycle lasting approximately 90 to 100 minutes. Most benzodiazepines reduce REM sleep but increase time spent in the intermediate stages. The patient may end up sleeping more but not feeling any more rested. In addition, some researchers believe that reducing REM sleep results in an REM rebound along with vivid dreams and nightmares after the medication is withdrawn. Another problem is that the use of these drugs for more than 1 to 2 weeks leads to tolerance to their effect on sleep. At least five benzodiazepines have been approved by the FDA for the treatment of insomnia. They seem to span all categories regarding duration of action. Triazolam is the shortest-acting drug but has been associated with rebound insomnia and excessive anterograde amnesia, as well as with confusion and bizarre behavior. The others are longer-acting drugs that lead to considerable daytime sedation, which is unacceptable to most patients. Zolpidem is actually a nonbenzodiazepine hypnotic that induces sleep at lower doses than the benzodiazepines with fewer effects on stage 4 and REM sleep. Less tolerance and less rebound insomnia are associated with this drug. It binds to the $GABA_A$ receptor but at a different site than the other drugs, so it lacks some of the properties of benzodiazepines. Zolpidem is devoid of the anticonvulsant, muscle relaxant, and antianxiety properties associated with the benzodiazepines.

Azapirones (Buspirone)

Buspirone is a drug for the treatment of anxiety.[5] It does not bind to the $GABA_A$ receptor but instead is a partial agonist at the $5\text{-}HT_{1A}$ receptor. The $5\text{-}HT_{1A}$ receptors are inhibitory presynaptic receptors and, when stimulated, actually reduce the firing of the serotonin neurons. Buspirone offers several advantages over the benzodiazepines because it does not produce sedation, amnesia, dependence, or tolerance.[93] However, it may take as long as 3 weeks to become active, and its effectiveness is not universal. Patients who have previously been treated with the benzodiazepines do not do as well when they take buspirone. In addition, buspirone is no better than placebo when used for the prevention of panic attacks and has only a modest impact on social phobia, although greater efficacy is seen when it is combined with an SSRI. Side effects are mild and consist of dizziness, headache, and lightheadedness.

SSRIs for Anxiety

The SSRIs are beginning to assume the leading role in the treatment of all types of anxiety, particularly when depression and anxiety occur together. They are the drugs of choice for the treatment of OCD and are good alternatives for treating anxiety in patients who have a history of substance abuse, panic, and social phobia.[94-96] In addition, they may be combined with a benzodiazepine for treatment of acute anxiety; and patients may then continue to take the SSRI while the benzodiazepine is withdrawn. They are particularly useful for treating anxiety in the elderly and for long-term anxiety management because these are cases in which benzodiazepines should be avoided.[60]

Venlafaxine for Anxiety

Venlafaxine extended-release has received approval for the long-term treatment of GAD.[97] It demonstrated efficacy for the treatment of GAD compared with placebo in a 6-month randomized controlled trial.[61,62] Further studies in which venlafaxine is compared with both SSRIs and Buspirone are needed.

ACTIVITIES 16

■ 1. A 32-year-old female patient has been attending physical therapy for the treatment of a herniated disk diagnosed 6 months ago. She has been in a great deal of pain and is depressed. Her husband brought her to your clinic today because she started displaying "odd behavior" this morning. He would like your opinion on what is going on and your advice on how to handle this situation. You are quite alarmed when you see the patient. She appears to be very agitated and unaware of where she is, and she may be having hallucinations. Her husband reports that she recently began taking an antidepressant (2 weeks ago), but he cannot remember which one or how much of the drug was prescribed. He also states that his wife was not responding to the medication. You take the patient's pulse and determine that there are cardiac irregularities.

Q Questions:

a. What is your immediate course of action?
b. What additional information should you obtain from the patient or her husband?
c. What do you think is happening?

■ 2. Given the side effects associated with sedative-hypnotic drugs, what nonpharmacological treatments can you offer a patient having difficulty falling asleep?

3. Many of our physical therapy patients receive prescriptions for benzodiazepines to reduce anxiety or to provide assistance for sleep. What side effects or adverse reactions should they be monitored for?

References

1. Wong ML, Licinio J. Research and treatment approaches to depression. *Nat Rev Neurosci.* 2001;2:343-351.
2. Lindeman S, Hamalainen J, Isometsa E, et al. The 12-month prevalence and risk factors for major depressive episode in Finland: representative sample of 5993 adults. *Acta Psychiatr Scand.* 2000;102(3):178-184.
3. Tomoda A, Mori K, Kimura M, Takahashi T, Kitamura T. One-year prevalence and incidence of depression among first-year university students in Japan: a preliminary study. *Psychiatry Clin Neurosci.* 2000;54:583-588.
4. Klein DN, Santiago NJ. Dysthymia and chronic depression: introduction, classification, risk factors, and course. *J Clin Psychol.* 2003;59(8):807-816.
5. Rang HP, Dale MM, Ritter JM, Moore JL. *Pharmacology.* 5th ed. New York: Churchill Livingstone; 2003.
6. Roose SP. Treatment of depression in patients with heart disease. *J Clin Psychol.* 2003;54(3):262-268.
7. Brown SE, Varghese FP, McEwen BS. Association of depression with medical illness: does cortisol play a role? *J Clin Psychol.* 2004;55(1):1-9.
8. Olfson M, Broadhead WE, Weissman MM, et al. Subthreshold psychiatric symptoms in a primary care group practice. *Arch Gen Psychiatry.* 1996;53(10):880-886.
9. Bell C, Abrams J, Nutt D. Tryptophan depletion and its implications for psychiatry. *Br J Psychiatry.* 2001;178(5):399-405.
10. Miller HL, Delgado PL, Salomon RM, et al. Clinical and biochemical effects of catecholamine depletion on antidepressant-induced remission of depression. *Arch Gen Psychiatry.* 1996;53(2):117-128.
11. Manji H, Drevets WC, Charney DS. The cellular neurobiology of depression. *Nat Med.* 2001;7(5):541-547.
12. Doris A, Ebmeier K, Shajahan P. Depressive illness. *Lancet.* 1999;354:1369-1375.
13. Dinan TG. Psychoneuroendocrinology of mood disorders. *Curr Opin Psychiatry.* 2001;14:51-55.
14. Manji H, Quiroz JA, Sporn J, et al. Enhancing neuronal plasticity and cellular resilience to develop novel, improved therapeutics for difficult-to-treat depression. *J Clin Psychol.* 2003;53(8):707-742.
15. Kramer MS, Cutler N, Feighner J, et al. Distinct mechanism for antidepressant activity by blockade of central substance P receptors. *Science.* 1998;281(5383):1640-1645.
16. Wahlestedt C. Reward for persistence in substance P research. *Science.* 1998;281(5383):1624-1625.
17. Joffe RT. Refractory depression: treatment strategies, with particular reference to the thyroid axis. *J Psychiatry Neurosci.* 1997;22(5):327-331.
18. Frazer A, Morilak DA. Drugs for the treatment of affective (mood) disorders. In: Brody MJ, Larner J, Minneman KP, eds. *Human Pharmacology: Molecular to Clinical.* 3rd ed. Philadelphia: Mosby; 1998:349-363.
19. Rampello LI, Nicoletti F, Nicoletti F. Dopamine and depression: therapeutic implications. *CNS Drugs.* 2000;13(1):35-45.
20. McCleane G. Pharmacological management of neuropathic pain. *CNS Drugs.* 2003;17(14):1031-1043.
21. Witchel HJ, Hancox JC, Nutt DJ. Psychotropic drugs, cardiac arrhythmia, and sudden death. *J Clin Psychopharmacol.* 2003;23(1):58-77.
22. Ray WA, Meredith S, Thapa PB, Hall K, Murray KT. Cyclic antidepressants and the risk of sudden cardiac death. *Clin Pharmacol Ther.* 2004;75(3):234-241.
23. Kerwin R, Travis MJ, Page C, et al. Drugs and the nervous system. In: Page C, Curtis MJ, Sutter MC, Walker MJ, Hoffman BB, eds. *Integrated Pharmacology.* 2nd ed. Philadelphia: Mosby; 2002:219-280.
24. Vaswani M, Linda FK, Ramesh S. Role of selective serotonin reuptake inhibitors in psychiatric disorders: a comprehensive review. *Prog Neuropsychopharmacol J Clin Psychol.* 2003;27:85-102.
25. Meyer JH, Kapur S, Eisfeld B, et al. The effect of paroxetine on 5-HT(2A) receptors in depression: an [(18)F] setoperone PET imaging study. *Am J Psychiatry.* 2001;158(1):78-85.
26. Benmansour S, Owens WA, Cecchi M, Morilak DA, Frazer A. Serotonin clearance in vivo is altered to a greater extent by antidepressant-induced downregulation of the serotonin transporter than by acute blockade of this transporter. *J Neurosci.* 2002;22(15):6766-6772.
27. Baumann P. Pharmacokinetic-pharmacodynamic relationship of the selective serotonin reuptake inhibitors. *Clin Pharmacokinet.* 1996;31:444-469.
28. Hirschfeld RM. Long-term side effects of SSRIs: sexual dysfunction and weight gain. *J Clin Psychiatry.* 2003;64(suppl 18):20-24.
29. Anderson IM. Selective serotonin reuptake inhibitors versus tricyclic antidepressants: a meta-analysis of efficacy and tolerability. *J Affect Disord.* 2000;58:19-36.

30. Geddes JR, Freemantile N, Mason J, Eccles MP, Boynton J. SSRIs versus other antidepressants for depressive disorder. *Cochrane Database Syst Rev.* 2000; 2(CD001851).

31. Song F, Freemantle N, Sheldon TA, Watson P, Long A, Mason J. Selective serotonin reuptake inhibitors: meta-analysis of efficacy and acceptability. *BMJ.* 1993; 306(6879):683-687.

32. Vythilingum B, Cartwright C, Hollander E. Pharmacotherapy of obsessive-compulsive disorder: experience with the selective serotonin reuptake inhibitors. *Int Clin Psychopharmacol.* 2000;15(suppl 2):S7-S13.

33. Mancini C, Van Ameringen M, Oakman JM, Farvolden P. Serotonergic agents in the treatment of social phobia in children and adolescents: a case series. *Depress Anxiety.* 1999;10(1):33-39.

34. Boyer W. Serotonin uptake inhibitors are superior to imipramine and alprazolam in alleviating panic attacks: a meta-analysis. *Int Clin Psychopharmacol.* 1995;10(1): 45-49.

35. Wilander I, Sundblad C, Andersch B. Citalopram in premenstrual dysphoria: is intermittent treatment during luteal phase more effective than continuous medication throughout the menstrual cycle? *J Clin Psychopharmacol.* 1998;18:390-398.

36. Berlant J. New drug development for post-traumatic stress disorder. *Curr Opin Invest Drugs.* 2003;4(1):37-41.

37. Kaye W, Gendall K, Strober M. Serotonin neuronal function and selective serotonin reuptake inhibitor treatment in anorexia and bulimia nervosa. *J Clin Psychol.* 1998;44(9):825-838.

38. de Jong JC, van den Berg PB, Tobi H, de Jong-van den Berg LT. Combined use of SSRIs and NSAIDs increases the risk of gastrointestinal adverse effects. *Br J Clin Pharmacol.* 2003;55(6):591-595.

39. Serebruany VL, Glassman AH, Malinin AI, et al. Selective serotonin reuptake inhibitors yield additional antiplatelet protection in patients with congestive heart failure treated with antecedent aspirin. *Eur J Heart Fail.* 2003;5(4):517-521.

40. Masand PS. Tolerability and adherence issues in antidepressant therapy. *Clin Ther.* 2003;25(8):2289-2304.

41. Arinzon ZH, Lehman YA, Fidelman ZG, Krasnyansky II. Delayed recurrent SIADH associated with SSRIs. *Ann Pharmacother.* 2002;36(7):1175-1177.

42. Which SSRI? *Med Lett Drugs Ther.* 2003;45(1170):93-95.

43. Gerber P, Lynd LD. Selective serotonin-reuptake inhibitor-induced movement disorders. *Ann Pharmacother.* 1998;32(6):692-698.

44. Jindal RD, Friedman ES, Berman SR, Fasiczka AL, Howland RH, Thase ME. Effects of sertraline on sleep architecture in patients with depression. *J Clin Psychopharmacol.* 2003;23(6):540-548.

45. Ditto KE. SSRI discontinuation syndrome. *Postgrad Med.* 2003;114(2):79-84.

46. Harvey BH, McEwen BS, Stein DJ. Neurobiology of antidepressant withdrawal: implications for the longitudinal outcome of depression. *J Clin Psychol.* 2003; 54(10):1105-1117.

47. Teicher MH, Glod C, Cole JO. Emergence of intense suicidal preoccupation during fluoxetine treatment. *Am J Psychiatry.* 1990;147:207-210.

48. Are SSRIs safe for children? *Med Lett Drugs Ther.* 2003; 45(1160)53-54.

49. Khan A, Khan S, Kolts R, Brown WM. Suicide rates in clinical trials of SSRIs, other antidepressants, and placebo: analysis of FDA reports. *Am J Psychiatry.* 2003; 160(4):790-792.

50. Healy D, Whitaker C. Antidepressants and suicide: risk-benefit conundrums. *J Psychiatry Neurosci.* 2003; 28(5):331-337.

51. Lapierre Y. Suicidality with selective serotonin reuptake inhibitors: valid claim? *J Psychiatry Neurosci.* 2003; 28(5):340-347.

52. Hall WD, Mant A, Mitchell PB, Rendle VA, Hickie IB, McManus P. Association between antidepressant prescribing and suicide in Australia, 1991-2000: trend analysis. *BMJ.* 2003;326:1008-1011.

53. Montgomery SA, Dunner DL, Dunbar GC. Reduction of suicidal thoughts with paroxetine in comparison with reference antidepressants and placebo. *Eur Neuropsychopharmacol.* 1995;5(1):5-13.

54. Wagner KD, Ambrosini P, Rynn M, et al. Efficacy of sertraline in the treatment of children and adolescents with major depressive disorder: two randomized controlled trials. *JAMA.* 2003;290(8):1033-1041.

55. Weintrob N, Cohen D, Klipper-Auerbach Y, Zadik Z, Dickerman Z. Decreased growth during therapy with selective serotonin reuptake inhibitors. *Arch Pediatr Adolesc Med.* 2002;156(7):696-701.

56. Loubinoux I, Pariente J, Rascol O, Celsis P, Chollet F. Selective serotonin reuptake inhibitor paroxetine modulates motor behavior through practice. A double-blind, placebo-controlled, multi-dose study in healthy subjects. *Neuropsychologia.* 2002;40:1815-1821.

57. Dam M, Tonin P, De Boni A, et al. Effects of fluoxetine and maprotiline on functional recovery in poststroke hemiplegic patients undergoing rehabilitation therapy. *Stroke.* 1996;27(7):1211-1214.

58. Pariente J, Loubinoux I, Carel C, et al. Fluoxetine modulates motor performance and cerebral activation of patients recovering from stroke. *Ann Neurol.* 2001; 50:718-729.

59. Guitierrez MA, Stimmel GL, Aiso JY. Venlafaxine: a 2003 update. *Clin Ther.* 2003;25(8):2138-2154.

60. Lydiard RB. An overview of generalized anxiety disorder: disease state-appropriate therapy. *Clin Ther.* 2000; 22(suppl A):A3-A24.

61. Gelenberg AJ, Lydiard RB, Rudolph RL, Aguiar L, Haskins JT, Salinas E. Efficacy of venlafaxine extended-release capsules in nondepressed outpatients with generalized anxiety disorder: a 6 month randomized controlled trial. *JAMA.* 2000;283(23):3082-3088.

62. Rickels K, Pollack MH, Sheehan DV, Haskins JT. Efficacy of extended-release venlafaxine in nondepressed outpatients with generalized anxiety disorder. *J Clin Psychiatry.* 2000;157(6):968-974.

63. Thase ME, Howland RH, Friedman ES. Treating antidepressant nonresponders with augmentation strategies: an overview. *J Clin Psychiatry.* 1998;59(suppl 5):5-12.

64. Entsuah AR, Huang H, Thase ME. Response and remission rates in different subpopulations with major depressive disorder administered venlafaxine, selective serotonin reuptake inhibitors, or placebo. *J Clin Psychiatry.* 2001;62:869-877.

65. Thase ME, Entsuah AR, Rudolph RL. Remission rates during treatment with venlafaxine or selective serotonin reuptake inhibitors. *Br J Psychiatry.* 2001;178:234-241.

66. Thase ME, Nierenberg AA, Keller MB, Panagides J. Efficacy of mirtazapine for prevention of depressive relapse: a placebo-controlled double-blind trial of recently remitted high-risk patients. *J Clin Psychiatry.* 2001; 62(10):782-788.

67. Nofzinger EA, Fasiczka AL, Berman SR, Thase ME. Bupropion SR reduces periodic limb movements associated with arousals from sleep in depressed patients with periodic limb movement disorder. *J Clin Psychiatry.* 2000;61(11):858-862.

68. Lenhart SE, Buysse DJ. Treatment of insomnia in hospitalized patients. *Ann Pharmacother.* 2001;35:1449-1457.

69. Nierenberg AA, Adler LA, Peselow E, Zornberg GL, Rosenthal M. Trazodone for antidepressant-associated insomnia. *Am J Psychiatry.* 1994;151:1069-1072.

70. Tanev K. Neuroimaging and neurocircuitry in post-traumatic stress disorder: what is currently known? *Curr Psychiatry Rep.* 2003;5(5):369-383.

71. Sandford JJ, Argyropoulos SV, Nutt DJ. The psychobiology of anxiolytic drugs. Part 1: Basic neurobiology. *Pharmacol Ther.* 2000;88:197-212.

72. Davidson RJ. Anxiety and affective style: role of prefrontal cortex and amygdala. *J Clin Psychol.* 2002;51:68-80.

73. Brunello N, Blier P, Judd LL, et al. Noradrenaline in mood and anxiety disorders: basic and clinical studies. *Int Clin Psychopharmacol.* 2003;18(4):191-202.

74. Lader M. Recent developments in the treatment of anxiety and depression. *Br J Clin Pharmacol.* 1996;41(5):356-358.

75. Bell CJ, Nutt DJ. Serotonin and panic. *Br J Psychiatry.* 1998;172(6):465-471.

76. Jenck R, Martin RJ, Moreau JL. Animal models of panic disorder—emphasis on face and predictive validity. *Eur Neuropsychopharmacol.* 1996;6(suppl 4):S4-S47.

77. Millan MJ. The neurobiology and control of anxious states. *Prog Neurobiol.* 2003;70:83-244.

78. Argyropoulos SV, Nutt D. The use of benzodiazepines in anxiety and other disorders. *Eur Neuropsychopharmacol.* 1999;9(suppl 6):S407-S412.

79. Rudolph U, Crestani F, Benke D, et al. Benzodiazepine actions mediated by specific γ-aminobutyric acid$_A$ receptor subtypes. *Nature.* 1999;401:796-800.

80. Atack JR. Anxioselective compound acting at the GABA(A) receptor benzodiazepine binding site. *Curr Drug Target CNS Neurol Disord.* 2003;2(4):213-232.

81. Bhagwagar Z, Wylezinska M, Taylor M, Jezzard P, Matthews PM, Cowen PJ. Increased brain GABA concentrations following acute administration of a selective serotonin reuptake inhibitor. *Am J Psychiatry.* 2004; 161(2):368-370.

82. Mohler H. Biochemical pharmacology of anti-anxiety drugs. *Br J Clin Pharmacol.* 1996;41(5):355-356.

83. Trevor AJ, Miller RD. General Anesthetics. In: Katzung BG, ed. *Basic and Clinical Pharmacology.* New York: McGraw Hill; 2001:419-435.

84. Trevor AJ, Way WL. Sedative-hypnotic drugs. In: Katzung BG, ed. *Basic and Clinical Pharmacology.* 8th ed. New York: McGraw Hill; 2001:364-381.

85. Karan LD, Benowitz NL. Substance abuse: dependence and treatment. In: Carruthers SG, Hoffman AR, Melmon KL, Nierenberg AA, eds. *Melmon and Morrelli's Clinical Pharmacology.* 4th ed. New York: McGraw-Hill; 2000:1053-1090.

86. Costa e Silva JA. Introduction: the implications for public health of controls on the benzodiazepines. *Eur Neuropsychopharmacol.* 1999;9(suppl 6):S391-S392.

87. Uhlenhuth EH, Balter MB, Ban TA, Yang BK. Trends in recommendations for the pharmacotherapy of anxiety disorders by an international expert panel, 1992-1997. *Eur Neuropsychopharmacol.* 1999;9(suppl 6):S393-S398.

88. Lader M. Limitations on the use of benzodiazepines in anxiety and insomnia: are they justified? *Eur Neuropsychopharmacol.* 1999;9(suppl 6):S399-S405.

89. Mattila MJ, Vanakoski J, Kalska H, Seppala T. Effects of alcohol, zolpidem, and some other sedatives and hypnotics on human performance and memory. *Pharmacol Biochem Behav.* 1998;59(4):917-923.

90. Verster JC, Volkerts ER. Clinical pharmacology, clinical efficacy, and behavioral toxicity of alprazolam: a review of the literature. *CNS Drug Rev.* 2004;10(1):45-76.

91. McKenry LM, Salerno E. Antianxiety, sedative, and hypnotic drugs. In: *Pharmacology in Nursing.* Philadelphia: Mosby; 2003:325-349.

92. Cumming RG, Le Couteur DG. Benzodiazepines and risk of hip fractures in older people: a review of the evidence. *CNS Drugs.* 2003;17(11):825-837.

93. Argyropoulos SV, Sandford JJ, Nutt D. The psychobiology of anxiolytic drugs. Part 2: Pharmacological treatments of anxiety. *Pharmacol Ther.* 2000;88:213-227.

94. Drugs for depression and anxiety. *Med Lett Drugs Ther.* 1999;41(1050):33-38.

95. Ninan PT. Obsessive-compulsive disorder: implications of the efficacy of an SSRI, paroxetine. *Psychopharmacol Bull.* 2003;37(suppl 1):89-96.

96. Blanco C, Raza MS, Schneier FR, Liebowitz MR. The evidence-based pharmacological treatment of social anxiety disorder. *Int J Neuropsychopharmacol.* 2003; 6(4):427-442.

97. Allgulander C, Bandelow B, Hollander E, et al. WCA recommendations for the long-term treatment of generalized anxiety disorder. *CNS Spectr.* 2003;8(suppl 1): 53-61.

CHAPTER 17

DRUG TREATMENT FOR SCHIZOPHRENIA AND BIPOLAR ILLNESS

ANTIPSYCHOTIC DRUGS AND SCHIZOPHRENIA

Antipsychotic drugs are also known as neuroleptic drugs, antischizophrenic drugs, or major tranquilizers. They are the main treatment intervention for schizophrenia and other psychoses and are characterized primarily by their dopamine receptor–blocking action. Although they are helpful for some patients, these drugs have some major shortcomings in terms of their effectiveness and side effect profile. Gradual improvements in drug treatment are being achieved, but major advances may have to wait until a more thorough understanding of this disease is obtained.

Etiology and Pathogenesis of Schizophrenia

Schizophrenia is a psychotic illness characterized by periods of psychosis (delusions and hallucinations) along with relatively chronic dysfunctions in mood, cognition, and social behavior.[1] It usually develops in adolescence or young adulthood and follows a relapsing and remitting course. Even though there are equal numbers of males and females affected, males tend to develop the disease earlier (by 2 to 4 years), to have more severe symptoms, and to be less responsive to medication than females.[2] In many cases, schizophrenia becomes chronic, progressive, and extremely disabling.

Symptoms of schizophrenia are characterized as either positive or negative, with the positive signs either a part of or signifying impending psychosis.[3] These include disturbances of reality and perception, bizarre behavior, hallucinations, and delusions. Hallucinations may be visual, olfactory, tactile, or auditory but are almost always auditory. In addition, there may be abnormal motor symptoms, echopraxia (imitation of another person's motor actions), posturing (assuming inappropriate or bizarre postures), and waxy flexibility (when the limbs are placed in a position by an observer and remain fixed by the patient for an extended period). Negative symptoms include diminished speech, flattened emotions, apathy, attention problems, impaired problem solving, difficulty with abstract reasoning, and social withdrawal. Anxiety and depression may also be experienced by the patient with schizophrenia. The relative balance between positive and negative symptoms varies greatly among individuals and may help determine which antipsychotic agent might be most effective.

The exact cause of schizophrenia has not been identified, but twin studies demonstrate some genetic predisposition, although prenatal and birth complications (hypoxia, infection, exposure to toxins) have also been implicated.[2] There is a 1% incidence of schizophrenia among the general population, but the incidence increases within families; the incidence is between 6% and 17% among first-degree relatives and as high as 50% among identical twins. Many investigators have classified this disease as a neurodevelopmental one, but others argue against this because its clinical onset is not until young adulthood. Closer scrutiny reveals a long premorbid course of subtle symptoms and behaviors, beginning with mild motor, social, and cognitive impairments in infancy and early childhood.[4] This period is followed by a prodromal phase, beginning around puberty, which is characterized by mood disturbances, impairments in attention and concentration, and suspicious thinking. During the premorbid course, the patient's personality may be cold, introverted, and aloof. This culminates in the onset of psychosis, followed by neuroprogressive deterioration. It is hypothesized that genetic abnormalities coupled with environmental insults produce defective connectivity between a number of brain regions, specifically, the midbrain, nucleus accumbens, thalamus, and temporo-limbic and prefrontal cortices. These functional deficits become unmasked during periods of stress and as a result of the hormonal influence on the central nervous system that occurs during puberty.

Imaging studies of the brains of patients with schizophrenia have shown some commonalities, but it has not always been easy to determine whether these structural abnormalities cause the disease or result from the disease. However, ventricular enlargement along with cortical gray matter volume reductions (greater in the mesial temporal, temporal neocortical, and prefrontal regions) are consistent findings present in patients with a recent diagnosis of schizophrenia.[5,6] In addition, these patients and those who have had the illness for some time show a reduction in blood flow in the prefrontal regions and a higher flow in the thalamus and cerebellum compared with healthy subjects.[7]

Neurochemical studies have implicated the dopamine and serotonin systems along with γ-aminobutyric acid (GABA) and glutamate. However, most of the current theory regarding the neurochemistry of schizophrenia resulted from analyzing effects of antipsychotic and pro-psychotic drugs rather than the neurochemistry itself. The dopamine hypothesis is based on the pharmacological evidence that dopamine agonists produce or exacerbate the positive symptoms of schizophrenia.[8] An example is amphetamine, which causes the release of dopamine in the brain, and in humans, produces a behavioral syndrome similar to an acute schizophrenic episode. In addition, dopamine D_2 receptor

agonists, such as bromocriptine, can produce similar effects in animals and exacerbate symptoms in patients who already have this disease. Drugs that block dopamine neural storage, such as reserpine, or drugs that act as dopamine antagonists are effective in reducing the positive symptoms of schizophrenia.

Dopamine is synthesized as a precursor to the catecholamines. It is metabolized by two enzymes, intraneurally by monoamine oxidase B and extraneuronally by catechol-o-methyl transferase. The final and primary metabolite of dopamine is homovanillic acid.

At least five types of dopamine receptors (D_1 to D_5) have been identified in the human brain.[9] D_1 and D_5 stimulate the formation of cyclic adenosine monophosphate by activating a stimulatory G-protein, whereas the other dopamine receptors activate an inhibitory G-protein. The dopamine pathways include the nigrostriatal tract, the mesolimbic/mesocortical tract, and the tuberoinfundibular tract (Figure 17-1). The nigrostriatal tract runs from the substantia nigra in the midbrain to the corpus striatum and is involved in motor control. The

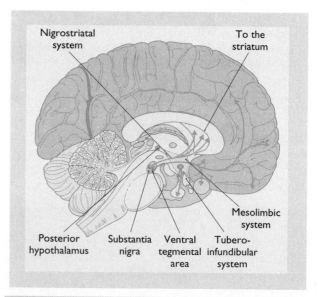

Figure 17-1

Dopamine pathways. These tracts include the nigrostriatal tract, the mesolimbic/mesocortical tract, and the tuberoinfundibular tract. (From Page C, Curtis MJ, Sutter MC, Walker MJ, Hoffman BB, eds. *Integrated Pharmacology.* 2nd ed. Philadelphia: Mosby; 2002.)

mesolimbic/mesocortical tract has cell bodies adjacent to the substantia nigra and runs to the limbic system and neocortex. It also supplies input to the medial surface of the frontal lobes and to the parahippocampus. This tract plays a crucial role in the regulation of behavior, particularly in the area of behaviors that are driven by reward. The tuberoinfundibular tract has cell bodies that lie in the arcuate nucleus and hypothalamus, projecting to the anterior pituitary. It is here that dopamine inhibits the release of prolactin. An overactivity in dopamine neurotransmission in the mesolimbic/mesocortical tract has been specifically implicated in schizophrenia.[2] However, the conclusion that there is an overabundance of dopamine should be avoided because schizophrenia may be associated with "dopamine dysregulation," meaning subcortical dopamine overactivity along with frontal dopamine underactivity.[10] In addition, there is no shortage of prolactin in patients with schizophrenia, which is what would be expected with an elevation of dopamine.

Patients with schizophrenia may have an increased density of D_2 receptors and show greater stimulation of these receptors after amphetamine challenge compared with healthy individuals.[10-12] Further studies with positron emission tomography and single-photon computerized emission tomography demonstrate that these manifestations are present at the onset of the disease and in patients who have not been treated with antipsychotic medications. In addition, when antipsychotic drugs occupy 65% to 70% of the D_2 receptors, a short-term clinical response is often achieved.[13]

Glutamate has also been implicated in the pathogenesis of schizophrenia, largely by studies of the behavioral effects of N-methyl-D-aspartate (NMDA) receptor antagonists.[2,14] Administration of ketamine and phencyclidine produces psychotic symptoms in healthy subjects and exacerbates symptoms in patients with schizophrenia. NMDA receptor hypofunction can result in decreased inhibition of dopamine neurons, resulting in increased mesolimbic dopamine release.[15]

More recently, the serotonin system has become the focus of many studies on schizophrenia.[16] There appears to be a reduction in the number of serotonin (5-hydroxytryptamine [$5-HT_{2A}$]) receptors in the prefrontal cortex of these patients and an increase in the number of $5-HT_{1A}$ receptors. In addition, there is evidence that the serotonin antagonist, ritanserin, is effective in reducing the negative symptoms of schizophrenia, as well as some of the side effects (extrapyramidal symptoms) of the typical antipsychotics. Further impetus to this theory comes from the fact that clozapine (an atypical antipsychotic agent) is an antagonist of the $5-HT_{2A}$ and $5-HT_{2C}$ receptors. Similar in some ways to the dopamine hypothesis, there may be a dysregulation in the serotoninergic system resulting in areas of hypoinnervation and hyperinnervation, starting with early damage in the dorsal raphe.

Neuropeptides have also been added to the list of chemicals considered to be responsible for schizophrenia.[17] Neurotensin is a peptide neurotransmitter that coexists with norepinephrine and dopamine in neurons. Studies have shown a decreased neurotensin concentration in the cerebrospinal fluid in some patients with schizophrenia, which normalizes with treatment. Drugs that affect neurotensin levels are currently being explored.

Antipsychotic Drugs (Typical Antipsychotic Agents)

Several different antipsychotic drugs are on the market today, but they basically fall into two categories. The main categories are the "typical antipsychotics" (including chlorpromazine, haloperidol, fluphenazine, thioridazine) and the "atypical antipsychotics" (clozapine, olanzapine, quetiapine, aripiprazole, and risperidone), which are more recent discoveries. The term *atypical* has several meanings; it is used to describe the antipsychotic agents that have a receptor profile different from that of the typical drugs, those that produce fewer side effects, and those agents that have some impact on the negative symptoms of schizophrenia.

Mechanism of Action of Antipsychotic Agents

As is the case for many drugs, the original antipsychotic agent was discovered serendipitously by a French surgeon testing different compounds to alleviate stress in surgical patients. He tested promethazine, which appeared to have a calming but not a sedating effect. From promethazine came chlorpromazine, the first antipsychotic agent.[1] Studies on chlorpromazine demonstrated that this drug blocked multiple receptor systems including the histamine, catecholamine, acetylcholine, and serotonin systems. It is now clear that the drug's ability to block the D_2 receptor is largely responsible for the reduction in the positive symptoms of schizophrenia.[8]

The typical agents have relative affinities for the D_2 receptor and block this receptor in the midbrain, mesolimbic system, and basal ganglia.[8] Potency of these agents is correlated with their D_2 receptor–blocking ability in the mesolimbic/mesocortical pathways, but their side effects are often correlated with activity in the basal ganglia region. They reduce the hallucinations and produce a calming effect without dulling intellectual function or impairing motor control. They are effective in reducing the positive symptoms of schizophrenia but less effective in relieving the negative symptoms. They may actually add to some of the negative symptoms by producing apathy and reducing initiative. The patient becomes slow to respond to external stimuli and may tend to fall asleep but is easily aroused. Because of their sedating effects, they are also used as tranquilizers to manage behavior in combative or agitated patients.

Other indications for the use of antipsychotic agents include nausea and vomiting, hiccups, Huntington's disease, and Tourette's syndrome.[18] Their antiemetic effect results from blocking the D_2 receptors in the chemoreceptor trigger zone in the medulla, and therefore they are often prescribed for nausea associated with anesthesia or chemotherapy. Chlorpromazine is also approved for the treatment of intractable hiccups and may be given orally, intramuscularly, or intravenously, depending on the severity. Pimozide is another conventional antipsychotic agent, which is approved by the Food and Drug Administration for the treatment of Tourette's syndrome. Tourette's syndrome is believed to be due to a hyperdopaminergic state and tends to respond to dopamine blockers. Like Tourette's syndrome, there is no cure for Huntington's disease, but the choreiform movements that characterize this illness are dampened by dopamine blockade. Lastly, these drugs may also be combined with narcotics to reduce chronic pain.

After diagnosis, patients are usually treated for a period of 4 to 6 weeks. If the response is positive, the patient may then be treated on a long-term basis with oral medications. Many patients become noncompliant as their condition improves, and depot preparations may then be necessary.[2] If treated properly early in the disease, many patients will experience a reduction in and maybe even a remission of psychotic behavior, although negative symptoms can persist. However, many patients discontinue drug therapy and will subsequently experience a relapse. Improvements result when drug therapy resumes, but full recovery grows increasingly more difficult to achieve with each exacerbation. Another reason for the 4- to 6-week trial dosing period is that several weeks are needed for a drug's effect to surface, even though evidence of its receptor-blocking ability is immediate. This suggests that an increase in the number of D_2 receptors as a result of up-regulation may be more important than the direct receptor-blocking ability.

Adverse Drug Reactions

Many side effects are associated with the antipsychotic agents because the classic drugs act as antagonists in four major neurotransmitter receptor systems: the dopamine receptor family (D_2, D_3, and D_4), muscarinic cholinergic receptors (M_1), α-adrenergic receptors (α_1 and α_2), and histamine receptors (H_1) (Table 17-1).[18] Lower-potency agents such as chlorpromazine require higher doses to achieve efficacy and therefore produce more side effects by interacting with the other receptor systems. This results in more antihistaminergic, anticholinergic, and antiadrenergic effects, but chlorpromazine has fewer D_2 receptor–related side effects. Higher-potency agents such as haloperidol have more D_2 receptor–related movement effects but produce considerably fewer effects on other receptor systems. In general, the anticholinergic action of these drugs leads to dry mouth, blurred vision, constipation, urinary retention, tachycardia, a prolonged QRS interval, confusion, and exacerbation of glaucoma. Blockade of the α_1 receptors is associated with orthostatic hypotension, prolongation of the QT interval, reflex tachycardia, dizziness, incontinence, and sedation. Histamine blockade leads to sedation and weight gain. Prescribing lower doses of these drugs, particularly if the D_2 receptor occupancies are in the therapeutic range, is recommended to minimize these effects, particularly for first-episode patients.[19]

Neuromuscular side effects are common and are due to the blockade of the D_2 receptors in the nigrostriatal dopaminergic pathway. These adverse drug reactions (ADRs) are known as extrapyramidal side effects (EPS) and include akathisia, parkinsonism, acute dystonias, and tardive dyskinesia.[20] Parkinsonism and the dystonias are associated with greater affinity for the D_2 receptor and are common

Table 17-1

Characteristics of Antipsychotic Drugs

Drug	Receptor Affinity					Main Side Effects				Notes
	D_1	D_2	α-adr	H_1	mACh	5-HT$_2$	EPS	Sed	Hypo	Other	
CLASSICAL											
Chlorpromazine	++	+++	–++	++	++	++	++	++	++	Increased prolactin (gynecomastia) Hypothermia Anticholinergic effects Hypersensitivity reactions Obstructive jaundice	Phenothiazine class **Fluphenazine and fluperazine** are similar but: • do not cause jaundice • less hypotension • more EPS Fluphenazine available as depot preparation
Thioridazine	+	++	–++	+	++	++	+	++	++	As chlorpromazine, but does not cause jaundice	Phenothiazine class First drug with lower EPS tendency
Haloperidol	+	+++	++	–	±	+	+++	–	++	As chlorpromazine, but does not cause jaundice	Butyrophenone class Widely used antipsychotic drug Strong EPS tendency
Flupenthixol	++	+++	++	++	–	+++	++	+	+	Fewer anticholinergic side effects Increased prolactin (gynecomastia) Restlessness	**Clopenthixol** is similar Available as depot preparations
ATYPICAL											
Sulpiride	–	+++	–	–	–	–	+	+	–	Increased prolactin (gynecomastia)	Benzamide class Selective D_2/D_3 antagonist Less EPS than haloperidol Poorly absorbed **Remoxipride and pimozide** (long acting) are similar

Continued

Table 17-1

Characteristics of Antipsychotic Drugs—cont'd

Drug	Receptor Affinity						Main Side Effects				Notes
	D_1	D_2	α-adr	H_1	mACh	5-HT$_2$	EPS	Sed	Hypo	Other	

ATYPICAL—cont'd

Drug	D_1	D_2	α-adr	H_1	mACh	5-HT$_2$	EPS	Sed	Hypo	Other	Notes
Clozapine	++	++	++	++	++	+++	−	++	+	Risk of agranulocytosis (~1%): regular blood counts required · Seizures · Sedation · Salivation · Anticholinergic side effects · Weight gain	Dibenzodiazepine class · Potent antagonist at D$_4$ receptors · No EPS · Shows efficacy in "treatment-resistant" patients · Effective against negative and positive symptoms · **Olanzapine** is similar, without risk of agranulocytosis
Risperidone	−	++	++	++	++	+++	+	++	+	Weight gain · EPS at high doses	Significant risk of EPS · ? Effective against negative symptoms
Sertindole	−	++	++	−	−	+++	+	+	++	Hypotension · Ventricular arrhythmias · (ECG checks advisable)	Potent on D$_4$ receptors · Long plasma half-life (~3 days) · ? Effective against negative symptoms
Quetiapine	−	+	+++	−	+	+	+	++	++	Weight gain · Nasal congestion · Tachycardia · Agitation · Dry mouth · Weight gain	Novel type, acting mainly on α-adrenoceptors · Not yet fully evaluated

From Rang HP, Dale MM, Ritter JM, Moore JL. *Pharmacology*. 5th ed. New York: Churchill Livingstone; 2003.

$D_{1/2}$, Types of dopamine receptor; *EPS*, extrapyramidal side effects; *Sed*, sedation; *Hypo*, hypotension; *adr*, adrenoreceptor; *mACh*, muscarine acetylcholine; *ECG*, electrocardiograph.

among the typical antipsychotics, particularly haloperidol.[13] EPS generally begin appearing when dopamine blockade at the D_2 receptor exceeds 75% to 80%.[21] The dystonias may appear as fixed muscle postures with involuntary spasms, clenched jaw, torticollis, protruding tongue, pharyngeal constriction, laryngospasm, or an oculogyric crisis (head back with mouth open and eyes staring upward).[20] Dystonia may begin early in treatment (within hours or days) and is more common in young male patients. The patient may also complain of tongue thickening, throat tightening, and difficulty speaking or swallowing. Such symptoms are treated immediately with an intravenous anticholinergic drug. Lowering the dose of the antipsychotic agent will then be necessary.

Pseudoparkinsonism may also appear early in the course of treatment.[1] It is more common in older patients, although it can occur at any age. Symptoms are identical to those of Parkinson's disease and can include muscle stiffness, shuffling gait, stooped posture, bradykinesia, resting tremor, and masked facies. These symptoms may be treated by dose reduction, addition of an anticholinergic drug, or switching to another drug that produces less motor involvement. Haloperidol and fluphenazine tend to produce more parkinsonian symptoms.

Akathisia is another early-onset side effect.[20] It refers to lower limb restlessness or the inability of a patient to stay still. It is also associated with repetitive, purposeless movements, such as finger tapping or pacing. It may be misdiagnosed as a worsening of psychosis and will become more pronounced if the antipsychotic dose is increased. Symptoms may be reduced by lowering the antipsychotic dose or adding an anticholinergic or a β-blocking drug. This is one of the most difficult EPS to treat.

Tardive dyskinesia is considered a late-onset EPS.[18] It is characterized by involuntary choreoathetoid movements of the head, limbs, and trunk. Lateral jaw movements and "fly-catching" motions of the tongue tend to be the most common early signs of this disorder. This condition is thought to result from up-regulation of postsynaptic dopamine receptors in the basal ganglia. However, one additional explanation that is growing in popularity relates to the rate at which the drugs dissociate from the D_2 receptors.[21] With a rapidly dissociating compound, a surge of dopamine can overcome the block (act competitively), but a slowly dissociating compound will not respond to this surge. Because the atypical agents dissociate rapidly from the D_2 receptors, it is thought that brief surges of dopamine prevent the motor ADRs while having no affect on the antipsychotic actions of the drugs. Tardive dyskinesia has been reported with almost every antipsychotic agent, although the typical agents account for most of the cases, providing support to this dissociation theory. Tardive dyskinesia is also more common in elderly patients, with an incidence as high as 25%.[22] Unfortunately, this condition can be irreversible, lasting long after the offending drug has been discontinued.

The EPS, particularly tardive dyskinesia, have been refractory to treatment. However, some additional pharmaceutical agents may offer some benefit.[23] Several drugs used in the treatment of Parkinson's disease have the potential to reduce EPS. These agents include anticholinergics (trihexyphenidyl), antihistaminics (diphenhydramine), and dopaminergic agents (amantadine). β-Blockers may also be effective for tremors; benzodiazepines, for akathisia; and botulinum toxin, for focal dystonias (see Chapter 19). Other options include reducing the dose of the antipsychotic agent, switching to a lower-potency neuroleptic, or administering clozapine, an atypical antipsychotic drug.

Neuroleptic malignant syndrome is another very serious side effect of these drugs.[18] It is a life-threatening event characterized by fever (101° F to 107° F), muscle rigidity, autonomic instability (hypotension or hypertension, tachycardia, diaphoresis), and loss of consciousness. Renal failure caused by rhabdomyolysis also occurs. Bromocriptine (a D_2 receptor agonist) is used to reverse this syndrome along with dantrolene to relax the skeletal muscles. The antipsychotic drug is also immediately withdrawn. This reaction may appear within a few days to weeks after treatment begins, but 80% of cases begin within the first 2 weeks. Risk factors include dehydration, poor nutrition, and the presence of mood disorders or organic brain syndromes. A 20% mortality rate is associated with neuroleptic malignant syndrome.

Additional side effects of the typical antipsychotic agents include dermatological, hematological, and endocrine dysfunction. Hypersensitivity rashes, most commonly maculopapular erythematous rashes on the trunk and face, and photosensitivity reactions that can lead to sunburn may be due to immune reactions.[18] Prolonged use of some of these drugs can lead to a blue-gray discoloration of the skin in areas exposed to sunlight. Hematological side effects, such as transient leukopenia and agranulocytosis, may also occur, although these are rare. Because dopamine is inhibitory to prolactin release, D_2 receptor blockade leads to unopposed secretion of this hormone. Prolactin in turn is responsible for amenorrhea, galactorrhea, infertility, osteoporosis, and gynecomastia. Lastly, antipsychotic agents are known to reduce the seizure threshold and to provoke epileptic seizures.[24]

Therapeutic Concerns with Typical Antipsychotic Agents

Patients who are taking antipsychotic agents should be considered at risk for cardiac abnormalities, as well as for obesity, diabetes, and high cholesterol.[25,26] Many of these agents produce tachycardia, electrocardiographic abnormalities, and cardiac arrhythmias. Prolongation of the QT interval and the associated torsades de pointes arrhythmia are particularly worrisome because they can lead to sudden death. These events are more common in patients taking moderate doses of antipsychotics, particularly thioridazine, as opposed to lower maintenance doses. Unfortunately, these issues have not been addressed clinically, but there is a call out to pharmacologists to evaluate potential antipsychotic agents for their effects on the ion channels involved in cardiac repolarization. For now, the clinical advice is to view these patients as having cardiac abnormalities and to monitor their vital signs and devise exercise protocols with this comorbidity in mind. In addition, because of the dermatological side effects, physical therapists must exercise extreme caution when using heat or light modalities. Use of UV light is contraindicated.

Other concerns with these drugs include heat intolerance and impaired thermoregulation.[27] The antipsychotic agents and the condition of schizophrenia itself are related to several hyperthermic syndromes, such as febrile catatonia, neuroleptic malignant syndrome, and heat stroke. These syndromes were recently studied when a group of patients were asked to ambulate on a treadmill at 3.2 mph at an ambient temperature of 40° C for 50 minutes. Rectal and skin temperatures were compared with those of healthy control subjects and were found to be statistically elevated. However, sweat production did not differ between the two groups, indicating that patients with schizophrenia

may have an impaired ability to conduct heat from the core of the body to the periphery. Initial signs of heat injury include faintness, nausea, vomiting, headache, piloerection, chills, hyperventilation, muscle cramps, and an unsteady gait.[28] During physical therapy, patients should be encouraged to maintain adequate fluid intake, and if performing strenuous exercise, they should drink water more frequently than thirst dictates. Physical therapists should be aware that mentally ill patients may not be thirsty, even though they are dehydrated; however, the opposite condition of water intoxication is common in patients with schizophrenia. Some patients may even need to be temporarily restrained to keep them away from water fountains. However, if hydration is necessary, it should be achieved with water or a hypotonic glucose-electrolyte solution (Gatorade). Salt tablets are not recommended because fluid losses during exercise are much greater than electrolyte losses. Exercise sessions should only be conducted in a cool environment. If heat stroke occurs, cooling measures should begin immediately. The extent of neurological damage is directly proportional to the duration and severity of the hyperthermia. Immersing the patient in ice and cold water or performing an ice massage can be quite helpful until emergency help arrives. Massage is necessary to counteract the vasoconstriction that occurs with cold application alone. Lastly, because the typical antipsychotic drugs have a high incidence of EPS, the physical therapist must be particularly diligent in observing for any change in motor function. The presence of any tremors, akathisia, or dystonias—particularly of the oral-facial region—should be recorded and reported to the patient's physician.

Antipsychotic Drugs (Atypical Antipsychotic Agents)

Atypical antipsychotic agents represent a new generation of antipsychotic drugs that have significantly fewer side effects, particularly a lower incidence of extrapyramidal effects and little hyperprolactinemia. On the whole, they have a lower affinity for the D_2 receptor and a higher affinity for the D_4 receptor.[29] The lower incidence of parkinsonism appears to be related to less activity at the D_2 receptor. There is also less tardive dyskinesia. In addition, many of these drugs have antagonistic activity at the $5-HT_{2A}$ receptor, which is why the drugs may improve the negative symptoms of schizophrenia more than the original antipsychotic agents.

Clozapine

The prototypic drug in this atypical or second-generation category is clozapine.[30] It was originally prescribed during the early 1970s; however, it was withdrawn soon after it appeared on the market as a result of several deaths caused by agranulocytosis. In the 1980s it was reintroduced in North America, but with restrictions. Only patients unresponsive to other neuroleptics (failed response to at least three antipsychotic drugs) or those who have severe extrapyramidal symptoms are considered eligible for treatment with this drug and only with mandatory blood monitoring on a regular basis.

Studies performed in patients with drug-resistant schizophrenia have demonstrated the superiority of clozapine in reducing both positive and negative symptoms as compared with both chlorpromazine with benztropine and haloperidol.[31] Patients given clozapine were also less likely to withdraw from these studies and had fewer relapses.[32] In fact, the recognition that this drug produced minimal EPS led to a reevaluation of the models used for developing antipsychotic drugs. Until this time, it was assumed that a good antipsychotic drug had to block D_2 receptors at high occupancy and that EPS would then be an expected outcome. However, clozapine challenged that belief when it was found to have a greater affinity for D_1 and D_4 receptors versus D_2 receptors. Clozapine appears effective in reducing psychosis when it occupies as few as 20% of the D_2 receptors. This property explains the reduction in EPS and also suggests that other receptors, not just the D_2 receptors, must be involved in reducing psychosis. A proposed role for the D_4 receptors in causing psychosis became an exciting concept, especially when it was determined that patients have a several-fold increase in the number of D_4 receptors.[33] However, experimental drugs with selective affinity for the D_4 receptor have not demonstrated any antipsychotic properties.[34]

Some researchers believe that clozapine's high affinity for the 5-HT_{2A} receptor compared with the D_2 receptor could be another reason for the drug's success.[29] Some data indicate that the 5-HT_{2A} system can modulate the effects of the D_2 system, and this is a favored theory among many researchers. How-ever, there are some gaps in this theory. Some of the typical antipsychotic agents also have high affinity for the 5-HT_{2A} receptors; pure 5-HT_2 receptor blockers have failed to reduce psychosis; and a new drug, amisulpride, which is a pure D_2/D_3 antagonist without 5-HT_2 properties, has been shown to be quite effective.

The last theory proposed for the success of clozapine and the other atypical agents is related to how fast the drug can be dissociated from the D_2 receptors.[21] As described earlier, a lower affinity for the D_2 receptor and a fast dissociation allow the drug to enter into a competitive relationship with endogenous dopamine, thus avoiding EPS and hyperprolactinemia.

Although clozapine appears to offer several advantages for patients with schizophrenia, it is plagued by many side effects. Agranulocytosis is defined as an absolute neutrophil count below 500 mm^3. In 1975, 17 cases of this illness were reported in Finland, which resulted in curtailment of the use of clozapine. When the drug was brought back onto the market in 1990, a Clozaril National Registry was established to keep track of patients' medical status while they were taking the drug. Between 1990 and 1994, more than 99,000 patients were registered, but only 382 (0.38%) had agranulocytosis.[35] This is obviously a very small percentage of patients, and the good news is that once the drug is discontinued, leukopenia resolves within 14 to 24 days.

Some of the cardiac issues that are present with the typical antipsychotic agents are also part of the side effect profile for clozapine.[32] Tachycardia, orthostatic hypotension, and even some cases of sudden death from ventricular arrhythmias have been reported. In fact, cardiac issues may be more worrisome with this drug and with the other second-generation drugs than they were for the original agents. This is because weight gain, new-onset diabetes, and dyslipidemia are common events with these drugs. The weight gain, in particular, is troublesome, with an average gain of 6.9 ± 0.8 kg in 6 months.[32,36,37] Of the atypical agents, clozapine appears to produce the most weight gain, followed by olanzapine. In addition, the distribution of the weight is greater in the abdomen than in the hips and also greater for male patients than female patients. The relative affinity for the H_1 receptor is to blame. Additional side effects include increased salivation and bedwetting.[38] The salivation is particularly problematic at night and necessitates frequent pillow case changes.

Olanzapine

Olanzapine is another second-generation antipsychotic agent.[39] Its chemical structure is very similar to that of clozapine, but it does not cause agranulocytosis. Specifically, this drug has affinity for D_2 and D_1 receptors, but the relative binding ratio is about 3:1, intermediate between haloperidol and clozapine. This reduced affinity for the D_2 receptor is responsible for fewer EPS. Olanzapine also has affinity for the 5-HT_2 receptors, similar to that of clozapine, and it has affinity for muscarinic (M_1 to M_5) receptors, as well as for the α_1-adrenergic and H_1 histaminic receptors. Hence, weight gain and subsequent diabetes occur frequently, with olanzapine rating second only to clozapine in terms of this side effect.[36] Postural hypotension, sedation, constipation, hyperlipidemia, dizziness, and akathisia also occur; but EPS are rare at therapeutic doses. Olanzapine has demonstrated efficacy similar to that of haloperidol in the treatment of first-episode psychosis and efficacy similar to that of clozapine in treatment-resistant schizophrenia; it is also associated with a slight adherence advantage over risperidone and the conventional antipsychotics.[40-42]

Quetiapine

Quetiapine also has a receptor binding profile similar to that of clozapine but with lower affinity for all the receptors, especially the muscarinic receptors.[43] Its efficacy is similar to that of the conventional antipsychotics, but the rates of EPS are significantly lower. This drug also has a lower potential to produce weight gain and does not increase prolactin levels. Major side effects include sedation and postural hypotension.

Aripiprazole

Aripiprazole represents a novel antipsychotic agent with a unique receptor profile that differs from those of the other agents. It exhibits partial agonist activity at the D_2, D_3, and 5-HT_{1A} receptors, but antagonist activity at the 5-HT_{2A} receptors.[44] A partial agonist minimizes excessive dopamine levels and increases low dopamine levels. Thus overactivity and underactivity are avoided. Aripiprazole also has strong affinity for the presynaptic dopamine autoreceptor, which then acts to reduce neuron firing. Because of this unique profile, it is being called

a dopamine-serotonin system stabilizer. Treatment with this drug is at least as effective as treatment with haloperidol but without EPS, electrocardiographic changes, prolactin elevation, weight gain, or abnormalities in glucose or lipid metabolism.[45,46] However, aripiprazole can cause akathisia, insomnia, anxiety, headache, nausea, constipation, and lightheadedness.

Other Second-Generation Antipsychotic Agents

Some other atypical agents include ziprasidone, amisulpride, and risperidone. Amisulpride is different from the other drugs in that it only blocks the D_2 and D_3 receptors.[1] It has efficacy similar to that of haloperidol, but at low doses, produces an excellent outcome for patients displaying only negative symptoms. This drug also produces less weight gain than the other atypical agents.

Risperidone and ziprasidone share many qualities. They both have a very high affinity for 5-HT_{2A} receptors and lower affinity for the D_2 receptor compared with clozapine. Risperidone is rather unique because it can reduce tardive dyskinesia more effectively than just discontinuing the incriminating antipsychotic drug.[47] However, risperidone still has all the other side effects—postural hypotension, constipation, dizziness, prolactin elevation, diabetes, and weight gain. Ziprasidone does not produce any increase in weight but does produce sedation and prolongation of the QT interval.[48]

Therapeutic Concerns with the Atypical Antipsychotic Agents

Concerns with the second-generation antipsychotic drugs rival or may even exceed those concerns with the first-generation drugs. The second-generation agents, with the exception of ziprasidone and aripiprazole, produce significant weight gain, hyperglycemia, and lipid abnormalities. Patients who regularly take these agents for schizophrenia need to be considered to be at risk for cardiac abnormalities, and appropriate monitoring is necessary. These drugs may also produce heat intolerance similar to the first-generation drugs, but this is less of a certainty.

Choice of Antipsychotics

For acute and first-episode psychosis, many psychiatrists still use a high-potency first-generation antipsychotic drug.[20] In cases of severe behavioral disturbances, a benzodiazepine can also be administered.

Current emphasis is on the early diagnosis and treatment of the first episode because recent studies (but not all) suggest that the longer the patient goes without treatment, the poorer the overall outcome will be.[49] In addition, it is believed that the antipsychotic drugs not only treat the symptoms of psychosis but also contribute to neuroplasticity of the adult brain and help reduce future relapses.[50] Discontinuation after remission of the first episode of psychosis is also controversial. Any decision regarding drug withdrawal needs to take into consideration side effects of the drugs, as well as high relapse rates—78% in the first year and 98% by the end of the second year without drug treatment.[51] Another study demonstrated that the relapse rate for patients who discontinued drug therapy is five times greater than that for patients who continue to receive medication.[52] If the decision to withdraw medication is made, discontinuation should be done very slowly, and the patient should be monitored carefully for an extended period. Because of the reduced incidence in EPS with the second-generation drugs, these drugs are becoming favored for use in maintenance therapy. Choice depends on the side effect profile because in terms of efficacy, with the exception of clozapine, they are all roughly equal.[20] Clozapine is the choice for treatment-resistant schizophrenia.

BIPOLAR DISORDER

Bipolar disorder is characterized by mood alterations that tend to fluctuate among recurrent episodes of mania, hypomania, and depression. Bipolar disorder is further divided into bipolar I disorder, in which one or more manic episodes are accompanied by a history of one or more major depressive episodes, and bipolar II disorder, in which major depressive episodes recur with one or more hypomanic or milder manic phases.[53] Specifically, a manic episode is defined as a period during which patients experience an abnormal, persistently elevated mood along with rapid speech, increased motor and speech activity, irritability, distractibility, decreased sleep, grandiose ideas, and possibly hallucinations and delusions. Hypomania is less well defined but consists of an elevated or irritable mood, lasting at least 4 days, and overactivity without psychotic thinking. A change in behavior must

be noticeable by others and must not be due to substance abuse. This criterion is currently being challenged, as is the duration of the hypomania. Overactivity with other hypomanic symptoms present for only 1 day may soon be accepted.[54]

More recently, efforts have been directed toward defining a continuum of bipolar phenotypes, ranging from mild depression with brief hypomania to severe rapid cycling, to help link the type of disorder to its most effective pharmacological agent. Additional terms involved in labeling of the variations include *mixed episodes* (characterized by a period of at least 1 week in which the patient displays symptoms of both mania and major depression), *rapid cycling* (in which four or more episodes of mania and depression occur in 1 year), and *very rapid cycling* (in which the fluctuations occur within days).[55]

Etiology and Pathophysiology

Bipolar disorder most commonly begins between the ages of 15 and 24 years, although there may be an extended period between the first episode and actual diagnosis and treatment.[55] Some patients are originally given a diagnosis of unipolar depression, only to have that diagnosis changed some time later after the induction of mania by a serotonin reuptake inhibitor.[56] Bipolar disorder affects men and women equally, with the exception of the very rapid cycling type, which is more prevalent in women. In addition, genetic factors are involved in this disorder, with a lifetime risk of 5% to 10% in first-degree relatives and a risk of 40% to 70% in monozygotic twins.

There are several theories on the pathophysiology of bipolar disorder, though none have been absolutely proven.[55] In the 1970s, the main theory was that this illness was caused by an imbalance between cholinergic and catecholaminergic activity. A lower concentration of choline (a precursor of acetylcholine) was found in the red blood cells of patients with bipolar disorder whose disease was primarily one of mania. Another theory was that levels of a serotonin metabolite were diminished, implicating the serotonergic system in this affective disorder. A third theory was that electrolyte fluxes caused by deficits in the Na^+/K^+-ATPase pump are responsible for bipolar disorder. Hormonal abnormalities, specifically abnormalities in the hypothalamic-pituitary-thyroid axis, are associated with major depression and bipolar disorder; and hypothyroidism is especially associated with the rapid cycling variant of bipolar illness.[57] The two major theories that are currently drawing the most attention are increased signaling via second-messenger systems in the circuitry between the prefrontal-subcortical and limbic areas and a decreased number of glial cells in the prefrontal cortex.[58]

Increased signal activity has been detected in both the cyclic adenosine monophosphate and phosphatidylinositol cascade along with elevations in G-proteins, particularly in the prefrontal cortex of patients with bipolar disorder.[58] Because G-proteins are involved with numerous neurotransmitter receptor families, multiple systems are affected, including dopamine receptors (D_1, D_2); adrenergic receptors (α_2, β_1, and β_2); a serotonin receptor (5-HT_1); a histamine receptor (H_2); GABA; and multiple peptide systems. It is unclear whether a reduction in glial cells causes the disorder or is an outcome of the disorder. Glial cells maintain metabolic and ionic homeostasis and also sequester glutamate; therefore their loss could lead to excitatory damage.[59] It is too early to exactly identify the significance of these findings, but because lithium (the major pharmacological agent used to treat bipolar disorder) appears to offer some neuroprotective function for glial cells and also reduces signal transduction intermediates, finding a connection between the two main themes regarding the pathophysiology of bipolar disorder has become prominent.[60]

Drug Treatment of Bipolar Disorder

The treatment of bipolar illness has traditionally involved immediate treatment of the affective episode (manic, mixed, or depressive) and prophylactic treatment to prevent relapses.[55] For improvement in the mental health of patients with this illness, a combination of drugs is usually necessary; exactly which ones depend on the major affective component present at the time. The term *mood stabilizer* has been adopted by psychiatrists to classify some of these drugs; however, there has been no consensus on the exact definition.[61] Some suggest that a drug is a mood stabilizer if it is effective in decreasing the severity and duration of a particular incident without cycling to the other polarity. Others have proposed that this term means that a drug is effective in treating both manic and depressive symptoms. A third proposition states

that for a drug to be classified as a mood stabilizer, it must have efficacy in four areas: treatment of acute mania, treatment of acute depression, prevention of mania, and prevention of depression. For the purposes of this book, the more liberal definition of the term will be used, that is improving the current condition while not facilitating the opposite affective profile. Thus the mood stabilizers are considered to be lithium, some antiepileptic agents, and the atypical antipsychotics.

Lithium

Lithium has been the main drug for the treatment of bipolar disorder for more than 50 years. It is used to treat acute mania and mixed episodes and to prevent relapse to either a manic or a depressive state; it is also used with other agents to treat the resistive depressive state.[9] It has superior efficacy compared with placebo for treatment of the acute manic state and has efficacy comparable to that of the other agents listed previously.[62] In addition, lithium treatment reduces the risk of relapse from 40% to 61%.[63] However, lithium appears to be more effective for those patients who have a more manic profile.

There are multiple theories regarding lithium's mechanism of action, but much research has been focused on its role as a noncompetitive inhibitor of inositol monophosphatase, depleting inositol in the frontal cortex.[64] Inositol is a major player in several signal transduction cascades, profoundly affecting many neurotransmitter systems in the brain. A reduction in inositol would subsequently reduce the synthesis of second messengers, such as diacylglycerol and inositol 1,4,5-triphosphate. It has been suggested that lithium only affects activated second-messenger systems so that basal release of inositol is not altered, and therefore there is no effect on control subjects. Another role for lithium is related to its neuroprotective properties over glial cells. Specifically, this drug reduces neurotoxicity by facilitating increased glutamate uptake into glial cells.[58]

Many side effects are associated with lithium treatment.[64] Patients report polydipsia, polyuria, nausea, diarrhea, and fine tremor. Other effects include weight gain, edema, and acne. Long-term effects include polyneuropathy, hypothyroidism, hyperparathyroidism, and diabetes insipidus. Lithium inhibits vasopressin action in the kidneys, so renal function must be monitored. In fact, baseline renal lab tests (blood urea nitrogen, creatinine level), as well as thyroid function tests and an electrocardiogram (for patients older than 40 years), are recommended. Renal function should be assessed every 2 to 3 months, and thyroid function should be assessed twice during the first 6 months of treatment. After the first 6 months, testing is recommended twice per year.

Lithium has a narrow therapeutic index, so plasma levels must be monitored frequently.[48,64] Levels should be checked every 5 days after a change in dose and every 2 to 3 months during maintenance therapy. Symptoms of lithium toxicosis include nausea, vomiting, coarse tremor, ataxia, dysarthria, confusion, and sedation. In later stages of toxicosis, when plasma levels increase further, side effects include impaired consciousness, nystagmus, muscle twitching, hyperreflexia, renal failure, and cardiac arrhythmias. If lithium toxicosis occurs, the drug should be stopped and measures such as dialysis should be taken to help facilitate elimination of the drug. Lithium is also involved in several drug-drug interactions. Nonsteroidal anti-inflammatory drugs except for aspirin increase plasma lithium levels by interfering with excretion. Diuretics act similarly. Cardiac drugs such as digoxin and angiotensin-converting inhibitors increase the risk of neurotoxic effects because of their electrical membrane effects.

Valproate and Divalproex Sodium
Divalproex and similar formulations of valproic acid have superior efficacy compared with placebo in the treatment of bipolar disorder and similar overall efficacy when compared with lithium.[62] These are antiseizure agents used primarily in the treatment of epilepsy; however, they deserve mention because they may be used in the treatment of bipolar disorder as either first-line agents or adjuncts in nonresponsive cases. They are particularly effective for patients who have experienced more depressive symptoms.[65] The exact mechanism of action is not fully understood, but it is thought that these agents stimulate glutamic acid decarboxylase, which is needed to synthesize GABA from glutamate, resulting in an increase in the concentration of GABA in the synapses.[66] In addition, they prevent reuptake of GABA and limit sodium entry into rapidly firing neurons.

Valproate is generally well tolerated during acute manic or mixed episodes.[62] Unlike lithium,

it has a high therapeutic index. Common side effects include gastrointestinal effects, sedation, ataxia, dysarthria, tremor, and a general cognitive slowing. Tremor may respond to β-blockers. Rare effects include pancreatitis, thrombocytopenia, and hepatic toxicity.

Carbamazepine
The anticonvulsant drug carbamazepine has been used to reduce mania and is considered an alternative agent for patients intolerant or nonresponsive to lithium or valproate.[67] Carbamazepine has a tricyclic structure similar to that of the tricyclic antidepressants but has markedly different neurochemical and side effect profiles. In terms of mechanism of action, it actually has many similarities to lithium. Carbamazepine inhibits inositol transport, thus affecting second-messenger systems. It also inhibits calcium influx through the NMDA receptors, blocks voltage-gated sodium channels, and increases limbic $GABA_B$ receptors.[68]

In several controlled trials, carbamazepine was found to be superior to placebo in its immediate antimanic efficacy, and it may have an overall response rate similar to that of lithium.[69,70] However, it appears to have a weaker antidepressant effect than lithium and is not as effective in preventing relapses in the classic bipolar disorder (bipolar type I).[70] Patients with an atypical or rapidly cycling disease may respond well to this drug.[71]

Adverse effects of carbamazepine include rash, drowsiness, blurred vision, ataxia, and occasional impairments in cognitive functioning.[68] Long-term use may produce agranulocytosis; thus any fever or infection should be reported immediately to the physician. This drug also induces its own metabolism, and therefore the patient may develop tolerance.

Other Agents
The atypical antipsychotic olanzapine is an effective treatment for acute bipolar mania, being superior to placebo and divalproex and equal in efficacy to lithium.[72-74] The drug also appears to be effective regardless of whether psychosis is present. More data on olanzapine's effectiveness during the depressive cycle and the overall effectiveness of the other atypical antipsychotic agents are needed.

The other drugs that are currently under study in bipolar illness include the newer antiseizure medications: lamotrigine, gabapentin, and topiramate.[62,75,76] Of these, lamotrigine appears worthy of further study, being effective in the treatment of bipolar depression.[77]

Treatment of Bipolar Disorder with Various Symptom Profiles

Manic and mixed episodes of bipolar illness are emergencies and require hospitalization. The primary goal during this phase is a rapid reduction in mania with lithium, divalproex, olanzapine, or carbamazepine, which all show efficacy as monotherapy for acute mania. A benzodiazepine may also be added to control hyperactivity. Most patients will show a response to this regimen, defined rather loosely as a >50% reduction in mania. However, only a few patients will reach complete remission within a 3- to 4-week period, and thus combination therapy is often recommended.[62] Popular initial combinations include an atypical antipsychotic along with lithium, divalproex, or carbamazepine.[55]

Treatment of an acute bipolar depressive episode is more challenging. There is a substantial risk of suicide in these patients and also the risk of switching to mania if the episode is treated solely with an antidepressant.[78] Until recently, recommendations were to administer lithium as monotherapy and to avoid antidepressants if possible. More recently, the selective serotonin reuptake inhibitors, bupropion, and venlafaxine have been recommended along with lithium as first-line agents.[79,80]

Because bipolar disorder is a recurrent and lifelong disease, maintenance therapy is recommended as soon as the first manic episode is under control.[62] In a meta-analysis of randomized, placebo-controlled trials that evaluated maintenance therapy, lithium was found to be more effective than placebo in preventing all types of relapses but with greater efficacy in preventing a manic relapse.[81] In the bipolar type II disorder, lithium and carbamazepine were equally effective, but the combination of lamotrigine and lithium might be superior.[77]

There is some concern regarding neural adaptation to long-term lithium treatment because of evidence that perfusion to the limbic area is altered during long-term lithium maintenance therapy.[82] If a patient who has been receiving lithium maintenance therapy for a while begins to experience side effects necessitating a reduction in dose, the ADR profile will improve, but the patient will be more likely to have a relapse. Therefore some patients may be switched to another regimen for maintenance after their illness stabilizes. For this reason, there is renewed interest in combination drug regimens.[83] The combination of divalproex and lithium offers some safety advantages because their pharmacokinetic profiles do not overlap and there is the potential for lower, better tolerated doses of lithium.[84] However, no matter what drug the patient is currently taking, if a switch is desired, the first drug must be discontinued slowly.

Therapeutic Concerns with Drugs for Bipolar Disorder

Because the majority of patients who have bipolar illness will be taking lithium, it is prudent for the physical therapist to become familiar with the side effects associated with this drug, as well as the indicators of lithium toxicosis. Easily discernable red flags include the presence of tremors, nystagmus, muscle weakness or twitching, and hyperreflexia. Because these manifestations are motor abnormalities, the physical therapist should be adept at identifying them early on. In addition, the physical therapist should be concerned about osteoporosis (resulting from hyperparathyroidism) in patients who have been taking lithium for an extended period.

Another concern is a worsening of the psychiatric condition. Because these patients cycle through different moods, keeping cognizant of the symptoms of depression, hypomania, and mania will be helpful so that the patients can be directed to their psychiatrists before the behavior becomes more difficult to manage.

ACTIVITES 17

■ 1. A significant number of side effects associated with the typical antipsychotic medications and some additional side effects of the atypical agents that will affect physical therapy may develop. List the ADRs for each type of drug and explain how they will affect treatment and how you should monitor for them.

■ 2. Scott and Pope[85] report that one in three patients with bipolar disorder do not adhere to their medication regimen and this non-adherence to treatment is a frequent cause of relapse necessitating hospitalization. Review the literature and identify factors that affect treatment adherence. What are some strategies that can be used to help improve treatment adherence?

References

1. Rang HP, Dale MM, Ritter JM, Moore JL. *Pharmacology.* 5th ed. New York: Churchill Livingstone; 2003.
2. Lewis DA, Lieberman JA. Catching up on schizophrenia: natural history and neurobiology. *Neuron.* 2000;28:325-334.
3. Pearlson GD. Neurobiology of schizophrenia. *Ann Neurol.* 2000;48:556-566.
4. Lieberman JA, Perkins D, Belger A, et al. The early stages of schizophrenia: speculations on pathogenesis, pathophysiology, and therapeutic approaches. *Biol Psychiatry.* 2001;50:884-897.
5. McCarley RW, Wible CG, Frumin M, et al. MRI anatomy of schizophrenia. *Biol Psychiatry.* 1999;45:1099-1119.
6. Goldstein JM, Goodman JM, Seidman LJ, et al. Cortical abnormalities in schizophrenia identified by structural magnetic resonance imaging. *Arch Gen Psychiatry.* 1999;56(6):537-547.
7. Kim JJ, Mohamed S, Andreasen NC, et al. Regional neural dysfunctions in chronic schizophrenia studied with positron emission tomography. *Am J Psychiatry.* 2000; 157(4):542-548.
8. Kapur S, Mamo D. Half a century of antipsychotics and still a central role for dopamine D2 receptors. *Prog Neuropsychopharmacol Biol Psychiatry.* 2003;27:1081-1090.
9. Kerwin R, Travis MJ, Page C, et al. Drugs and the nervous system. In: Page C, Curtis MJ, Sutter MC, Walker MJ, Hoffman BB, eds. *Integrated Pharmacology.* 2nd ed. Philadelphia: Mosby; 2002.
10. Laruelle M, Abi-Dargham A, Gil R, Kegeles L, Innis R. Increased dopamine transmission in schizophrenia: relationship to illness phases. *Biol Psychiatry.* 1999; 46:56-72.
11. Abi-Dargham A, Rodenhiser J, Printz D, et al. Increased baseline occupancy of D2 receptors by dopamine in schizophrenia. *Proc Natl Acad Sci U S A.* 2000;97(14): 8104-8109.
12. Breier A, Su TP, Saunders R, et al. Schizophrenia is associated with elevated amphetamine-induced synaptic dopamine concentrations: evidence from a novel positron emission tomography method. *Proc Natl Acad Sci U S A.* 1997;94:2569-2574.
13. Kapur S, Zipursky R, Jones C, Remington G, Houle S. Relationship between dopamine D2 occupancy, clinical response, and side effects: a double-blind PET study of first-episode schizophrenia. *Am J Psychiatry.* 2000; 157(4):514-520.
14. Tsai G, Coyle JT. Glutamatergic mechanisms in schizophrenia. *Annu Rev Pharmacol Toxicol.* 2003;42: 165-179.
15. Kegeles L, Abi-Dargham A, Zea-Ponce Y, et al. Modulation of amphetamine-induced striatal dopamine release by ketamine in humans: implications for schizophrenia. *Biol Psychiatry.* 2000;48(7):627-640.
16. Brunello N, Masotto C, Steardo L, Markstein R, Racagni G. New insights into the biology of schizophrenia through the mechanism of action of clozapine. *Neuropsychopharmacology.* 1995;13(3):177-213.
17. Binder EB, Kinkead B, Owens MJ, Nemeroff CB. The role of neurotensin in the pathophysiology of schizophrenia and the mechanism of action of antipsychotic drugs. *Biol Psychiatry.* 2001;50:856-872.
18. Wilkaitis J, Mulvihill T, Nasrallah HA. Classic antipsychotic medications. In: Schatzberg AF, Nemeroff CB, eds. *Textbook of Psychopharmacology.* 3rd ed. Washington, DC: American Psychiatric Publishing, Inc.; 2004:425-441.
19. Kapur S, Remington G, Jones C, et al. High levels of dopamine D2 receptor occupancy with low-dose haloperidol treatment: a PET study. *Am J Psychiatry.* 1996;153(7):948-950.
20. Woo TU, Zimmet SV, Wojcik J, Canuso CM, Green AI. Treatment of schizophrenia. In: Schatzberg AF, Nemeroff CB, eds. *Textbook of Psychopharmacology.* 3rd ed. Washington, DC: American Psychiatric Publishing, Inc.; 2004:885-912.
21. Kapur S, Seeman P. Does fast dissociation from the dopamine d(2) receptor explain the action of atypical antipsychotics? A new hypothesis. *Am J Psychiatry.* 2001;158(3):360-369.
22. Jeste DV, Lacro JP, Palmer B, Rockwell E, Harris MJ, Caligiuri MP. Incidence of tardive dyskinesia in early stages of low-dose treatment with typical neuroleptics in older patients. *Am J Psychiatry.* 1999; 156(2):309-311.

23. Stanilla JK, Simpson GM. Drugs to treat extrapyramidal side effects. In: Schatzberg AF, Nemeroff CB, eds. *Textbook of Psychopharmacology*. 3rd ed. Washington, DC: American Psychiatric Publishing; 2004:519-544.

24. Pisani F, Oteri G, Costa C, Di Raimondo G, Di Perri R. Effect of psychotropic drugs on seizure threshold. *Drug Saf*. 2002;25(2):91-110.

25. Witchel HJ, Hancox JC, Nutt DJ. Psychotropic drugs, cardiac arrhythmia, and sudden death. *J Clin Psychopharmacol*. 2003;23(1):58-77.

26. Cavazzoni P, Mukhopadhyay N, Carlson C, Breier A, Buse J. Retrospective analysis of risk factors in patients with treatment-emergent diabetes during clinical trials of antipsychotic medications. *Br J Psychiatry*. 2004; 47(suppl):S94-S101.

27. Hermesh H, Shiloh R, Epstein Y, Manaim H, Weizman A, Munitz H. Heat intolerance in patients with chronic schizophrenia maintained with antipsychotic drugs. *Am J Psychiatry*. 2000;157(8):1327-1329.

28. Prevention and treatment of heat injury. *Med Lett Drugs Ther*. 2003; 45(1161):58-60.

29. Remington G. Understanding antipsychotic "atypicality": a clinical and pharmacological moving target. *J Psychiatry Neurosci*. 2003;28(4):275-284.

30. Kapur S, Remington G. Atypical antipsychotics: new directions and new challenges in the treatment of schizophrenia. *Annu Rev Med*. 2001;52:503-517.

31. Geddes JR, Freemantle N, Harrison P, Bebbington P. Atypical antipsychotics in the treatment of schizophrenia: systematic overview and meta-regression analysis. *BMJ*. 2000;321:1371-1376.

32. Marder SR, Wirshing DA. Clozapine. In: Schatzberg AF, Nemeroff CB, eds. *Textbook of Psychopharmacology*. 3rd ed. Washington, DC: American Psychiatric Publishing; 2004:443-456.

33. Wong AHC, Van Tol HHM. The dopamine D4 receptors and mechanisms of antipsychotic atypicality. *Prog Neuropsychopharmacol Biol Psychiatry*. 2003;27: 1091-1099.

34. Kramer MS, Last B, Getson A, Reines SA. The effects of a selective D4 dopamine receptor antagonist (L-745,870) in acutely psychotic inpatients with schizophrenia. *Arch Gen Psychiatry*. 1997;54:567-572.

35. Honigfeld G. Effects of the clozapine national registry system on incidence of deaths. *Psychiatr Serv*. 1996; 47(1):52-56.

36. Wirshing DA, Wirshing WC, Kysar L, et al. Novel antipsychotics: comparison of weight gain liabilities. *J Clin Psychiatry*. 1999;60(6):358-363.

37. Lindenmayer JP, Czobor P, Volavka J, et al. Changes in glucose and cholesterol levels in patients with schizophrenia treated with typical or atypical antipsychotics. *Am J Psychiatry*. 2003;160(2):290-296.

38. Choice of an antipsychotic. *Med Lett Drugs Ther*. 2003; 45(1172):102-104.

39. Schulz SC, Olson S, Kotlyar M. Olanzapine. In: Schatzberg AF, Nemeroff CB, eds. *Textbook of Psychopharmacology*. 3rd ed. Washington, DC: American Psychiatric Publishing; 2004:457-472.

40. Diaz E, Neuse E, Sullivan MC, Pearsall HR, Woods SW. Adherence to conventional and atypical antipsychotics after hospital discharge. *J Clin Psychiatry*. 2004;65(3): 354-360.

41. Bitter I, Dossenbach MR, Brook S, et al. Olanzapine versus clozapine in treatment-resistant or treatment-intolerant schizophrenia. *Prog Neuropsychopharmacol Biol Psychiatry*. 2004;28(1):173-180.

42. Lieberman JA, Tollefson G, Tohen M, et al. Comparative efficacy and safety of atypical and conventional antipsychotic drugs in first-episode psychosis: a randomized, double-blind trial of olanzapine versus haloperidol. *Am J Psychiatry*. 2003;160(8):1396-1404.

43. Lieberman JA. Quetiapine. In: Schatzberg AF, Nemeroff CB, eds. *Textbook of Psychopharmacology*. 3rd ed. Washington, DC: American Psychiatric Publishing; 2004:473-486.

44. Yokoi F, Grunder G, Biziere K, et al. Dopamine D_2 and D_3 receptor occupancy in normal humans treated with the antipsychotic drug aripiprazole (OPC 14597): a study using positron emission tomography and [^{11}C]Raclopride. *Neuropsychopharmacology*. 2002;27(2):248-259.

45. Kasper S, Lerman MN, McQuade RD, et al. Efficacy and safety of aripiprazole vs. haloperidol for long-term maintenance treatment following acute relapse of schizophrenia. *Int J Neuropsychopharmacol*. 2003;6(4):325-337.

46. Pigott TA, Carson WH, Saha AR, Torbeyns AF, Stock EG, Ingenito GG. Aripiprazole for the prevention of relapse in stabilized patients with chronic schizophrenia: a placebo-controlled 26-week study. *J Clin Psychiatry*. 2003;64(9):1048-1056.

47. Bai YM, Yu SC, Lin CC. Risperidone for severe tardive dyskinesia: a 12-week randomized, double-blind, placebo-controlled study. *J Clin Psychiatry*. 2003;64(11):1342-1348.

48. Drugs for psychiatric disorders. *Treat Guidel Med Lett*. 2003;1(11)69-76.

49. Wyatt RJ, Damiani LM, Henter ID. First episode schizophrenia: early intervention and medication discontinuation in the context of course and treatment. *Br J Psychiatry*. 1998;172(suppl 33):77-83.

50. Konradi C, Heckers S. Antipsychotic drugs and neuroplasticity: insights into the treatment and neurobiology of schizophrenia. *Biol Psychiatry*. 2001;50:729-742.

51. Gitlin M, Nuechterlein K, Subotnik KL, et al. Clinical outcome following neuroleptic discontinuation in patients with remitted recent-onset schizophrenia. *Am J Psychiatry*. 2001;158(11):1835-1842.

52. Robinson DG, Woerner MG, Alvir JM, et al. Predictors of treatment response from a first episode of schizophrenia or schizoaffective disorder. *Am J Psychiatry*. 1999; 156(4):544-549.

53. Angst J, Gamma A, Benzazzi F, Ajdacic V, Eich D, Rossler W. Diagnostic issues in bipolar disorder. *Eur Neuropsychopharmacol*. 2003;13:S43-S50.

54. Tillman R, Geller B. Definitions of rapid, ultrarapid, and ultradian cycling and of episode duration in pediatric and adult bipolar disorders: a proposal to distinguish episodes from cycles. *J Child Adolesc Psychopharmacol*. 2003;13(3):267-271.

55. Muller-Oerlinghausen B, Berghofer A, Bauer M. Bipolar disorder. *Lancet*. 2002;359:241-247.

56. Howland RH. Induction of mania with serotonin reuptake inhibitors. *J Clin Psychopharmacol*. 1996;16(6):425-427.

57. Bauer M, London ED, Silverman DH, Rasgon N, Kirchheiner J, Whybrow PC. Thyroid, brain and mood modulation in affective disorder: insights from molecular research and functional brain imaging. *Pharmacopsychiatry*. 2003;36(suppl 3):S215-S221.

58. Vawter MP, Freed WJ, Kleinman JE. Neuropathology of bipolar disorder. *Biol Psychiatry.* 2000;48(6):486-504.

59. Sheline YI. Neuroimaging studies of mood disorder effects on the brain. *Biol Psychiatry.* 2003;54:338-352.

60. Bauer M, Alda M, Priller J, Young LT, International Group for the Study of Lithium Treated Patients (IGSLI). Implications of the neuroprotective effects of lithium for the treatment of bipolar and neurodegenerative disorders. *Pharmacopsychiatry.* 2003;36(suppl 3):S250-S254.

61. Bauer MS, Mitchner L. What is a "mood stabilizer"? An evidence-based response. *Am J Psychiatry.* 2004; 161(1):3-18.

62. Keck PE, McElroy SL. Treatment of bipolar disorder. In: Schatzberg AF, Nemeroff CB, eds. *Textbook of Psychopharmacology.* 3rd ed. Washington, DC: American Psychiatric Publishing; 2004:865-884.

63. Geddes JR, Burgess S, Hawton KD, Jamison K, Goodwin GM. Long-term lithium therapy for bipolar disorder: systematic review and meta-analysis of randomized controlled trials. *Am J Psychiatry.* 2004; 161(2):217-222.

64. Freeman MP, Wiegand C, Gelenberg AJ. Lithium. In: Schatzberg AF, Nemeroff CB, eds. *Textbook of Psychopharmacology.* 3rd ed. Washington, DC: American Psychiatric Publishing; 2004:547-561.

65. Freeman TW, Clothier JL, Pazzaglia P, Lesem MD, Swann AC. A double-blind comparison of valproate and lithium in the treatment of acute mania. *Am J Psychiatry.* 1992;149(1):108-111.

66. Bowden CL. Valproate. In: Schatzberg AF, Nemeroff CB, eds. *Textbook of Psychopharmacology.* 3rd ed. Washington, DC: American Psychiatric Publishing; 2004:567-579.

67. Hartong EG, Moleman P, Hoogduin CA, Broekman TG, Nolen WA. Prophylactic efficacy of lithium versus carbamazepine in treatment-naive bipolar patients. *J Clin Psychiatry.* 2003;64(2):144-151.

68. Ketter TA, Wang PW, Post RM. Carbamazepine and oxcarbazepine. In: Schatzberg AF, Nemeroff CB, eds. *Textbook of Psychopharmacology.* 3rd ed. Washington, DC: American Psychiatric Publishing; 2004:581-606.

69. Weisler RH, Kalali AH, Ketter TA. A multicenter, randomized, double-blind, placebo-controlled trial of extended-release carbamazepine capsules as mono-therapy for bipolar disorder patients with manic or mixed episodes. *J Clin Psychiatry.* 2004;65(4):478-484.

70. Small JG, Klapper MH, Milstein V, et al. Carbamazepine compared with lithium in the treatment of mania. *Arch Gen Psychiatry.* 1991;48(10):915-921.

71. Greil W, Kleindienst N, Erazo N, Muller-Oerlinghausen B. Differential response to lithium and carbamazepine in the prophylaxis of bipolar disorder. *J Clin Psychopharmacol.* 1998;18(6):455-460.

72. Tohen M, Baker RW, Altshuler LL, et al. Olanzapine versus divalproex in the treatment of acute mania. *Am J Psychiatry.* 2002;159(6):1011-1017.

73. Tohen M, Jacobs TG, Grundy SL, et al. Efficacy of olanzapine in acute bipolar mania: a double-blind, placebo-controlled study. The Olanzapine HGGW Study Group. *Arch Gen Psychiatry.* 2000;57(9):841-849.

74. Berk M, Ichim L, Brook S. Olanzapine compared to lithium in mania: a double-blind randomized controlled trial. *Int Clin Psychopharmacol.* 1999;14(6):339-343.

75. Keck PE. Treatment advances in bipolar disorder—making up for lost time. *Biol Psychiatry.* 2000;48:430-432.

76. Calabrese JR, Vieta E, Shelton MD. Latest maintenance data on lamotrigine in bipolar disorder. *Eur Neuropsychopharmacol.* 2003;13:S57-S66.

77. Calabrese JR, Bowden CL, Sachs GS, et al. A placebo-controlled 18 month trial of lamotrigine and lithium maintenance treatment in recently depressed patients with bipolar I disorder. *J Clin Psychiatry.* 2003;64(9):1013-1024.

78. Keck PE, Nelson EB, McElroy SL. Advances in the pharmacologic treatment of bipolar depression. *Biol Psychiatry.* 2003;53(8):671-679.

79. Thase ME, Sachs GS. Bipolar depression: pharmaco-therapy and related therapeutic strategies. *Biol Psychiatry.* 2000;48:558-572.

80. Shelton RC. The combination of olanzapine and fluoxetine in mood disorders. *Expert Opin Pharmacother.* 2003;4(7):1175-1183.

81. Goodwin GM, Geddes DM. Latest maintenance data on lithium in bipolar disorder. *Eur Neuropsychopharmacol.* 2003;13:S51-S55.

82. Perlis RH, Sachs GS, Lafer B, et al. Effect of abrupt change from standard to low serum levels of lithium: a reanalysis of double-blind lithium maintenance data. *Am J Psychiatry.* 2002;159(7):1155-1159.

83. Grof P. Selecting effective long-term treatment for bipolar patients: monotherapy and combinations. *J Clin Psychiatry.* 2003;64(suppl 5):53-61.

84. Bowden CL. Clinical correlates of therapeutic response in bipolar disorder. *J Affect Disord.* 2001;67:257-265.

85. Scott J, Pope M. Self-reported adherence to treatment with mood stabilizers, plasma levels, and psychiatric hospitalization. *Am J Psychiatry.* 2002;159(11):1927-1929.

7
SECTION

Drugs Affecting
the Nervous System

CHAPTER 18

Drugs for Epilepsy and Attention-Deficit/Hyperactivity Disorder

OVERVIEW OF EPILEPSY

Epilepsy is a disorder characterized by seizures, which may appear in various forms, depending on the locations affected in the brain.[1] A seizure is the outward expression of a sudden excessive electrical discharge of neurons, with firing rates between 200 and 900 Hz, many times the activity of normal neurons. A seizure may appear as a brief lapse in attention or as a convulsive episode lasting for several minutes. Seizures involving the motor cortex produce convulsions, those involving the hypothalamus produce autonomic changes, and those involving the reticular formation in the brainstem produce a loss of consciousness.

Seizures may occur as a result of fever, alcohol withdrawal, head trauma, stroke, a brain tumor, central nervous system (CNS) infections, or epilepsy.[1] Epilepsy, however, is the only disorder characterized by recurrent spontaneous seizures. In more than 50% of cases of epilepsy, the cause is unknown, and this is called *primary* or *idiopathic epilepsy*. Epilepsy related to a particular event is called *secondary epilepsy*. The principal causes of secondary epilepsy in children are injury at birth and metabolic disease. Traumatic brain injury is the primary cause in adults.

Diagnosis of epilepsy requires careful clinical observation of the seizure in progress, an adequate patient history, and an electroencephalogram, which detects excessive electrical discharges in the brain (Figure 18-1).[2] A computed tomography or magnetic resonance imaging scan may also assist in the diagnosis, particularly if a structural lesion is present.

Types of Epilepsy

Epileptic seizures are divided into two main classes: partial seizures and generalized seizures (Box 18-1).[2] They are further divided into simple seizures, if consciousness remains intact, or complex seizures, if consciousness is lost.

Partial seizures originate in a localized area of one cerebral hemisphere. The discharge begins locally and ends locally. The simple partial seizure has a primary sensory component (odor or taste), or some autonomic discharge, without loss of consciousness. However, there may be some focal motor symptoms, depending on the anatomical region affected. In the complex partial seizure, loss of consciousness may occur. If the anatomical insult is in the motor cortex, it is called *Jacksonian epilepsy*. This consists of repetitive jerking movements of a specific muscle group, which can, on occasion, spread to involve much of the body. The psychomotor seizure often has its foci in the temporal lobe and may show stereotypical purposive movements or automatisms (e.g., chewing movements, hand rubbing, patting movements, or hair combing). This type of seizure may last for a few minutes, and the patient has no memory of it when he or she recovers.

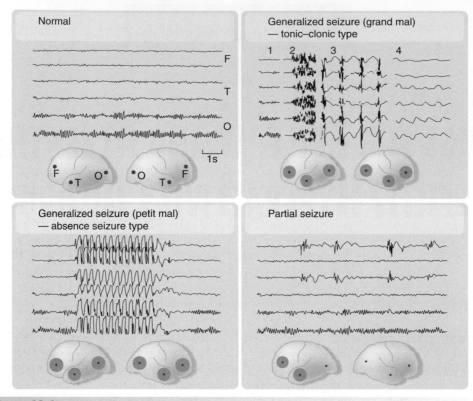

Figure 18-1

Electroencephalograph (EEG) records in epilepsy. **A,** Normal EEG recorded from frontal (*F*), temporal (*T*), and occipital (*O*) sites on both sides, as shown in the inset diagram. The α-rhythm (10/s) can be seen in the occipital region. **B,** Sections of EEG recorded during a generalized tonic-clonic (grand mal) seizure. *1,* Normal record; *2,* onset of tonic phase; *3,* clonic phase; *4,* postconvulsive coma. **C,** Generalized absence seizure (petit mal) showing sudden brief episode of 3/s "spike and wave" discharge. **D,** Partial seizure with synchronous abnormal discharges in left frontal and temporal regions. (From Eliasson SG et al. *Neurological Pathophysiology.* 2nd ed. New York: Oxford University Press; 1978.) (From Rang HP, Dale DC, Ritter JM, Moore JL. Antiepileptic drugs. In: *Pharmacology.* New York: Churchill Livingstone; 2003.)

In generalized seizures, the neuronal discharge involves both cerebral hemispheres. Immediate loss of consciousness occurs as a result of involvement of the reticular formation. There are six types of generalized seizures. The most common type is the tonic-clonic seizure. This seizure begins with a sudden rigid extensor spasm, causing the patient to fall to the ground, with rigidity lasting for 10 to 30 seconds. Respiration ceases; and defecation, micturition, or salivation may occur. This is followed by the clonic phase in which there is a rhythmic flexor spasm lasting 2 to 4 minutes. The spasm gradually lessens, but the patient may remain unconscious for a few more minutes. Alertness occurs slowly, with the patient feeling ill and confused at first. Tonic seizures consist of tonic contractions of certain muscle groups and altered consciousness, but no progression to the clonic phase. Clonic seizures are characterized by repetitive clonic jerks without a tonic component. Both types of seizures last only seconds.

Absence seizures occur most often in children. They are less dramatic in presentation but may occur more frequently than tonic-clonic seizures. An absence seizure consists of an abrupt, brief loss of consciousness with amnesia. The patient suddenly stops whatever he or she is doing, even ceasing to finish a sentence, and stares blankly for a few seconds. Some mild clonic movements, such as eye blinking and slight changes in postural tone, may occur. The patient recovers quickly with no ill feeling.

International Classification of Seizures

Partial seizures

Description

Short alterations in consciousness, repetitive unusual movements (chewing or swallowing movements), psychologic changes, and confusion.

Simple seizures

- No impaired consciousness
- Motor symptoms (most commonly face, arm or leg)
- Hallucinations of sight, hearing, or taste along with somatosensory changes (tingling)
- Autonomic nervous system responses
- Personality changes

Complex seizures

- Impaired consciousness
- Memory impairment
- Behavioral effects
- Purposeless behaviors
- Aura, chewing and swallowing movements, unreal feelings, bizarre behavior
- Tonic, clonic, or tonic-clonic seizures

Generalized seizures

Description

Most often seen in children and commonly characterized by temporary lapses in consciousness lasting a few seconds. Staring off into space, daydreaming, and inattentive look are common symptoms. Patients may exhibit rhythmic movements of their eyes, head, or hands but do not convulse. May have several attacks per day.

- Both cerebral hemispheres involved
- Tonic, clonic, myotonic, atonic, or tonic-clonic seizures and infantile spasms possible
- Brief loss of consciousness for a few seconds with no confusion
- Head-drop or falling-down symptoms

From Lilley LL, Harrington D, Snyder JS. Antiepileptic agents. In: *Pharmacology and the Nursing Process.* 4th ed. St Louis: Mosby; 2005.

There are few other kinds of generalized seizures. Atonic seizures, also known as drop attacks, are characterized by a sudden reduction in muscle tone of selective muscle groups, leading to head dropping or dropping of a limb. Duration is 10 to 30 seconds. Myoclonic seizures are characterized by a single contraction or multiple sudden, brief, con-

tractions confined to the face, trunk, or extremities, again lasting only seconds.

Neural Mechanisms and Models of Epilepsy

The underlying neuronal mechanism of epilepsy is not well understood. It is thought that excitation of neurons will spread unless normally prevented from doing so by inhibitory devices. Thus a seizure can occur if excitation is increased or inhibition is reduced. Glutamate, an excitatory amino acid that activates N-methyl-D-aspartate receptors, is believed to be increased in areas where seizures originate.

Animal models are available, but none match the human form of epilepsy exactly.[1] There are mice that convulse briefly in response to certain sounds, baboons that show seizures in response to certain visual stimuli, and a group of beagles with an inherited disorder that resembles the human form of epilepsy. In addition, chemical and electrical means can be used to produce a seizure in an animal. Local application of penicillin crystals in the brain may result in a partial seizure, and the convulsant drug, pentylenetetrazol, can produce a generalized seizure. It has been found that drugs that inhibit these convulsions are effective against absence seizures and drugs that inhibit electrically induced seizures are helpful for tonic-clonic seizures. There is also a kindling model that may evoke seizures that more closely resemble the human versions more than the drug or chemical model.[3] Low-intensity electrical stimulation is applied to the amygdala with implanted electrodes. Normally, this would not evoke a seizure, except that when the stimulation is repeated daily for several days, seizures may begin to occur spontaneously. The seizures are blocked by glutamate antagonists.

ANTIEPILEPTIC DRUGS

The main mechanisms of action of the current antiepileptic drugs (AEDs) are the augmentation of γ-aminobutyric acid (GABA) activity and the blockade of sodium or calcium channels.[1] Like drugs for cardiac arrhythmias, the purpose of AEDs is to prevent abnormal and excessive discharge without inhibiting normal transmission.

Many of the AEDs have multiple effects on neuronal activity; however, some predominant effects for each drug can be delineated (Table 18-1).[4]

Table 18-1

Ion Channel Activity of Antiepileptic Drugs				
Drug	Na$^+$ Channels	Ca^{2+} Channels	K$^+$ Channel	Inhibitory Transmission
Phenytoin	+++	+		
Carbamazepine	+++			
Valproate	+	+		++
Ethosuximide		+++		
Phenobarbital		+		+++
Lamotrigine	+++	+		
Zonisamide	++	++		
Gabapentin				++
Topiramate	++	++		++

Adapted from Brodie MJ, Kwan P. Staged approach to epilepsy management. *Neurology.* 2002; 58(suppl 5):S2-S8. *Na$^+$*, Sodium; *Ca^{2+}*, calcium; *K$^+$*, potassium; +++, primary action; ++, probable action; +, possible action.

Many drugs control seizures by acting on voltage-gated sodium channels and are particularly effective for tonic-clonic seizures and complex partial seizures. Other drugs act on voltage-gated calcium channels in the thalamus and are effective against absence seizures. Additionally, the benzodiazepines and barbiturates act at the GABA-gated chloride channel to provide some inhibition of the spreading excitation. Some newer drugs target glutamate receptors directly.

AEDs may produce changes in the brain that provide neuroprotection from seizure damage in addition to action on specific ion channels and neurotransmitters.[5] It has been believed for years that seizure activity can facilitate additional seizures by producing abnormal structural and neurochemical processes. It is also known that status epilepticus can result in hippocampal and cerebral damage, although it is not certain that tonic-clonic and complex partial seizures cause brain damage. Animal models are currently being used to determine whether the drugs are anti-epileptogenic, neuroprotective, or both.

Relatively few drugs are available for the treatment or control of seizures compared with drugs for treatment of conditions such as hypertension and angina. In fact, before 1990, only six major AEDs were available to treat all forms of epilepsy.[6] These older AEDs include carbamazepine, phenobarbital, phenytoin, primidone, valproic acid, and ethosuximide. Although they are helpful for some, many patients have seizures that are refractory to

treatment or require combination therapies for effectiveness. The other problem with these drugs is that several are hepatic enzyme inducers, resulting in numerous drug-drug interactions, namely with warfarin, oral contraceptives, calcium channel antagonists, and some chemotherapeutic agents; these drugs also affect how sex steroids and vitamin D are metabolized.[7]

The problems in pharmacokinetics and effectiveness with the older AEDs have led investigators to the discovery of at least seven new AEDs within the past 10 years. However, the majority of the new AEDs are approved only for adjunctive treatment.[8] This is because the studies evaluated by the Food and Drug Administration were conducted with patients who had refractory seizures and continued to receive their original antiseizure medication but were given either placebo or study drug as an adjunct. These studies, for the most part, are flawed because they were conducted with patients whose seizures were refractory to their original medicines and thus would be presumed to be more difficult to treat. Additionally, these patients do not represent the patient with a new diagnosis of epilepsy seeking first-time help from a neurologist. Nevertheless, many clinical investigators are using the new AEDs off-label as monotherapy.

Phenytoin

Phenytoin is one of the primary drugs for controlling all seizures with the exception of absence seizures. It alters conductance at potassium and calcium channels, but its primary action is blocking of the sodium current. It is also used in the treatment of trigeminal neuralgia and related neuralgias.

Adverse effects from phenytoin include rashes, hirsutism, hepatitis, gingival hyperplasia, and a coarsening of facial features. The hirsutism and changes in facial features may be due to elevated androgen levels produced by the drug. The gingival hyperplasia occurs only in portions of the gum that have teeth. Good oral hygiene may help to minimize this effect and periodontal disease as well. Endocrine effects such as hyperglycemia and osteomalacia may also occur. The hyperglycemia is due to inhibition of insulin secretion, and the osteomalacia is due to inhibition of calcium absorption through the intestines and accelerated hydroxylation of vitamin D to its inactive forms.[9] Dysrhythmias and hypotension can also occur and are adverse effects related to the drug's action on sodium channels in the heart. Phenytoin also has an excitatory effect on the cerebellar-vestibular system, resulting in nystagmus, ataxia, and dizziness. These effects plus additional CNS effects—including blurred vision, hyperactivity, silliness, confusion, sedation, and coma—are dose related. Long-term use may produce megaloblastic anemia and hypoprothrombinemia and hemorrhage caused by vitamin K deficiency. Many of the drug-drug interactions are connected to phenytoin's metabolism. Some drugs decrease its effects by inducing hepatic microsomal enzymes, and other drugs, such as alcohol, stimulate the enzymes, producing a decrease in antiseizure activity. Excessive or long-term consumption of alcohol can significantly reduce phenytoin's effectiveness. Phenytoin itself is an enzyme inducer. Other drugs increase phenytoin's effect by displacing the drug from its protein-binding sites.

Barbiturates (Phenobarbital, Primidone)

Barbiturates inhibit seizure activity by increasing the threshold for neuronal firing. They also enhance inhibition by activating the GABA receptors. Primidone is a prodrug that is metabolized in the liver to phenobarbital and phenylethylmalonamide, both of which have antiseizure properties. These drugs provide effective treatment for tonic-clonic

and partial seizures, but their laundry list of side effects prevents them from being chosen as first-line agents.

The majority of side effects are related to CNS depression. These drugs usually produce drowsiness, depression, inattention, confusion, and ataxia; but in some cases, they cause excitation. They may also cause skin rashes and hematological effects such as megaloblastic anemia and osteomalacia, similar to the side effects of phenytoin. They should not be taken during pregnancy because they can produce congenital malformations and coagulation problems in the newborn. Also, lower intelligence scores have been noted in children whose mothers took phenobarbital during pregnancy. Phenobarbital is a P450 enzyme inducer, so not only does some tolerance develop with this drug, but it is also affected by other enzyme-inducing drugs. This drug is as effective as phenytoin for the treatment of generalized tonic-clonic seizures but less effective for partial seizures. It continues to be used as a third-line agent. The only advantage to using this drug is that it has the longest half-life of all the older AEDs, allowing for once-a-day dosing.

Carbamazepine

Carbamazepine has a structure similar to that of the tricyclic antidepressants, although pharmacologically it resembles phenytoin by blocking voltage-gated sodium channels. This drug is highly effective in the treatment of all partial seizures, including complex partial seizures and tonic-clonic seizures, and it is currently the second most commonly prescribed AED after phenytoin.

Drowsiness, fatigue, vertigo, ataxia, diplopia, hyperirritability, and respiratory depression are related to the depressive effects on the CNS. Gastrointestinal (GI) reactions may also occur and include nausea, vomiting, and dry mouth. Dry mouth is related to the anticholinergic effects of carbamazepine. More severe reactions involve the skin, cardiovascular, and hematological systems. Skin reactions include rashes, urticaria, photosensitivity, and altered skin pigmentation. The cardiovascular reactions include congestive heart failure, syncope, hypertension, and hypotension. These symptoms may be related to excessive secretion of antidiuretic hormone with concomitant hyponatremia. The hematological reactions include aplastic anemia, agranulocytosis, and thrombocytopenia. Lastly, this drug is an enzyme inducer, so when it is taken with other drugs, it may make them less effective.

Valproic Acid (Sodium Valproate)

Valproic acid stimulates glutamic acid decarboxylase, which is needed to synthesize GABA from glutamate, resulting in an increase in the concentration of GABA in the synapses.[10] In addition, it prevents reuptake of GABA and limits sodium entry into rapidly firing neurons. Valproic acid is very effective for many types of seizures (tonic-clonic, atonic, and myoclonic) and is the drug of choice for absence seizures. It is also used for migraine prophylaxis.

The CNS depressive effects of valproic acid are less severe than those of the other antiseizure agents. However, side effects still include drowsiness, sedation, headache, dizziness, ataxia, confusion, and some visual disturbances. Valproic acid also produces thinning of the hair in about 10% of patients.[1] Hematological reactions occur as a result of inhibition of platelet aggregation and lead to bleeding, and there are also some reports of liver damage. GI disturbances are common but may be minimized by administration with food.

Ethosuximide

Ethosuximide works by increasing the seizure threshold by blocking the T-type calcium currents in the thalamus. This type of current controls the depolarization threshold and may be intimately involved with the generation of absence seizures; however, more studies are needed.[11] Ethosuximide is well tolerated, having few side effects with the exception of headache, fatigue, and some GI problems. Agranulocytosis has been reported.

Lamotrigine

The exact mechanism of action of lamotrigine is unknown, but it is believed to block sodium channels, reduce calcium influx, and inhibit the release of excitatory amino acids, glutamate, and aspartate.[12] It is approved as adjunctive therapy, usually administered with carbamazepine or phenytoin for the treatment of partial seizures. Although it has been approved for monotherapy in the United Kingdom because some studies have shown similar efficacy and better tolerability compared with carbamazepine, it is mostly used as an add-on drug for generalized seizures, with

significant efficacy for absence seizures. This drug is also being studied for use in depression and bipolar disorder. Lamotrigine does not induce or inhibit the P450 enzymes, so it can be used safely with a variety of drugs. Adverse drug reactions include dizziness, diplopia, ataxia, headache, and rashes.

Gabapentin

Gabapentin acts on a unique receptor that has not yet been identified.[13] It is structurally related to GABA but has no affinity for the GABA, glutamate, N-methyl-D-aspartate, kainate, glycine, cholinergic, dopamine (D_1 or D_2), 5-hydroxytryptamine (5-HT), opiate, voltage-gated calcium, or sodium channel receptors. Gabapentin is used as an adjunct in the treatment of partial and tonic-clonic seizures and is also used to reduce pain in neuropathic pain syndromes.[14]

Side effects of gabapentin are relatively minor and include sedation and ataxia. Patients also might experience dizziness and nystagmus. Because this drug does not undergo metabolism, it does not interfere with the breakdown of any other antiseizure medications.

Levetiracetam

Levetiracetam belongs to a new class of antiseizure medications recently approved by the Food and Drug Administration.[15] The mechanism of action is unknown, and it does not seem to be similar to that of the other medications previously discussed. It is approved for use as an adjunct in the treatment of partial onset seizures.

This drug is well tolerated but has side effects resulting from CNS depression similar to those of the other antiseizure medications (i.e., dizziness, headache, and fatigue). Studies show a higher rate of rhinitis during treatment with this drug compared with placebo in clinical trials, but it is not known whether this adverse effect is related to the drug. Levetiracetam is not metabolized by the cytochrome P450 enzymes, and therefore fewer drug-drug interactions may be expected.

Oxcarbazepine

Oxcarbazepine is a new drug to the U.S. market that became available in 1999.[15] It is structurally related to carbamazepine with similar action.

Oxcarbazepine is a prodrug that is converted into the primary active metabolite, monohydroxy derivative, which is not metabolized by the P450 enzymes as carbamazepine, so there is less potential for drug interactions. It is approved for monotherapy and adjunctive use in the treatment of partial seizures in adults and for adjunctive therapy in children. This drug produces side effects similar to those of carbamazepine, but they are less frequent and milder. Hepatic and hematological problems have not been reported, but the CNS effects of dizziness and sedation are present.

Additional Antiepileptic Drugs

Topiramate, tiagabine, and zonisamide were approved for use in the United States in the late 1990s and early 2000s.[1] Topiramate appears to be the "jack-of-all-trades" of antiseizure medications. It blocks sodium channels, enhances the action of GABA, and inhibits glutamate activity. Tiagabine is an analog of GABA that can advance through the blood-brain barrier. It also functions to inhibit the reuptake of GABA. Last, zonisamide is a new drug to the United States but has been approved in Japan since 1989. The exact mechanism of action is unknown.

GENERAL APPROACH TO THE MANAGEMENT OF EPILEPSY

Patients with epilepsy start with one drug and then increase the dose gradually until they are either free of seizures or the side effects become intolerable.[4]

If the first drug fails to control the seizures or the patient cannot tolerate the side effects, either another drug is tried or the dose of the first is lowered and a second drug is added. The choice of drug depends on the seizure type, age of the patient, psychiatric history, other disease states, and concomitant use of other medication (Table 18-2). Most patients with a partial-onset seizure disorder are initially given drugs that block voltage-dependent sodium channels such as phenytoin, carbamazepine, and oxcarbazepine.[16] Second-line choices and add-ons include gabapentin, lamotrigine, levetiracetam, valproic acid, and the other newer agents. Drugs commonly used for generalized seizures include lamotrigine and valproic acid, with lamotrigine being favored because of fewer adverse effects, and ethosuximide or valproate for absence seizures.

Approximately 60% to 70% of patients become free of seizures with a first- or second-choice antiseizure medication as monotherapy.[4] The remainder of patients have difficult-to-control seizures but may respond to combination therapy, particularly when drugs with different mechanisms of action are used. Some effective combinations include valproate with ethosuximide for absence seizures, valproate with lamotrigine for partial and generalized seizures, and lamotrigine with topiramate for a variety of atypical seizures. However, some patients have epilepsy that remains refractory to their combination medications. These patients may be candidates for epilepsy surgery or a vagus nerve stimulator. In addition, because current technology can be used to identify the site of seizure onset in some patients and can detect an impending seizure, it may be

Table 18-2

Efficacy of Selected Antiepileptic Drugs for Different Seizures

Drug	Partial	Tonic-clonic	Absence	Myoclonic	Atonic
Phenobarbital	+	+	0	?	?
Phenytoin	+	+	−	−	0
Carbamazepine	+	+	−	−	0
Valproate	+	+	+	+	+
Ethosuximide	0	0	+	0	0
Gabapentin	+	+	−	−	0
Lamotrigine	+	+	+	+	+
Topiramate	+	+	?	+	+

Adapted from Brodie MJ, Kwan P. Staged approach to epilepsy management. *Neurology*. 2002;58(suppl 5):S2-S8.
+, Efficacy; 0, ineffective; −, negative effect (enhances seizure activity); ?, unknown efficacy.

possible in the future to deliver small amounts of antiseizure medications directly to the site of origin to avert an episode.

Regular blood level monitoring of the AEDs is not only necessary for minimizing toxic effects but also represents another management tool. Monitoring the plasma concentration is necessary for maximizing therapeutic effects, and the plasma concentration is important information to have before a second or even a third drug is added to the regimen.

When to begin treatment with AEDs is controversial.[17,18] The seizure recurrence rate has been reported to be 20% and 80%. After two tonic-clonic seizures, the risk of a third seizure may be as high as 85%. Factors that lead to recurrence are a family history of seizures, neurological deficit, cognitive dysfunction, and abnormal findings on an electroencephalogram. Head trauma accounts for 5% of epilepsy and 20% of the symptomatic cases. This has provoked studies to determine whether the prophylactic use of AEDs after trauma can reduce the occurrence of epilepsy.[19] Using animals, investigators were able to determine that administering valproic acid 20 to 30 minutes after head trauma on a one-time basis reduced the incidence of post-traumatic epilepsy. Early administration of the drug was critical to its success.

Certain types of seizures are also more likely to recur. An unprovoked, single, prolonged seizure is likely to be repeated and require medication, but a febrile seizure does not need treatment. Partial seizures are also more likely to recur. Noncompliance with the drug program after a single seizure is high, but patients show greater compliance after the second seizure experience and are more willing to take medication.

When to withdraw medication is also a difficult decision.[20] Most physicians prefer a seizure-free interval of 2 to 5 years, absence of abnormalities on an electroencephalogram, and normal findings on a neurological exam before medication is withdrawn. Withdrawal must be accomplished slowly because sudden withdrawal may result in status epilepticus. Most recurrences, however, develop within the first 6 months after withdrawal and many are observed within the first year. Childhood-onset epilepsy has a better prognosis than adult-onset epilepsy. Reasons to withdraw medications include a desired pregnancy (because many of the drugs are teratogenic) or intolerable side effects such as sedation in school-age children or adolescents. Seizure control with medication is desired in cases in which the patient cannot risk seizure activity, for example, a person who needs to drive to work or operate dangerous equipment. Drug withdrawal is performed slowly over a period of 3 to 6 months to avoid recurrence, but epilepsy of long duration (more than 6 years) before control may warrant continuation of therapy.

Poor compliance with the drug regimen is a problem that leads to recurrence of seizure activity.[21] Many of these drugs must be taken multiple times per day. This is disruptive to a person's lifestyle, particularly for a child who must be removed from the classroom for dosing. New extended-release formulations exist for carbamazepine, phenytoin, and valproic acid, and are expected to improve compliance.

Treatment of Status Epilepticus

Status epilepticus is defined as a function of time. The clinical presentation is 30 minutes of continuous seizure activity or two or more seizures within this time frame without regaining full consciousness.[22] Lorazepam is the first-line treatment for status epilepticus and is given along with a loading dose of phenytoin.[5] Both are given intravenously. Fosphenytoin is a prodrug of phenytoin and is a good alternative. It is water soluble, making infusion easier and faster. If the seizure is refractory to these drugs, intravenous midazolam or propofol may be added. Supportive care is also given in the form of maintaining an airway, providing ventilation, and ensuring that the patient is safe.

Is There a Superior Antiepileptic Agent?

Neurologists and patients were pleased when the newer AED agents were released on the market. They were expected to be superior to the traditional drugs in efficacy and side effect profile, especially for patients who continued to experience breakthrough seizures. However, there has been a lack of clinical trials in which the new agents are compared with the older ones. Gabapentin, lamotrigine, and oxcarbazepine have each been compared with carbamazepine as monotherapy for partial seizures and found to be more tolerable but no more or less effective.[6,23,24] The newer agents do not affect the

Table 18-3

Factors Associated with Seizure Activity

Pre-Seizure (Possible Provoking Stimuli)	Activity During Seizure	Post-Seizure Events
Emotional stress	Aura	Confusion
Sleep deprivation	Rhythmic behavior of face or extremities in a partial seizure	Fatigue
Flashing lights	Tonic movements or posturing observed as stiffening	Focal weakness or diminished sensation
Recent illness	Clonic movements	Headache
Drugs	Incontinence	Physical injury
Alcohol withdrawal	Tongue biting	
Fever	Rhythmic flexion and extension of limbs	
Hypoglycemia		

Adapted from Brodie MJ, Kwan P. Staged approach to epilepsy management. *Neurology.* 2002;58(suppl 5):S2-S8.

hepatic enzymes and therefore produce fewer drug-drug interactions and side effects than the older agents. Of the newer agents, only felbamate, which is used infrequently for only the most refractory seizure disorders, is associated with serious organ toxicity. However, in terms of efficacy, there seems to be little difference between the newer and older drugs.

Therapeutic Concerns

The major side effects that will affect physical therapy intervention and attainment of goals include sedation, dizziness, and ataxia. Some of these drugs also produce a moderate amount of cognitive slowing, particularly topiramate.[25] Patients may develop some tolerance for the sedating qualities, but if seizures are difficult to control, a patient may be receiving such a high dose of medication that this tolerance may not be recognized. Another side effect that needs to be recognized is the presence of skin rashes. In most cases, the drug will be withdrawn, but if the patient is allowed to continue using the medication, skin care is important. Realize that modalities and massage may exacerbate the condition. Because bone marrow depression and vitamin K deficiency, which leads to depression of clotting factors, may occur with some antiseizure agents, the presence of bruising or bleeding must be reported. Infection control and careful handling must be instituted.

There are special concerns for women taking AEDs. Negative interactions between the drugs and endocrine system may affect ovarian function, produce polycystic ovary disease, increase weight, and reduce fertility.[26] If a woman taking these drugs becomes pregnant, there is a 4% to 6% greater risk of the infant having a neural tube defect.[27] In addition, the effect of these drugs on bone health is a real concern, particularly for postmenopausal women.

Physical therapists should also be able to recognize seizures and maintain a record of the number and quality of events witnessed during a therapy session.[17] See Table 18-3 for important observations to be recorded when a seizure is witnessed. In some therapy centers, an incident report may need to be completed, especially if a fall was involved.

ATTENTION-DEFICIT/ HYPERACTIVITY DISORDER

Attention-deficit/hyperactivity disorder (ADHD) is present in 3% to 10% of children, with a percentage continuing to have this disorder into adulthood.[28] ADHD commonly occurs with a variety of behavioral disorders including conduct disorder, oppositional defiant disorder, depression, anxiety, and many developmental disorders. The American Academy of Pediatrics uses criteria from *The Diagnostic and Statistical Manual of Mental Disorders,* 4th ed. (*DSM-IV*) for identifying ADHD. This manual defines ADHD as consisting of a triad of symptoms (inattention, impulsivity, and hyperactivity) that must appear together in at least two different environments, such as home and school. This *DSM-IV* criteria goes on to define three subtypes of ADHD: the inattentive type, the hyperactive-impulsive type, and the combined type.

The etiology of ADHD is most likely a combination of environmental, genetic, and biological factors.[29] Prenatal and perinatal exposure to cigarettes or alcohol increases the risk of ADHD two to three times. Having a parent with ADHD increases the risk eight times. In a study of dizygotic and monozygotic twins, genetics accounted for a 75% contribution.

There appears to be a plethora of information regarding the behavioral aspects of ADHD but little information on the neurochemical or anatomical anomalies associated with this disorder. Brain imaging and electroencephalography studies have not shown clear differences between control subjects and children with ADHD, nor is there a particular defect solely associated with this disorder.[28] Structural magnetic resonance imaging studies have shown that children with ADHD have a reduced brain volume, especially in the corpus callosum, caudate, and cerebellar areas [30] Despite aggressive treatment, there is no reversal of this abnormality. However, there are some neurochemical explanations for this disorder. Dopamine dysfunction in the prefrontal cortex, particularly decreased activity of dihydroxyphenylalanine (DOPA) decarboxylase, has been seen in adults with ADHD.[31] However, researchers are not sure whether this dysfunction is responsible for the ADHD or represents a secondary change caused by the ADHD experienced in childhood. An extension of this dopamine dysfunction theory includes mention of a defect in glutamate-stimulated release of dopamine in the nucleus accumbens that results in dopamine hypofunction.[32] Other investigators are looking for a candidate gene, possibly one involved with expression of the dopamine (D_4) receptor to describe the neurobiology of the subtype of ADHD that continues into adulthood.[33] Increased expression of dopamine transporters has been observed in adults with ADHD.[34] It has also been determined that dopamine, epinephrine, and norepinephrine all have activity at the D_4 receptor sites, which helps explain the usefulness of some drugs in treating this disorder. Specifically, it has been found that therapeutic doses of methylphenidate (a commonly used medication

for ADHD) blocks more than half of the dopamine transporters, thus increasing extracellular dopamine levels.[35] A further complication to our understanding of ADHD is related to the theory that the motor (hyperactivity) and cognitive (inattention) predominance of symptoms may represent two separate dysfunctions with insult in different parts of the brain.[36] Specifically, the hyperactivity may result from dysfunction at subcortical sites in which insufficient dopamine produces a "reverse parkinsonism" or excessive motor output through loss of inhibition. The lack of attention and diminished memory might relate to lesions in the prefrontal cortex. This is further supported clinically by the divergence of dose-response curves for motor and cognitive effects produced by the stimulant agents. The theories are complicated by the fact that little reference has been made to the role of presynaptic autoreceptors and how increased dopaminergic activity affects them. Clearly, understanding of this disorder is in its infant stage.

Drug Treatment for ADHD

Medications are the foundation of treatment for children and adults with ADHD in addition to support groups, specialized educational planning, and focused therapies.[33] Stimulants, antidepressants, and antihypertensive medications are among the most commonly used agents for this disorder, and the stimulants in particular are considered to be first-line agents.

Stimulant Therapy (Methylphenidate, Amphetamine)
CNS stimulants are used to reduce the hyperactivity, impulsivity, and inattentiveness that characterize ADHD behavior. At first, the use of these agents for hyperactivity seems counterintuitive. These drugs are sympathomimetic, producing increased mental alertness and wakefulness and decreased fatigue. However, they also produce nervousness and heightened motor activity, symptoms that are already seen in the ADHD population. As mentioned previously, explanations are uncertain, but what is clear is that stimulants significantly improve behavior as judged by both parents and teachers.[36] In addition, they reduce restless behavior and improve memory, although to a greater extent in subjects who do not have comorbid symptoms such as anxiety.[37,38]

Both D-amphetamine and methylphenidate bind to the dopamine and norepinephrine transporters, blocking reuptake of dopamine. In addition D-amphetamine facilitates release of dopamine.[36] These drugs are used to treat ADHD in both children and adults.[39] However, outcomes are variable, and approximately 30% of patients do not respond to the medication or cannot tolerate the side effects. Children with tic symptoms may experience a worsening of this condition.[40]

Short-term side effects include reduced appetite, insomnia, nervousness, and GI dysfunction. In adults, hypertension is a problem, and D-amphetamine and methylphenidate should not be prescribed for an individual with borderline or above-normal blood pressure.

There have been increasing concerns over possible long-term consequences of stimulant use. The first is that use of stimulant medication in early childhood will lead to the development of substance abuse later in life.[41] However, a meta-analysis of six studies that included 674 patients receiving medication and 360 control subjects indicated that the children who were treated for ADHD with stimulants had a reduction in substance abuse. Another concern is the possibility of growth retardation with stimulant therapy.[40] Unfortunately, the studies that address this issue have some intrinsic flaws, and the question remains. Some retrospective studies have shown a height reduction of 3 to 4 cm after 3 years of treatment when patients were matched with untreated siblings. However, a prospective study performed with females demonstrated that methylphenidate had no effect on height. In none of these studies was final adult height examined.

Methylphenidate and D-amphetamine are both short-acting compounds with onset of action in about 30 to 60 minutes. Peak effect occurs in 1 to 2 hours and lasts for 2 to 5 hours. New extended-release preparations of both drugs prolong the duration of action to between 8 and 12 hours.[42-44] These preparations eliminate dosing during the school hours while covering late afternoon homework time. In addition, they eliminate some of the moodiness and headaches associated with peaks in plasma level reported by patients taking drugs with short durations of action.

The effects of the stimulant drugs used for ADHD resemble the actions of cocaine, and therefore these drugs present a risk of abuse when they are taken in an unauthorized manner.[45,46] They are listed as schedule II controlled substances. Because many children and adults take a stimulant drug for ADHD, it is widely available and can be obtained easily, although illegally. Some reports in the literature have documented the abuse of methylphenidate. When methylphenidate is used for recreational purposes, the tablets are often crushed and the powder is then sniffed. In other cases, the powder has been mixed with liquid and administered intravenously. Under these conditions, the drug creates euphoria with a very high abuse potential.

Antidepressants for the Treatment of ADHD

Tricyclic antidepressants have been shown to be effective in treating ADHD but not superior to the stimulants. Their mechanism of action in ADHD relates to their action of catecholamine reuptake. The advantages to the tricyclic antidepressants include reducing comorbid mood disorders, a longer half-life, and a low abuse potential. In addition, they do not exacerbate tic disorders. The disadvantages of tricyclic antidepressants are their anticholinergic side effects and cardiac effects. Other antidepressants under study for ADHD include venlafaxine and bupropion (see Chapter 16).[40,47] Both appear to be effective in patients with comorbid mood disorders.

α$_2$-Noradrenergic Agonists (Clonidine, Lofexidine)

α$_2$-Agonists have been used for years in the treatment of ADHD. Clonidine has been used as monotherapy or in conjunction with methylphenidate in children with both ADHD and tic disorder.[40] Lofexidine is a new α$_2$-agonist that has action similar to that of clonidine but is much less sedating, making it more inviting for use in children. In three small trials, lofexidine was significantly superior to placebo according to teacher and clinician ADHD rating scales. Side effects were no different from those of placebo. More studies are needed to determine its efficacy compared with methylphenidate.

Atomoxetine

Atomoxetine is a new drug approved for use in children 6 years of age and older, as well as in adults. It is a very selective presynaptic norepinephrine reuptake inhibitor and thus has little influence over other neurotransmitters, limiting its side effects. It is the first nonstimulant drug to be approved by the Food and Drug Administration for ADHD. Several small trials have shown that atomoxetine is superior to placebo and equal to methylphenidate in efficacy.[48-50] Side effects of atomoxetine include abdominal pain, decreased appetite, dizziness, and vomiting. Some growth disturbances may also be associated with this drug because mean height and weight declined in children treated with this drug for more than 18 months. As for most new drugs, further study is warranted.

Therapeutic Concerns with Drugs for ADHD

When patients with ADHD are receiving physical therapy, it is particularly important for therapists to assess behavior and attention span. This assessment is not only important because the patient must be cooperative and follow instructions for therapy to be successful but also because therapists must determine whether the patient is taking the medication properly. Because methylphenidate is a CNS stimulant and has recently become a drug of abuse, some patients may decide to sell their drugs rather than take them. If this becomes a concern, the therapist can discuss this with the prescribing physician by framing the conversation in terms of the patient's inattentive or impulsive behavior.

Other assessments that should be performed include measurement of resting and exercise blood pressure and heart rate. Vital signs may be elevated, especially in adults, as a result of stimulant therapy. In addition, questioning the patient about angina is important. Angina may occur if the patient combines the stimulants with caffeine or other sympathomimetic agents and exercise. Other side effects to look for are loss of appetite and insomnia. Physical therapists are uniquely qualified to offer suggestions for combating insomnia. Biofeedback and relaxation exercises, as well as proper positioning for sleep, can be helpful.

Therapists should consult with the patient's physician and teacher about providing the same structure during physical therapy sessions as that provided in the school setting. Therapy can complement the educational goals outlined for the classroom, and therapists can follow through with the same reward system to foster successful behavior.

ACTIVITIES 18

■ 1. You are treating a 16-year-old boy for chondromalacia patella. He is performing a sitting knee extension exercise when he begins to have a tonic-clonic seizure. Describe what you are witnessing. Construct a seizure diary for the patient and family to assist them in recording seizure activity.

■ 2. Interview a pediatric therapist who has worked with children with epilepsy. Discuss what impact seizure medication has had on a particular patient he or she has treated.

References

1. Lilley LL, Harrington D, Snyder JS. Antiepileptic agents. In: *Pharmacology and the Nursing Process*. 4th ed. St Louis: Mosby; 2005:204-219.

2. Rang HP, Dale DC, Ritter JM, Moore JL. Antiepileptic drugs. In: *Pharmacology*. New York: Churchill Livingstone; 2003:550-561.

3. Post RM. Neurobiology of seizures and behavioral abnormalities. *Epilepsia*. 2004;45(suppl 2):5-14.

4. Brodie MJ, Kwan P. Staged approach to epilepsy management. *Neurology*. 2002;58(suppl 5):S2-S8.

5. Duncan JS. The promise of new antiepileptic drugs. *Br J Clin Pharmacol*. 2002;53(2):123-131.

6. French JA, Kanner AM, Bautista J, et al. Efficacy and tolerability of the new antiepileptic drugs, I: Treatment of new-onset epilepsy: report of the TTA and QSS Subcommittees of the American Academy of Neurology and the American Epilepsy Society. *Epilepsia*. 2004;45(5):401-409.

7. Patsalos PN, Froscher W, Pisani F, Van Rijn C. The importance of drug interactions in epilepsy therapy. *Epilepsia*. 2002;43(4):365-385.

8. LaRoche SM, Helmers SL. The new antiepileptic drugs. *JAMA*. 2004;291(5):605-614.

9. Ali II, Schuh L, Barkley GL, Gates JR. Antiepileptic drugs and reduced bone mineral density. *Epilepsy Behav*. 2004;5:296-300.

10. Johannessen CU, Johannessen SI. Valproate: past, present, and future. *CNS Drug Rev*. 2003;9(2):199-216.

11. Posner EB, Mohamed K, Marson AG. Ethosuximide, sodium valproate or lamotrigine for absence seizures in children and adolescents. *Cochrane Database Syst Rev*. 2003;3(CD003032).

12. Hurley SC. Lamotrigine update and its use in mood disorders. *Ann Pharmacother*. 2002;36(5):860-873.

13. McLean MJ, Gidal BE. Gabapentin dosing in the treatment of epilepsy. *Clin Ther*. 2003;25(5):1382-1406.

14. Pappagallo M. Newer antiepileptic drugs: possible uses in the treatment of neuropathic pain and migraine. *Clin Ther*. 2003;25(10):2506-2538.

15. McAuley JW, Biederman TS, Smith JC, Moore JL. Newer therapies in the drug treatment of epilepsy. *Ann Pharmacother*. 2002;36:119-129.

16. Beydoun A, Passaro EA. Appropriate use of medications for seizures. *Postgrad Med*. 2002;111(1):69-82.

17. Prego-Lopez M, Devinsky O. Evaluation of a first seizure. *Postgrad Med*. 2002;111(1):34-48.

18. Sirven JL. Antiepileptic drug therapy for adults: when to initiate and how to choose. *Mayo Clin Proc*. 2002;77(12):1367-1375.

19. Benardo LS. Prevention of epilepsy after head trauma: do we need new drugs or a new approach? *Epilepsia*. 2003;44(suppl 10):27-33.

20. Specchio LM, Beghi E. Should antiepileptic drugs be withdrawn in seizure-free patients? *CNS Drugs*. 2004;18(4):201-212.

21. Pellock JM, Smith MC, Cloyd JC, Uthman B, Wilder BJ. Extended-release formulations: simplifying strategies in the management of antiepileptic drug therapy. *Epilepsy Behav*. 2004;5:301-307.

22. Manno EM. New management strategies in the treatment of status epilepticus. *Mayo Clin Proc*. 2003;78(4):508-518.

23. Brodie MJ, Richen A, Yuen AWC. Double-blind comparison of lamotrigine and carbamazepine in newly diagnosed epilepsy. *Lancet*. 1995;345:476-479.

24. Dam M, Ekberg R, Loyning Y, Waltimo O, Jakobsen K. A double-blind study comparing oxcarbazepine and carbamazepine in patients with newly diagnosed, previously untreated epilepsy. *Epilepsy Res*. 1989;3(1):70-76.

25. Loring DW, Meador KJ. Cognitive side effects of antiepileptic drugs in children. *Neurology*. 2004;62:872-877.

26. Tatum WO, Liporace J, Benbadis SR, Kaplan PW. Updates on the treatment of epilepsy in women. *Arch Intern Med*. 2004;164:137-145.

27. Yerby MS. Management issues for women with epilepsy: neural tube defects and folic acid supplementation. *Neurology*. 2003;61(6 suppl 2):S23-S26.

28. Clinical practice guideline: diagnosis and evaluation of the child with attention-deficit/hyperactivity disorder. American Academy of Pediatrics. *Pediatrics*. 2000;105:1158-1170.

29. Spencer TJ, Biederman J, Wilens TE, Faraone SV. Overview and neurobiology of attention-deficit/hyperactivity disorder. *J Clin Psychiatry*. 2002;63(suppl 12):3-9.

30. Zametkin A, Liotta W. The neurobiology of attention-deficit/hyperactivity disorder. *J Clin Psychiatry*. 1998;59:17-23.

31. Ernst M, Zametkin A, Matochik JA, Jons PH, Cohen RM. DOPA decarboxylase activity in attention deficit hyperactivity disorder adults. A [fluorine-18] fluorodopa positron emission tomographic study. *J Neurosci*. 1998;18(15):5901-5907.

32. Russell VA. Dopamine hypofunction possibly results from a defect in glutamate-stimulated release of dopamine in the nucleus accumbens shell of a rat model for attention deficit hyperactivity disorder—the spontaneously hypertensive rat. *Neurosci Biobehav Rev*. 2003(27):671-682.

33. Wilens TE, Biederman J, Spencer TJ. Attention deficit/hyperactivity disorder across the lifespan. *Ann Rev Med*. 2002;53:113-131.

34. Madras BK, Miller GM, Fischman AJ. The dopamine transporter: relevance to attention deficit hyperactivity disorder (ADHD). *Behav Brain Res*. 2002;130:57-63.

35. Sergeant JA, Geurts H, Huijbregts S, Scheres A, Oosterlaan J. The top and the bottom of ADHD: a neuropsychological perspective. *Neurosci Biobehav Rev*. 2003;27:583-592.

36. Solanto MV. Dopamine dysfunction in AD/HD: integrating clinical and basic neuroscience research. *Behav Brain Res*. 2002;130:65-71.

37. Tannock R, Ickowicz A, Schachar R. Differential effects of methylphenidate on working memory in ADHD children with and without comorbid anxiety. *J Am Acad Child Adolesc Psychiatry*. 1995;34(7):886-896.

38. Waxmonsky J. Assessment and treatment of attention deficit hyperactivity disorder in children with comorbid psychiatric illness. *Curr Opin Pediatr*. 2003;15(5):476-482.

39. Lutton ME, Leach L, Triezenberg D. Does stimulant therapy help adult ADHD? *J Fam Pract*. 2003;52(11):888-889.

40. Daley KC. Update on attention-deficit/hyperactivity disorder. *Curr Opin Pediatr*. 2004;16(2):217-226.

41. Wilens TE, Faraone SV, Biederman J, Gunawardene BS. Does stimulant therapy of attention-deficit/hyperactivity disorder beget later substance abuse? A meta-analytic review of the literature. *Pediatrics*. 2003;111(1):179-185.

42. McCracken JT, Biederman J, Greenhill LL, et al. Analog classroom assessment of a once-daily mixed amphetamine formulation, SLI381 (Adderall XR), in children with ADHD. *J Am Acad Child Adolesc Psychiatry*. 2003; 42(6):673-683.

43. Dexmethylphenidate (Focalin) for ADHD. *Med Lett Drugs Ther*. 2002;44(1130):45-46.

44. A new long-acting methylphenidate (Concerta). *Med Lett Drugs Ther*. 2000;42(1086):80-81.

45. Swanson JM, Volkow ND. Serum and brain concentrations of methylphenidate: implications for use and abuse. *Neurosci Biobehav Rev*. 2003;27:615-621.

46. Volkow ND, Fowler JS, Wang GJ, Ding YS, Gatley SJ. Role of dopamine in the therapeutic and reinforcing effects of methylphenidate in humans: results from imaging studies. *Eur Neuropsychopharmacol*. 2002; 12:557-566.

47. Hornig-Rohan M, Amsterdam JD. Venlafaxine versus stimulant therapy in patients with dual diagnosis ADD and depression. *Prog Neuropsychopharmacol Biol Psychiatry*. 2002;26:585-589.

48. Atomoxetine (Strattera) for ADHD. *Med Lett Drugs Ther*. 2003;45(1149):11-12.

49. Kratochvil CJ, Heiligenstein JH, Dittmann R, et al. Atomoxetine and methylphenidate treatment in children with ADHD: a prospective, randomized, open-label trial. *J Am Acad Child Adolesc Psychiatry*. 2002;41(7):776-784.

50. Eiland L, Guest AL. Atomoxetine treatment of attention-deficit/hyperactivity disorder. *Ann Pharmacother*. 2004; 38:86-90.

CHAPTER 19

ANTISPASTICITY MEDICATIONS AND SKELETAL MUSCLE RELAXANTS

Several pharmacological agents are available for patients with spasticity who have upper motor neuron syndrome and also who have muscle spasms. This chapter is organized first to review the neurophysiology of muscle tone and spasms, followed by a description of agents commonly used to treat spasticity. Because spasticity is present in any upper motor neuron disease, such as stroke, spinal cord injury (SCI), or cerebral palsy (CP), this section is not focused on one diagnostic group selectively.

PHYSIOLOGY OF SPASTICITY AND MUSCLE SPASMS

A widely accepted definition of spasticity is a velocity-dependent increased resistance to passive stretch.[1] Although the pathophysiology of spasticity is poorly understood, the final common pathway is overactivity of the alpha motor neuron.[2] This is unlike dystonia, which is not dependent on sensory input, but rather on supraspinal output or efferents not involved in the reflex arc.[3] In 2001, the National Institutes of Health defined spasticity, through an interdisciplinary workshop, as hypertonia with resistance to externally imposed movement that increases with increasing speed and varies with the direction of joint movement and/or is above a threshold speed or joint angle. Spasticity results from a lesion along the path of the corticospinal tracts. These pyramidal tracts include the motor pathways of the cortex, basal ganglia, thalamus, cerebellum, brainstem, central white matter, and spinal cord.[4] The term *parapyramidal* can be used to describe upper motor neuron fibers that travel near the pyramidal fibers, modulating tone and movement.[5] The term *extrapyramidal* refers to fibers associated with the basal ganglia and clinical findings of Parkinson's disease.[4] Spasticity is a result of an imbalance between the afferent excitatory and descending inhibitory pathways after central nervous system (CNS) damage.[6]

SPASTICITY

Medications to resolve excessive muscle tone are numerous, but few have been established to reduce disability. Adverse effects, or negative effects, of a drug should be considered when the effect of a drug on a patient is evaluated. The mechanisms and anatomical site of action are not well understood. The consensus is that they either alter function of neurotransmitters or neuromodulators in the CNS or have an action on the peripheral neuromuscular sites. The CNS function could include suppression of excitation through glutamate or by enhancement of inhibition either through γ-aminobutyric acid (GABA) or glycine.[7]

Pharmacotherapy for spasticity is generally initiated at low doses and then gradually increased to avoid potential adverse effects. Ideally, therapy is optimal at the lowest dose. Baclofen, diazepam, tizanidine, and dantrolene are currently approved for use in patients with spasticity. In addition, clonidine (usually as combination therapy), gabapentin, and botulinum toxin have shown efficacy; however, more studies are needed to confirm their efficacy. Intrathecal baclofen, administered via a surgically implanted pump and reservoir, may provide relief for patients with severe refractory spasticity.[2]

Centrally Acting Agents for Spasticity

Examples of centrally acting agents include diazepam, baclofen, and tizanidine. Their mechanisms of action are dissimilar, and therefore they are described separately. However, all three are useful in reducing spasticity of spinal origin (spinal cord and multiple sclerosis [MS]) in which there is less sensitivity to their sedating effects.

Diazepam (Valium)

Diazepam is indicated for the management of anxiety disorders or for the short-term relief of the symptoms of anxiety.[8] However, it is also a useful adjunct for the relief of skeletal muscle spasms caused by reflex spasms of a local pathological condition (such as inflammation of the muscles or joints or trauma injury); spasticity caused by upper motor neuron disorders (such as CP and paraplegia); athetosis; stiff-person syndrome; and tetanus (Table 19-1). Stiff-person syndrome is a rare neurological disorder with autoimmune features. It is characterized by progressive, severe muscle rigidity or stiffness, most prominently affecting the spine and lower extremities.[9] In addition, injectable diazepam is a useful adjunct in status epilepticus and severe recurrent convulsive seizures.[8]

The antispasticity effects of benzodiazepines are achieved by binding to the $GABA_A$-gated chloride channel.[8] Diazepam binds in the brainstem, reticular formation, and spinal pathways with particular predilection for the higher pathways. It is considered to be an intermediate-acting to long-acting benzodiazepine because of its half-life of 20 to 80 hours. The duration of its half-life is dependent on metabolism of one active intermediate, desmethyldiazepam, and two minor active metabolites. In animals, diazepam appears to act on parts of the limbic system, the thalamus and hypothalamus, and induces calming effects. It has no demonstrable peripheral autonomic blocking action, nor does it produce extrapyramidal side effects; however, at

Table 19-1

Efficacy of Selected Antispasticity Medications and Adverse Effects						
	MS	SCI	Stroke	TBI	CP	Adverse Effects
Dantrolene	+	+	++		+	Decreased walking speed, muscle weakness, hepatotoxicity
Oral baclofen	++	+	+/−			Decreased walking speed, muscle weakness, sedation, lowered threshold for seizures
Intrathecal baclofen	+	+	+	?	?	Decreased walking speed, muscle weakness, sedation, lowered threshold for seizures, pump malfunction
Diazepam	+	+	+/−		+	Decreased walking speed, marked sedation, cognitive slowing, hypotension
Tizanidine	++	+	+	?		Minor muscular weakness, sedation, dry mouth, dizziness, hypotension, liver dysfunction

+, Effective in a double-blind study; ++, demonstrated effectiveness in a double-blind comparative study; +/−, effectiveness was modulated by annoying side effects; ?, effectiveness established in open trials; *empty block,* indicates lack of information up to 1997; *MS,* multiple sclerosis; *SCI,* spinal cord injury; *TBI,* traumatic brain injury; *CP,* cerebral palsy.
Adapted from Gracies J, Nance P, McGuire J, Simpson DM. General pharmacological treatments for spasticity part II: General and regional treatments. *Muscle Nerve.* 1997;(suppl 6):S61-S92.

higher doses, transient ataxia can occur. Diazepam was found to have transient cardiovascular depressor effects in animals.[8]

Side effects most commonly reported are drowsiness, fatigue, and ataxia. Infrequently encountered are confusion, constipation, depression, diplopia, dysarthria, headache, hypotension, incontinence, jaundice, changes in libido, nausea, changes in salivation, skin rash, slurred speech, tremor, urinary retention, vertigo, and blurred vision. Cutson et al.[10] examined the effect of a single dose of diazepam on a spectrum of balance measures in healthy older subjects and found that benzodiazepines affect neuromuscular processing related to balance control. They observed increased muscle latency in response to sudden perturbations, which are suggested to have an effect on the oligosynaptic spinal reflex distinct from the sedation.[10]

Paradoxical reactions such as acute hyperexcited states, anxiety, hallucinations, increased muscle spasticity, insomnia, rage, and sleep disturbances have been reported; should these occur, use of the drug should be discontinued.[8] Because of isolated reports of neutropenia and jaundice, periodic blood counts and liver function tests are advisable during long-term therapy. Minor changes in electroencephalographic patterns, usually low-voltage fast activity, have been observed in patients during and after diazepam therapy and are of no known significance.

Concomitant use of barbiturates, alcohol, or other CNS depressants increases CNS depression with increased risk of apnea.[8] If diazepam is to be combined with other psychotropic agents or anticonvulsant drugs, careful consideration should be given to the pharmacology of the agents to be used—particularly known compounds that may potentiate the action of diazepam, such as phenothiazines, narcotics, barbiturates, and antidepressants.

Benzodiazepines have a hypotensive effect. Kitajima et al.[11] found that after diazepam administration, systolic and mean blood pressure decreased significantly; they concluded that the hypotensive effect of diazepam is mainly due to the central mechanism rather than an alteration in autonomic cardiovascular control. The protein binding characteristic of the pharmacology of diazepam is clinically significant in SCI and stroke because a low serum albumin level is often associated with these conditions. Consequently, diazepam could be more toxic in these circumstances.[7]

As always, dosing depends on the indication and severity and is adjusted to achieve the maximal benefit with the lowest dose. Lower doses with gradual increases should be given to the elderly or those taking other sedatives (2 to 5 mg).[8] Spasticity associated with local pathological conditions, CP, athetosis, stiff-person syndrome, or tetanus may be treated with 5 to 10 mg of diazepam, administered via the intravenous route initially; then 5 to 10 mg may be administered in 3 to 4 hours, at which time the intramuscular route could be used, if necessary.[8] If diazepam is administered to infants or young children for tetanus spasm, respiratory assistance should be available in case breathing is depressed.

Withdrawal symptoms, similar in character to those noted with barbiturates and alcohol (convulsions, tremor, abdominal and muscle cramps, vomiting, and sweating), have occurred after abrupt discontinuation of diazepam.[8] The more severe withdrawal symptoms have usually been limited to those patients who had received excessive doses over an extended period. Generally, milder withdrawal symptoms (e.g., dysphoria and insomnia) have been reported after abrupt discontinuation of benzodiazepines taken continuously at therapeutic levels for several months. Consequently, after extended therapy, abrupt discontinuation should generally be avoided, and a gradual dose tapering schedule should be followed.

Beard et al.[12] conducted a systematic review to identify the drug treatments currently available for the management of spasticity and pain in MS and evaluated their clinical effectiveness and cost-effectiveness. Evidence of the effectiveness of oral diazepam for treatment of spasticity is limited. Many of the interventions identified are not approved for the alleviation of pain or spasticity in MS, and the lack of evidence relating to their effectiveness may also limit their widespread use. Diazepam is widely prescribed for persons with SCI to treat muscular spasticity.[13] Because diazepam binds in both the reticular formation and spinal polysynaptic pathways, it appears to produce a lesser response in patients with complete SCI.[14]

Drugs Affecting Skeletal Muscle and Calcium Stores

Agents that act at the skeletal muscle level affect change peripherally instead of at the neural level. Dantrolene is the only agent in this category that has been approved as a general pharmacological treatment for spasticity. It is used when muscle over-activity is diffuse or when the number of muscles affected precludes local treatment.

Dantrolene Sodium (Dantrium)

Dantrolene produces relaxation of the muscle at the myoneural junction. Most likely, it interferes with calcium flux at the sarcoplasmic reticulum, thereby interfering with the excitation-contraction coupling process. Dantrolene generally affects skeletal muscle fast twitch fibers to a greater extent than the slow twitch fibers, but it will affect both fiber types.[8] It does not appear to affect the neural input to the muscle, the neuromuscular junction, or the excitable muscle membranes themselves.[15] Indirect CNS effects sometimes cause drowsiness, dizziness, and generalized weakness. The duration of dantrolene depends on the dose. Its biological half-life is 8.7 hours after a 100-mg dose. The metabolic patterns appear to be similar in adults and children.[8]

In chronic disability when upper motor neuron disease or injury is present, dantrolene is used when spasticity has limited rehabilitation goals. A reduction in spasticity can enhance function, nursing care, and use of braces and can reduce painful clonus that may disturb sleep. Dantrolene is not indicated for skeletal muscle spasms in rheumatic disorders.

The dose of dantrolene should be maintained for at least 4 to 7 days to determine the patient's response. Some patients do not respond until higher doses are used. Dosing should begin with 25 to 50 mg once a day and progress to 25 mg three times a day (tid), 50 mg tid, and 100 mg tid. Doses higher than 100 mg four times daily (qid) should not be used. Pediatric doses are 5 mg once daily, progressed to 0.5 mg tid, 1 mg tid, and 2 mg tid or 12 mg/kg/day. If no benefits are derived within 45 days, administration of dantrolene should be discontinued.[8]

Dantrolene is contraindicated when spasticity is required for upright posture, balance, or locomotion.[15] In such cases, reduction in spasticity would result in loss of function. Spasticity of spinal origin responds less favorably to dantrolene because of the resultant weakness. Few studies have evaluated this effect. One study of patients with spasticity of spinal origin demonstrated a decrease in severity of spasticity; however, the reduction in strength outweighed the benefit.[16]

The most frequently occurring side effects of dantrolene are drowsiness, dizziness, weakness, general malaise, fatigue, and diarrhea.[8] These are generally transient, occurring early in treatment, and can often be obviated by beginning with a low dose and increasing the dose gradually until an optimal regimen is established. Diarrhea may be severe and may necessitate temporary withdrawal. If diarrhea recurs on re-administration of dantrolene, therapy should probably be discontinued permanently. Dantrolene has the advantage of having minimal cognitive side effects and modest interactions.[17]

Several precautions should be taken when patients are prescribed dantrolene. Patients should not use dantrolene when they have pulmonary dysfunction such as chronic obstructive pulmonary disease, severe cardiac dysfunction such as myocardial disease, or certain forms of liver disease. Because of the potential for hepatotoxicity, dantrolene should be used with caution, and liver function should be monitored.[17,18] The risk for hepatotoxicity appears greatest for women 35 years and older and patients taking more than 300 mg daily. The risk can be increased when dantrolene is combined with some other medications.

Dantrolene is used for patients with stroke, CP, and MS and may be preferable for these indications because sensitivity in terms of sedation appears to be higher in spasticity of cerebral origin (stroke) (Table 19-1). Steinberg et al.[19] found a decrease in clonus in patients treated with dantrolene for hemiparetic spasticity. This was accompanied by improvements in gait and personal care abilities. Less improvement was noted in resistance to passive stretch. A study in which oral agents for treatment of spasticity in CP were compared indicated that dantrolene compared favorably with diazepam and baclofen in reducing spasticity.[20] A brief withdrawal of dantrolene for a period of up to 2 days should result in exacerbation of symptoms and confirm the clinical impression or patient self-report of symptoms of spasticity. In one study, when patients with hemiparesis stopped taking dantrolene, a significant decrement in motor performance occurred, suggesting the benefit of dantrolene for spasticity of central origin.[21] Some studies indicate that dantrolene acts favorably in combination with other agents. Dantrolene was compared with diazepam in a double-blind study of children with spasticity. The combination of the two drugs was suggested to be most effective.[21]

Drugs Acting on the γ-Aminobutyric Acid_B Receptors

The pharmacological control of spasticity is believed to result from the reduction of inhibitory mechanisms, namely GABA-mediated or glycine-mediated antagonism of excitatory mechanisms, or both. GABA receptor sites are widely present in the CNS and therefore are amenable to pharmacological manipulation.[6]

Baclofen (Lioresal)

Baclofen is a structural analog of GABA but does not bind to the $GABA_A$ receptor but rather to the more recently identified $GABA_B$ receptor, both presynaptically and postsynaptically. When the drug binds to the GABAergic interneuron, membrane hyperpolarization blocks influx of calcium into the presynaptic terminal, thus reducing neurotransmitter release.[8] Postsynaptic binding of the drug on the Ia sensory afferent terminal also produces hyperpolarization and increases potassium influx so that inhibition is enhanced. $GABA_B$ receptors may inhibit gamma motor neuron activity and reduce muscle spindle sensitivity. The net effect is inhibition of monosynaptic and polysynaptic spinal reflexes.

Baclofen is useful for the alleviation of spasticity resulting from MS, particularly for the relief of flexor spasms and associated pain, clonus, and muscle rigidity.[7] Patients should have reversible spasticity so that baclofen treatment will aid in restoring residual function. Baclofen may also be of some value for patients with spinal cord injuries and spinal diseases, but it is not indicated in the treatment of skeletal muscle spasm resulting from rheumatic disorders.

Very few double-blind, placebo-controlled studies of baclofen have been performed.[22] However, the efficacy of oral baclofen has been established for MS and SCI, and the efficacy of intrathecal baclofen has been established for MS, SCI, and stroke (Table 19-1). This is not to say that these medications are not effective for other conditions associated with spasticity, but only that placebo-controlled studies have not been performed in patients with other conditions.

The optimal oral dose of baclofen requires titration. Therapy should be started at a low dose and increased gradually until optimum effect is achieved (usually between 40 and 80 mg daily).[7] The following dosage schedule is suggested: 5 mg tid for 3 days increasing to 5 mg every 3 days. Thereafter, additional increases may be necessary, but the total daily dose should not exceed 80 mg (20 mg qid). As always, the lowest dose compatible with an optimal response is recommended. If benefits are not evident after a reasonable trial period, the drug should be slowly withdrawn. Baclofen has general CNS depressant properties as evidenced by increases in somnolence, ataxia, and cardiac and respiratory depression. Baclofen may also impair attention and memory and produce confusion, particularly in elderly patients and patients with brain injuries.[23] Baclofen can also interfere with neural recovery because of its GABA central pathways, can lower the seizure threshold, and cause withdrawal syndrome.[21-24] Patients should be cautioned about the additive effects of baclofen and alcohol and other CNS depressants. Like other antispasticity drugs, baclofen should not be used when spasticity is needed to maintain upright function.[25] In general, patients who have had a stroke do not tolerate the drug well.[21]

Another central effect may be hallucinations.[8] Baclofen also induces muscle weakness, which may be a more significant problem for the functional patient than the patient with severe impairment.[7] Increased gait disturbances have been reported in patients with MS receiving baclofen, presumably as a result of induced weakness or underlying weakness that becomes apparent after spasticity is reduced or removed.[26,27] Sudden withdrawal of oral baclofen may result in seizures, hallucinations, and rebound spasticity with fever.

Intrathecal Baclofen

For spasticity of spinal cord origin, long-term infusion of baclofen may be prescribed for patients with severe spasticity that is unresponsive to oral antispasticity medication or for those who experience intolerable CNS side effects at effective doses.[28] Patients with spasticity caused by traumatic brain injury should wait at least 1 year after the injury before long-term intrathecal baclofen therapy is considered.

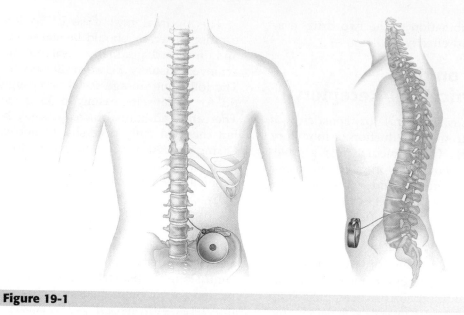

Figure 19-1

The pump is surgically implanted in the abdominal region (*front view*). The pump is connected to a catheter that is tunneled under the skin, around to the spine, and enters the intrathecal space (*side view*). (Courtesy Medtronic, Inc.)

Long-term intrathecal administration of baclofen entails the subcutaneous implantation of a pump in the abdominal wall with the catheter tip placed in the subarachnoid space[29] (Figure 19-1). Usually, the tip is placed between T12 and L1, but if a patient has significant upper extremity spasticity, the tip may be placed in the midthoracic area. Because the drug is delivered directly into the spinal cord, higher concentrations are placed in the target area with lower doses than those used with the oral route so that overall systemic effects are reduced. The intrathecal dose is only 1% of the oral dose. The pumps can be programmed to infuse the drug at a constant rate or can be titrated according to the patient's individual needs; for example, a patient may be given a greater concentration at night to relieve night spasms (Figure 19-2).

Before pump insertion, patients must demonstrate a positive clinical response to a baclofen screening injection of a bolus dose.[29] For this "intrathecal baclofen screening trial," patients are usually admitted to the hospital for 1 to 3 days. The trial begins with an initial Ashworth screening, often performed by the physical therapist, followed by a 50-μg intrathecal injection. The therapist returns after 1 hour to repeat the Ashworth screening and

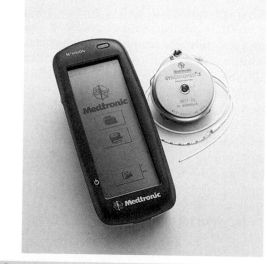

Figure 19-2

SynchroMed programmable infusion pump (*foreground*). (Courtesy Medtronic, Inc.)

then every 2 hours for the next 8 hours. If Ashworth scores do not drop, a higher dose (75 μg) is administered on the next day. If scores remain the same, a 100-μg dose may be given on the third day. The goal of each injection is a decrease in the

Ashworth score of 1 point and maintenance of this score over two consecutive assessments. Hypotonia, even if greater than desired, is a positive result on the screening test.[29] If this goal is achieved without respiratory or other complications, then the pump is offered to the patient.

The onset of action of an intrathecal bolus dose of baclofen in adults is generally $\frac{1}{2}$ hour to 1 hour after injection.[8] The peak spasmolytic effect is seen at approximately 4 hours after dosing, and effects may last 4 to 8 hours; however, this may vary, depending on the dose and severity of symptoms. Similar responses are seen in pediatric patients.

The pharmacokinetics of cerebrospinal fluid (CSF) clearance of baclofen injection calculated from intrathecal bolus or continuous infusion studies approximates CSF turnover.[8] After a bolus lumbar injection of 50 or 100 µg or intrathecal infusion of baclofen injection, the average CSF clearance is approximately 30 mL/hr. Limited pharmacokinetic data suggest that a lumbar cisternal concentration gradient of about 4:1 is established along the neuraxis during baclofen infusion. Absorption may be dose dependent, being reduced with increasing doses. Mean absorption and half-life of baclofen is 3.5 hours.[7]

After the pump is implanted, the patient will stay in the hospital for a few days.[29] Often, the patient is required to remain supine in bed for the first 2 to 3 days to prevent headaches and CSF leaks With continuous infusion using the pump, baclofen injection's antispastic action is first seen at 6 to 8 hours after initiation of infusion. Maximum activity is observed in 24 to 48 hours. If swelling occurs over either the pump incision or back incision, an Ace bandage is fitted around the abdomen. An abdominal binder may be used when the patient sits up for the first few weeks. At this point, the patient must be instructed that transfers and mobility will feel very different. Transfer training should begin with the family members for low-functioning patients, and training with assistive devices should begin for ambulatory patients, but actual rehabilitation will be on hold for a few weeks until healing occurs.

The intensity and frequency of therapy depend on underlying weakness, motor control, and in the real world, insurance coverage. A thorough evaluation performed after pump implantation will likely show that the patient has very different impairments and functional limitations than he or she did before implantation.[29] Splints and seating systems will need to be reassessed, and new assistive devices may be considered. New goals will be established, and depending on the patient, may range from feeding and oral motor skills to wheelchair mobility or even driving and sport activities. However, for any patient, balance and safety issues are paramount as the patient learns to adjust to new tone. Modalities such as ultrasound and electrical stimulation may be used but not over or near the pump site.

The postimplantation titration period requires the determination of the initial total daily dose. This dose should be double the screening dose that produced the positive clinical effect delivered over 24 hours.[7] Adult patients with SCI or stroke should have the daily dose increased by 10% to 30% (SCI) or 5% to 15% (stroke) after the first 24 hours until the desired clinical effect is achieved. Maintenance therapy requires periodic refills in which the daily dose for a patient with SCI may increase by 10% to 40%, then be reduced if the patient experiences side effects. The allowable increase in daily dose for a patient with stroke or brain injury is less and should only be increased by 5% to 20%, then reduced if any side effects occur.

For most patients, the dose must be gradually increased over time to maintain effectiveness.[7] A sudden requirement for an increase in dose usually means a kink in the catheter or a pump malfunction. Dose adjustment may be titrated to maintain some degree of spasms for circulation and to prevent deep vein thrombosis. Concomitant administration of oral baclofen should be decreased and eliminated to avoid overdose.

The pump will need to be refilled approximately every 3 months, and refilling takes about 30 to 45 minutes.[28] A syringe is inserted through the subcutaneous tissue into the pump. The pump should emit a soft beep when the volume decreases to a certain level to warn the patient when the drug level is low. A beeping sound will also occur when the battery gets low, which usually occurs between 4 and 5 years.

Complications associated with the pump include infection, dislodgment, kinking or blocking of the catheter, and pump failure.[7,28,29] With the exception of infection, any of these complications may produce symptoms of overdose or withdrawal. All medical personnel and caregivers should be instructed in the signs and symptoms of overdose, the procedures to follow if there are signs of an overdose, and ways to manage the pump and injection site. Signs of overdose include sedation, confusion, hypotonia, urinary hesitancy, respiratory depression, and even coma. Signs associated with withdrawal include increased spasticity and dystonia, hyperthermia, pruritus, agitation, hallucinations, multiple organ system failure, and death. Death is rare but has been seen with sudden withdrawal, caused by the pump running out of baclofen or a clogged catheter. Patients and caregivers should be diligent in keeping appointments for programming and monitoring of the infusion system and pump alarms and refilling the pump to avoid the risk of withdrawal.

Baclofen has been used for the treatment of spasticity in persons with SCI, CP, MS, stroke, and brain injury. The majority of studies have demonstrated efficacy in the reduction of hypertonicity in patients with SCI and MS; however, improvement in physical functions, such as ambulation or activities of daily living, has not been demonstrated.[22] In a Scandinavian study of patients with MS, no significant functional improvement was observed among those treated with baclofen.[27] This agent seems most effective for those with spasticity of spinal pathogenesis. There is no doubt that baclofen decreases spasticity and painful spasms in a variety of neurological conditions; however, many studies have failed to demonstrate improvement in gait and activities of daily living. This lack of functional gain may be due to variations in study design and the difficulty in making comparisons between studies because of the wide variety of outcome measures used. The outcome measures themselves may be the problem in that they do not always identify the specific daily activity that the patient deems most important in terms of individual improvement. Others have reported that limitation in functional gains could be due to muscle weakness that overrides the gains in reduction in stiffness from baclofen.[22]

Drugs Acting on the α_2 Receptor

The centrally acting α_2 adrenoceptor agonists are primarily used to reduce blood pressure. However, because they interact with these receptors both spinally and supraspinally, they can also be used to reduce tone.

Tizanidine (Zanaflex)

Tizanidine is a centrally acting α_2-adrenergic agonist that presumably decreases spasticity by increasing presynaptic inhibition of spinal motor neurons. It acts on the group II sensory afferents, decreases the impact on excitatory transmission, and facilitates glycine.[30] The effect is greatest on polysynaptic pathways rather than monosynaptic spinal reflexes, skeletal muscle, or the neuromuscular junction. Therefore presynaptic inhibition occurs. Clonidine is another drug in this category that is primarily used for lowering blood pressure.

Tizanidine tablets and capsules are bioequivalent to each other under fasting conditions, but not under fed conditions, as determined by changing the plasma concentrations.[8] Food also increases the extent of absorption for both the tablets and capsules. The amount absorbed with food for the tablet is significantly greater than that for the capsule.

Those sensitive to the ingredients of tizanidine should not use it and should use it with caution if renal or hepatic disease is present. Monitoring of aminotransferase levels is recommended during the first 6 months of treatment (e.g., baseline, 1, 3, and 6 months) and periodically thereafter, based on clinical status. Because of the potential toxic hepatic effect of tizanidine, the drug should be used only with extreme caution in patients with impaired hepatic function.[8]

Tizanidine's peak plasma concentration occurs 1.0 to 2.0 hours after dosing, and its half-life is 2.5 hours.[8] The starting dose for tizanidine is 2 to 4 mg at bedtime, increasing to a maximum of 36 mg/day. A slow titration program is often best tolerated.

Commonly reported side effects include somnolence, asthenia, dizziness, dry mouth, and hypotension.[8] Hypotension can be seen within 1 hour after dosing and peaks 2 to 3 hours after dosing; it can also be associated, at times, with bradycardia, orthostatic hypotension, light-headedness or dizziness, and rarely, syncope. The hypotensive effect has been measured after administration of single doses of 2 mg; therefore advancement of doses should be based on hypotensive signs and symptoms. Tizanidine can also produce sedation that appears to be dose related; sedation may be noted approximately 30 minutes after dosing and peaks at 1.5 hours afterward. Tizanidine use has been associated with hallucinations. Formed, visual hallucinations or delusions have been reported. Additionally, tizanidine can have cardiovascular effects. Caution is advised when tizanidine is to be administered to patients receiving concurrent antihypertensive therapy and should not be used with other α_2-adrenergic agonists. Prolongation of the QT interval and bradycardia were noted in patients with chronic toxicosis. Still, studies comparing tizanidine with other agents suggest that it is better tolerated than baclofen and diazepam.[31] It is less likely to weaken muscles but is still of concern because it may slow neural recovery in patients with brain injury.[21]

The therapeutic profile of antispastic drugs must be evaluated in comparison with existing drugs. Lataste et al.[32] reviewed the efficacy and tolerability of tizanidine with those of baclofen and diazepam, the most widely used antispastic agents, for a variety of diagnoses and target symptoms associated with spasticity. More than 20 double-blind, comparative studies between 1977 and 1987 included a total of 777 patients with spasticity from various causes. Tizanidine emerged as a valuable drug in the treatment of spasticity related to cerebral and spinal disorders. Groves et al.[33] conducted a meta-analysis of the antispastic efficacy and tolerability of tizanidine compared with baclofen or diazepam. As measured by Ashworth scores, tizanidine had spasticity-reducing effects similar to those of both baclofen and diazepam. Muscle strength was affected less by tizanidine than by either comparator, and tizanidine was judged to have greater tolerability.

The efficacy of tizanidine has been shown in MS. In a multicenter trial, there was a significant decrease in spasticity as measured by the Ashworth scale and the knee swing pendulum test compared with placebo.[34] A good reduction in tone was seen in stroke-related and traumatic brain injury–related spasticity without effects on the strength of muscle force, tendon reflexes, or clonus.[31]

Therapeutic Concerns Regarding the Use of Oral Antispasticity Medications

Baclofen, dantrolene, diazepam, and tizanidine continue to be the most commonly used oral systemic agents in the treatment of spasticity.[7] These are all nonspecific and produce a variety of side effects. The most troublesome effects are related to sedation and weakness, both of which interfere with therapeutic intervention and attainment of functional goals. Fine tuning the dose often takes time because drug benefit in terms of reducing tone must be balanced against the sedating or weakening effects of the drug.

The other issue is the less than optimal spasticity rating scales that are used to determine drug efficacy.[22] Often, a reduction in tone is achieved but without improvement in results of standardized tests of gross motor or functional performance. The test may not address the specific individual's improvements, or perhaps, there are simply not enough functional gains achieved with the medication. More likely, it is a problem with the standardized tests because patient caregiver reports often indicate improvements with medication.

The third issue to consider before a drug trial is proper patient selection.[29] Are there severe contractures that would still require orthopedic surgery if drug therapy were instituted and is this available to the patient? Does the patient have adequate underlying strength, particularly trunk strength? Does the patient need tone for function? Patients who ambulate in hip and knee flexion and ankle dorsiflexion may not benefit from drug intervention. In addition, intensive physical therapy is also needed along with drug therapy to help the patient develop new motor patterns and functional abilities. So there are many factors to consider, especially if the patient opts for intrathecal drug application.

Drugs Affecting the Neuromuscular Junction and Nerve Fibers

Local treatments for spasticity are those agents that are administered directly to the region of interest.[35] Several agents can be administered for chemodenervation, a method of injection directly into the muscle or nerve for the intended treatment effect. Two local treatments for spasticity are discussed: botulinum toxins and alcohols including ethanol and phenol.

Chemodenervation

Pharmacological neuromuscular blockades, such as botulinum toxins and alcohol injections, are collectively defined as chemodenervation.[35] These interventions are used to produce focal effects rather than the systemic effects that oral medications may have.

Chemical Neurolysis

Reports of the use of phenol to perform peripheral and intramuscular nerve blocks were published in the 1960s.[36] A nerve block is the application of a chemical to impair nerve function, either for the short term or permanently. A percutaneous block of a peripheral nerve trunk produces a chemical neurolysis and damage to the nerve by demyelinating it, thereby weakening the muscle.[37] Ethanol can also be used for nerve blocks to produce neurolysis (Table 19-2).

Ethyl alcohol is a powerful drug, causing extraction of lipids from the neuron and precipitation of proteins.[37] One hundred percent alcohol is used, which can cause edema of the Schwann cells and axons with separation of the myelin sheath. Eventually, wallerian degeneration begins without differential action on specific nerve roots.[36] Phenol injections or nerve blocks are often used for their clinical effect on larger proximal muscle groups because the nerve injected often supplies multiple muscles and therefore can have a greater effect for a given dose.[38]

Neurolysis to reduce spasticity is preferable to use of other agents when there is no hope of recovery of function in the injected muscle.[37] If a person with SCI is not expected to have a return of function, either because of the neurological completeness or the chronicity of the injury, neurolysis may be chosen so that several muscles could benefit from a

Table 19-2

Local Treatments for Spasticity

Drug	Mechanism	Site of Injection	Structure Blocked	Onset	Duration	Adverse Effects
Ethyl alcohol (>10%)	Tissue destruction	Intramuscular, perineural	Sensory and motor nerves; muscle; neuromuscular junction	<1 hr	2-36 mo	Pain at intramuscular injection site; pain and dysesthesia perineurally; microcirculatory damage; permanent nerve palsy; tissue necrosis
Phenol (>3%)	Tissue destruction	Intramuscular, perineural	Sensory and motor nerves; muscle; neuromuscular junction	<1 hr	2-36 mo	Pain at intramuscular injection site; pain and dysesthesia perineurally; microcirculatory damage; pain and dysesthesia perineurally; permanent nerve palsy; tissue necrosis
Botulinum toxin	Blocks acetylcholine release	Intramuscular	Neuromuscular junction	24-72 hr	3-6 mo	Rarely, distant paralysis; otherwise, no major risk

Adapted from Gracies J, Nance P, McGuire J, Simpson DM. Traditional pharmacological treatments for spasticity Part I: Local treatments. *Muscle Nerve Suppl.* 1997;6:S61-S92.

permanent reduction in activation. Alternatively, a combination of neurolysis and botulinum toxin may produce more desirable effects when there is significant spasticity in many muscles. Botulinum toxin decreases spasticity by affecting the fusimotor system and muscle spindle, whereas phenol decreases spasticity by affecting the α-motor fibers within the fusimotor system.[38-42]

Injection of phenol and alcohol chemoneurolysis require great skill and a cooperative patient. The injection techniques for neurolytic blocks involve use of small portable stimulators.[43] The anode is attached behind the limb, and the cathode is a hollow Teflon-coated needle that is attached to the stimulator. The bare needle tip serves to localize the stimulation site to which the neurolytic agent, such as phenol or alcohol, flows. The needle is directed toward the nerve trunk or at an electrically active site. In locations where the current can be reduced to approximately 0.5 mA while still producing a palpable contraction, the phenol is then injected. Initially, after the limb is injected, it may be erythematic and warm as a result of the sympathetic block in the nerve distribution. The sites of neurolytic blocks could include mixed sensorimotor nerves, such as the musculocutaneous nerve to decrease elbow flexion and the median nerve to decrease finger flexion. Other examples are injection of the obturator nerve to decrease hip adduction, injection of the sciatic nerve to address the hamstrings, and injection of the tibial nerve to decrease clonus and equinus at the ankle.[43] The clinical implications of these sites are improvement in hygiene or functional mobility.

Clinical experience indicates that caution should be used when injections are performed on patients who are receiving anticoagulation therapy because of the potential for bleeding at the injection site. Another factor to consider is that if patients already demonstrate significant weakness or flaccidity, the use of this modality may decrease function instead of improving it.[35] Careful assessment is needed because mild weakness may be overshadowed by spastic musculature. Chemodenervation could further weaken these muscles, potentially reducing function. Therefore other muscles must be capable of compensating for the functional control of the muscles weakened by injection.

Finally, if there are joint deformities or other restrictions located where the muscle to be injected crosses, there will likely be few gains.[35] Reducing muscle spasticity cannot increase limb mobility if the restriction is primarily orthopedic in nature. Additionally, although not substantiated in the literature, in cases in which significant, chronic muscle shortening is present, the mobility gains from chemodenervation are likely to be more protracted compared with cases in which muscle shortening is limited or spasticity is acute.

If a nerve trunk is selected for neurolytic injection to produce a more complete block of muscle activity, there is a greater risk of partially involving the sensory nerves causing dysesthesias. Where there is complete sensory loss such as in SCI with American Spinal Injury Association A classification, complete neurolysis may be less likely to produce dysesthesias.[44] Treatments for dysesthesias include oral glucocorticoids such as prednisone, tricyclic antidepressants, carbamazepine, and gabapentin; transcutaneous electrical nerve stimulation; and repeat blocks.[44,45] A repeat block may be helpful because the dysesthesia may be caused by an incomplete initial block of sensory fibers. However, chemical neurolysis with alcohol or phenol is often unsuccessful when the procedure is repeated more than a few times, theoretically because of fibrous tissue formation at the injection site.[46] There is also an increased risk of dysesthesias and phlebitis when more distal and deeper muscles are injected with phenol.[39]

In general, adverse effects associated with neurolytic blocks include painful injections, chronic dysesthesia, necrosis of muscle, and necrosis of the intimal lining of arteries. The disadvantage to both drugs is the sensory involvement that may occur. A positive result from these injections is that stretch reflexes tend to be more affected than strength, unless muscle necrosis is present. Because studies on both alcohol and phenol injections are limited, many clinicians today prefer to treat local muscle overactivity with botulinum toxin.

Botulinum Toxin

There are seven neurotoxins produced by *Clostridium botulinum* designated by the letters A through G.[35,47] They are genetically distinct but have overlapping sequences of homology. Botulinum toxin type A (BTX-A) has been used for years to reduce muscle overactivity, and more recently, BTX-B has been introduced. BTX-A blocks peripheral nerve cholinergic synaptic transmission. Axonal conduction is unaffected. The toxin blocks the release of acetylcholine by binding to the presynaptic nerve ending, followed by an internalization of the toxin by endocytosis, thereby blocking exostosis or the release of neurotransmitter. The mechanism for neurotransmitter blockade is not completely understood, but botulinum toxin selectively cleaves a protein called *SNAP-25,* which is responsible for the fusion of neurotransmitter vesicles at the nerve terminal. The complexity of this mechanism may explain why there is a relatively slow onset of action of BTX. The effect of BTX on individual nerve terminals is irreversible; therefore recovery of neuromuscular control occurs only when nerve sprouting creates new terminal formation. If symptoms recur, re-injection is necessary.[38]

BTX is packaged in glass vials containing 100 units.[35] A unit is not a measure of weight but of potency. One unit of BTX-A is equivalent to the amount of toxin that can kill 50% of a group of 18- to 20-gram female Swiss-Webster mice. Two types of BTX-A are available: Botox manufactured by Allergan, Inc. in the United States and Dysport, manufactured by Speywood Pharmaceuticals in England and available in Europe. Botox is the more potent preparation. Doses must be adjusted depending on the type of toxin injected. In addition, the dose of botulinum toxin is based on adjusted patient weight, muscle size, and desired effect. The onset of action is 24 to 72 hours, although the clinical effect is seen more often in 2 to 3 days.[36] The maximum recommended dose for humans is 300 to 400 U of Botox in any one session and no more than 400 U over a 3-month period (Table 19-3). The median lethal dose (LD_{50}) in humans is not known, but it has been determined in monkeys and is approximately 40 U/kg with either intramuscular or intravenous administration. An antitoxin is available if complications occur.

BTX should be diluted with preservative-free 0.9% saline solution and used within 4 hours.[40] Dilution, needle size, and injection sites per muscles vary according to clinician preference. BTX injections can be guided by muscle palpation, with electromyography, or by electrical stimulation with a Teflon-coated needle. Some have suggested that injecting near the motor end plate produces greater denervation, but these areas can be difficult to locate because of variability of location.[39,41] Electromyography can be used to help determine the injection sites, especially during complex activities such as gait to identify where muscles are overactive.

Deeper muscles or muscles not under volitional control can demonstrate improved clinical benefit when identified with electrical stimulation.[42] Typically, when the needle is inserted to locate the muscle by using electrical stimulation, the same site is used for the insertion of the needle for BTX injections. When BTX is injected into proximal muscles, a much larger dose is needed to have a clinical effect, based on muscle size, compared with that needed for smaller muscles. Because there is a limited safe dosage of the total BTX allowable every 3 months, the clinician can use the entire dosage on one or two larger proximal muscles.

After numerous injections of BTX, some patients may develop antibodies, thereby rendering the injections ineffective. However, if only the minimum dose of 400 units is used and injections are given at 3-month intervals, this can be minimized.[35] Swelling can occur at or around the injection site, especially in the lower leg, and should be treated with cold compresses and an elastic wrap to minimize it. Dysphagia has also been reported to be a side effect of BTX in the treatment of cervical dystonia, presumed to be related to toxin diffusion from an injection into the sternocleidomastoid muscle.[48] Weakness, however, is the most common adverse effect with the use of BTX. The toxin does spread to neighboring muscles and possibly into the CNS by retrograde transmission. This may be of concern when large muscles that may be needed for functional tasks are injected. Therefore it is important, when treatment with BTX is considered, to make sure that loss of muscle function will not limit functional capacity. For example, in the quadriceps group, injection of the rectus femoris may decrease knee extension during the swing phase of gait while still preserving knee extension during stance through the action of the other recti. Because of potential loss of hip flexion after injection of the rectus femoris, sufficient strength of the iliopsoas muscles must be available to compensate.

Long-term effects of BTX injections have been reported, but they are isolated and distinct problems without an overall pattern.[35] Gallbladder emptying has been slowed by these injections. There have also been reports of brachial plexus problems after sternocleidomastoid injections and a report of urinary incontinence after injections for lower extremity spasticity. Changes in muscle fiber size have also been reported but seem to have little clinical significance.

Table 19-3

Botulinum Toxin A Dosing Recommendations: A Comparison Between Adult and Pediatric Doses					
Abnormal Pattern	Muscles Involved	Botox Pediatric Dosing (units/kg)	No. of Injection Sites/Muscle (Pediatrics)	Botox Adult Dosing (units/visit)	No. of Injection Sites/Muscle (Adult)
Adducted/internally rotated shoulder	Pectoralis major and minor	2	2-3	75-150	4
	Latissimus dorsi	2	2	50-150	4
	Teres major	2	1-2		
Flexed elbow	Brachioradialis	1	1	25-75	2
	Biceps	2	2-3	50-200	4
	Brachialis	2	1-2	25-75	2
Flexed wrist	Flexor carpi radialis	1-2	1	25-100	2
	Flexor carpi ulnaris	1-2	1	10-50	2
Fist	Flexor digitorum superficialis	1-2	1-2	25-75	4
	Flexor digitorum profundus	1-2	1-2	25-100	2
Flexed hip	Iliacus	1-2	1-2	50-150	2
	Rectus femoris	3-4	2	75-200	3
Flexed knee	Medial hamstrings	3-6	3-4	50-150	3
	Gastrocnemius	3-6	2-4	50-150	4
	Lateral hamstrings	2-3	1-2	100-200	3
Adducted Thighs	Adductor brevis/longus/ magnus	3-6	1-2	75-300	6/leg
Equinovarus foot	Medial and lateral gastrocnemius	3-6	1-2	50-200	4
		2-3	1-2	50-100	2
	Soleus	1-3	1	50-150	3
	Tibialis Anterior	1-2	1	50-200	2
	Tibialis Posterior	1-2	1	50-100	4
	Flexor digitorum longus/brevis				

Adapted from Russman BS, Tilton A, Gormley ME. Cerebral palsy: a rational approach to a treatment protocol and the role of botulinum toxin in treatment. *Muscle Nerve Suppl.* 1997; 6:S181-S206; and Brin MF, and the Spasticity Study Group. Dosing, administration, and a treatment algorithm for use of botulinum toxin A for adult-onset spasticity. *Muscle Nerve Suppl.* 1997; 6:S208-S220.

Dosing Guidelines: 400 units = total maximum dose per visit for adults; 400 units or <12 units/kg = total maximum dose per visit for children; 50 units = maximum dose per injection site.

Hyman et al.[49] reported the two most frequent adverse events of patients treated with BTX were hypertonia (new or worsening spasticity after the drug wears off) of injected and/or noninjected muscles and weakness of noninjected muscles caused by spread of the drug. The authors report that this could have been attributed to normal variation in the disease state in the study sample (patients with MS).

BTX is used for a variety of conditions that produce muscle overactivity.[35,49] The list is long and includes strabismus, blepharospasm, hemi-facial spasm, cervical dystonia, writer's cramp, tremors, tics, and of course, spasticity related to CNS injury or disease. The Food and Drug Administration has recently approved Botox under the label of Botox Cosmetic for the treatment of frown lines.

Intramuscular injections of botulinum toxin have been found to reduce extremity muscle tone of patients with stroke, brain injury, SCI, neurodegenerative diseases, and MS. Richardson et al.[50] conducted a randomized, placebo-controlled trial of BTX in the upper and lower limbs for patients with stroke, head injury, incomplete SCI, tumors, and CP. The authors identified improvements in Ashworth scale of spasticity severity, passive range of motion (ROM), motor scores, and subjective ratings of severity. This underscores the notion that BTX can alleviate spasticity, regardless of cause.

In the cases in which functional recovery cannot be reasonably expected, BTX has been demonstrated to be effective in increasing mobility to improve personal care and hygiene. Examples include reducing adductor spasticity for improved hygiene in the genital region and in positional flexor spasticity for improved hand hygiene and dressing.[49-54]

There are numerous reports of reduction in tone after an injection of BTX for a variety of diagnoses. In patients with SCI, Keren et al.[55] found that the injection of 200 to 300 units of BTX into the lower limbs was effective in reducing spasticity and improving gait. Wilson et al.[56] performed a three-dimensional gait analysis on a single subject with traumatic brain injury who received BTX in the ankle plantar flexors. The subject demonstrated improved kinematic angles, such as knee extension and ankle dorsiflexion, throughout the gait cycle. Additionally, increased stride time and gait velocity were exhibited. Yablon et al.[52] studied the effect of BTX on upper limb spasticity in 21 patients with traumatic brain injury, categorized as either acute or chronic. Chemodenervation combined with physical therapy exercises such as passive ROM exercises and modalities significantly improved ROM and significantly reduced spasticity as measured by the Ashworth scale of spasticity severity.

Wissel et al.[57] evaluated two doses, a high dose and a low dose, of BTX in a randomized double-blind study of children and teenagers with spastic gait caused by CP. Both the high-dose group and the low-dose group demonstrated significant improvement in muscle spasticity and knee ROM, but a high dose was needed for significance in ankle ROM, gait velocity, and stride length after injection. However, 200 units of BTX distributed to four to five muscles per leg was better than 100 units without significant side effects. Koman et al.[58] conducted a randomized, double-blind, placebo-controlled clinical trial on BTX for lower limb spasticity in CP. Approximately 50% to 60% of the children with CP in the BTX group demonstrated significantly higher physician rating scores (specifically the ankle component of gait), greater ROM (increased between

3 and 7 degrees), and a significant reduction in the M response.

BTX has also been shown to reduce spasticity in neurodegenerative diseases. Spasticity resulting from MS was evaluated by Hyman et al.[49] who studied adductor spasticity. After 4 weeks, the authors found that 1500 units of Dysport resulted in a statistically significant improvement in maximal distance between the knees, indicating reduced adductor muscle tone. Hyman et al.[49] recommended that the clinical dose of 500 to 1000 units, divided between both legs, was best because the group that received 1500 units sometimes demonstrated too much weakness. Giladi and Honigman[59] reported on a single case of BTX injection into one leg of a patient with Parkinson's disease to alleviate freezing of gait. The freezing of gait was determined to have been due to focal foot dystonia. After injections to the extensor hallicis longus and gastrocnemius, the patient reported almost complete reduction in gait hesitation.

Hesse et al.[60] studied 12 patients with stroke and chronic hemiparesis using electronic goniometry and electromyography and found that approximately 75% of these patients demonstrated a more normal temporal pattern of muscle activity with a prominent reduction in premature activity of the plantar flexors after BTX injection. Brashear et al.[61] performed a placebo-controlled clinical trial of 126 patients with stroke and upper-limb spasticity. The injections produced a significant decrease in wrist and finger muscle tone as measured by the Ashworth scale of spasticity severity, especially during week 4 of a 12-week protocol.

Considerations for the Physical Therapist

The physical therapist should expect that the patient may show diminished function initially after a BTX injection as a result of uncovering of weakness in the antagonist muscles. The therapist should pay particular attention to safety issues while the patient adapts to the new reduced tone. Use of modalities over the injection site is contraindicated for at least 10 days.

MUSCLE RELAXANTS

Muscle relaxants are drugs typically used for relaxation of spasms caused by musculoskeletal injury. The two agents covered in this section are cyclobenzaprine, an oral agent, and the topical agent, dichlorodifluoromethane. These drugs are typically used for the treatment of low back pain resulting from muscle spasms, certain types of pain resulting from tight muscles such as the hamstrings, headache related to muscle tension and referred pain caused by trigger points.

Cyclobenzaprine Hydrochloride (Flexeril)

Cyclobenzaprine improves the signs and symptoms of skeletal muscle spasm. Additional improvements can be seen in the reduction of local pain and tenderness, increased ROM, and less restriction in activities of daily living. Improvements can be seen as early as the first day of therapy.

Cyclobenzaprine relieves skeletal muscle spasm locally without interfering with muscle function and therefore is ineffective in treating spasms of CNS origin. Animal studies show that cyclobenzaprine acts at the brainstem rather than the spinal cord. The net effect of cyclobenzaprine is a reduction of tonic somatic motor activity, influencing both gamma (γ) and alpha (α) motor systems.[8] Orally administered cyclobenzaprine is well absorbed but has a lengthy elimination time. Its half-life is between 1 and 3 days.

Cyclobenzaprine is used as an adjunct to physical therapy and rest for the treatment of muscle spasms, which are most often caused by an acute musculoskeletal injury. Its benefit is indicated by a reduction of pain and tenderness, increased ROM, and an improvement in activities of daily living. Cyclobenzaprine should only be used for a short period, about 2 to 3 weeks. There is inadequate evidence of long-term use because it is beneficial for acute injuries.

Cyclobenzaprine is contraindicated during the immediate recovery phase of myocardial infarction, arrhythmias, heart block or other conduction disturbances, or congestive heart failure. Additionally, the drug should not be used if hyperthyroidism is present because of its atropine-like action. Similarly, cyclobenzaprine should be used with caution in patients with a history of urinary retention, in patients with glaucoma or increased intraocular pressure, and in patients taking anticholinergic medication.[8] Cyclobenzaprine can enhance the effects of alcohol and barbiturates and other CNS depressants.

The usual dosage of cyclobenzaprine is 10 mg three times a day, with a range of 20 to 40 mg a day in divided doses. Dose should not exceed 60 mg a day. Use of cyclobenzaprine for periods longer than 2 or 3 weeks is not recommended.[8]

The most common side effects reported by patients who take cyclobenzaprine are drowsiness, dry mouth, and dizziness. Less frequent side effects are fatigue/tiredness, asthenia, nausea, constipation, dyspepsia, unpleasant taste, blurred vision, headache, nervousness, and confusion.

Cyclobenzaprine was compared with diazepam and placebo in double-blind trials for efficacy in treating spasms and pain in the neck and low back. Clinical improvement over 2 weeks was statistically significant in all treatment groups with a preference for cyclobenzaprine. The most striking improvements recorded were in the electromyographic findings, which showed statistically significant changes for this group.[62] Borenstein and Korn[63] conducted randomized controlled trials to assess the efficacy and tolerability of cyclobenzaprine 2.5, 5, and 10 mg tid compared with placebo in patients with acute musculoskeletal spasm. Neither study included a nonsteroidal antiinflammatory drug as an active control, which is frequently prescribed along with cyclobenzaprine by physicians. Cyclobenzaprine 2.5 mg tid was not significantly more effective than placebo, but the cyclobenzaprine 5- and 10-mg tid regimens were associated with significantly higher mean efficacy scores compared with placebo. Cyclobenzaprine 5 mg tid was as effective as 10 mg tid and was associated with a lower incidence of sedation. Katz and Dube[64] reported that cyclobenzaprine was found to have a more rapid onset of action than diazepam and was associated with few serious adverse experiences. The authors concluded that cyclobenzaprine represents a cost-effective approach to the management of acute muscle spasms, primarily because of the rapid symptomatic relief that it provides.

Dichlorodifluoromethane: Trichloromonofluoromethane (Fluori-Methane)

Dichlorodifluoromethane is a vapocoolant spray intended for topical use.[65] It is used for the management of pain and muscle spasms and myofascial pain and for the prevention of pain before muscular injections. In the case of muscle spasms, the spray sweeps should move from the muscle origin to insertion. In the case of a trigger point, sweeping the target and referral zone is advisable. During the spraying procedure, the muscle is passively stretched, and stretch is gradually increased with successive sweeps. As this is continued, a new resting length of the muscle is achieved. This new resting length should eliminate muscle spasms and trigger point pain. After the muscle has been rewarmed, the spraying procedure can be repeated again until the pain is significantly reduced or eliminated. The technique can be followed with the application of a heat pack to enhance the warming. Postural and relaxation exercises or any other therapeutic technique to reduce the primary source of the muscle spasms and pain should be applied.[8]

Dichlorodifluoromethane spray can also be used as a pre-injection analgesia. The spray is applied to minimize cutaneous sensation before injection and has been demonstrated to be a useful technique in the treatment of children to reduce the anxiety associated with injections.[65]

This product should not be used for individuals who are hypersensitive to dichlorodifluoromethane or trichloromonofluoromethane. It is especially contraindicated for individuals with vascular insufficiencies because the drop in surface temperature may result in further vessel constriction. Dichlorodifluoromethane should be used with caution to avoid inhalation of vapors, especially when applied around the face and neck, such as

when it is used for facial neuralgia.[65] Contact with the eyes should be avoided, and use should never take a region to the frost point. It must be remembered that the contents of the bottle are under pressure and therefore should be stored in a cool dry place (not over 120° F) away from high-frequency ultrasound equipment.

The application of dichlorodifluoromethane for myofascial pain involves three steps: evaluation, spraying, and stretching—which if performed in the proper sequence—produce optimal results.[66] Evaluation is done to determine whether the pain is due to muscle spasms or a trigger point. The spraying phase involves positioning the patient in a comfortable position and covering the eyes and nose if spraying will be done near the face. The spraying technique involves inverting the bottle at least 12 inches (30 to 45 cm) away from the target area and pressing the valve to release a stream of vapocoolant spray. The stream should be applied at an oblique angle parallel to the muscle belly fibers in rows of about 2 to 3 cm apart and at a rate of 10 cm/sec until the entire muscle is covered. Passive stretching then is performed.

Though extremely rare, cutaneous sensitization is possible. Also rare is a discoloration or pigment change. Otherwise, there are relatively few side effects of the topical treatment as long as the nose and eyes are protected when dichlorodifluoromethane is applied around the face.

ACTIVITIES 19

■ 1. Review the literature on botulinum toxin (BTX) and discuss the advantages BTX has over alcohol and phenol injections. Discuss patient selection issues.

■ 2. A 12-year-old boy with a diagnosis of CP (spastic quadriplegia) has been taking baclofen for the past 6 months. After careful titration, a dosage of 20 mg qid (oral) was determined to be optimum. At this dosage the patient needed only minimal assistance for dressing and was independent in both transfers and hygiene. In addition, the patient progressed to independent

ambulation with a rolling walker. However, over the last several weeks, there has been an increase in rigidity and spasticity of the lower extremities. The patient now requires moderate assistance for all dressing and hygiene activities, and ambulation is now too slow to be functional. The patient's mother reports that he is very distressed over his loss of function. Today, however, his condition has worsened and appears to be different than it was in previous weeks. She brings him to the emergency department because he is confused, weak, and very lethargic.

Questions

a. Why did this patient develop increased spasticity after 6 months of improved function?

b. Are the patient's current symptoms due to adverse effects of the drug, drug withdrawal, or drug overdose?

c. How should this patient's spasticity be managed without producing drowsiness or muscular weakness?

d. Describe the role of the physical therapist in an "intrathecal baclofen screening trial."

References

1. Lance JW. *Spasticity: Disordered Motor Control.* Chicago: Yearbook Medical Publishers; 1980.
2. Kita M, Goodkin DE. Drugs used to treat spasticity. *Drugs.* 2000;59:487-495.
3. Denny-Brown D, Feldman RG. Historical aspects of the relation of spasticity to movement. In: Feldman RG, Young RR, Koella WP, eds. *Spasticity: Disordered Motor Control.* Chicago: Yearbook Medical Publishers; 1980.
4. Ivanhoe CB, Reistetter TA. Spasticity: the misunderstood part of upper motor neuron syndrome. *Am J Phys Med Rehabil.* 2004;83:S3-S9.
5. Sehgal N, McGuire JR. Beyond Ashworth: electrophysiologic quantification of spasticity. *Phys Med Rehabil Clin N Am.* 1998;9:949-979.
6. Francisco GE, Kothari S, Huls C. GABA agonists and gabapentin for spastic hypertonia. *Phys Med Rehabil Clin N Am.* 2001;12:875-888, viii.
7. Gracies JM, Nance P, Elovic E, McGuire J, Simpson DM. Traditional pharmacological treatments for spasticity. Part II: General and regional treatments. *Muscle Nerve Suppl.* 1997;6:S92-S120.
8. Mosby. *Mosby's Drug Consult.* St Louis: Mosby; 2005.
9. Murinson BB. Stiff-person syndrome. *Neurologist.* 2004;10:131-137.
10. Cutson TM, Gray SL, Hughes MA, Carson SW, Hanlon JT. Effect of a single dose of diazepam on balance measures in older people. *J Am Geriatr Soc.* 1997;45:435-440.
11. Kitajima T, Kanbayashi T, Saito Y, et al. Diazepam reduces both arterial blood pressure and muscle sympathetic nerve activity in human. *Neurosci Lett.* 2004;355:77-80.
12. Beard S, Hunn A, Wight J. Treatments for spasticity and pain in multiple sclerosis: a systematic review. *Health Technol Assess.* 2003;7:iii, ix-x, 1-111.
13. Broderick CP, Radnitz CL, Bauman WA. Diazepam usage in veterans with spinal cord injury. *J Spinal Cord Med.* 1997;20:406-409.
14. Davidoff RA. Antispasticity drugs: mechanisms of action. *Ann Neurol.* 1985;17:107-116.
15. Elovic E. Principles of pharmaceutical management of spastic hypertonia. *Phys Med Rehabil Clin N Am.* 2001;12:793-816.
16. Glass A, Hannah A. A comparison of dantrolene sodium and diazepam in the treatment of spasticity. *Paraplegia.* 1974;12:170-176.
17. Zafonte R, Lombard L, Elovic E. Antispasticity medications: uses and limitations of enteral therapy. *Am J Phys Med Rehabil.* 2004;83:S50-S58.
18. Chan CH. Dantrolene sodium and hepatic injury. *Neurology.* 1990;40:1427-1432.
19. Steinberg F, Ferguson K. Effect of dantrolene sodium on spasticity associated with hemiplegia. *J Am Geriatr Soc.* 1975;23:70-73.
20. Krach L. Pharmacotherapy of spasticity: oral medications and intrathecal baclofen. *J Child Neurol.* 2001;16:31-36.
21. Ketel W, Kolb M. Long term treatment with dantrolene sodium of stroke patients with spasticity limiting return of function. *Curr Med Res Opinion.* 1984;9:161-169.
22. Pierson SH. Outcome measures in spasticity management. *Muscle Nerve Suppl.* 1997; 6:S36-S60.
23. Castellano C, Brioni JD, McGaugh JL. Post-training systemic and intra-amygdala administration of the GABA-B agonist baclofen impairs retention. *Behav Neurol Biol.* 1989;52(2):170-179.
24. Terrence CF, Fromm GH, Roussan MS. Baclofen. Its effect on seizure frequency. *Arch Neurol.* 1983;40:28-29.
25. Taricco M, Adone R, Pagliacci C. Pharmacological interventions for spasticity following spinal cord injury. *Cochrane Database Syst Rev.* 2000;2:CD001131.
26. Nielsen JF, Sinkjaer T. Peripheral and central effect of baclofen on ankle joint stiffness in multiple sclerosis. *Muscle Nerve.* 2000;23:98-105.
27. Orsnes G, Sorensen P, Larsen T. Effect of baclofen on gait in spastic MS patients. *Acta Neurol Scand.* 2000; 101:244-248.
28. Meythaler JM, Guin-Renfroe S, Brunner RC, Hadley MN. Intrathecal baclofen for spastic hypertonia from stroke. *Stroke.* 2001;32(9):2099-2109.
29. Barry MJ, Shultz BL. Intrathecal baclofen therapy and the role of the physical therapist. *Pediatr Phys Ther.* 2000; 12:77-86.
30. Skoog B. A comparison of the effects of two antispastic drugs, tizanidine and baclofen, on synaptic transmission from muscle spindle afferents to spinal interneurons in cats. *Acta Physiol Scand.* 1996;156:81-90.
31. Wallace JD. Summary of combined clinical analysis of controlled clinical trials with tizanidine. *Neurology.* 1994; 44:S60-S68; discussion S68-S69.
32. Lataste X, Emre M, Davis C, Groves L. Comparative profile of tizanidine in the management of spasticity. *Neurology.* 1994;44:S53-S59.
33. Groves L, Shellenberger MK, Davis CS. Tizanidine treatment of spasticity: a meta-analysis of controlled, double-blind, comparative studies with baclofen and diazepam. *Adv Ther.* 1998;15:241-251.
34. Nance PW, Sheremata WA, Lynch SG, et al. Relationship of the antispasticity effect of tizanidine to plasma concentration in patients with multiple sclerosis. *Arch Neurol.* 1997;54:731-736.
35. Gracies JM, Elovic E, McGuire J, Simpson DM. Traditional pharmacological treatments for spasticity. Part I: Local treatments. *Muscle Nerve Suppl.* 1997;6:S61-S90.

36. Little JW, Micklesen P, Umlauf R, Britell C. Lower extremity manifestations of spasticity in chronic spinal cord injury. *Am J Phys Med Rehabil*. 1989;68:32-36.

37. Bell KR. The use of neurolytic blocks for the management of spasticity. *Phys Med Rehabil Clin N Am*. 1995;6:885-895.

38. On AY, Kirazli Y, Kismali B, Aksit R. Mechanisms of action of phenol block and botulinus toxin type A in relieving spasticity: electrophysiologic investigation and follow-up. *Am J Phys Med Rehabil*. 1999;78:344-349.

39. McGuire JR. Effective use of chemodenervation and chemical neurolysis in the management of poststroke spasticity. *Top Stroke Rehabil*. 2001;8:47-55.

40. O'Brien CF. Injection techniques for botulinum toxin using electromyography and electrical stimulation. *Muscle Nerve Suppl*. 1997;6:S176-S180.

41. Shaari CM, Sanders I. Quantifying how location and dose of botulinum toxin injections affect muscle paralysis. *Muscle Nerve*. 1993;16:964-969.

42. Comella CL, Buchman AS, Tanner CM, Brown-Toms NC, Goetz CG. Botulinum toxin injection for spasmodic torticollis: increased magnitude of benefit with electromyographic assistance. *Neurology*. 1992;42(4):878-882.

43. Bell KR. The use of neurolytic blocks for the management of spasticity. *Phys Med Rehabil Clin N Am*. 1995;6:885-895.

44. Glenn MWJ. Practical management of spasticity in children and adults. In: Glenn M, ed. *Nerve Blocks*. Philadelphia: Lea & Febiger; 1990:227-258.

45. Kirshblum S. Treatment alternatives for spinal cord injury related spasticity. *J Spinal Cord Med*. 1999;22:199-217.

46. Bakheit A. Management of muscle spasticity. *Crit Rev Phys Med Rehabil*. 1996;8:235-252.

47. Brin MF. Botulinum toxin: chemistry, pharmacology, toxicity, and immunology. *Muscle Nerve Suppl*. 1997;6:S146-S168.

48. Jankovic J, Schwartz K, Donovan DT. Botulinum toxin treatment of cranial-cervical dystonia, spasmodic dysphonia, other focal dystonias and hemifacial spasm. *J Neurol Neurosurg Psychiatry*. 1990;53:633-639.

49. Hyman N, Barnes M, Bhakta B, et al. Botulinum toxin (Dysport) treatment of hip adductor spasticity in multiple sclerosis: a prospective, randomised, double blind, placebo controlled, dose ranging study. *J Neurol Neurosurg Psychiatry*. 2000;68:707-712.

50. Richardson D, Sheean G, Werring D, et al. Evaluating the role of botulinum toxin in the management of focal hypertonia in adults. *J Neurol Neurosurg Psychiatry*. 2000;69:499-506.

51. Snow BJ, Tsui JK, Bhatt MH, Varelas M, Hashimoto SA, Calne DB. Treatment of spasticity with botulinum toxin: a double-blind study. *Ann Neurol*. 1990;28:512-515.

52. Yablon SA, Agana BT, Ivanhoe CB, Boake C. Botulinum toxin in severe upper extremity spasticity among patients with traumatic brain injury: an open-labeled trial. *Neurology*. 1996;47(4):939-944.

53. Bakheit AM, Pittock S, Moore AP, et al. A randomized, double-blind, placebo-controlled study of the efficacy and safety of botulinum toxin type A in upper limb spasticity in patients with stroke. *Eur J Neurol*. 2001;8:559-565.

54. Bhakta BB, Cozens JA, Chamberlain MA, Bamford JM. Impact of botulinum toxin type A on disability and caregiver burden due to arm spasticity after stroke: a randomised double blind placebo controlled trial. *J Neurol Neurosurg Psychiatry*. 2000;69:217-221.

55. Keren O, Shinberg F, Catz A, Giladi N. Botulin toxin for spasticity in spinal cord damage by treating the motor endplate [in Hebrew]. *Harefuah*. 2000;138:204-208, 270.

56. Wilson DJ, Childers MK, Cooke DL, Smith BK. Kinematic changes following botulinum toxin injection after traumatic brain injury. *Brain Inj*. 1997;11:157-167.

57. Wissel J, Heinen F, Schenkel A, et al. Botulinum toxin A in the management of spastic gait disorders in children and young adults with cerebral palsy: a randomized, double-blind study of "high-dose" versus "low-dose" treatment. *Neuropediatrics*. 1999;30:120-124.

58. Koman LA, Mooney JF III, Smith BP, Walker F, Leon JM. Botulinum toxin type A neuromuscular blockade in the treatment of lower extremity spasticity in cerebral palsy: a randomized, double-blind, placebo-controlled trial. BOTOX Study Group. *J Pediatr Orthop*. 2000;20:108-115.

59. Giladi N, Honigman S. Botulinum toxin injections to one leg alleviates freezing of gait in a patient with Parkinson's disease. *Mov Disord*. 1997;12:1085-1086.

60. Hesse S, Krajnik J, Luecke D, Jahnke MT, Gregoric M, Mauritz KH. Ankle muscle activity before and after botulinum toxin therapy for lower limb extensor spasticity in chronic hemiparetic patients. *Stroke*. 1996;27:455-460.

61. Brashear A, Gordon MF, Elovic E, et al. Intramuscular injection of botulinum toxin for the treatment of wrist and finger spasticity after a stroke. *N Engl J Med*. 2002;347:395-400.

62. Basmajian JV. Cyclobenzaprine hydrochloride effect on skeletal muscle spasm in the lumbar region and neck: two double-blind controlled clinical and laboratory studies. *Arch Phys Med Rehabil*. 1978;59:58-63.

63. Borenstein DG, Korn S. Efficacy of a low-dose regimen of cyclobenzaprine hydrochloride in acute skeletal muscle spasm: results of two placebo-controlled trials. *Clin Ther*. 2003;25:1056-1073.

64. Katz WA, Dube J. Cyclobenzaprine in the treatment of acute muscle spasm: review of a decade of clinical experience. *Clin Ther*. 1988;10:216-228.

65. Cohen Reis E, Holubkov R. Vapocoolant spray is equally effective as EMLA cream in reducing immunization pain in school-aged children. *Pediatrics*. 1997;100:E5.

66. Travell J. Identification of myofascial trigger point syndromes: a case of atypical facial neuralgia. *Arch Phys Med Rehabil*. 1981;62:100-106.

CHAPTER 20

PHARMACOLOGICAL MANAGEMENT OF DEGENERATIVE NEUROLOGICAL DISORDERS

INTRODUCTION

The focus of this chapter is on degenerative diseases of the nervous system. Although great time and detail could be spent on the wide spectrum of neurodegenerative disorders, the discussion in this chapter is limited to three specific pathologic conditions. The three conditions covered here—Parkinson's disease (PD), multiple sclerosis (MS), and Alzheimer's disease (AD)—all have unclear etiologies, although a genetic predisposition and environmental exposure appear to play a part in all three cases.

Because no distinct causative agent has been identified in any of these conditions, the current pharmacological management focuses on addressing body system abnormalities imposed by the disease (neurotransmitter dysfunction in PD and AD and immune system dysfunction in MS). In addition, because these conditions are progressive, the needs for pharmacological management may change over time. The sections on each of these disorders include discussions of basic epidemiology and pathology, followed by coverage of treatments targeted at the impaired system. Given the unclear etiologies of these three disorders, in each section, a discussion of treatments targeted at slowing neuronal loss (neuroprotection) is provided for each of the three conditions.

PARKINSON'S DISEASE: EPIDEMIOLOGY AND PATHOLOGY

PD is common among older people, affecting more than 1 in every 100 people over the age of 75 years and 1 in every 1000 people over the age of 65 years.[1] Globally, it is estimated that 10 million older people have PD.[2] As a result of an increasing proportion of the population being older than 60 years, it has been estimated that by the year 2020, more than 40 million people in the world will have PD.

The primary movement deficits associated with PD are akinesia (delayed initiation of movement), bradykinesia (slowness of movement), postural instability, rigidity, and tremor.[2] The neurochemical origin of these movement disturbances is a neurotransmitter imbalance in the basal ganglia, a region of the brain thought to be critical in the production of voluntary movement (specifically the execution of well-learned automatic movements). The neurotransmitter imbalance develops in the motor circuit from the frontal lobe to the basal ganglia to the motor cortex as a result of progressive death of dopamine-producing neurons in the substantia nigra pars compacta of the basal ganglia. The cause of the selective neuronal death that occurs is not known, although current theories support the interaction of environmental exposure and a genetic predisposition to PD. Considerable evidence suggests that the interplay of genetics and the environment leads to mitochondrial dysfunction and oxidative damage, which contribute to neuronal death. The result of dopaminergic cell loss is a disruption of the fine balance of dopamine, acetylcholine, γ-aminobutyric acid, and other neurotransmitters in the basal ganglia and in the projections of the basal ganglia throughout the central nervous system (CNS).[2]

Despite little knowledge regarding the cause of the neurotransmitter imbalance, medical management of PD does result in improved movement abilities and reductions in most of the primary movement deficits. Pharmacological management of PD can be divided into several categories: (1) dopamine replacement, (2) increasing dopamine stimulation, and (3) modulation of nondopaminergic systems. Treatments targeted at these categories strive to restore a neurochemical balance in the basal ganglia and its functionally connected areas. The following sections describe the pharmacological mechanisms of action and the positive and negative effects of these medications. This section on PD ends with a discussion of the effects of the medications on movement abilities and a discussion of pharmacological treatments targeted toward neuroprotection, slowing the degradation of the neurons within the basal ganglia.

Dopamine Replacement

In 1960, studies of cadaveric brains of individuals with extrapyramidal movement disorders suggested that the loss of dopamine in a portion of the basal ganglia was characteristic for persons with PD.[3,4] This neuroanatomical finding led to experimentation with dopamine replacement as a means of treating persons with PD. Although dopamine was determined to be the neurotransmitter that is deficient in the basal ganglia in patients with PD, dopamine did not cross the blood-brain barrier and therefore was ineffective in reducing the cardinal symptoms associated with PD (the motor impairments of bradykinesia, tremor, rigidity, and postural instability). However, the utility of the dopamine precursor levodopa (L-dopa) was studied and found to be effective.[5] As opposed to dopamine, L-dopa is able to cross the blood-brain barrier, and it then undergoes enzymatic conversion to dopamine.[6-8] At present, dopamine replacement with L-dopa is the most effective and widely used treatment for PD.[9-11]

Levodopa is available as an oral medication that is coupled with a dopamine decarboxylase inhibitor (carbidopa or benserazide) to minimize metabolism outside of the CNS (Figure 20-1).

Positive Effects of Dopamine Replacement on Movement Tasks

The majority of studies describe the benefits of pharmacological therapy in PD in terms of outcomes on the Unified Parkinson's Disease Rating Scale (UPDRS).[12,13] Although the UPDRS is the primary outcome measure used to judge symptomatic relief in studies of dopamine agonists and other medications, studies of L-dopa have included more sensitive measures of bradykinesia, tremor, rigidity, and postural instability.[13,14]

Dopamine replacement results in substantial increases in overall movement velocity as compared with the off-medication state. This improved movement velocity appears to be due in part to the improved magnitude of agonist muscle action potentials as determined by electromyography (EMG). Although dopamine replacement improves the magnitude of the initial agonist EMG bursts, dopamine replacement appears to have little effect on temporal aspects (burst duration, multiple agonist bursts, timing of antagonist bursts) of EMG control.[15-34] Therefore dopamine replacement may preferentially affect only one of the determinants of force generation and is limited in its ability to improve muscle activation in patients with PD.[33,35-41]

Studies in which the effects of dopamine replacement on tremor have demonstrated a 50% reduction in tremor amplitude.[42-44] Although results of these studies support the effectiveness of dopamine replacement in reduction of tremor, other reports have indicated little or no response to dopamine replacement and better responses to other medications (e.g., anticholinergics). Such findings suggest that tremor associated with PD may have multiple causes with contributions from dopaminergic and nondopaminergic pathways.[42]

Studies in which PD rigidity was examined consistently demonstrate reductions in tonic EMG activity as a result of dopamine replacement. Such findings suggest that the active muscle contribution to rigidity is diminished by dopamine replacement.[26,27, 44,45]

Although force production and coordination of anticipatory postural tasks have been shown to

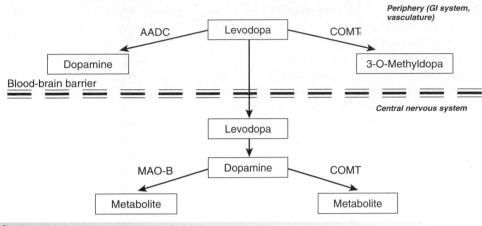

Figure 20-1

Orally ingested levodopa can be broken down in the periphery (gastrointestinal system or blood) by amino acid decarboxylase *(AADC)* or catechol-O-methyl transferase *(COMT)*. Such breakdown will lead to adverse effects of nausea, vomiting, diarrhea, and orthostatic hypotension and will decrease the effective dose reaching the brain. Coupling of levodopa with carbidopa (an AADC inhibitor) diminishes peripheral side effects and increases the effective dose reaching the brain. In addition, once levodopa enters the brain, inhibition of monoamine oxidase B and COMT will slow the synaptic breakdown of dopamine.

improve in response to dopamine replacement, control of the center of mass during reactive postural control tasks is adversely affected.[46-49] Specifically, dopamine replacement appears to diminish distal lower extremity background postural tone and lower the magnitude of reactive EMG bursts in response to support surface displacements. The functional consequences of this abnormality are that dopamine replacement may reduce the ability of a patient with PD to react appropriately and catch his or her balance if pushed off balance.[47-56]

Negative Effects of Dopamine Replacement on Movement Tasks

Although the positive effects of dopamine replacement are well documented, it is not a benign medication. Despite its widespread use and effectiveness, dopamine replacement can cause significant adverse effects.

Immediate effects of dopamine replacement. Stimulation of dopamine receptors within the gastrointestinal system and the vasculature can immediately lead to nausea, vomiting, and anorexia and hypotension, respectively. The oversupply of dopamine to nondeficient areas within the CNS contributes to the gastrointestinal effects (through stimulation of the chemoreceptor trigger zone) and

can also lead to adverse cognitive and psychiatric effects (anxiety, insomnia, psychoses, nightmares, hallucinations, paranoia, and confusion).[57]

Long-term effects of dopamine replacement. Chronic exposure to exogenous sources of dopamine may contribute to the advent of movement-related complications. The most common types of movement-related complications are dyskinesias and motor fluctuations (wearing-off and on-off phenomena).[58,59]

Dyskinesias are dynamic involuntary movements that are classically choreoathetotic in nature. The functional impact of dyskinesias can vary from negligible to completely disabling.[60,61] A thorough discussion of dyskinesias and other motor fluctuations is beyond the scope of this chapter. For additional information, readers are referred to recent journal supplements dealing specifically with dyskinesias (Movement Disorders, 1999; *Annals of Neurology*, 2000).[62,63]

Dyskinesias and motor fluctuations have been reported in as many as 84% of individuals with PD.[57,64] Although these problems are typically not observed on initiation of dopamine replacement, some authors have reported the onset after as few as 18 to 28 months of dopamine replacement therapy. Clinical observations indicate that the majority of patients with PD will experience dyskinesias and motor fluctuations after more than 5 years of dopamine replacement therapy.[65,66]

The pathophysiology of dyskinesias and motor fluctuations is thought to result from chronic exposure to the nonphysiological stimulation of dopamine receptors.[58,59] Under normal neural functioning, dopamine release within the basal ganglia is a tonic process with intermittent changes in synaptic concentrations. With the advance of PD, dopaminergic transmission within the basal ganglia becomes a more phasic process, dependent on exogenous sources of dopamine via L-dopa, which results in neurophysiological abnormalities in pathways through the basal ganglia.[11,67-69]

Recent research has suggested that persons with dyskinesias undergo a conversion in the way that the basal ganglia respond to dopamine replacement compared with those without dyskinesias. As a result, dopamine receptors become supersensitized, creating an altered functional state of the basal ganglia that allows overactivity of connections from the basal ganglia to the frontal lobe.[70,71]

As the severity of PD progresses, the therapeutic effect of each L-dopa dose lasts a progressively shorter time[72] (Figure 20-2). Patients with PD must resort to taking L-dopa more often for the same level of relief from symptoms. The dose that previously gave them relief from their motor symptoms for several hours becomes effective for progressively shorter periods (what is referred to as the "wearing off" phenomenon"). Initially, these "wearing off" periods may occur on a predictable schedule, such as end-of-dose deteriorations. With additional disease progression, the response to L-dopa becomes more unpredictable, and patients with PD may fluctuate between an effective medication state for management of motor symptoms (the "on-medication state") and complete ineffectiveness of the medication and immobility (the "off-medication state") in a matter of minutes. The motor manifestations of these off-medication periods are often freezing, falls, stiffness, and bradykinesia. Because these motor fluctuations are often related to overall L-dopa dose, pharmacological management of these movement-related complications involves the manipulation of other antiparkinsonian medications (dopamine agonists, enzymatic inhibitors, anticholinergics). Through careful, individually determined combinations of medications, neurologists

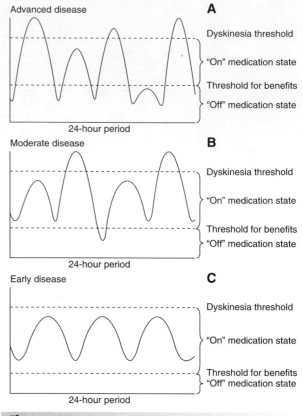

Figure 20-2

Schematic of the relationship between levodopa dosage and the clinical effects as Parkinson's disease (PD) progresses. **A,** In early PD, there is a prolonged therapeutic response to a given dose without exceeding the dyskinetic threshold, and no off-medication times are present. **B,** In moderate PD, the duration of therapeutic effect for a given dose may narrow. Thus more frequent dosing for the same clinical effect is necessary. Variability in medication responses may begin with intermittent but often predictable off-medication periods and dyskinesias. **C,** In severe PD, variability of response may be the rule rather then the exception. There may be periods of ineffective response, followed by dyskinetic responses at the same dose. The duration of effective therapeutic response may be greatly narrowed and often will be accompanied by dyskinesias.

can maximize function while minimizing the L-dopa dosage.[72]

Despite consistent exposure to pulsatile dosing, not all persons with PD experience dyskinesias and motor fluctuations.[66,73] Factors identified in the literature as playing a role in the development of dyskinesias and motor fluctuations include the following: the severity of PD when dopamine replacement is initiated (patients with more functional involvement, at Hoehn and Yahr stage III, are more likely to have dyskinesias and motor fluctuations); the duration of dopamine replacement therapy (more than 5 years of therapy is associated with a greater likelihood of dyskinesias and motor fluctuations); the age at diagnosis (age less than 60 years is associated with a greater likelihood of dyskinesias and motor fluctuations); the cumulative L-dopa dose; and a large initial dopamine replacement response.[57,59,63,65,66,72,73]

Although the presence of dyskinesias and motor fluctuations complicates the clinical treatment of the patient with PD, dyskinesias and motor fluctuations may have positive aspects. In a recent longitudinal study, the authors report that the development of dyskinesias is associated with a better long-term prognosis for functional independence because individuals with dyskinesia have a greater capacity to respond to pharmacological treatment.[73]

The composite effects of disease progression and the long-term effects of dopamine replacement may eventually limit the clinical usefulness of L-dopa in many individuals. Despite these negative effects, in some cases, the reduction in cardinal movement impairments far exceeds the problems. For this reason, many patients with PD choose to endure any short- or long-term negative effects in exchange for the improved movement abilities and lessened disability.[10,11,74,75]

Increasing Dopamine Receptor Stimulation

Two classes of medications work to increase the stimulation of postsynaptic dopamine receptors (Table 20-1). The first (dopamine agonists) operate through the direct stimulation of dopamine receptors, whereas the second class of drugs (enzymatic inhibitors) exert their action through reduced breakdown of dopamine within the synapse.[74,75]

Dopamine Receptor Agonists
Dopamine agonists produce their symptomatic effects in PD by binding directly with the postsynaptic dopamine receptors.[75] This class of drugs includes bromocriptine mesylate, pergolide mesylate, pramipexole, and ropinirole hydrochloride

(Table 20-2). They are currently used in early PD as monotherapy and in late PD as a means of lowering L-dopa doses and therefore minimizing dyskinesias and motor fluctuations.[76-82] Recently, they have gained popularity because they have a much longer half-life than L-dopa, which creates more sustained stimulation of dopamine receptors and less phasic stimulation. Given the theorized role of pulsatile stimulation of dopamine receptors in the generation of dyskinesias, this may reduce the progression of motor complications.[76-82]

Short-term studies have shown that dopamine agonists are effective in early and later stages of PD, both as monotherapy and as adjuncts to L-dopa.[11,76-82] Pramipexole and ropinirole have an advantage over older dopamine agonists in that they do not stimulate serotonin receptors and thus do not cause some of the side effects of the other dopamine agonists. All dopamine agonists can cause symptoms similar to those of L-dopa, but these are usually transient.[83] This class of drugs must be used with caution in elderly patients, who may have CNS effects, such as confusion and cognitive impairment.

Enzymatic Inhibitors
Enzymatic inhibitors inhibit monoamine oxidase type B (MAOB) and catechol-O-methyl transferase (COMT), resulting in greater serum L-dopa levels. This increases the amount of time available for L-dopa to cross the blood-brain barrier. The bioavailability of L-dopa is approximately doubled in combination with these drugs.

Selegiline hydrochloride, is an MAOB inhibitor that acts clinically by inhibiting dopamine metabolism in the brain.[75] Selegiline improves motor performance, activities of daily living, and total scores on the UPDRS. In addition, it reduces the incidence of motor fluctuations, and in some studies, has delayed the need for L-dopa therapy. Although selegiline does not stop the progression of PD, the delay in the need for L-dopa that it causes has been interpreted by some as a sign of a neuroprotective benefit. Selegiline may be used early in the illness because of its potential neuroprotective effects. As patients with PD begin to take L-dopa, selegiline can be used as an adjunct to L-dopa, especially for those experiencing wearing off effects. Its effectiveness, when combined with low doses of L-dopa, is comparable to that of a higher

Table 20-1

Common Drugs Used for Parkinson's Disease

Drug	Primary PD Deficits Addressed	Common Side Effects	Starting Dosage
DOPAMINE REPLACEMENT			
Levodopa-carbidopa (Sinemet)	Bradykinesia, tremor, rigidity	Dizziness, nausea, psychiatric, dyskinesias	25/100 mg three times daily
INCREASING DOPAMINE RECEPTOR STIMULATION			
Bromocriptine (Parlodel)	Bradykinesia, tremor, rigidity	See Table 20-2	1.25 mg twice daily
Pergolide (Permax)	Bradykinesia, tremor, rigidity	See Table 20-2	0.05 mg at bedtime
Pramipexole (Mirapex)	Bradykinesia, tremor, rigidity	See Table 20-2	0.125 mg three times daily
Ropinirole (Requip)	Bradykinesia, tremor, rigidity	See Table 20-2	0.25 mg three times daily
Selegiline (Eldepryl)	Bradykinesia, tremor, rigidity	Insomnia, headaches, sweating, dyskinesias	5 mg twice daily
Tolcapone (Tasmar)	Bradykinesia, tremor, rigidity	Dizziness, orthostasis, diarrhea, dyskinesias	100 mg three times daily
Entacapone (Comtan)	Bradykinesia, tremor, rigidity	Dizziness, orthostasis, diarrhea, dyskinesias	200 mg
MODULATING NONDOPAMINERGIC SYSTEMS			
Amantadine (Symmetrel)	Bradykinesia, rigidity	Confusion, nausea, hallucination	100 mg twice daily
Trihexyphenidyl (Artane)	Tremor, rigidity	Confusion, dry mouth, nausea	0.5 to 1 mg twice daily
Biperiden (Akineton)	Tremor, rigidity	Confusion, dry mouth, nausea	
Procyclidine (Kemadrin)	Tremor, rigidity	Confusion, dry mouth, nausea	
Benztropine (Cogentin)	Tremor, rigidity	Confusion, dry mouth, nausea	1 to 2 mg twice daily

L-dopa dose and also to doses given at more frequent intervals.[75,80,84]

Selegiline is generally well tolerated, although the production of amphetamine metabolites may predispose patients to insomnia, so it is most commonly taken in the morning.[75,80,84] There are few dietary restrictions compared with the nonselective monoamine oxidase inhibitors (see discussion of monoamine oxidase inhibitors in Chapter 16. Gastrointestinal side effects and exacerbation of peptic ulcers may occur. When selegiline is administered with L-dopa, dopaminergic side effects are often increased (e.g., hallucinations, nausea, orthostatic hypotension). In addition,

because of the role of MAOB in the metabolism of serotonin, selegiline cannot be given in conjunction with tricyclic antidepressants and selective serotonin reuptake inhibitors. Because of its CNS effects, it must be used with caution in elderly patients.[80,84]

The COMT inhibitors are one of the newest classes of drugs for PD and include entacapone and tolcapone.[75,84-88] In addition, there is a combination formulation available, Stalevo, which is L-dopa, carbidopa, and entacapone. The COMT inhibitors reduce L-dopa breakdown to 3-O-methyldopa, mainly in the periphery, and increase the amount crossing the blood-brain barrier. Thus when given in conjunction with L-dopa, COMT inhibitors may

Table 20-2

Dopamine Agonists Used in Parkinson's Disease: Properties and Side Effects				
	Bromocriptine (Parlodel)	**Pergolide (Permax)**	**Pramipexole (Mirapex)**	**Ropinirole (Requip)**
Initial dosage	1.25 mg bid	0.05 mg	0.125 mg tid	0.25 mg tid
Half-life	10 to 12 hours	16 to 24 hours	8 hours	6 hours
POTENTIAL SIDE EFFECTS				
Somnolence	+	++	+++	++
Insomnia	+	++	++++	+
Dizziness or lightheadedness	+++	+++	+++	++
Hallucinations or confusion	+++	++	++	++
Headache	+++	+++		++
Orthostasis	+++	+++	++	+++
Nausea	++++	++++	++++	++
Constipation		++	++	

bid, Two times per day; *tid,* three times per day; +, incidence of 1% to 5%; ++, incidence of 6% to 15%; +++, incidence of 16% to 25%; ++++, incidence of greater than 25%.

increase CNS delivery of dopamine and therefore reduce the L-dopa dose necessary for a given clinical effect. Pharmacokinetic studies have shown that they increase the area under the plasma L-dopa concentration-time curve but not peak levels of L-dopa. They also provide a more controlled concentration of L-dopa, thereby decreasing pulsatility. Such a mechanism is potentially ideal for patients with peak dose dyskinesias and motor fluctuations.[75,84-88] Currently, these drugs appear particularly useful for patients with "brittle" PD (i.e., those who fluctuate between off-medication and on-medication states frequently throughout the day). Research is ongoing to determine whether this will reduce progression of motor complications and to determine whether these drugs are indicated for both early and fluctuating PD.[75,84-88]

Because COMT inhibitors work by improving and prolonging dopamine stimulation, the side effects are similar to those seen with L-dopa. These drugs may trigger dyskinesias or produce cognitive impairments (e.g., hallucinations). Nausea and diarrhea are also common side effects. In addition, there have been a number of reports of fatal liver damage with tolcapone, which has led to its withdrawal in Europe. In the United States, the Food and Drug Administration (FDA), as well as the drug manufacturers, require monitoring of liver function and have changed the package labeling to state that the drug should be reserved for patients who have severe movement abnormalities and who are not appropriate candidates for other available pharmacological therapy[75,84-88]

Modulating Nondopaminergic Systems

In addition to drugs that primarily interact with the dopaminergic system, there are several medications that seek to normalize the unopposed actions of other neurotransmitter systems. These may be used as monotherapy or in conjunction with drugs that modulate the dopaminergic system.

Amantadine

The antiinfluenza drug amantadine was serendipitously discovered to have antiparkinsonian effects in 1969[43,75,84] (Table 20-1). The exact mechanism of action has not been determined, but it probably acts as a glutamate antagonist. In addition, it may exert its effect through enhanced release of stored dopamine, inhibition of presynaptic reuptake, or dopamine receptor agonism. It is commonly used as monotherapy in early, mild PD, and it appears to be most effective in patients whose bradykinesia, akinesia, or rigidity is more prominent than tremor.

Because amantadine has an additive effect with L-dopa, it can be used in combination with L-dopa for patients with moderate PD who are experiencing "wearing off" effects. The side effects include nausea, insomnia, hallucinations, and autonomic symptoms.[43,75,84]

Anticholinergics

Before the discovery of L-dopa, anticholinergics were the only drugs available to treat PD.[43,75,89] This class of drugs includes trihexyphenidyl, benztropine mesylate, procyclidine, biperiden, and diphenhydramine. Anticholinergics reduce the relative cholinergic excess produced by dopamine deficiency, thereby counterbalancing the reduced dopaminergic influence on the basal ganglia output neurons. They are most effective in patients with mild PD whose tremor is more prominent than rigidity or akinesia.[43,75,89] They appear to have little effect on bradykinesia. Although anticholinergics can be beneficial for some patients, the side effects are significant. Mucosal secretions may be inhibited, causing dry mouth and skin. Because they antagonize the cardiac cholinergic receptors, tachycardia is another adverse effect. Other anticholinergic side effects include dilation of the pupils, increased intraocular pressure, and gastrointestinal and genitourinary motility inhibition. Urine retention, especially in men with prostatic hypertrophy, is often a problem.[43,75,89]

Neuroprotection

Considerable evidence suggests that mitochondrial dysfunction and oxidative damage may play a role in the pathogenesis of PD.[80,90-91] One area of intense research interest is the search for compounds that can modulate cellular energy metabolism and exert antioxidative effects. The aim of neuroprotective therapy is to prevent further dopaminergic cell death, thereby slowing or halting disease progression. The objective of neuroprotection trials is to prove decreased loss of dopaminergic neurons from the basal ganglia in patients receiving the potentially neuroprotective agent. This type of proof is impossible to obtain in vivo, so researchers currently use outcome measures, such as clinical rating scales (e.g., the UPDRS), time to clinical endpoints (e.g., time until L-dopa therapy is required in previously untreated patients), radionuclide imaging (i.e., single photon emission computed tomography and

positron emission tomography), and mortality rates.[80,90-91]

Recently, The Committee to Identify Neuroprotective Agents in Parkinson's (a committee formed by the United States National Institute of Neurologic Disorders and Stroke) reviewed potential neuroprotective agents for PD.[75,80,90-91] The committee concluded that at least a dozen compounds should be candidates for further clinical trials. These included but were not limited to MAOB inhibitors (selegiline, rasagiline), dopamine agonists (ropinirole, pramipexole), and coenzyme Q-10. Two groups of prescription medications (MAOB inhibitors and dopamine agonists) and two supplements (vitamin E and coenzyme Q-10) are discussed in terms of their potential neuroprotective abilities.[80,90-91]

Monoamine Oxidase Type B Inhibitors

The MAOB inhibitor selegiline inhibits production of a free radical metabolite and has been found to be neuroprotective in an animal model.[9,10] To examine the potential neuroprotective abilities of selegiline and vitamin E, the Deprenyl and Tocopherol Antioxidative Therapy of Parkinsonism Trial included a comparison of selegiline with placebo in persons with untreated PD.[80,90-91] Although a 9-month delay in the need for L-dopa in selegiline-treated patients was observed, follow-up interpretation determined this benefit to be due to the drug's symptomatic effects. With long-term follow-up (10 years), no difference in mortality rate between the two treatment groups was seen. Subsequent studies have demonstrated equivocal or conflicting results. In fact, a recent meta-analysis of the results of all selegiline trials in early PD showed no statistically significant increase in the mortality rate among those treated with selegiline. Currently, selegiline is considered to have a limited neuroprotective benefit. The neuroprotective abilities of another MAOB inhibitor, rasagiline, are currently being examined.[80,90-91]

Dopamine Agonists

Recent evidence from in vitro and animal models of PD suggests that dopamine agonists have neuroprotective effects. As follow-up to these observations, two studies have examined the neuroprotective effects of two dopamine agonists (ropinirole and pramipexole) through the use of radionuclide imaging.[91a,92b] The findings of these studies showed reduced decline in radionucleotide markers of dopamine function in the dopamine agonist groups. These findings were initially interpreted to indicate neuroprotective effects. However, subsequent evaluation of the findings has called the methods into question, and at this time, none of the dopamine agonist drugs are indicated for slowing of disease progression.[75,80-82,90-91]

Vitamin E and Coenzyme Q-10

Epidemiological researchers have examined the associations between dietary intake of vitamin E and the risk of PD.[80,90-91] In two large longitudinal studies conducted in the United States, there was no evidence that the use of vitamin E reduced the risk of PD. However, higher intake of dietary vitamin E was associated with a significantly lower risk of PD. Because of the inherent weaknesses of epidemiological methods for determining cause and effect, the lower risk of PD should be interpreted cautiously and may be due to other unidentified dietary or lifestyle factors. As mentioned earlier, the Deprenyl and Tocopherol Antioxidative Therapy of Parkinsonism Trial examined the effects of selegiline and vitamin E on early PD over a 5-year period. The benefits of vitamin E could not be confirmed by this trial.[90,91]

In addition to vitamin E, coenzyme Q-10 has received recent attention as a potential neuroprotective agent. In a recent multicenter, placebo-controlled trial, participants taking 1200 mg of coenzyme Q-10 were found to have developed less disability than those receiving placebo (as measured by the UPDRS). Further studies are needed with larger samples, long-term follow-up, and a broader range of outcome measures to confirm these preliminary findings.[90,91]

Changes in Pharmacological Management with Disease Progression

Generally, PD signs and symptoms appear to decrease as a result of use of medications such as dopamine agonists; however, the most potent effect on movement abilities is from dopamine replacement. Although dopamine replacement will result in reductions in the cardinal movement impairments associated with PD, it will not restore movement control to normal levels, and the response to dopamine replacement may vary among individuals. Specifically, bradykinesia, tremor, and rigidity are all reduced to variable degrees.[9-11,75,78,79,86]

After being treated with L-dopa for more than 5 years, the majority of individuals will demonstrate some form of movement-related complications, such as dyskinesias and wearing-off phenomena.[65-66,73] As a result of these complications, pharmacological treatment of these individuals may be changed. Patients with PD who begin experiencing movement-related complications may be switched to controlled-release formulations of dopamine replacement medications in an effort to provide more prolonged stimulation to dopamine receptors. Other options are treatment with dopamine agonists, enzymatic inhibitors, or other medications as a means of lowering the overall L-dopa dose.[9-11,75,78,79,86]

Clinical Practice Considerations

Given the fact that medications for the treatment of PD produce a profound effect on the motor system, there are therapeutic concerns regarding the drugs and physical therapy practice. Obviously, the timing of physical therapy services is important to consider because intervention would be useless if it did not take place during peak effect of the drug. However, there are also some concerns that exercising the patient who is taking dopamine may negatively affect absorption.

Timing of Physical Therapy Treatment with Medications

Despite the lack of specific examinations of the effects of medications on responses to exercise, research demonstrating improvements in UPDRS items related to activities of daily living implies that exercise/rehabilitation training should take place while patients with PD are in an on-medication state.[92] Most individuals with mild to moderate PD demonstrate improved movement competencies within 1 to 1.5 hours of taking their dopamine replacement medication. If physical therapy is scheduled during optimal medication effects, the improved movement competencies seen during on-medication states should allow patients with PD to participate to a greater degree in rehabilitative efforts.[92]

Effect of Exercise on Dopamine Pharmacotherapeutics

An additional clinical concern is the relationship of exercise to L-dopa absorption, utilization, and subsequent motor effects. Physical therapists will likely treat patients with PD who experience a variety of effects of exercise on the physiological effect of their dopamine replacement medications (in some, exercise improves medication effects; in others, exercise decreases medication effects).[93-96] Synthesis of the results of the few studies that have examined this issue suggests that as a result of aerobic exercise, L-dopa absorption improves. However, in the literature there is a lack of agreement regarding whether there is an increased demand for L-dopa during exercise. One study demonstrated a decrease in the duration and severity of dyskinesias during exercise.[93] Large intersubject variability and small sample sizes limit the conclusions that can be drawn from this research.[93-96] Additional research with larger samples, control for severity and subtype of PD (tremor predominate vs akinetic rigid predominate), and comparison of exercise types (aerobic training vs strength training) is needed to better understand this issue.

MULTIPLE SCLEROSIS: PATHOLOGY AND CLINICAL PRESENTATION

MS is an inflammatory, degenerative disease of the CNS, which is usually progressive and eventually results in permanent neurological damage and disability.[97,98] The onset of MS is often very gradual, and the wide variety of symptoms that can occur overlap to some extent with those of other neurological disorders. For this reason, establishing a definitive diagnosis of MS is not straightforward, and there is often a significant period of latency between the onset of clinical signs and symptoms and the point at which clinically definite MS is diagnosed.[99,100] Relative to many neurodegenerative diseases, the average age of onset for MS is early (20 to 40 years), and there is generally a 2:1 predominance in women over men.[101-102]

The clinical presentation of MS is generally characterized by periods of impaired neurological function interspersed with periods of complete or partial recovery. Such disease behavior has led MS to be categorized according to the pattern and progression of neurological function. In the majority of patients (up to 85%) with MS, the disease will initially follow a relapsing-remitting course (i.e., relapses separated by periods of remission). Of these patients, approximately 50% to 60% will have secondary progressive MS within 10 to 15 years.[97] A small percentage (15%) of patients with MS will

experience a gradual worsening of neurological function from the outset. This form of the disease is known as primary progressive MS.[103,104] Exacerbations typically develop slowly over hours to several days, persist for several days or weeks, and then gradually remit.

The development of MS lesions is thought to be a consequence of alterations in normal immune regulation, leading to the development and proliferation of T cells that react to myelin and/or oligodendrocytes. These activated T cells cross the blood-brain barrier and enter the CNS, where they encounter the antigen (i.e., myelin). An inflammatory process is initiated, and this process involves the release of inflammatory mediators, generation of acute edema, and neural tissue injury.[105]

Recent research is challenging the classic descriptions of the pathogenesis and progression of MS. MS is no longer considered to be simply an autoimmune demyelinating disease. Although autoimmune processes are critical to the development of the neuronal lesions, a genetic predisposition coupled with environmental exposures (perhaps mediated by a viral or other infectious disease vector) contribute to the development of the disease.[105-108] In addition to the classically described demyelination, it is now clear that substantial axonal injury within active MS lesions is a central pathological feature. Within the past decade, clinical and laboratory studies have demonstrated that axonal injury occurs very early in the disease process and appears to contribute significantly to the accumulation of disability associated with disease progression. It is now theorized that axonal transection is the pathological correlate of the irreversible neurological impairment seen in MS. The relationship between axonal damage and other components of the pathological features, such as demyelination and remyelination, are the focus of current research.[109-112]

Examination of CNS tissue of individuals with MS reveals multiple sharply demarcated plaques.[98] The demyelinating lesions and axonal damage of MS can occur in the white matter throughout the CNS but most commonly occur in the optic nerves, white matter tracts of the periventricular regions, brainstem, cerebellar tracts, and spinal cord. The consequences of demyelination for neuronal conduction reflect the functional anatomy of impaired saltatory conduction at affected sites and account for many of the observed signs and symptoms.

Common signs and symptoms may include blurred vision, upper motor neuron signs (spastic muscle weakness, hyperreflexia, positive Babinski response), nystagmus, dysarthria, ataxia, autonomic dysfunction, and sensory abnormalities (from internal capsule or spinal cord lesions).

Outcome Measures Used for Multiple Sclerosis Drug Studies

In human studies of MS medications, several different outcome measures are used. These include magnetic resonance imaging (MRI), relapse rate, and the Kurtzke Expanded Disability Severity Scale (EDSS)[113,114] (Table 20-3). There appears to be a relationship between these outcome measures in that MRI activity and relapse rate during the initial phase of the disease have been found to correlate to some extent with the degree of long-term disability.[115,116]

Magnetic Resonance Imaging
MRI is used to visualize MS lesions and to distinguish between old lesions (from previous MS exacerbations) and new or active lesions (where inflammation and demyelination are ongoing).[117] Typically used with the contrast agent gadolinium, MRI has proved to be highly valuable in assessing the effects of potential disease-modifying drugs. The use of MRI in the monitoring of disease progression has led to the understanding that disease activity is likely present in the absence of corresponding clinical symptoms (on the order of 5 to 10 times more new or active lesions than the number of clinical relapses observed).[118,119]

Relapse Rate
The frequency of exacerbations/relapses is used to determine whether medications reduce the progression of disease activity. The initial studies of interferon beta-1a in MS involved the evaluation of change in the exacerbation rate.[116]

Expanded Disability Severity Scale
For most studies, significant progression of disability has been defined as an increase of one or more points on the Kurtzke EDSS, a standard measure of disability used in clinical studies of MS, sustained for at least 6 months.[113] The EDSS quantifies disability in eight functional systems and allows neurologists to assign a functional system score in each of these. The functional systems are pyramidal, cerebellar, brainstem, sensory, bowel and bladder, visual, cerebral, and other.

Disease-Modifying Drug Therapies

Pharmacological therapies developed for the treatment of MS can be divided into two main categories: drugs for the treatment of acute relapses (corticosteroids) and drugs that affect the disease course (collectively termed *disease-modifying drugs*). The latter group can be subdivided into those with broad immunosuppressive effects (e.g., methotrexate and mitoxantrone) and those with immunomodulatory effects (interferon beta and glatiramer acetate [GA]). At this time, the class of medications considered to be disease-modifying drugs include three commonly used interferon medications (two types of interferon beta-1a, one type of interferon beta-1b), one medication that modifies the immune response to myelin basic protein (GA), and one chemotherapeutic agent (mitoxantrone).

Interferons
The belief that MS had a virus-mediated component contributed to the study of interferons in reducing the number of exacerbations in specific groups of patients with MS. First studied for efficacy in the late 1970s, interferon beta has subsequently been shown to have antiviral, antiinflammatory, and immunomodulatory properties.[120] Evidence in support of an immunomodulatory mechanism of action comes from both laboratory and clinical studies, which have shown that interferon beta has dose-dependent actions on a variety of mediators that inhibit MS disease activity. These processes include the inhibition of proinflammatory cytokines and stimulation of the production of the antiinflammatory cytokines.[121,122]

Phase III drug trials of all of the available interferon medications have shown these medications to be effective in reducing lesion accumulation, relapse frequency, and progression of disability. However, questions remain regarding the relative merits of different types of interferons, the most effective route of delivery, the frequency of dosing, and the dose-response relationship for individual interferon medications[123-127] (Table 20-4).

In recent years, it has become increasingly apparent that the demyelination and axonal damage

Table 20-3

Kurtzke Expanded Disability Status Scale

Score	Description
0.0	Normal neurological examination
1.0	No disability, minimal signs in one FS
1.5	No disability, minimal signs in more than one FS
2.0	Minimal disability in one FS
2.5	Mild disability in one FS or minimal disability in two FS
3.0	Moderate disability in one FS or mild disability in three or four FS; fully ambulatory
3.5	Fully ambulatory but with moderate disability in one FS and more than minimal disability in several others
4.0	Fully ambulatory without aid, self-sufficient, up and about some 12 hours a day despite relatively severe disability; able to walk without aid or rest some 500 meters
4.5	Fully ambulatory without aid, up and about much of the day, able to work a full day, may otherwise have some limitation of full activity or require minimal assistance; characterized by relatively severe disability; able to walk without aid or rest some 300 meters
5.0	Ambulatory without aid or rest for about 200 meters; disability severe enough to impair full daily activities (work a full day without special provisions)
5.5	Ambulatory without aid or rest for about 100 meters; disability severe enough to preclude full daily activities
6.0	Intermittent or unilateral constant assistance (cane, crutch, brace) required to walk about 100 meters with or without resting
6.5	Constant bilateral assistance (canes, crutches, braces) required to walk about 20 meters without resting
7.0	Unable to walk beyond approximately 5 meters even with aid, essentially restricted to wheelchair; wheels self in standard wheelchair and transfers alone; up and about in wheelchair some 12 hours a day
7.5	Unable to take more than a few steps; restricted to wheelchair; may need aid in transfer; wheels self but cannot carry on in standard wheelchair a full day; may require motorized wheelchair
8.0	Essentially restricted to bed or chair or perambulated in wheelchair but may be out of bed itself much of the day; retains many self-care functions; generally has effective use of arms
8.5	Essentially restricted to bed much of day; has some effective use of arms; retains some self-care functions
9.0	Confined to bed; can still communicate and eat
9.5	Totally helpless, bed-ridden patient; unable to communicate effectively or eat/swallow
10.0	Death due to MS

From Kurtzke JF. Rating neurologic impairment in multiple sclerosis: an expanded disability status scale (EDSS). *Neurology.* 1983;33(11):1444–1452. Available at www.nationalmssociety.org. Accessed June 17, 2005.
EDSS steps 1.0 to 4.5 refer to people with MS who are fully ambulatory.
EDSS steps 5.0 to 9.5 are defined by the impairment to ambulation.
FS, Functional system; *MS,* multiple sclerosis.

that appear to lead to irreversible disability actually begin very early in the course of the disease. For this reason, it has been suggested that in order to prevent axonal damage, interferon therapy be initiated as soon as possible after the diagnosis of MS is made. There is also emerging evidence that initiation of interferon treatment with signs of clinically silent MRI lesions (subclinical demyelination) may slow the progression to clinically definite MS.[128-131]

Glatiramer Acetate

GA is a synthetic protein mixture of random polymers containing glutamic acid, tyrosine, lysine, and alanine. It appears to simulate myelin basic protein, a component of the myelin that insulates nerve fibers in the brain and spinal cord. Through a mechanism that is not completely understood, this drug seems to block myelin-damaging T cells by acting as a myelin decoy. Potential mechanisms of

Table 20-4

Drugs Approved for Treatment of Multiple Sclerosis				
Drug Name (Trade Name)	Class of Medication	Common Side Effects	Type of MS Indicated	Dosage/Frequency Route of Administration
Interferon beta-1a (Avonex)	Immunomodulator	Flu-like symptoms (fever, chills, sweating, muscle aches, and tiredness)	RRMS	30 µg/once per week/ intramuscular injection
Interferon beta-1a (Rebif)	Immunomodulator	Flu-like symptoms (fever, chills, sweating, muscle aches, and tiredness)	RRMS	44 µg/3 times per week/subcutaneous injection
Interferon beta-1b (Betaseron)	Immunomodulator	Flu-like symptoms (fever, chills, sweating, muscle aches, and tiredness)	RRMS	250 µg/every other day/subcutaneous injection
Glatiramer acetate (Copaxone)	Immunomodulator	Skin reactions (itching, inflammation), nausea, upset stomach, muscle weakness or stiffness, flushing, chest/joint pain	RRMS	20 mg/every day/subcutaneous injection
Mitoxantrone (Novantrone)	Antineoplastic	Immunosuppression, heart muscle damage*	SPMS, PRMS, worsening RRMS	Four times a year by IV infusion in a medical facility. Lifetime limit of 8-12 doses (12 mg/m^2 every 3 months)

MS, Multiple sclerosis; *RRMS*, relapsing remitting multiple sclerosis; *SPMS*, secondary progressive MS; *PRMS*, progressive, relapsing MS.

*The total lifetime dose of mitoxantrone is limited to avoid possible heart damage. Patients taking mitoxantrone should have regular tests of their heart function. Mitoxantrone cannot be used by patients with preexisting heart problems, liver disease, and certain blood disorders.

action suggested for GA include the alteration of immune function and reduction of inflammation via a T-cell receptor pathway and/or a neuroregenerative/protective action.[132-135]

In controlled clinical trials with relapsing-remitting MS, GA appears to have positive effects on MRI measures (reduction of new lesions, prevention of re-enhancement of old lesions, and potentiation of reparative mechanisms), as well as effects on clinical measures (reduction of relapses and slowing disability) compared with placebo.[136-141]

Although the mechanisms of action of GA and interferon beta are not completely understood,

multiple lines of research suggest that they work through different immunological pathways. For this reason, if a patient with MS does not respond to interferon beta, it is possible that he or she will respond to GA and vice versa. When GA is compared with interferon beta, the advantage of GA treatment is the absence of important side effects (flu-like symptoms), but the disadvantage is the need for daily administration.

Mitoxantrone

Mitoxantrone belongs to the general group of medicines called *antineoplastics*. Before its approval for use in MS, it was used only to treat certain forms of cancer. It acts in MS by suppressing the activity of T cells and other immune system cell types thought to be involved in the degradation of the myelin sheath and axonal damage.

The use of mitoxantrone for the treatment of MS was evaluated in a series of studies in Europe during the 1990s. The results of these studies indicate that mitoxantrone delays the time to first treated relapse and time to disability progression and also reduces the number of treated relapses and number of new lesions detected by MRI.

Based on findings from these studies, the United States Food and Drug Administration approved mitoxantrone in October 2000 for reducing neurological disability and/or the frequency of clinical relapses (attacks). Because of its significant side effect profile, the indications are limited to specific subgroups of patients. These groups are as follows[142-144]:

1. Patients with secondary progressive MS (MS that has changed from relapsing-remitting MS to progressive MS at a variable rate)
2. Progressive-relapsing MS (disease characterized by a gradual increase in disability from onset with clear, acute relapses along the way)
3. Worsening relapsing-remitting MS (disease characterized by clinical attacks without complete remission, resulting in a stepwise worsening of disability)

As with other chemotherapeutic drugs, there are potential adverse side effects of mitoxantrone on healthy tissues in the body. These include cardiotoxicity, liver dysfunction, and treatment-related acute leukemia.[145,146]

Because of these side effects, monitoring for potential cardiac, hematological, and hepatic complications is necessary. The potential for cardiac complications dictates that mitoxantrone be prescribed only for patients with normal cardiac function, and evaluation of cardiac output is necessary before treatment is started. In addition, periodic cardiac monitoring is required throughout the treatment period. The lifetime cumulative dose is limited to 140 mg/m^2 (approximately 8 to 12 doses over 2 to 3 years). Because mitoxantrone can increase the risk of infection (by decreasing the number of protective white blood cells) and damage the liver, blood counts and liver enzyme levels are determined before each dose is given.

Emerging Medications

Recent evidence has emerged that statins, a class of drugs originally indicated for hypercholesteremia, have immunomodulatory effects. Recent reports showed that statins prevent and reverse tissue damage in an animal model of MS (experimental autoimmune encephalomyelitis).[147] In addition, laboratory studies with human immune cells have shown immunomodulatory abilities of statins comparable to those of interferon beta. Clinically, a nonblinded clinical trial of a specific statin (simvastatin) in patients with MS revealed a significant decrease in the number and volume of new lesions detected by MRI and a favorable safety profile.[148]

Despite the initial positive clinical findings, many issues remain to determine the utility of statins in the treatment of MS. These include which of the available statins might be the best potential therapy for MS and whether the high doses used in recent studies are safe and effective over longer periods. Currently, there is no indication that the use of statins at the doses generally used for lowering cholesterol are of any value in the treatment of MS, and there are no data to suggest that individuals with MS who use statins to control cholesterol levels have experienced benefits. Larger, randomized, placebo-controlled trials are required to determine the safety and effectiveness of this class of medications for treatment of MS. Such trials are currently in process.

Monoclonal Antibodies

The monoclonal antibody natalizumab was recently approved by the United States FDA for reduction in the frequency of clinical relapses in relapsing forms of MS.[149,150] In the initial analyses of the ongoing trials, natalizumab reduced the relapse rate by up to 66% and reduced the development of new MRI-detected brain lesions. In addition, a greater proportion of patients receiving natalizumab remained relapse free compared with those receiving the control drug. However, because of adverse reactions in several patients receiving both natalizumab and interferon beta-1a, the manufacturer has voluntarily suspended its use pending further study.

Natalizumab is given every 4 weeks by infusion into a vein. It is designed to interfere with the movement of T cells across the blood-brain barrier and into the brain and spinal cord. The most common side effects included headache, fatigue, urinary tract infection, depression, lower respiratory tract infection, joint pain, and abdominal discomfort. Currently, no information on long-term safety is available. Additional research examining the effects of monoclonal antibodies (alemtuzumab, natalizumab) on MS is needed. The trials that demonstrated the initial positive results for natalizumab are still underway.

Symptomatic Treatment

Two of the most common complaints of patients with MS are the presence of abnormal fatigue (estimated to be present in nearly 90% of patients with MS) and motor signs such as spasticity (estimated to be present in more than 60% of patients with MS). Although treatments of spasticity are discussed elsewhere in this text, pharmacological treatment of fatigue warrants further discussion.[151-153]

Fatigue is one of the most common symptoms of MS and is often rated by patients with MS as the most disabling symptom.[153] Fatigue is especially bothersome in MS because it can potentiate other symptoms: it may reduce cognition, increase depression, or further limit physical abilities. Several drugs have been examined to determine their effect on what is thought to be CNS-mediated fatigue in patients with MS. Although no medications have been approved by the United States FDA for the treatment of MS-related fatigue, in an expert opinion paper from the United States National Multiple Sclerosis Society the off-label uses of four specific drugs (modafinil, amantadine, pemoline, and methylphenidate) are discussed.[153a]

Modafinil is a CNS α-adrenergic receptor agonist with wakefulness-promoting properties. Its FDA-approved use is for the treatment of excessive daytime sleepiness in persons with narcolepsy. Studies in patients with MS-related fatigue demonstrate reductions in fatigue severity scale scores and improvements in self-rated feelings of fatigue, quality of life, and overall satisfaction with treatment.[154] The typical prescription of modafinil is for 50 to 100 mg to be taken in the morning. The dose is then gradually increased to achieve optimal benefit with minimal side effects (which include appetite suppression, headache, insomnia, nervousness, and restlessness). The recommended daily dose is 400 mg.[154,155]

Amantadine is an antiviral agent whose primary use is as an antiparkinsonian drug. It has been used to treat MS-related fatigue for approximately 20 years.[153] More than 20% of mild to moderately disabled patients with MS experience significant reductions in fatigue while taking amantadine. The recommended dose of amantadine is 100 mg in the morning and 100 mg in the early afternoon.

Two specific CNS stimulants have been used to treat MS-related fatigue.[156-158] Pemoline is preferred to other stimulants because it appears to be less addictive; however, it is not recommended as a first-line therapy for MS-related fatigue because of its limited efficacy and the high risk of adverse effects (e.g., irritability, anxiety, hyperactivity, anorexia, and liver dysfunction). Although study results have been contradictory, pemoline may be an effective therapy for patients with MS that do not respond to amantadine or modafinil. Lastly, the stimulant methylphenidate has been used. Although methylphenidate's primary use is for the treatment of attention disorders in children, it appears to be effective and well tolerated with few side effects. The patient should be observed for overstimulation side effects such as anxiety and tachycardia, which are possible with methylphenidate.

ALZHEIMER'S DISEASE: PATHOLOGY AND EPIDEMIOLOGY

AD is a progressive, neurodegenerative disease characterized by protein abnormalities in the brain. The damage associated with AD begins in the entorhinal cortex, which is near the hippocampus and has direct connections to it. It then proceeds to the hippocampus, a structure deep in the brain that helps to encode memories, and then to other areas of the cerebral cortex that are used in thinking and making decisions.

The characteristic symptoms of AD include memory loss, language deterioration, impaired ability to mentally manipulate visual information, poor judgment, confusion, restlessness, and mood swings. Eventually AD destroys cognition, personality, and the ability to function. The early symptoms of AD, which include forgetfulness and loss of concentration, are often missed because they resemble natural signs of aging. AD is clinically characterized by a global decline of cognitive function that cannot be accounted for by acute delirium or depression. In comparison with other potential causes of decreased cognition, AD progresses slowly but consistently and leaves patients in the end stage of the disease bedridden, incontinent, and dependent on custodial care. Death occurs, on average, 9 years after diagnosis.

More than 12 million individuals worldwide have AD, and AD accounts for most cases of dementia that are diagnosed after the age of 60. AD is the most common cause of dementia among people age 65 and older, and it is estimated that up to 4 million people now have AD. For every 5-year age group beyond 65, the percentage of people with AD doubles. By 2050, 14 million older Americans are expected to have AD.[159-164]

An understanding of the neuronal pathophysiology associated with AD is critical to the understanding of current treatments, potential neuroprotective agents, and emerging lines of pharmacological management. A broad view of the etiology and pathology of AD is that AD arises from a series of genetic and/or environmental cellular stressors that increase with age. These stressors can include but may not be limited to inherited genetic mutations, free radical oxidative stress, reduced energy metabolism, excitotoxicity, and mitochondrial dysfunction. Regardless of the original causes, a cascade of biochemical abnormalities leads to cellular dysfunction, failure of neurotransmission, cell death, and a common clinical outcome. The defining neuropathological hallmarks of AD are extracellular plaques containing the β-amyloid peptide and intracellular neurofibrillary tangles containing abnormally phosphorylated tau protein grouped into filaments.[165,166]

Amyloid Plaques and Neurofibrillary Tangles

In AD, amyloid plaques accumulate in the critical parietal, temporal cortex, and hippocampus areas associated with memory and learning functions. In a manner similar to atherosclerotic plaques in arteries, amyloid deposits can develop into β-amyloid plaques that damage the cell walls of neurons.[167] These plaques trigger an inflammatory cascade, which ultimately results in loss of synapses, pruning of dendrites, decreased neurotransmitter release (especially acetylcholine), and cell death.

Healthy neurons have an internal support structure made up in part of microtubules. These microtubules act to guide molecules from the neuronal cell body to the axon terminals and back. A specific protein, tau, makes these microtubules stable. In AD, tau is chemically altered and begins to pair with other tau threads, and they become tangled up together. When this happens, the microtubules disintegrate, collapsing the neuron's transport system. This may result first in malfunctions in communication between neurons and later in the death of the cells.

Neuronal Cell Death and Neurotransmitter Depletion

Although it is not clear whether β-amyloid plaques and neurofibrillary tangles themselves cause AD or whether they are a by-product of the AD process, they appear critical in the process, given that the load and distribution of these protein abnormalities correlate with the severity and manifestation of AD.[168,169] The intracellular and extracellular abnormalities caused by β-amyloid plaques and neurofibrillary tangles are associated with loss of synaptic density and neuronal death. Degeneration of neurons dramatically reduces the production of the neurotransmitter acetylcholine. A loss of 60% to 90% of acetylcholine activity results in memory impairment. Other neurotransmitters depleted in AD include serotonin, somatostatin, and norepinephrine. Receptors for these neurotransmitters are also reduced.

Symptomatic treatment of AD focuses on manipulation of neurotransmission. The greatest success has been obtained by blocking the enzyme acetylcholinesterase.[170] More recently, one medication that targets an N-methyl-D-aspartate (NMDA) pathway has become available.

Treatment of Mild to Moderate Alzheimer's Disease

Cholinergic neurotransmission within the cerebrum plays an important role in cognition. In AD, the central cholinergic system, particularly in the hippocampus and entorhinal cortex, has reduced functional capacity, as well as loss of neurons. This has led to the hope that improving the remaining cholinergic neurotransmission would minimize symptoms of AD.[171] Acetylcholinesterase inhibitors (AChEIs) appear to do this through their inhibition of acetylcholinesterase, the major enzyme that degrades acetylcholine.

This class of drugs may help delay or prevent symptoms from becoming worse for a limited time and may help control some behavioral symptoms.[171] However, as AD progresses, the brain produces progressively less acetylcholine; therefore AChEIs may eventually lose their effect. The AChEI medications currently approved for use in the United States are tacrine, donepezil, rivastigmine, and galanthamine (Table 20-5).

In virtually all randomized placebo-controlled trials of AChEIs versus placebos, untreated patients showed significant decline in cognition and function. In contrast, treated patients tended not to show this response. This preservation of function is an important therapeutic outcome. Although all AChEIs would be considered "beneficial" for treatment of AD, at this time studies in which different AChEIs were directly compared showed no evidence of superiority of one agent over another with cognitive, behavioral, or functional outcomes.[172,173] In addition, it should be noted that although AChEIs appear to delay admission to nursing homes, they are not neuroprotective and offer little clinical improvement when the Mini-Mental Status Examination score drops below 12.[174]

Treatment of Moderate to Severe Alzheimer's Disease

One NMDA antagonist, memantine, is approved for the treatment of moderate to severe AD. The apparent mechanism of action of memantine involves

Table 20-5

Drugs Approved for Treatment of Alzheimer's Disease				
Drug Name (Trade Name)	Class of Medication	Common Side Effects	Possible Drug Interactions	Recommended Dosage
Tacrine* (Cognex)	Cholinesterase inhibitor	Liver damage nausea, indigestion, vomiting, diarrhea, skin rash	Drugs with anticholinergic action[†]	40-160 mg/day
Donepezil (Aricept)	Cholinesterase inhibitor	Headache, generalized pain, fatigue, dizziness, nausea, vomiting, diarrhea, insomnia, increased frequency of urination.	Drugs with anticholinergic action[†]	5-10 mg/day
Galantamine (Reminyl)	Cholinesterase inhibitor	Nausea, vomiting, diarrhea, weight loss	Drugs with anticholinergic action[†]	8-24 mg/day
Rivastigmine (Exelon)	Cholinesterase inhibitor	Nausea, vomiting, weight loss, upset stomach, muscle weakness	Drugs with anticholinergic action[†]	1.5-6 mg/day
Memantine (Namenda)	NMDA antagonist	Dizziness, headache, constipation, confusion	Other NMDA antagonists such as amantadine, dextromethorphan	5-20 mg

NMDA, N-methyl-D-aspartate.
*Tacrine has a higher incidence of gastrointestinal side effects than the other marketed agents. In addition, it produces significant liver toxicity in a small percentage of patients. For these reasons, tacrine is no longer actively marketed by the manufacturer.
[†]These drugs include: atropine, benztropine, trihexyphenidyl, paroxetine, amitriptyline, fluoxetine, fluvoxamine

regulation of glutamate concentrations, thereby reducing excitotoxic neuronal injury. Memantine appears to delay the progression of cognitive and physical functioning deficits associated with moderate to severe AD. Because NMDA antagonists work very differently from cholinesterase inhibitors, the two types of drugs can be prescribed in combination. Combining memantine with other AD drugs may be more effective than any single therapy, and in fact, one controlled clinical trial has demonstrated that patients receiving donepezil plus memantine perform better on cognitive and physical functioning measures than patients receiving donepezil alone. Recent studies of persons with moderate to severe AD have demonstrated functional improvement, slowing of the rate of cognitive decline, and a reduction in care dependence.[175-179]

Neuroprotective Strategies

Neuroprotection has been suggested as a means of preventing or slowing the progression of AD. Two specific classes of prescription drugs have been suggested as a means of neuroprotection for patients with AD. These are nonsteroidal antiinflammatory drugs (NSAIDs) and statins.

Nonsteroidal Antiinflammatory Drugs

Epidemiological research suggests that the inflammatory response is a significant component of the pathogenesis in AD.[180] In these studies, NSAIDs have been associated with risk reduction and slower progression but only if they are started in the preclinical phase and used for a minimum of 2 years. Prospective examination of efficacy of NSAIDs in AD has produced conflicting results.[181,182]

Statins

Several recent epidemiological studies have suggested a link between cardiovascular disease and AD. People with systolic high blood pressure, elevated low-density lipoprotein levels, or elevated apolipoprotein E levels in midlife have three times the risk of AD in later life.[183-186] Epidemiological studies have demonstrated that statin medications used to control hyperlipidemia are associated with a 60% lower incidence of AD. There is also mounting evidence that lowering serum cholesterol levels retards the onset of AD.[187] The hypothesized mechanism of action of the statin medications is the alteration of amyloid regulation. Research is cur-

rently underway to explore this potential treatment in greater detail.

Antiamyloid Strategies

Animal studies of antiamyloid treatments initially generated excitement when it was observed that long-term immunization of a mouse model of AD resulted in much less β-amyloid being deposited in the brains of the mice. Similar transgenic mice that had been immunized also performed better on memory tests than did a group of these mice that had not been immunized.[188-190]

These results led to preliminary studies in humans to test the safety and effectiveness of the vaccine. However, initial studies of the immune response in β-amyloid vaccine had to be stopped because of a high incidence of encephalitis in treatment subjects. Research examining this line of treatment continues.

Symptomatic Management

Because AD affects memory and mental abilities, it begins to change a person's emotions and behaviors. More than 70% of patients with AD eventually have one or more behavioral symptoms that contribute substantially to patient morbidity and caregiver distress. The common behavioral symptoms include sleeplessness, wandering and pacing, aggression, agitation, anger, depression, hallucinations, psychosis, and delusions. Some of these symptoms may become worse in the evening, a phenomenon called *sundowning,* or during daily routines, especially bathing. A variety of medication classes are used to treat behavioral symptoms. Antipsychotic, antiseizure, and selective serotonin reuptake inhibitor medications are used to treat psychosis and other psychiatric or behavioral symptoms in AD, although treatment guidelines are not well defined. Anecdotally, medications in these classes have been shown to reduce psychosis and behavioral symptoms in patients with AD, although the evidence is inconclusive for many medications. Side effects vary substantially across these medication classes. A full discussion of the pharmacological management of AD behavioral symptoms with noncholinergic medications is beyond the scope of this chapter, and readers should refer to recent reviews for more in-depth discussion of this topic.[191,192]

ACTIVITIES 20

■ 1. There are several symptoms associated with MS that have devastating effects on patients' quality of life. These symptoms include fatigue, bowel and bladder dysfunction, sexual dysfunction, weakness, visual problems, psychiatric issues, pain, spasticity, and tremor. Review the literature and discuss pharmacological and nonpharmacological methods for reducing these symptoms.

■ 2. Ms. C is a 65-year-old woman who has been referred to physical therapy for evaluation and treatment of her right knee. She reported that she was rushing to cross the street and tripped at the curb and fell. She was transported to University Hospital by ambulance and subsequently seen in the emergency department for an evaluation. X-ray films showed no fracture but did reveal moderate joint narrowing. Ms. C was sent home with an Ace wrap and instructed to ice and elevate the leg for the next 24 hours. She was also given aspirin to take every 4 to 6 hours for pain. One week later, she went to see her general practitioner for further evaluation. Her right knee continued to be swollen and painful and therefore she asked to see a physical therapist.

Medical history
Hypertension × 5 years

Social History
Married, two grown children, homemaker, no smoking or alcohol abuse

Meds
Hydrochlorothiazide, aspirin

Physical Therapy Exam
The patient presents with swelling in the right knee with limited range of motion (ROM) (30-80/20-85). The left knee is slightly limited (10-100/10-110). She is ambulating with a cane in her right hand. It was borrowed from a friend and is too long. In general, her gait is very slow with decreased movements in the lower limbs, hip, knee, and ankles bilaterally.

As you proceed with your evaluation, you notice resting tremors of the hands. When you ask the patient about this, she reports that they developed about 1 year ago but have gotten much worse since the fall. You complete the evaluation and call the physician to discuss the tremors.

The patient returns to the clinic 1 week later. She reported having a full neurological workup, which revealed early Parkinson's disease (PD). She began receiving selegiline. The patient continued with physical therapy for 2 more weeks on a program of electrical stimulation, active and passive range of motion, and gait training. ROM of the right knee improved and was equal in range to the left.

Questions

a. What symptoms of PD were displayed by this patient?
b. What are the goals of drug therapy in PD?
c. Given the diagnosis of PD, what other interventions might be helpful?
d. Is there any problem with the drug combination that she is currently receiving?

Two years later, Ms. C returns to your clinic with the chief complaint that her PD has worsened. She reports having some good days, but the majority are bad. She has difficulty performing her chores, continues to have resting tremors, and now shows rigidity of the right upper extremity and general difficulty in initiating movements. Further evaluation shows a shuffling gait with decreased trunk and arm movements.

Questions

e. What should be your goals for physical therapy?
f. Considering her current level of functioning with selegiline therapy, what drug therapy would you recommend at this time?
g. How are you going to schedule physical therapy treatment, given the possibility of drug-related fluctuations in function?

h. What information should you regularly send to the neurologist that would help in determining what combination of medicines Ms. C should be receiving as maintenance therapy?

■ 3. You periodically follow a patient for assessment of his Alzheimer's disease. What questions should you ask the patient and family that might assist you in determining the effectiveness of his drug therapy?

References

1. Shoenberg BS. Epidemiology of movement disorders. In: Marsden CD, Fahn S, eds. *Movement Disorders 2*. London, England: Butterworth, 1987:17-32.
2. Marsden CD. Parkinson's disease. *J Neurol Neurosurg Psychiatry*. 1994;57:672-681.
3. Hornykiewicz O. Historical aspects and frontiers of Parkinson's disease research. *Adv Exp Med Biol*. 1977; 90:1-20.
4. Hornykiewicz O. How L-DOPA was discovered as a drug for Parkinson's disease 40 years ago. *Wien Klin Wochenschr*. 2001;113(22):855-862.
5. Cotzias GC, Papavasiliou PS, Gellene R. Experimental treatment of parkinsonism with L-dopa. *Neurology*. 1968;18(3):276-277.
6. Cotzias GC. L-dopa for parkinsonism. *N Engl J Med*. 1968;278(11):630-631.
7. Cotzias GC, Papavasiliou PS, Gellene R. Modification of parkinsonism: chronic treatment with L-dopa. *N Engl J Med*. 1969;280(7):337-345.
8. Cotzias GC, Papavasiliou PS, Gellene R. L-dopa in Parkinson's syndrome. *N Engl J Med*. 1969;281(5):272.
9. Lang AE, Lozano AM. Parkinson's disease. First of two parts. *N Engl J Med*. 1998;339(15):1044-1053.
10. Lang AE, Lozano AM. Parkinson's disease. Second of two parts. *N Engl J Med*. 1998;339(16):1130-1143.
11. Metman LV, Konitsiotis S, Chase TN. Pathophysiology of motor response complications in Parkinson's disease: hypotheses on the why, where, and what. *Mov Disord*. 2000;15(1):3-8.
12. Ramaker C, Marinus J, Stiggelbout AM, Van Hilten BJ. Systematic evaluation of rating scales for impairment and disability in Parkinson's disease. *Mov Disord*. 2002;17(5):867-876.
13. Gordon AM, Reilmann R. Getting a grasp on research: does treatment taint testing of parkinsonian patients? *Brain*. 1999;122 (Pt 8):1597-1598.
14. Berardelli A, Rothwell JC, Thompson PD, Hallett M. Pathophysiology of bradykinesia in Parkinson's disease. *Brain*. 2001;124(Pt 11):2131-2146.
15. Berardelli A, Dick JP, Rothwell JC, Day BL, Marsden CD. Scaling of the size of the first agonist EMG burst during rapid wrist movements in patients with Parkinson's disease. *J Neurol Neurosurg Psychiatry*. 1986;49(11): 1273-1279.
16. Blin O, Ferrandez AM, Pailhous J, Serratrice G. Dopa-sensitive and dopa-resistant gait parameters in Parkinson's disease. *J Neurol Sci*. 1991;103(1):51-54.
17. Ferrandez AM, Blin O. A comparison between the effect of intentional modulations and the action of L-dopa on gait in Parkinson's disease. *Behav Brain Res*. 1991; 45(2):177-183.
18. O'Sullivan JD, Said CM, Dillon LC, Hoffman M, Hughes AJ. Gait analysis in patients with Parkinson's disease and motor fluctuations: influence of levodopa and comparison with other measures of motor function. *Mov Disord*. 1998;13(6):900-906.
19. Robertson LT, Hammerstad JP. Jaw movement dysfunction related to Parkinson's disease and partially modified by levodopa. *J Neurol Neurosurg Psychiatry*. 1996;60(1):41-50.
20. Shan DE, Lee SJ, Chao LY, Yeh SI. Gait analysis in advanced Parkinson's disease: effect of levodopa and tolcapone. *Can J Neurol Sci*. 2001;28(1):70-75.
21. Baroni A, Benvenuti F, Fantini L, Pantaleo T, Urbani F. Human ballistic arm abduction movements: effects of L-dopa treatment in Parkinson's disease. *Neurology*. 1984;34(7):868-876.
22. Burleigh-Jacobs A, Horak FB, Nutt JG, Obeso JA. Step initiation in Parkinson's disease: influence of levodopa and external sensory triggers. *Mov Disord*. 1997; 12(2):206-215.
23. Cioni M, Richards CL, Malouin F, Bedard PJ, Lemieux R. Characteristics of the electromyographic patterns of lower limb muscles during gait in patients with Parkinson's disease when OFF and ON L-Dopa treatment. *Ital J Neurol Sci*. 1997;18(4):195-208.
24. Corcos DM, Chen CM, Quinn NP, McAuley J, Rothwell JC. Strength in Parkinson's disease: relationship to rate of force generation and clinical status. *Ann Neurol*. 1996;39(1):79-88.
25. Forssberg H, Johnels B, Steg G. Is parkinsonian gait caused by a regression to an immature walking pattern? *Adv Neurol*. 1984;40:375-379.
26. Johnson MT, Mendez A, Kipnis AN, Silverstein P, Zwiebel F, Ebner TJ. Acute effects of levodopa on wrist movement in Parkinson's disease. Kinematics, volitional EMG modulation and reflex amplitude modulation. *Brain*. 1994;117 (Pt 6):1409-1422.
27. Johnson MT, Kipnis AN, Coltz JD, et al. Effects of levodopa and viscosity on the velocity and accuracy of visually guided tracking in Parkinson's disease. *Brain*. 1996;119 (Pt 3):801-813.
28. Morris M, Iansek R, Matyas T, Summers J. The pathogenesis of gait hypokinesia in Parkinson's disease. *Brain*. 1994;117:1169-1181.
29. Morris M, Iansek R, Matyas T, Summers J. Stride length regulation in Parkinson's disease. Normalization strategies and underlying mechanisms. *Brain*. 1996;119:551-568.
30. Morris M, Iansek R. Characteristics of motor disturbance in Parkinson's disease and strategies for movement rehabilitation. *J Human Mov Sci*. 1996;15(5):649-669.
31. Morris ME, Matyas TA, Iansek R, Summers JJ. Temporal stability of gait in Parkinson's disease. *Phys Ther*. 1996;76(7):763-777; discussion 778-780.

32. Murray M, Sepic S, Gardner G, Downs W. Walking patterns of men with parkinsonism. *Am J Phys Med.* 1978;57:278-294.

33. Robichaud JA, Pfann KD, Comella CL, Corcos DM. Effect of medication on EMG patterns in individuals with Parkinson's disease. *Mov Disord.* 2002;17(5):950-960.

34. Weinrich M, Koch K, Garcia F, Angel RW. Axial versus distal motor impairment in Parkinson's disease. *Neurology.* 1988;38(4):540-545.

35. Pastor MA, Jahanshahi M, Artieda J, Obeso JA. Performance of repetitive wrist movements in Parkinson's disease. *Brain.* 1992;115 (Pt 3):875-891.

36. Glendinning DS, Enoka RM. Motor unit behavior in Parkinson's disease. *Phys Ther.* 1994;74(1):61-70.

37. Kakinuma S, Nogaki H, Pramanik B, Morimatsu M. Muscle weakness in Parkinson's disease: isokinetic study of the lower limbs. *Eur Neurol.* 1998;39(4):218-222.

38. Nogaki H, Fukusako T, Sasabe F, Negoro K, Morimatsu M. Muscle strength in early Parkinson's disease. *Mov Disord.* 1995;10(2):225-226.

39. Nogaki H, Kakinuma S, Morimatsu M. Muscle weakness in Parkinson's disease: a follow-up study. *Parkinsonism Relat Disord.* 2001;8(1):57-62.

40. McAuley JH, Corcos DM, Rothwell JC, Quinn NP, Marsden CD. Levodopa reversible loss of the Piper frequency oscillation component in Parkinson's disease. *J Neurol Neurosurg Psychiatry.* 2001;70(4):471-476.

41. Pedersen SW, Oberg B. Dynamic strength in Parkinson's disease. Quantitative measurements following withdrawal of medication. *Eur Neurol.* 1993;33(2):97-102.

42. Deuschl G, Raethjen J, Baron R, Lindemann M, Wilms H, Krack P. The pathophysiology of parkinsonian tremor: a review. *J Neurol.* 2000;247(suppl 5):V33-V48.

43. Koller WC. Pharmacologic treatment of parkinsonian tremor. *Arch Neurol.* 1986;43(2):126-127.

44. Burleigh A, Horak F, Nutt J, Frank J. Levodopa reduces muscle tone and lower extremity tremor in Parkinson's disease. *Can J Neurol Sci.* 1995;22(4):280-285.

45. Dietz V. Neurophysiology of gait disorders: present and future applications. *Electroencephalogr Clin Neurophysiol.* 1997;103(3):333-355.

46. Rogers MW. Motor control problems in Parkinson's disease. *Contemporary Management of motor control problems: Proceedings of the II Step Conference.* Alexandria, Va: American Physical Therapy Association; 1991:195-208.

47. Horak FB, Frank J, Nutt J. Effects of dopamine on postural control in parkinsonian subjects: scaling, set, and tone. *J Neurophysiol.* 1996;75(6):2380-2396.

48. Frank JS, Horak FB, Nutt J. Centrally initiated postural adjustments in parkinsonian patients on and off levodopa. *J Neurophysiol.* 2000;84(5):2440-2448.

49. Johnson MT, Kipnis AN, Lee MC, Loewenson RB, Ebner TJ. Modulation of the stretch reflex during volitional sinusoidal tracking in Parkinson's disease. *Brain.* 1991; 114 (Pt 1B):443-460.

50. Benecke R, Rothwell JC, Dick JP, Day BL, Marsden CD. Simple and complex movements off and on treatment in patients with Parkinson's disease. *J Neurol Neurosurg Psychiatry.* 1987;50(3):296-303.

51. Fattapposta F, Pierelli F, Traversa G, et al. Preprogramming and control activity of bimanual self-paced motor task in Parkinson's disease. *Clin Neurophysiol.* 2000; 111(5):873-883.

52. Fattapposta F, Pierelli F, My F, et al. L-dopa effects on preprogramming and control activity in a skilled motor act in Parkinson's disease. *Clin Neurophysiol.* 2002; 113(2):243-253.

53. Ingvarsson P, Johnels B, Lund S, Steg G. Coordination of manual, postural, and locomotor movements during simple goal-directed motor tasks in parkinsonian off and on states. *Adv Neurol.* 1987;45:375-382.

54. Ingvarsson PE, Johnels B, Steg G, Olsson T. Objective assessment in Parkinson's disease: optoelectronic movement and force analysis in clinical routine and research. *Adv Neurol.* 1999;80:447-458.

55. Johnels B, Ingvarsson PE, Steg G, Olsson T. The Posturo-Locomotion-Manual Test. A simple method for the characterization of neurological movement disturbances. *Adv Neurol.* 2001;87:91-100.

56. Johnels B, Ingvarsson PE, Matousek M, Steg G, Heinonen EH. Optoelectronic movement analysis in Parkinson's disease: effect of selegiline on the disability in de novo parkinsonian patients—a pilot study. *Acta Neurol Scand Suppl.* 1991;136:40-43.

57. Rajput AH, Fenton ME, Birdi S, et al. Clinical-pathological study of levodopa complications. *Mov Disord.* 2002;17(2):289-296.

58. Bedard PJ, Blanchet PJ, Levesque D, et al. Pathophysiology of L-dopa-induced dyskinesias. *Mov Disord.* 1999;14(suppl 1):4-8.

59. Kostic V, Przedborski S, Flaster E, Sternic N. Early development of levodopa-induced dyskinesias and response fluctuations in young-onset Parkinson's disease. *Neurology.* 1991;41(2 (Pt 1):202-205.

60. Linazasoro G. Physiopathology of parkinsonism and dyskinesias: lessons from surgical observations [in Spanish]. *Neurologia.* 2001;16(1):17-29.

61. Nutt JG, Gancher ST. Parkinson's disease dyskinesias. *Neurology.* 1994;44(6):1187; author reply 1187-1188.

62. Obeso JA, Rodriguez-Oroz MC, Rodriguez M, DeLong MR, Olanow CW. Pathophysiology of levodopa-induced dyskinesias in Parkinson's disease: problems with the current model. *Ann Neurol.* 2000;47(4 suppl 1): S22-S32; discussion S32-S24.

63. Rascol O. L-dopa-induced peak-dose dyskinesias in patients with Parkinson's disease: a clinical pharmacologic approach. *Mov Disord.* 1999;14(suppl 1):19-32.

64. Chase TN, Mouradian MM, Engber TM. Motor response complications and the function of striatal efferent systems. *Neurology.* 1993;43(12 suppl 6):S23-S27.

65. Rascol O, Brooks DJ, Korczyn AD, De Deyn PP, Clarke CE, Lang AE. A five-year study of the incidence of dyskinesia in patients with early Parkinson's disease who were treated with ropinirole or levodopa. 056 Study Group. *N Engl J Med.* 2000; 342(20):1484-1491.

66. Reardon KA, Shiff M, Kempster PA. Evolution of motor fluctuations in Parkinson's disease: a longitudinal study over 6 years. *Mov Disord.* 1999;14(1):605-611.

67. Wenzelburger R, Zhang BR, Poepping M, et al. Dyskinesias and grip control in Parkinson's disease are normalized by chronic stimulation of the subthalamic nucleus. *Ann Neurol.* 2002;52(2):240-243.

68. Wenzelburger R, Zhang BR, Pohle S, et al. Force overflow and levodopa-induced dyskinesias in Parkinson's disease. *Brain.* 2002;125(Pt 4):871-879.

69. Nutt JG, Gancher ST, Woodward WR. Does an inhibitory action of levodopa contribute to motor fluctuations? *Neurology.* 1988;38(10):1553-1557.

70. Blanchet PJ, Calon F, Morissette M, et al. Regulation of dopamine receptors and motor behavior following pulsatile and continuous dopaminergic replacement strategies in the MPTP primate model. *Adv Neurol.* 2001;86:337-344.

71. Rascol O, Sabatini U, Brefel C, et al. Cortical motor overactivation in parkinsonian patients with L-dopa-induced peak-dose dyskinesia. *Brain.* 1998;121 (Pt 3): 527-533.

72. de Jong GJ, Meerwaldt JD, Schmitz PI. Factors that influence the occurrence of response variations in Parkinson's disease. *Ann Neurol.* 1987;22(1):4-7.

73. McColl CD, Reardon KA, Shiff M, Kempster PA. Motor response to levodopa and the evolution of motor fluctuations in the first decade of treatment of Parkinson's disease. *Mov Disord.* 2002;17(6):1227-1234.

74. Levodopa: management of Parkinson's disease. *Mov Disord.* 2002;17(suppl 4):S23-S37

75. Tintner R, Jankovic J. Treatment options for Parkinson's disease. *Curr Opin Neurol.* 2002;15(4):467-476.

76. Clarke CE. Dopamine agonist monotherapy in early Parkinson's disease. *Hosp Med.* 2003;64(1):8-11.

77. Gerlach M, Double K, Reichmann H, Riederer P. Arguments for the use of dopamine receptor agonists in clinical and preclinical Parkinson's disease. *J Neural Transm Suppl.* 2003(65):167-183.

78. Grimes DA, Lang AE. Treatment of early Parkinson's disease. *Can J Neurol Sci.* 1999;26(suppl 2):S39-S44.

79. Mendis T, Suchowersky O, Lang A, Gauthier S. Management of Parkinson's disease: a review of current and new therapies. *Can J Neurol Sci.* 1999;26(2):89-103.

80. Schreck J, Kelsberg G, Rich J. What is the best initial treatment of Parkinson's disease? *J Fam Pract.* 2003; 52(11):897-899.

81. Schwarz J. Rationale for dopamine agonist use as monotherapy in Parkinson's disease. *Curr Opin Neurol.* 2003;16(suppl 1):S27-S33.

82. Tintner R, Jankovic J. Dopamine agonists in Parkinson's disease. *Expert Opin Investig Drugs.* 2003;12(11):1803-1820.

83. Stocchi F, Vacca L, Onofrj M. Are there clinically significant differences between dopamine agonists? *Adv Neurol.* 2003;91:259-266.

84. Romrell J, Fernandez HH, Okun MS. Rationale for current therapies in Parkinson's disease. *Expert Opin Pharmacother.* 2003;4(10):1747-1761.

85. Gordin A, Kaakkola S, Teravainen H. Position of COMT inhibition in the treatment of Parkinson's disease. *Adv Neurol.* 2003;91:237-250.

86. Melamed E, Zoldan J, Galili-Mosberg R, Ziv I, Djaldetti R. Current management of motor fluctuations in patients with advanced Parkinson's disease treated chronically with levodopa. *J Neural Transm Suppl.* 1999;56:173-183.

87. Rinne JO, Ulmanen I, Lee MS. Catechol-O-methyl transferase (COMT) inhibitors in patients with Parkinson's disease: is COMT genotype a useful indicator of clinical efficacy? *Am J Pharmacogenomics.* 2003;3(1):11-15.

88. Tolosa E. Advances in the pharmacological management of Parkinson disease. *J Neural Transm Suppl.* 2003(64):65-78.

89. Wasielewski PG, Burns JM, Koller WC. Pharmacologic treatment of tremor. *Mov Disord.* 1998;13(suppl 3): 90-100.

90. Mandel S, Grunblatt E, Riederer P, Gerlach M, Levites Y, Youdim MB. Neuroprotective strategies in Parkinson's disease: an update on progress. *CNS Drugs.* 2003;17(10):729-762.

91. Stocchi F, Olanow CW. Neuroprotection in Parkinson's disease: clinical trials. *Ann Neurol.* 2003;53(suppl 3): S87-S97.

91a. Whone AL, Watts RL, Stoessl AJ, et al., REAL-PET Study Group. Slower progression of Parkinson's disease with ropinirole versus levodopa: the REAL-PET study. *Ann Neurol.* 2003;54:93–101.

91b. Parkinson Study Group. Dopamine transporter brain imaging to access the effects of promixpexole vs levodopa on Parkinson disease progression. *JAMA.* 2002;287:1653–1661.

92. Morris ME. Movement disorders in people with Parkinson disease: a model for physical therapy. *Phys Ther.* 2000;80(6):578-597.

93. Reuter I, Harder S, Engelhardt M, Baas H. The effect of exercise on pharmacokinetics and pharmacodynamics of levodopa. *Mov Disord.* 2000;15(5):862-868.

94. Goetz CG, Thelen JA, MacLeod CM, Carvey PM, Bartley EA, Stebbins GT. Blood levodopa levels and unified Parkinson's disease rating scale function: with and without exercise. *Neurology.* 1993;43(5): 1040-1042.

95. Mouradian MM, Juncos JL, Serrati C, Fabbrini G, Palmeri S, Chase TN. Exercise and the anti-parkinsonian response to levodopa. *Clin Neuropharmacol.* 1987; 10(4):351-355.

96. Carter JH, Nutt JG, Woodward WR. The effect of exercise on levodopa absorption. *Neurology.* 1992; 42(10):2042-2045.

97. Weinshenker B. The natural history of multiple sclerosis. *Neurol Clin.* 1995;13: 119-146.

98. Keegan B, Noseworthy J. Multiple sclerosis. *Annu Rev Med.* 2002;53: 285-302.

99. McDonald W, Compston A, Edan G, et al. Recommended diagnostic criteria for multiple sclerosis: guidelines from the International Panel on the Diagnosis of Multiple Sclerosis. *Ann Neurol.* 2001;50:121-127.

100. Poser C, Brinar V. Diagnostic criteria for multiple sclerosis. *Clin Neurol Neurosurg.* 2001;103:1-11.

101. Confavreux C, Aimard G, Devic M. Course and prognosis of multiple sclerosis assessed by the computerized data processing of 349 patients. *Brain.* 1980;103:281-300.

102. Weinshenker B, Bass B, Rice G, et al. The natural history of multiple sclerosis: a geographically based study. I. Clinical course and disability. *Brain.* 1989; 112:133-146.

103. Sweeney V, Sadovnick A, Brandejs V. Prevalence of multiple sclerosis in British Columbia. *Can J Neurol Sci.* 1986;13:47-51.

104. Thompson A, Polman C, Miller D, et al. Primary progressive multiple sclerosis. *Brain.* 1997;120:1085-1096.

105. Compston A, Coles A. Multiple sclerosis. *Lancet.* 2002; 359:1221-1231.

106. Skegg D. Multiple sclerosis: nature or nurture? *BMJ.* 1991;302:846-847.

107. Wingerchuk D, Weinshenker B. Multiple sclerosis: epidemiology, genetics, classification, natural history, and clinical outcome measures. *Neuroimaging Clin N Am.* 2000;10:611-624.

108. Compston A, Sawcer S. Genetic analysis of multiple sclerosis. *Curr Neurol Neurosci Rep.* 2002; 2:259-266.

109. Trapp BD, Peterson J, Ransohoff RM, Rudick R, Mork S, Bo L. Axonal transection in the lesions of multiple sclerosis. *N Engl J Med.* 1998;338:278-285.

110. Trapp B, Ransohoff R, Rudick R. Axonal pathology in multiple sclerosis: relationship to neurologic disability. *Curr Opin Neurol.* 1999; 12:295-302.

111. Trapp B, Ransohoff R, Fischer E, Rudick R. Neurodegeneration in multiple sclerosis: relationship to neurological disability. *Neuroscientist.* 1999; 5:48-57.

112. De Stefano N, Narayanan S, Francis G, et al. Evidence of axonal damage in the early stages of multiple sclerosis and its relevance to disability. *Arch Neurol.* 2001; 58: 65-70.

113. Kurtzke JF. Rating neurologic impairment in multiple sclerosis: an expanded disability status scale (EDSS). *Neurology.* 1982;33(11):1444-1452.

114. Hobart J, Freeman J, Thompson A. Kurtzke scales revisited. *Brain.* 2000;123(Pt 5):1027-1040.

115. O'Riordan J, Thompson A, Kingsley D, et al. The prognostic value of brain MRI in clinically isolated syndromes of the CNS. A 10-year follow-up. *Brain.* 1998; 121:495-503.

116. Brex P, Ciccarelli O, O'Riordan J, Sailer M, Thompson A, Miller D. A longitudinal study of abnormalities on MRI and disability from multiple sclerosis. *N Engl J Med.* 2002;346:158-164.

117. Rovaris M, Filippi M. Contrast enhancement and the acute lesion in multiple sclerosis. *Neuroimaging Clin N Am.* 2000;10: 705-715.

118. McFarland H, Frank J, Albert P, et al. Using gadolinium-enhanced magnetic resonance imaging lesions to monitor disease activity in multiple sclerosis. *Ann Neurol.* 1992;32: 758-766.

119. Miller D, Albert P, Barkhof F, et al. Guidelines for the use of magnetic resonance techniques in monitoring the treatment of multiple sclerosis. US National MS Society Task Force. *Ann Neurol.* 1996;39: 6-16.

120. Cook S, Dowling P. Multiple sclerosis and viruses: an overview. *Neurology.* 1980;30: 80-91.

121. Revel M, Chebath J, Mangelus M, Harroch S, Moviglia G. Antagonism of interferon beta on interferon gamma: inhibition of signal transduction in vitro and reduction of serum levels in multiple sclerosis patients. *Mult Scler.* 1995;1(suppl 1):S5-S11.

122. Hohlfeld R. Biotechnological agents for the immunotherapy of multiple sclerosis. Principles, problems and perspectives. *Brain.* 1997;120:865-916.

123. Durelli L, Verdun E, Barbero P, et al. Independent Comparison of Interferon (INCOMIN) Trial Study Group. Every-other-day interferon beta-1b versus once-weekly interferon beta-1a for multiple sclerosis: results of a 2-year prospective randomised multicentre study (INCOMIN). *Lancet.* 2002;359:1453-1460.

124. Durelli L, Verdun E, Barbero P, Bergui M, Versino E, Ghezzi A, Montanari E, Zaffaroni M; Independent Comparison of Interferon (INCOMIN) Trial Study Group. Every-other-day interferon beta-1b versus once-weekly interferon beta-1a for multiple sclerosis: results of a 2-year prospective randomised multicentre study (INCOMIN). *Lancet.* 2002 Apr 27;359(9316):1453-1460.

125. Benatar M. Interferon beta-1a and beta-1b for treatment of multiple sclerosis. *Lancet.* 2002;360:1428; author reply 1428-1429.

126. Panitch H, Goodin DS, Francis G, et al. Randomized, comparative study of interferon beta-1a treatment regimens in MS: the EVIDENCE Trial. *Neurology.* 2002; 59:1496-1506.

127. Clanet M, Radue EW, Kappos L, et al. A randomized, double-blind, dose-comparison study of weekly interferon beta-1a in relapsing MS. *Neurology.* 2002;59: 1507-1517.

128. Jacobs LD, Beck RW, Simon JH, et al. Intramuscular interferon beta-1a therapy initiated during a first demyelinating event in multiple sclerosis. CHAMPS Study Group. *N Engl J Med.* 2000;343:898-904.

129. Comi G, Filippi M, Barkhof F, et al. Effect of early interferon treatment on conversion to definite multiple sclerosis: a randomised study. *Lancet.* 2001;357:1576-1582.

130. Beck RW, Chandler DL, Cole SR, et al. Interferon beta-1a for early multiple sclerosis: CHAMPS trial subgroup analyses. *Ann Neurol.* 2002;51:481-490.

131. Barkhof F, Filippi M, Miller DH, et al. Comparison of MRI criteria at first presentation to predict conversion to clinically definite multiple sclerosis. *Brain.* 1997; 120:2059-2069.

132. Duda PW, Schmied MC, Cook SL, Krieger JI, Hafler D. Glatiramer acetate (Copaxone) induces degenerate, Th2-polarized immune responses in patients with multiple sclerosis. *J Clin Invest.* 2000;105: 967-976.

133. Chen M, Gran B, Costello K, Johnson K, Martin R, Dhib-Jalbut S. Glatiramer acetate induces a Th2-biased response and crossreactivity with myelin basic protein in patients with MS. *Mult Scler.* 2001; 7: 209-219.

134. Schori H, Kipnis J, Yoles E, et al. Vaccination for protection of retinal ganglion cells against death from glutamate cytotoxicity and ocular hypertension: implications for glaucoma. *Proc Natl Acad Sci.* 2001;98: 3398-3403.

135. Schwartz M. Physiological approaches to neuroprotection. Boosting of protective autoimmunity. *Surv Ophthalmol.* 2001; 45(suppl 3): S256-S260; discussion, S273-S276.

136. Bornstein M, Miller A, Slagle S, et al. A pilot trial of Cop 1 in exacerbating-remitting multiple sclerosis. *N Engl J Med.* 1987;317(7):408-414.

137. Johnson KP, Brooks BR, Cohen JA, et al. Copolymer 1 reduces relapse rate and improves disability in relapsing-remitting multiple sclerosis: results of a phase III multicenter, double-blind placebo-controlled trial. The Copolymer 1 Multiple Sclerosis Study Group. *Neurology.* 1995;45(7):1268-1276.

138. Johnson KP, Brooks BR, Cohen JA, et al. Extended use of glatiramer acetate (Copaxone) is well tolerated and maintains its clinical effect on multiple sclerosis relapse rate and degree of disability. Copolymer 1 Multiple Sclerosis Study Group. *Neurology.* 1998;50(3):701-708.

139. Johnson KP, Brooks BR, Cohen JA, et al. Sustained clinical benefits of glatiramer acetate in relapsing multiple sclerosis patients observed for 6 years. Copolymer 1 Multiple Sclerosis Study Group. *Mult Scler.* 2000;6(4):255-266.

140. Wolinsky JS, Narayana PA, Johnson KP. United States open-label glatiramer acetate extension trial for relapsing multiple sclerosis: MRI and clinical correlates. Multiple Sclerosis Study Group and the MRI Analysis Center. *Mult Scler.* 2001;7(1):33-41.

141. Comi G, Filippi M, Wolinsky JS. European/Canadian multicenter, double-blind, randomized, placebo-controlled study of the effects of glatiramer acetate on magnetic resonance imaging–measured disease activity and burden in patients with relapsing multiple sclerosis. European/Canadian Glatiramer Acetate Study Group. *Ann Neurol.* 2001;49(3):290-297.

142. Hartung HP, Gonsette R, Konig N, et al. Mitoxantrone in progressive multiple sclerosis: a placebo-controlled, double-blind, randomised, multicentre trial. *Lancet.* 2002;360:2018-2025.

143. Hartung HP, Gonsette R, Konig N, et al. Therapeutic effect of mitoxantrone combined with methylprednisolone in multiple sclerosis: a randomised multicentre study of active disease using MRI and clinical criteria. *J Neurol Neurosurg Psychiatry.* 1997; 62:112-118.

144. Hartung HP, Gonsette R, Konig N, et al. Randomized placebo-controlled trial of mitoxantrone in relapsing-remitting multiple sclerosis: 24-month clinical and MRI outcome. *J Neurol.* 1997;244:153-159.

145. Ghalie RG, Mauch E, Edan G, et al. A study of therapy-related acute leukaemia after mitoxantrone therapy for multiple sclerosis. *Mult Scler.* 2002;8: 441-445.

146. Ghalie RG, Edan G, Laurent M, et al. Cardiac adverse effects associated with mitoxantrone (Novantrone) therapy in patients with MS. *Neurology.* 2002;59: 909-913.

147. Youssef S, Stuve O, Patarroyo JC, et al., The HMG-CoA reductase inhibitor, atorvastatin, promotes a Th2 bias and reverses paralysis in central nervous system autoimmune disease. *Nature.* 2002;420(6911):78-84.

148. Vollmer T, Key L, Durkalski V, et al. Oral simvastatin treatment in relapsing-remitting multiple sclerosis. *Lancet.* 2004;363:1607-1608.

149. Kappos L, Kuhle J, Gass A, Achtnichts L, Radue CW. Alternatives to current disease-modifying treatment in MS: what do we need and what can we expect in the future? *J Neurol.* 2004;251(suppl 5):V57-V64.

150. Natalizumab (Tysabri) for relapsing multiple sclerosis. *Med Lett Drugs Ther.* 2005;47(1202):13-15.

151. Miller A, Bourdette D, Cohen JA, et al. Multiple sclerosis. *Continuum.* 1999;5:120-133.

152. Krupp LB, Rizvi SA. Symptomatic therapy for under-recognized manifestations of multiple sclerosis. *Neurology.* 2002;58 (suppl 4): S32-S39.

153. Krupp LB. Mechanisms, measurement, and management of fatigue in multiple sclerosis. In: Thompson AJ, Polman C, Hohfeld R, eds. *Multiple sclerosis: clinical challenges and controversies.* London: Martin Dunitz; 1997:283-294.

153a. Medical Advisory Board of the National Multiple Sclerosis Society. Expert opinion paper: treatment recommendations for physicians—Management of MS-related fatigue. New York: National Multiple Sclerosis Society, 2002. Available at: http://www.nationalmssociety.org/pdf/forpros/Expert_fatigue.pdf. Accessed June 14, 2005.

154. Zifko UA, Rupp M, Schwarz S, Zipko HT, Maida EM. Modafinil in treatment of fatigue in multiple sclerosis. Results of an open-label study. *J Neurol.* 2002;249: 983-987.

155. Rammohan KW, Rosenberg JH, Lynn DJ, et al. Efficacy and safety of modafinil (Provigil®) for the treatment of fatigue in multiple sclerosis: a two center phase 2 study. *J Neurol Neurosurg Psychiatry.* 2002;72:179-183.

156. Weinshenker BG, Penman M, Bass B, Ebers GC, Rice GPA. A double-blind, randomized, crossover trial of pemoline in fatigue associated with multiple sclerosis. *Neurology.* 1992;42:1468-1471.

157. Steinman L, Martin R, Bernard C, et al. Multiple sclerosis: deeper understanding of its pathogenesis reveals new targets for therapy. *Annu Rev Neurosci.* 2002;25:491-505.

158. Wiendl H, Kieseier BC. Disease modifying therapies in multiple sclerosis: an update on recent and ongoing trials and future strategies. *Exp Opin Invest Drugs.* 2003; 12:689-712.

159. Bachman DL, Wolf PA, Linn RT, et al. Incidence of dementia and probable Alzheimer disease in a general population: the Framingham Study. *Neurology.* 1993; 43:515-519.

160. Jorm AF, Jolley D. The incidence of dementia: a meta-analysis. *Neurology.* 1998;51:728-733.

161. Kawas C, Gray S, Brookmeyer R, et al. Age-specific incidence rates of Alzheimer disease: the Baltimore Longitudinal Study of Aging. *Neurology.* 2000;54: 2072-2077.

162. Brookmeyer R, Gray S, Kawas C. Projections of Alzheimer disease in the United States and the public health impact of delaying disease onset. *Am J Public Health.* 1998;88:1337-1342.

163. Ernst RL, Hay JW. Economic research on Alzheimer disease: a review of the literature. *Alzheimer Dis Assoc Disord.* 1997;11(suppl 6):135-145.

164. McKhann G, Drachman D, Folstein M, et al. Clinical diagnosis of Alzheimer disease: report of the NINCDS-ADRDA Work Group under the auspices of Department of Health and Human Services Task Force on Alzheimer Disease. *Neurology.* 1984;34:939-944.

165. Cotman CW, Anderson AJ. A potential role for apoptosis in neurodegeneration and Alzheimer's disease. *Mol Neurobiol.* 1995;10:19-45.

166. Mattson MP, Bruce AJ, Mark RJ. Amyloid cytotoxicity and Alzheimer's disease: roles of membrane oxidation and perturbed ion homeostasis. In: Brioni JD, ed. *Pharmacological treatment of Alzheimer's disease: molecular and neurobiological foundations.* New York: Wiley-Liss; 1997:239-285.

167. Selkoe DJ. The genetics and molecular pathology of Alzheimer's disease: roles of amyloid and the presenilins. *Neurol Clin.* 2000;18:903-922.

168. Arriagada PV, Growdon JH, Hedley-Whyte ET, et al. Neurofibrillary tangles but not senile plaques parallel duration and severity of Alzheimer's disease. *Neurology.* 1992;42:631-639.

169. Giannakopoulos P, Hof PR, Michel JP, et al. Cerebral cortex pathology in aging and Alzheimer's disease: a quantitative survey of large hospital-based geriatric and psychiatric cohorts. *Brain Res Brain Res Rev.* 1997; 25:217-245.

170. Francis PT, Palmer AM, Snape M, Wilcock GK. The cholinergic hypothesis of Alzheimer's disease: a review of progress. *J Neurol Neurosurg Psychiatry.* 1999;66: 137-147.

171. Mayeux R, Sano M. Treatment of Alzheimer's disease. *N Engl J Med.* 1999;341:1670-1679.

172. Mohs RC, Doody RS, Morris JC, et al. A 1-year, placebo-controlled preservation of function survival study of donepezil in AD patients. *Neurology.* 2001;57:481-488.

173. Winblad B, Engedal K, Soininen H, et al. A 1-year, randomized, placebo-controlled study of donepezil in patients with mild to moderate AD. *Neurology.* 2001; 57:489-495.

174. O'Brien JT, Ballard CG. Drugs for Alzheimer's disease. *BMJ.* 2001;323:123-124.

175. Winblad B, Poritis N. Memantine in severe dementia: results of the M-BEST study (benefit and efficacy in severely demented patients during treatment with memantine). *Int J Geriatr Psychiatry.* 1999;14:135-146.

176. Reisberg B, Doody R, Stöffler A, et al. Memantine in moderate-to-severe Alzheimer's disease. *N Engl J Med.* 2003;348:1333-1341.

177. Ferris SH, Schmitt FA, Doody RS, et al. Long-term treatment with the NMDA antagonist, memantine: results of a 24-week, open-label extension study in moderate to severe Alzheimer's disease [abstract]. *Neurology.* 2003;60(suppl 1):A414.

178. Farlow MR, Tariot PN, Grossberg GT, et al. Memantine/donepezil dual-therapy is superior to placebo/donepezil therapy for treatment of moderate to severe Alzheimer's disease [abstract]. *Neurology.* 2003; 60(suppl 1):A412.

179. Hartmann S, Möbius HJ. Tolerability of memantine in combination with cholinesterase inhibitors in dementia therapy. *Int Clin Psychopharmacol.* 2003;18:81-85.

180. McGeer PL, Schulzer M, McGeer EG. Arthritis and anti-inflammatory agents as possible protective factors for Alzheimer disease: a review of 17 epidemiologic studies. *Neurology.* 1996;47:425-432.

181. Pasinetti GM. From epidemiology to therapeutic trials with anti-inflammatory drugs in Alzheimer disease: the role of NSAIDs and cyclooxygenase in beta-amyloidosis and clinical dementia. *J Alzheimers Dis.* 2002;4:435-445.

182. Moore AH, O'Banion MK. Neuroinflammation and anti-inflammatory therapy for Alzheimer's disease. *Adv Drug Deliv Rev.* 2002;54:1627-1656.

183. Kivipelto M, Helkala EL, Laakso MP, et al. Midlife vascular risk factors and Alzheimer's disease in later life: longitudinal, population based study. *BMJ.* 2001; 322:1447-1451

184. Moroney JT, Tang MX, Berglund L, et al. Low-density lipoprotein cholesterol and the risk of dementia with stroke. *JAMA.* 1999;282:254-260.

185. Wolozin B, Kellman W, Ruosseau P, Celesia GG, Siegel G. Decreased prevalence of Alzheimer disease associated with 3-hydroxy-3-methyglutaryl coenzyme A reductase inhibitors. *Arch Neurol.* 2000;57:1439-1443;

186. Yaffe K, Barrett-Connor E, Lin F, Grady D. Serum lipoprotein levels, statin use, and cognitive function in older women. *Arch Neurol.* 2002;59:378-384.

187. Scott HD, Laake K. Statins for the prevention of Alzheimer's disease. *Cochrane Database Syst Rev.* 2001;(4):CD003160.

188. Schenk D, Barbour R, Dunn W, et al. Immunization with amyloid-beta attenuates Alzheimer-disease-like pathology in the PDAPP mouse. *Nature.* 1999;400:173-177

189. Younkin SG. Amyloid beta vaccination: reduced plaques and improved cognition. *Nat Med.* 2001;7:18-19.

190. Weiner HL, Lemere CA, Maron R, et al. Nasal administration of amyloid-beta peptide decreases cerebral amyloid burden in a mouse model of Alzheimer's disease. *Ann Neurol.* 2000;48:567-579.

191. Sultzer DL. Psychosis and antipsychotic medications in Alzheimer's disease: clinical management and research perspectives. *Dement Geriatr Cogn Disord.* 2004;17:78-90.

192. Kindermann SS, Dolder CR, Bailey A, Katz IR, Jeste DV. Pharmacological treatment of psychosis and agitation in elderly patients with dementia: four decades of experience. *Drugs Aging.* 2002;19:257-276.

Additional Resources

The following references are comprehensive resources with greater specificity than were able to be provided in this chapter.

Fillit HM, O'Connell AW. *Drug discovery and development for Alzheimer's disease.* New York: Springer; 2000.

Fillit HM, O'Connell AW, Refolo LM. Drug discovery in Alzheimer's disease. *J Mol Neurosci.* 2002;19:1-245.

Qizilbash N, Schneider LS. Practical recommendations and opinions on therapies for cognitive symptoms and prognosis modification. In: Qizilbash N, Schneider LS, Chui H, et al, eds. *Evidence-based dementia practice.* London: Blackwell; 2002:560-588.

Schneider LS, Tariot PN. Cognitive enhancers and treatments for Alzheimer's disease. In: Tasman A, Kay J, Lieberman JA, eds. *Psychiatry.* 2nd ed. London: John Wiley and Sons; 2003.

Zlokovic BV. Alzheimer's disease (AD) has been classified and treated as a neurodegenerative disorder. *Adv Drug Deliv Rev.* 2002;54:1533-1537.

Zlokovic BV. Vascular disorder in Alzheimer's disease: role in pathogenesis of dementia and therapeutic targets. *Adv Drug Deliv Rev.* 2002;54:1553-1559.

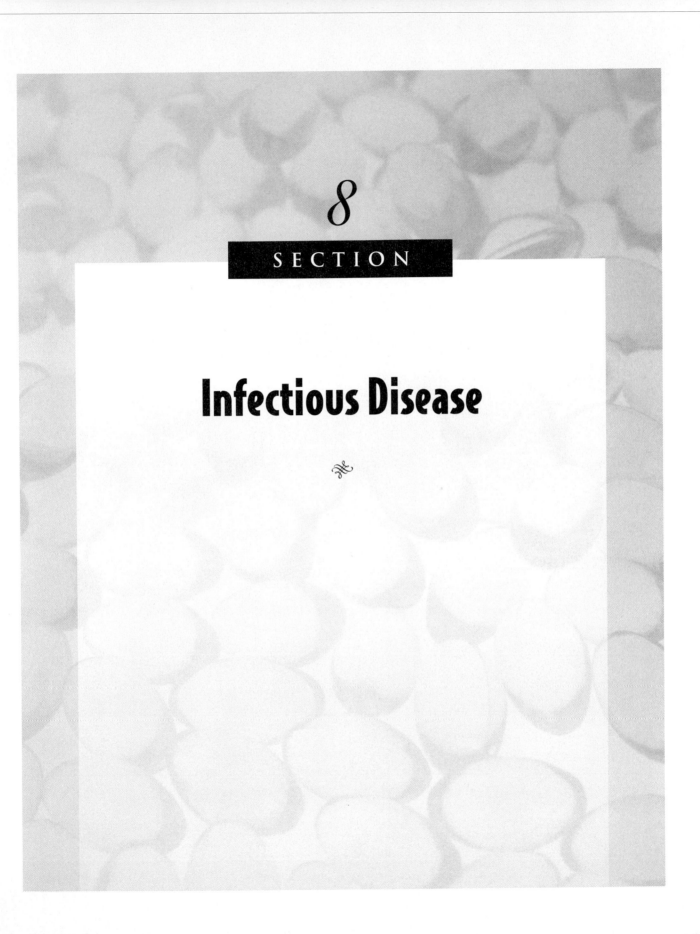

8

SECTION

Infectious Disease

CHAPTER 21

ANTIMICROBIAL AGENTS

CHARACTERISTICS AND CLASSIFICATION OF BACTERIA

Bacteria cause more infectious diseases than any other parasite, and bacterial infections cause substantial morbidity and mortality.[1] Therefore antibacterial drugs are among the most important groups of medicines that we possess, having substantially reduced or changed the course of many illnesses. In actuality, antibacterial agents belong to a larger group of drugs called *chemotherapeutic drugs,* defined as agents that have selective toxicity to invading parasites. In more recent times, the term *chemotherapy* has been used to refer to the treatment of cancer rather than infectious diseases, and antibacterial agents and antibiotics are substances that destroy or inhibit the growth and multiplication of microorganisms.

Although a detailed description of microbes is beyond the scope of this book, a brief review of bacteria and their classification is warranted. Bacteria are unicellular microorganisms that usually possess a rigid cell wall. They lack a true cell nucleus but do contain the basic subcellular organelles to make proteins. They rely on their host for metabolic substrates such as amino acids and glucose. Bacteria exert harmful effects through a variety of mechanisms. They may release toxic substances or compete with the host for essential nutrients. They may also invade organ systems and create an inflammatory or immune response and interfere with normal function.

Classifying Bacteria

Bacteria are classified according to their shape and histological staining.[2,3] Gram's stain assists in the classification of bacteria by differentiating the bacteria with thick cell walls (gram-positive) from those with alcohol-labile or acetone-labile outer membranes (gram-negative) based on their susceptibility to staining with a combination of dyes. Gram-positive organisms stain purple or black, and gram-negative organisms stain pink. See Table 21-1 for the classification of many bacterial organisms.

In general, most gram-positive organisms are cocci, and most gram-negative organisms are rods. See Table 21-2 for the most common microorganisms and the infections they produce.

Bacterial Cell Wall Structure

Not only does the bacterial cell wall assist in classifying the organism as gram-positive or gram-negative, it plays an integral role in determining which antimicrobial agents will be effective (i.e., those that can successfully penetrate it).[1] The bacterial cell wall is somewhat rigid owing to the presence of polysaccharide structures called *peptidoglycans* (Figure 21-1). Gram-positive organisms have many layers of peptidoglycan strands and are also polar, having a negative charge. This strongly polar and charged layer favors the penetration of positively charged compounds.

Table 21-1

Classifications of Bacterial Microorganisms

Type	Shape	Examples
Gram-positive cocci	Spherical	*Staphylococcus aureus, Streptococcus pneumoniae*
Gram-negative cocci	Spherical	*Neisseria gonorrhoeae, Neisseria meningitidis*
Gram-positive bacilli	Rod shaped	*Clostridium tetani, Listeria* spp., *Clostridium perfringens, Clostridium difficile*
Gram-negative bacilli	Rod shaped	*Escherichia coli, Klebsiella pneumoniae, Pseudomonas aeruginosa, Shigella* spp., *Salmonella* spp., *Legionella* spp. (legionnaires' disease)
Acid fast bacilli	Rod shaped; retain color of certain stains even when exposed to acid; appears pink or red	*Mycobacterium tuberculosis, Mycobacterium leprae* (leprosy)
Spirochetes	Corkscrew shaped organisms that are able to move without flagella	*Borrelia burgdorferi* (Lyme disease), *Treponema pallidum* (syphilis)
Mycoplasma	Spherical shaped organisms that lack a rigid cell wall	*Mycoplasma pneumoniae*
Rickettsiae	Intracellular bacterial parasites that appear like small gram-negative bacilli	*Rickettsia rickettsii* (Rocky Mountain spotted fever)
Actinomycetes	Gram-positive collection of microfilament rods	*Actinomyces israelii, Nocardia* spp.
Chlamydia	Atypical bacteria that stains similarly to *Mycobacterium tuberculosis*	—

Each peptidoglycan layer consists of multiple amino sugars that are cross-linked by short peptide side chains to form a latticework.[1] The cross-links are different for each type of bacteria. Synthesis of the peptidoglycan layer presents a challenge to the bacterium because it must use cytoplasmic materials to build a large insoluble wall that sits on the outside of the cell membrane. The bacterium constructs pieces of the hydrophilic wall intracellularly and then transports them via a large lipid carrier across the membrane. The synthesis, including the cross-linking, can be blocked at several stages by antibiotics. Specifically, the β-lactam antibiotics (penicillin) work by preventing the cross-linking peptides from binding to the amino sugar (Figure 21-2).

Within and directly below the peptidoglycan layer are the penicillin-binding proteins that offer a binding site for the drugs. However, also within the peptidoglycan strands are β-lactamases, which provide a barrier to drug entry into the bacterium. β-Lactamases are produced by the bacterium and behave like enzymes to inactivate the antimicrobial agent.

The gram-negative organisms have an outer membrane containing lipopolysaccharide structures and also an inner cytoplasmic membrane.[1] The space between the two membranes is the periplasmic space, and it contains β-lactamases. The presence of these two membranes offers quite a bit of resistance to drug entry. In fact, many drugs can only enter the bacterium through specialized aqueous pores existing in the cell wall. Thus, in general, it is more difficult to kill a gram-negative organism than a gram-positive organism.[4]

PROPERTIES OF ANTIBIOTICS

Properties of antibiotics, such as whether a drug is bacteriocidal or bacteriostatic and its antimicrobial spectrum of activity, help guide the physician in choosing the appropriate drug with which to treat an infection.

Table 21-2

Common Microorganisms Causing Infections

Body Site	Microorganisms	Gram's Stain	Body Site	Microorganisms	Gram's Stain
Eyes	*Neisseria gonorrhoeae*	–	Ears	*Haemophilus influenzae*	–
	Chlamydia trachomatis			*Streptococcus pneumoniae*	+
	Staphylococcus aureus	+		*Moraxella catarrhalis*	–
	Haemophilus spp.	–		*Streptococcus pyogenes*	+
	Streptococcus pneumoniae	+	Larynx-	Respiratory viruses	
	Pseudomonas aeruginosa	–	trachea	*Streptococcus pneumoniae*	+
	Fungi			*Moraxella catarrhalis*	–
	Herpes		Lungs	*Streptococcus pneumoniae*	+
	Adenoviruses			*Haemophilus influenzae*	–
Oral cavity	Herpes			*Staphylococcus aureus*	+
	Candida			*Mycoplasma pneumoniae*	
	Actinomyces	+		*Legionella* spp	
	Anaerobic cocci	+		*Chlamydia psittaci*	
	Fusobacterium spp.	–		*Mycobacterium tuberculosis*	
Throat	*Streptococcus pyogenes*	+		Enterobacteriaceae*	–
	Corynebacterium diphtheriae	+	Bone	*Staphylococcus aureus*	+
	Arcanobacterium	+	(osteomyelitis)	*Salmonella* spp.	–
	haemolyticum			*Haemophilus influenzae*	–
	Neisseria gonorrhoeae	–		*Pseudomonas aeruginosa*	–
	Pseudomonas spp.	–		*Escherichia coli*	–
	Staphylococcus aureus	+	Urinary tract	*Staphylococcus saprophyticus*	+
Lung	Anaerobic bacteria			Enterobacteriaceae	–
(abscesses)	*Staphylococcus aureus*	+		Enterococci	+
	Mycobacterium tuberculosis			*Pseudomonas aeruginosa*	–
	Fungi		Peritoneum	Enterobacteriaceae	
Heart	Viridans group streptococci	+	(peritonitis)	*Bacteroides* spp.	
	Staphylococcus aureus	+		Anaerobic streptococci	+
	Enterococci	+		Enterococci	+
	Streptococcus agalactiae	+		*Clostridium* spp.	+
Meninges	*Escherichia coli*	–	Skin	*Staphylococcus aureus*	+
	Streptococcus pneumoniae	+		Herpes simplex	
	Haemophilus influenzae	–		*Clostridium perfringens*	+
	Neisseria meningitidis	–		*Pseudomonas* spp.	–
	Listeria monocytogenes	+		*Bacteroides* spp.	–
Brain	Anaerobic bacteria	–/+		Enterobacteriaceae*	–
(abscesses)	*Nocardia*	+		Fungi	
	Staphylococcus aureus	+	Bloodstream	*Staphylococcus aureus*	+
	Streptococci	+	(septicemia)	*Streptococcus pyogenes*	+
Sinuses	*Haemophilus influenzae*	–		Enterobacteriaceae*	–
	Moraxella catarrhalis	–		*Pseudomonas aeruginosa*	–
	Streptococcus pneumoniae	+		*Staphylococcus epidermidis*	+
	Streptococcus pyogenes	+		*Candida albicans*	
	Anaerobic streptococci	+		*Haemophilus influenzae*	–
	Rhinoviruses			*Streptococcus pneumoniae*	+
	Coronaviruses			*Neisseria meningitidis*	–

From Brody MJ, Larner J, Minneman KP, eds. *Human Pharmacology: Molecular to Clinical.* 3rd ed. Philadelphia: Mosby; 1998.
+, Positive; –, negative.
E. coli, Klebsiella, Enterobacter, Serratia species

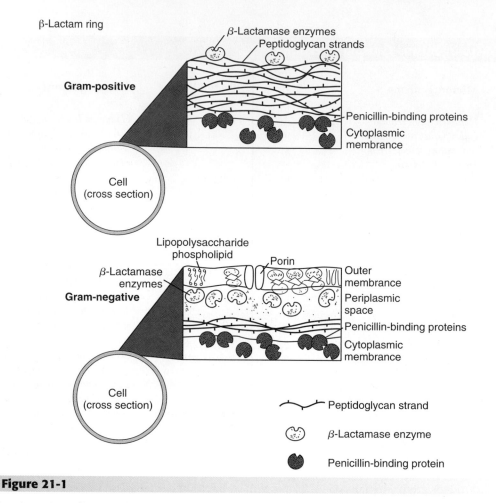

β-Lactam ring

β-Lactamase enzymes
Peptidoglycan strands

Gram-positive

Penicillin-binding proteins
Cytoplasmic membrane

Cell
(cross section)

Lipopolysaccharide
phospholipid

β-Lactamase enzymes

Porin

Gram-negative

Outer membrane
Periplasmic space
Penicillin-binding proteins
Cytoplasmic membrane

Cell
(cross section)

Peptidoglycan strand

β-Lactamase enzyme

Penicillin-binding protein

Figure 21-1

Outer coating of gram-positive (20 to 30 strands) and gram-negative bacteria showing a thinner (three to five strands) rigid peptidoglycan structure but an added outer membrane for gram-negative cells. β-Lactam drugs act by inhibiting the synthesis of the rigid peptidoglycan part of the cell wall. (from Brody MJ, Larner J, Minneman KP, eds. *Human Pharmacology: Molecular to Clinical.* 3rd ed. Philadelphia: Mosby; 1998.)

Selective Toxicity

Antibiotics possess selective toxicity because they have influence over the function of bacteria but little effect on the host. Scientists have exploited the differences between bacteria and human cells to design drugs to attack targets that exist solely within the bacteria. For example, some of the drugs inhibit production of the cell wall as mentioned previously. These drugs will have little effect on the host because human cells do not contain the same rigid walls. Some other drugs target the bacterial ribosome, but this organelle is sufficiently different from human ribosomes. This selective toxicity enables antibiotics to have a high therapeutic index.

Bactericidal or Bacteriostatic

Antibiotics can be classified as either bacteriostatic or bacteriocidal.[5] Bacteriostatic drugs inhibit bacterial growth but do not actually kill the organisms (Figure 21-3). They depend on the body's immune system for that action. Bactericidal drugs will attain a high enough concentration in the body to kill the organisms. Which type of drug is used depends on the bacteria and certain host factors.

A bacteriostatic drug may be adequate to eradicate a simple infection in a healthy host but fail in a patient with a compromised immune system.[6] Tetracyclines are bacteriostatic agents that inhibit growth of pneumococci; the actual destruction of

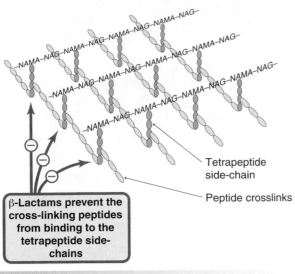

β-Lactams prevent the cross-linking peptides from binding to the tetrapeptide side-chains

Tetrapeptide side-chain

Peptide crosslinks

Figure 21-2

Schematic diagram of a single layer of peptidoglycan from a bacterial cell (e.g., *Staphylococcus aureus*) showing the site of action of the β-lactam antibiotics. In *S. aureus* the peptide cross-links consist of five glycine residues. Gram-positive bacteria have several layers of peptidoglycan. *NAMA*, N-acetylmuramic acid; *NAG*, N-acetylglucosamine. (From Rang HP, Dale MM, Ritter JM, Moore JL. *Pharmacology*. 5th ed. New York: Churchill Livingstone; 2003.)

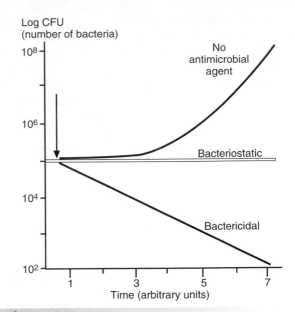

Figure 21-3

Bactericidal versus bacteriostatic antimicrobial agents. A typical culture is started at 10^5 colony-forming units *(CFU)* and incubated at 37°C for various times (time in arbitrary units). In the absence of an antimicrobial agent, cell growth occurs. With a bacteriostatic agent added, no growth occurs, but the existing cells are not killed. If the added agent is bactericidal, 99.9% of the cells are killed during the standardized time. (From Brody MJ, Larner J, Minneman KP, eds. *Human Pharmacology: Molecular to Clinical*. 3rd ed. Philadelphia: Mosby; 1998.)

the bacteria requires action of macrophages and neutrophils, which is unachievable in a patient with a low neutrophil count. The site of infection also influences the choice of bactericidal versus bacteriostatic agent. Certain sites are considered relatively protected from the host's immune responses. Bacteriostatic agents are associated with a high failure rate when used to treat infections in the cerebrospinal fluid, endocarditic vegetations, or another site that is difficult for the drug or immune system to access.

Bactericidal drugs are less dependent on the body's natural defenses, but they are effective in either a concentration-dependent or time-dependent manner.[7] Time-dependent killing depends on the drug concentration being maintained above a certain level for the majority of the dosing interval, whereas concentration-dependent killing depends on achieving a specific high concentration. Concentration-dependent drugs also exhibit a postantibiotic effect. This refers to a period in which growth of the bacteria ceases even after the antibiotic is withdrawn. The duration of the post-antibiotic effect is directly proportional to the

concentration of drug entering the bacteria. This phenomenon allows flexible dosing and longer dosing intervals than those used with most other drugs. It also allows pulse dosing, which is the administration of a large concentration (much greater than needed to kill bacteria) at dosing intervals longer than the drug's half-life. This is different from what is done with most other drugs, particularly antiseizure medications, which are often given every half-life. Antibiotics may be given every 12 half-lives with no reduction in efficacy. The main reasons for this are the host's ability to tolerate high levels of antibiotics without significant toxic effects (i.e., a high therapeutic index) and the concentration-dependent killing.

Antimicrobial Spectrum of Activity

Antibiotics that have activity against many different bacteria are called *broad-spectrum agents*. Those with activity against only a few organisms are called *narrow-spectrum*. In practice, broad-spectrum drugs are usually prescribed first, followed by a narrow-spectrum drug after the identity of the infecting organism is known. The initial drug choice is empiric and depends on the symptoms and location of infection. The exact identity, or a bacteria's susceptibility to a drug, is usually not known until 18 to 24 hours after an initial culture has been done.

One way to determine bacterial susceptibility to a drug is the disk diffusion method (Figure 21-4).[5] Paper disks impregnated with different antimicrobial agents are incubated in an Agar plate along with unknown bacteria obtained from a patient. The amount of drug placed on the disk is that which will provide a bacteria-free zone around the drug if the organism is susceptible. A bacteria-free zone of 14 mm or more implies that the organism is susceptible to the drug, whereas a zone of 11 mm or less implies some resistance.

DRUG-RESISTANT BACTERIA

Almost since the very beginning of antibiotic development, drug-resistant organisms have been emerging. To scientists who study evolution, this is no accident. Organisms frequently make biochemical or genetic changes to adapt to their environment.[1] Bacteria can multiply in as little as 20 minutes. Given this rapid rate of reproduction, it is conceivable that in a few hours there might be several generations of bacteria, and many may have undergone genetic mutations, making them less resistant to drugs. Repeated courses of antibiotics kill off the susceptible organisms but leave the more resistant strains.

Resistance to antibiotics can be either innate or acquired.[1] Some bacteria lack the transport mechanism that allows the antibiotic to enter the cell, making the drug useless in fighting infection. This is an example of innate resistance. Acquired resistance occurs when gene mutations, either single or multiple, prevent the drug from entering the cell. The probability of a spontaneous mutation is 1 per 10^6 to 10^8, which is low, but many more cells are present in an infection so that the probability of a mutation is actually higher.

Another form of acquired resistance involves extrachromosomal genetic material that exists in the cytoplasm called *plasmids,* and plasmids containing genes for resistance are referred to as *R plasmids.*[8] These R plasmids can exchange genetic information

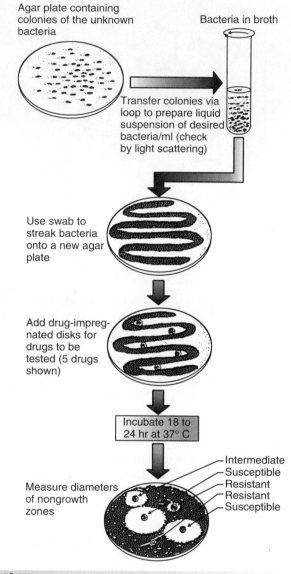

Figure 21-4

Disk diffusion method for testing bacteria for susceptibility to specific antimicrobial agents. (Redrawn from Brody MJ, Larner J, Minneman KP, eds. *Human Pharmacology: Molecular to Clinical.* 3rd ed. Philadelphia: Mosby; 1998.)

with DNA segments, and subsequently, these can be transferred to another bacterial cell.

The results of the previously mentioned genetic mutations produce several biochemical and physical alterations in bacteria that ultimately reduce the efficacy of antimicrobial agents. A significant example of resistance produced by genetic mutation is inactivation of the β-lactam antibiotics by the production of destructive enzymes.[9] These β-lactamases cleave the β-lactam ring of penicillins and cephalosporins. Staphylococci are the chief bacteria that produce β-lactamase through genes coding on plasmids. Synthesis of these enzymes is inducible, meaning that it occurs only in the presence of a drug. Once produced, the enzymes can pass through the bacterial wall to inactivate antibiotic molecules in the surrounding medium. Scientists have developed some drugs to inactivate these β-lactamases, and in part, some of the problem has been solved by the development of semisynthetic penicillins (methicillin) and new β-lactam antibiotics (monobactams and carbapenems).

Gram-negative organisms also produce β-lactamases via chromosomal genes or plasmid genes. The enzymes, however, are not free to enter the substrate; they remain fixed within the cell wall but still represent a formidable challenge to drugs by blocking access to the binding site. Another challenge is that production of these enzymes does not depend on the presence of drug.

Another form of resistance occurs when the genetic mutation alters the drug-binding site. Obviously, if the drug cannot bind to its receptor, it will be unable to carry out the purpose for which it was intended. Gaining access to the binding site is critical for its function. Another mutation can actually produce a membrane transporter that actively pumps the antibiotic out of the cell.[4] This phenomenon has been seen in both gram-negative and gram-positive organisms.[10]

The main cause of antimicrobial resistance is overuse or inappropriate use of antibiotics.[11] Bacteria face an onslaught of antibacterial agents so that the genetic mutations that have developed can be viewed as the organisms' acquired survival mechanism. The attacks from these drugs do not occur only in response to an illness or prophylactic treatment before surgery but are ubiquitous across the food chain and in the general environment. Antibiotics are commonly given to animals both as growth enhancers and treatment for infection. Molecules are then passed down to offspring, appear in feed, and end up on dinner tables. In addition, efforts to sterilize the environment by destroying bacteria indiscriminately with antibacterial soaps and cleaners are adding to the problem.

Control of antimicrobial resistance can be achieved but not without money, research, and cooperation from those who care for the ill. The number one way to reduce resistance is to decrease antibiotic consumption. Accurate and rapid diagnostic equipment is needed to identify a bacterial organism so that treatment can begin with the appropriate drug.[12] As mentioned earlier, treatment is usually begun with a broad-spectrum agent until the bacteria are identified, followed by switching the patient to a narrow-spectrum agent. It would be more effective to start treatment with a narrow but appropriate agent. Major efforts need to be directed toward surveillance of resistant bacterial, especially bacteria affecting the respiratory tract, because about 80% of antibiotic use in the community is related to respiratory tract infections.[13] Being able to differentiate a viral infection from a bacterial infection is also paramount. The second major way to reduce infection is through hygienic measures. This is particularly important for hospitals because bacteria can be transferred from one patient to another by health care workers. Each hospital needs an active infection control team to closely monitor hygiene practices and cleanup and sterilizing procedures, as well as the typical and atypical pathogens found in the facility.

FACTORS TO CONSIDER IN THE CHOICE OF AN ANTIMICROBIAL AGENT

One of the major factors to consider in the choice of an antimicrobial agent is the identity of the bacteria causing the infection. Often, the offending agent is not known, but a knowledgeable physician may be able to make an educated guess. For example, a urinary tract infection in a sexually active woman may be due to *Escherichia coli*. Cellulitis is often caused by *Streptococcus pyogenes* or *Staphylococcus aureus*.

Several host factors also influence antibiotic choice (Table 21-3).[7] Allergies to certain drugs dictate that these medications be avoided. Hepatic and renal function also need to be considered. Antibiotics are cleared by either the liver or the kidneys, and loss of function in either of these organs means that higher serum levels will be observed. Another factor is the age of the patient. Although most antibiotics are safe, some are contraindicated for infants and children and also for pregnant women. Site of infection represents another important host factor. Brain infections are difficult to treat because only a

Table 21-3

Bacterial, Host, and Drug Factors That Must Be Considered in Selection of Antibiotic Therapy		
Bug Factors	**Host Factors**	**Drug Factors**
Identity of pathogens*	Site of infection	Activity against pathogen(s)*
Susceptibility of pathogens*	Allergies	Ability to get to site of infection
	Renal function	Potential for drug interactions
	Hepatic function	Available routs of administration
	Neutropenia	Dosing frequency (for outpatients)
	Digestive tract function	Taste (for liquid formulations)
	Other underlying diseases	Stability at different temperatures (for liquid formulations)
	Concomitant medication	Cost
	Pregnancy	
	Desired route of administration	

From Page C, Curtis MJ, Sutter MC, Walker MJ, Hoffman BB, eds. *Integrated Pharmacology.* 2nd ed. Philadelphia: Mosby; 2002.
*Often not known at the start of therapy.

few antibiotics are able to enter the central nervous system in the required concentrations. Penicillins and cephalosporins only cross into the brain when the meninges are inflamed. This problem also exists for the prostate gland, and infection in the prostate gland tends to require weeks to months of therapy. Kidney infections must be treated with antibiotics that remain in the active form so that they are effective as they travel through the kidneys into the bladder and urethra.

MAJOR ANTIMICROBIAL AGENTS

Antibiotics may be classified in a variety of ways. Some are classified according to their chemical structure, bacterial spectrum, or pharmacokinetic properties. However, most are classified according to the most common mechanisms of actions

Bacterial Cell Wall Inhibitors

The class of drugs known as the bacterial cell wall inhibitors is made up of the β-lactams (penicillins, cephalosporins, carbapenems, and monobactams) and glycopeptides. The β-lactam antibiotics have a four-member nitrogen-containing β-lactam ring (Figure 21-5). They bind to the penicillin-binding proteins and inhibit the linking of the peptide chains to the bacterial cell wall. These drugs are bactericidal and kill in a time-dependent manner.

Penicillins
Penicillins consist of the β-lactam ring attached to a five-member thiazolidine ring.[14] Alterations of the side chains result in different antibacterial properties and thus different drugs. There are four types of penicillin drugs: naturally occurring penicillin G and V, antistaphylococcal penicillins, aminopenicillins, and antipseudomonal penicillins (Table 21-4).

Penicillin G is given parenterally, and penicillin V is given orally. Penicillin G will enter the cerebrospinal fluid when given in high doses to treat neurosyphilis and meningitis. However, these two drugs have a narrow spectrum and are active only against a few gram-positive and gram-negative cocci. They are useful for some streptococcal and meningococcal infections and syphilis, but resistance is growing, particularly for *Streptococcus pneumoniae*. In fact, shortly after the introduction of penicillin, many strains of staphylococci became resistant, primarily through the bacteria's production of β-lactamase. Resistance is also due to modification of target penicillin-binding proteins.

Antistaphylococcal Penicillins
Antistaphylococcal penicillins specifically target the staphylococcal β-lactamase. Methicillin was the first antistaphylococcal drug developed; however, it is seldom used today because of a high incidence of allergic interstitial nephritis and the development of resistance. This particular resistance represents such

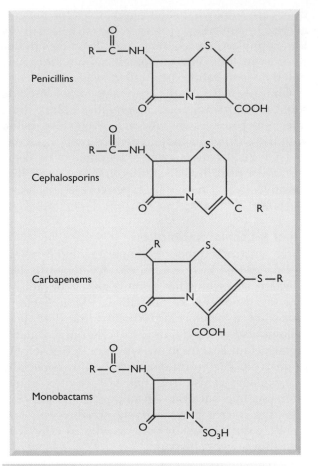

Figure 21-5

Basic chemical structures of the four main classes of β-lactam antibiotics. *R* denotes sites where chemical substitutions are made to create individual drugs. (From Page C, Curtis MJ, Sutter MC, Walker MJ, Hoffman BB, eds. *Integrated Pharmacology.* 2nd ed. Philadelphia: Mosby; 2002.)

a serious problem for infectious disease specialists that it is known as methicillin-resistant *Staphylococcal aureus* (MRSA) (see discussion of MRSA).

Aminopenicillins

Aminopenicillins are made by addition of an amino group to the penicillin side chain. This enhances the activity of these drugs against gram-negative bacilli while still maintaining activity for the cocci such as the other penicillins. Specifically, the aminopenicillins show activity against *E. coli, Proteus mirabilis,* and some strains of *Salmonella* and *Shigella.* The two most common aminopenicillins are ampicillin and amoxicillin. These drugs are also prescribed for respiratory tract infections because of their action

Table 21-4

Classification of Penicillins	
Classification	**Examples**
Standard penicillins	Penicillin G
	Penicillin V
Antistaphylococcal	Methicillin
	Nafcillin
	Oxacillin
	Cloxacillin
	Dicloxacillin
Aminopenicillins	Ampicillin
	Amoxicillin
Antipseudomonal	Carbenicillin
	Ticarcillin
	Piperacillin
	Mezlocillin

against *Streptococcus pneumoniae* and *Haemophilus influenzae.*

Antipseudomonal Penicillins

Antipseudomonal penicillins have actions similar to those of the aminopenicillins but with extended activity against more gram-negative bacilli including pseudomonads. A few have activity against anaerobic bacteria. However, none of the aminopenicillins or the antipseudomonal drugs has stable activity against staphylococcal β-lactamase.

β-Lactamase Inhibitors

Some drugs have been developed that lack antimicrobial activity but are strong inhibitors of β-lactamases.[15] These include clavulanate, sulbactam, and tazobactam. They are administered in combination with some antibiotic drugs; for example, clavulanate plus amoxicillin is called *augmentin.*[16,17] However, despite these advances, several strains of streptococci and staphylococci, including MRSA, remain resistant to the penicillins.

Clinical Uses for Penicillins

Penicillins are the first-choice drugs for many infections. In general, they are active against many gram-positive and gram-negative cocci and some gram-negative bacilli. Penicillins are commonly used to treat bacterial meningitis caused by *Neisseria meningitidis* and *Streptococcus pneumoniae;* skin and soft tissue infections caused by *Streptococcus pyogenes* or *Staphylococcus aureus;* urinary tract infections caused by *E. coli;* and otitis media caused by *Streptococcus pyogenes* or *H. influenzae;* they are also used for the treatment of gonorrhea and syphilis. It is important to realize that this list is far from complete.

Adverse Drug Reactions Associated with Penicillins

The side effects of penicillins are relatively minor for most individuals compared with those of other drugs. They include gastrointestinal (GI) discomfort and symptoms related to allergy, urticaria, joint swelling, and respiratory problems. However, if a patient is allergic to one of the penicillins, he or she is allergic to all of them because they are all cross-sensitizing. Penicillins also have cross-sensitivity with the cephalosporins for anaphylaxis.

Cephalosporins

Cephalosporins are similar in structure to the penicillins except they have a six-member ring attached to the β-lactam ring (Figure 21-5).[7] They are also classified as first-, second-, and third-generation drugs according to their activity. The first-generation drugs are active against gram-positive cocci and some gram-negative bacilli. Specifically, they fight streptococci, staphylococci, *E. coli, P. mirabilis,* and *Klebsiella pneumoniae.* They also perform well against skin and soft tissue infections caused by *Streptococcus pyogenes* and *Staphylococcus aureus.* They are favored among surgeons for prophylaxis against infection after surgery. Examples include cefadroxil, cefazolin, and cephalexin.

The second-generation cephalosporins have activity against gram-positive cocci but are more effective than the first group against gram-negative bacteria. Some have action against *H. influenzae, Bacteroides fragilis,* and even some anaerobic organisms that are found in the GI tract. Examples include cefaclor, cefotetan, and cefoxitin.

The third-generation cephalosporins have the most activity against gram-negative bacilli, especially the Enterobacteriaceae, *Pseudomonas aeruginosa,* and *H. influenzae.* However, they have reduced activity against *Staphylococcus aureus.* Some advantages of these drugs include being able to enter the central nervous system at concentrations high enough to treat bacterial meningeal infections and limited cross-reactivity (10%) with the penicillins, even though they are structurally related. Therefore these

drugs are somewhat safer alternatives for patients allergic to penicillin. However, the cross-sensitivity for anaphylactic reactions is high. Examples in this category include ceftriaxone, ceftazidime, and a new oral third-generation drug called *cefditoren.*[18]

Clinical uses of the cephalosporins include septicemia, pneumonia, meningitis, biliary tract infection, and sinusitis. Adverse events associated with these drugs include hypersensitivity reactions and GI disturbances, which are similar to those seen with penicillin. In addition, a few penicillin-sensitive individuals will experience some cross-reactions.

Other β-Lactam Antibiotics

Carbapenems and monobactams are other β-lactam antibiotics that were specifically developed to treat β-lactamase–producing gram-negative organisms that are resistant to penicillins.[1] Monobactams consist of a single ring structure attached to a sulfonic acid group (Figure 21-5). The only available monobactam is aztreonam, which only has activity against aerobic gram-negative bacilli, especially *P. aeruginosa.* This drug has no activity against gram-positive bacteria. An important property of this drug is that it is relatively nonallergenic and therefore can be used by patients who are allergic to penicillin or cephalosporin.[19]

Carbapenems have a very broad spectrum of activity against gram-positive, gram-negative, and some anaerobic organisms.[20] In addition, their activity is stable against many β-lactamases. Because of their broad effects, these drugs can be used to treat polymicrobial infections instead of two or more different antibiotics. Examples include imipenem, meropenem, and a new agent called *ertapenem.*

Glycopeptides

Vancomycin and teicoplanin are very potent bacterial cell wall inhibitors that lack a β-lactam ring.[1] These drugs act by binding to the terminal two alanine amino acids at one end of the peptidoglycan backbone, thus blocking elongation. Because they do not bind to the penicillin-binding proteins and do not have a β-lactam ring, they are not broken down by β-lactamase. The glycopeptides are active against gram-positive bacteria and are especially active against many resistant forms of streptococci and staphylococci. They are the drug of choice for methicillin-resistant staphylococci, penicillin-resistant pneumococci, and *Clostridium difficile.*[21] Vancomycin is given orally for the treatment of *C. difficile* because the drug cannot be absorbed from the GI tract, thus producing a high concentration at the target organ. Otherwise the drug is given intravenously.

Vancomycin is an extremely important arsenal in our war against bacteria. So far, only a few cases of resistance to vancomycin have been reported: *Enterococcus faecium* and a genetically based neonatal MRSA.[22,23] Because of its importance, indiscriminate use is discouraged. However, it is an excellent substitute treatment for patients with β-lactam allergy because there is no cross-reactivity between vancomycin and the β-lactam antibiotics.

The major side effect of vancomycin is an erythematous rash that is confined to the neck and upper trunk, called *red man syndrome*.[1] This reaction occurs when the drug is infused too quickly, creating a histamine reaction.

Inhibitors of Bacterial Cell Membrane Functioning

Polymyxin B and polymyxin E are drugs that injure the plasma membrane of gram-negative bacteria. Because they are quite toxic (neurotoxicity and nephrotoxicity), their use is limited to skin infections that allow topical application of the drugs.[7]

Antibiotics That Inhibit Bacterial Protein Synthesis

Bacterial protein synthesis takes place in the ribosomes.[1] The other structures involved in protein synthesis include messenger RNA (mRNA), which provides the instructions for protein synthesis, and transfer RNA (tRNA), which physically brings the amino acids to the ribosome (Figure 21-6). Because the bacterial ribosome is sufficiently different in structure from the mammalian ribosome, it represents a good target for drug action.

Aminoglycosides

Streptomycin, gentamicin, neomycin, and other aminoglycosides bind to bacterial ribosomes, causing misreadings of the mRNA genetic code.[1] These drugs enter the bacterial cells with the help of an oxygen-dependent transport system, which is not present in anaerobic bacteria or streptococci. They are active against many gram-negative bacilli, staphylococci, and mycobacteria. They are especially used for gram-negative enteric organisms in the

treatment of sepsis. Resistance to these agents is becoming more problematic and develops by alterations in the bacterial cell wall or by the synthesis of aminoglycoside-modifying enzymes. These drugs are both nephrotoxic and ototoxic, depending on duration of use. The nephrotoxic effect is reversible, but the ototoxicity can be permanent. Because of these side effects, use is limited to *P. aeruginosa* and the Enterobacteriaceae.

Macrolides

Macrolides are primarily used to treat respiratory tract infections and are the drugs of choice for community-acquired pneumonia.[24] They work by binding to specific parts of the ribosome and inhibiting formation of peptide bonds between amino acids and tRNA. They are active against streptococci, staphylococci, pneumococci, *Mycoplasma pneumoniae*, *Bordetella pertussis,* and legionellae. They are also the drugs of choice for treatment of *Chlamydia* infections during pregnancy because tetracyclines are contraindicated. Erythromycin is the prototypic drug, but because it may cause excessive nausea and vomiting, it is poorly tolerated. Clarithromycin and azithromycin produce less severe GI effects.

Tetracyclines

Tetracyclines consist of four fused cyclic rings that bind to the ribosome in a manner that blocks binding of the tRNA to the mRNA-ribosome complex (Figure 21-7).[7] Thus the growing peptide chain is terminated. They offer broad activity against chlamydiae, mycoplasmas, spirochetes, rickettsiae, and legionellae. They have traditionally been used for the treatment of acne vulgaris. They bind strongly to developing bone, impairing growth, and also produce yellowing of teeth. They are contraindicated in pregnant and breast-feeding women and also in children younger than 8 years. Examples include tetracycline, doxycycline, and minocycline.

Streptogramins

Quinupristin and dalfopristin are members of a new family of antibiotics called *streptogramins*.[1] When administered individually, they show minimal antimicrobial action, but when given together intravenously, they are quite potent against gram-positive bacteria. Dalfopristin binds to the 50S subunit of the bacterial ribosome, changing its configuration and facilitating quinupristin binding. These drugs are new alternatives to the standard

The elements involved in protein synthesis are shown: a ribosome (with 3 binding sites for transfer RNA [tRNA]: the P, A, and E sites), messenger RNA (mRNA) and tRNA. The different mRNA codons (triplets of 3 nucleotides that code for specific amino acids) are represented by dots, dashes, and straight or wavy lines and are shown in different colors. A tRNA with the growing peptide chain (consisting so far of Met–Leu–Trp: MLT) is in the P site, bound by codon:anticodon recognition (i.e., by complementary base-pairing). The incoming tRNA carries valine (V), covalently linked.

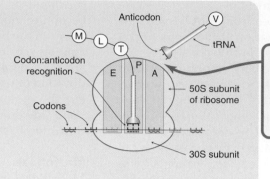

Competition with tRNA for the A site, e.g., tetracyclines; selectivity largely through selective uptake by active transport into prokaryotic cells

The incoming tRNA binds to the A site by complementary base-pairing.

Abnormal codon:anticodon leads to misreading of the message, e.g., aminoglycosides, gentamycin, amikacin, etc.

Transpeptidation occurs, i.e., the peptide chain on the tRNA in the P site is transferred to the tRNA on the A site. The peptide chain attached to the tRNA in the A site now consists of Met–Leu–Trp–Val (MLTV). The tRNA in the P site has been "discharged," i.e., has lost its peptide.

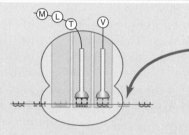

Inhibition of transpeptidation, e.g., chloramphenicol

Premature termination of peptide chain, e.g., puromycin, which resembles the amino acid end of tRNA (it also affects mammalian cells; used as an experimental tool)

The discharged tRNA is now transferred from the P site to the E site; the tRNA with the growing peptide chain is translocated from the A site to the P site, and the ribosome moves on one codon, relative to the messenger.

Inhibition of translocation, e.g., erythromycin (also spectinomycin, fusidic acid)

The tRNA from which the peptide chain has been removed is ejected. A new tRNA, with amino acid (M) attached and with the relevant anticodon, now moves into the A site, and the whole process is repeated.

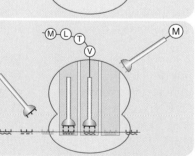

Figure 21-6

Schematic diagram of bacterial protein synthesis indicating the points at which antibiotics inhibit the process. (From Rang HP, Dale MM, Ritter JM, Moore JL. *Pharmacology.* 5th ed. New York: Churchill Livingstone; 2003.)

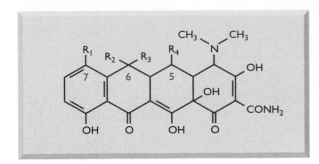

Figure 21-7

Chemical structure of tetracyclines. Substitutions at positions five, six, and seven result in different drugs, including the three common agents tetracycline, doxycycline, and minocycline. (From Page C, Curtis MJ, Sutter MC, Walker MJ, Hoffman BB, eds. *Integrated Pharmacology.* 2nd ed. Philadelphia: Mosby; 2002.)

treatment for infections caused by multiresistant gram-positive bacteria so they are quite important. When combined with other agents such as ampicillin or doxycycline, they mount an impressive attack against vancomycin-resistant *Enterococcus faecium,* another very resistant and dangerous organism.[25] Studies are ongoing to determine their effectiveness alone and in combination with other agents against MRSA. Adverse drug reactions include inflammation at the infusion site, GI effects, myalgias, and arthralgias.

Oxazolidinones

Linezolid is the first drug in a new category, the oxazolidinones, that inhibits bacterial protein synthesis at a step earlier than the other antimicrobials. Linezolid attaches to the 50S subunit at a position that interferes with tRNA binding.[26] It is active against penicillin-resistant pneumococci and *Staphylococcus aureus,* resistant staphylococci including MRSA, and methicillin-resistant *Staphylococcus epidermidis.* [27,28] So far, only rare resistance has been reported.

Antibiotics That Inhibit Bacterial DNA Synthesis

Each strand of DNA consists of a series of sugars (deoxyribose) and phosphate molecules as the backbone, with either a purine (adenine [A] or guanine [G]) or a pyrimidine (cytosine [C] or thymine [T]) base attached.[1] The base, sugar, and phosphate form the nucleotide. Two DNA strands are coiled together and held in place by hydrogen bonds link-

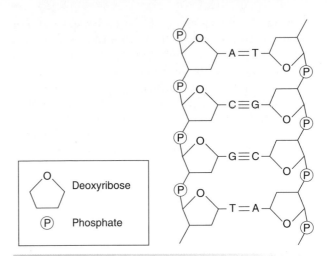

Figure 21-8

Structure of DNA. Each strand of DNA consists of a sugar-phosphate backbone with purine or pyrimidine bases attached. The purines are adenine (A) or guanine (G), and the pyrimidines are cytosine (C) or thymine (T). The sugar is deoxyribose. Complementarity between the two strands of DNA is maintained by hydrogen bonds (either two or three) between bases. (From Rang HP, Dale MM, Ritter JM, Moore JL. *Pharmacology.* 5th ed. New York: Churchill Livingstone; 2003.)

ing purine and pyrimidine bases between G and C and between A and T on each strand (Figure 21-8). During DNA synthesis, each original DNA strand serves as a template for the formation of a new strand. The enzyme DNA polymerase copies the DNA strand by complementary base pairing.[29] Before this can occur, DNA gyrase, also known as topoisomerase II, produces a double-strand break in the DNA helix necessary for the separation of the two strands. The same enzyme is responsible for resealing the breaks and preventing tangling problems. If this enzyme is deactivated, the chromosomes remain intertwined during mitosis and are unable to separate. Inhibition of DNA gyrase is an important target for the fluoroquinolone antibiotics.

Fluoroquinolones

Fluoroquinolones inhibit DNA synthesis by blocking DNA gyrase.[1] They are active against aerobic gram-negative bacilli such as pseudomonads and gram-negative cocci. They can also penetrate difficult-to-reach areas such as the prostate gland. The most commonly used fluoroquinolone is ciprofloxacin. Cipro, as it is more commonly known, received attention in 2001 when it was used to treat anthrax infections.[30] It has a somewhat broader spectrum of activity than the other fluoroquinolones and has excellent activity against the Enterobacteriaceae; gram-negative bacilli; and many organisms that are resistant to penicillins, cephalosporins, and aminoglycosides. Some clinical uses include complicated urinary tract infections, respiratory tract infections and otitis produced by pseudomonads, gonorrhea, bacterial prostatitis, cervicitis, and anthrax. Side effects associated with these drugs include cystic lesions in articular cartilage, spontaneous tendon ruptures, dizziness, headaches, and visual disturbances. Two other fluoroquinolones are gatifloxacin and moxifloxacin.[31]

Nitroimidazoles

Metronidazole is active against anaerobic bacteria, especially *B. fragilis*, *C. difficile*, and certain protozoa (*Giardia lamblia*, *Entamoeba histolytica*, and *Trichomonas* species). It is the drug of choice for bacterial vaginosis and *C. difficile* and is also used in Crohn's disease. Side effects include numbness in the hands and a disulfiram-like effect (vomiting with alcohol intake).

Antifolates

Antifolates interfere with the production of folate, which is necessary for the production of purine, and subsequently, DNA.[7] Humans can utilize folate obtained from dietary sources, but bacteria must synthesize folate from para-aminobenzoic acid. These antibiotics block enzymes involved in this pathway (Figure 21-9). Sulfonamides are used to treat bacterial conjunctivitis, urinary tract infections, inflammatory bowel disease; and they are applied topically to prevent infection associated with burns. Because they are quire allergenic, producing a pruritic maculopapular rash, and have a high rate of bacterial resistance, they are rarely used. However, silver sulfadiazine and sulfamethoxazole are still used. In fact, sulfamethoxazole is combined with a drug that blocks another step in this folate biosynthetic pathway called *trimethoprim*. The combination is called *trimethoprim-sulfamethoxazole (TMP-SMZ)* and is also known as *co-trimoxazole*. This combination is effective against several gram-negative bacilli including *E. coli*, the Enterobacteriaceae, and *P. mirabilis*. TMP-SMZ is the drug of choice for urinary tract infections.

Silver sulfadiazine is a topical sulfonamide compound of silver nitrate and sodium sulfadiazine.

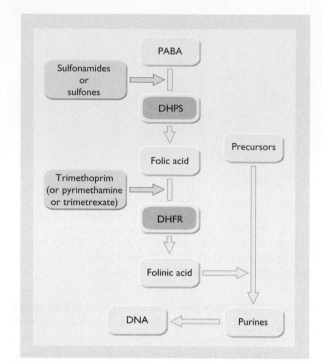

Figure 21-9

The folate biosynthetic pathway. Sulfonamides and sulfones compete with para-aminobenzoic acid (*PABA*) for dihydropteroate synthetase. Trimethoprim and the antiprotozoal drugs pyrimethamine and trimetrexate inhibit dihydrofolate reductase (*DHFR*). (From Page C, Curtis MJ, Sutter MC, Walker MJ, Hoffman BB, eds. *Integrated Pharmacology.* 2nd ed. Philadelphia: Mosby; 2002.)

It is useful against a wide range of gram-negative bacteria, especially *E. coli* and *P. aeruginosa*, and also against gram-positive bacteria such as *Staphylococcus aureus* and *Candida* species. It is most useful as a topical agent for deep partial-thickness and full-thickness burns or large superficial partial-thickness injuries. In addition to its antimicrobial effect, it may accelerate wound healing.[32] It is applied with a gloved hand thickly enough that the wound cannot be seen. Dry gauze is then applied over the cream.

Antimycobacterial Drugs

Tuberculosis (TB) in its active form is estimated to affect 8 million people, resulting in 2 million deaths every year.[33] In addition, it is estimated that more than 2 billion people have been infected with *Mycobacterium tuberculosis,* and many are not even aware of it because the bacteria can persist asymptomatically for long periods, finally causing an active infection years later (latent TB). Most individuals control the initial infection by mounting a cell-mediated immune response that prevents the disease but may leave some viable mycobacteria, resulting in clinical disease in 5% to 10% of cases. Primary disease can develop later in life, either by reactivation of the bacteria remaining from the initial infection or by the development of a subsequent infection.

The risk of developing TB is highly dependent on the host's immune status. Co-infection with HIV markedly increases the development of symptoms of both diseases.[34] In the year 2000, it was estimated that 11 million people were co-infected with HIV and *M. tuberculosis,* and in the same year, there were 500,000 new cases of active TB associated with HIV. The interaction between the two diseases appears to be synergistic in that each increases the pathogenesis of the other. HIV promotes progression to active TB in people with latent or recently acquired infection, and TB increases HIV viremia.

M. tuberculosis is transmitted by airborne particles in respiratory secretions when an infected person coughs, sneezes, or speaks. The bacteria are inhaled deep into the lungs and into the alveoli where they are engulfed by macrophages. However, the thick wall of the mycobacterium provides some resistance against the bacterial fighting mechanisms of the macrophages. The macrophages launch their own attack, with the result being *M. tuberculosis* uptake by the phagocytes into an immature phagosomal compartment, allowing the bacteria to replicate inside the macrophages.[35-37] At this point, the infection is controlled, and there are no clinical symptoms. However, the infection site can be identified by the presence of small granulomas characterized by a central area of mycobacteria-infected cells surrounded by other noninfected phagocytic cells and foamy giant cells (giant macrophages containing lipids). Lymphocytes are found around the periphery. The granuloma is sealed off from other tissue by a fibrotic capsule. The material is at first solid but becomes liquefied because of the continued multiplication of the bacilli. The liquefied granuloma may open up into a bronchus and infect the sputum. At this point, the patient is very infectious. Bacilli are ingested by macrophages and transported via the bloodstream and lymphatics to other areas. Eventually, fibrosis and calcification of the tissues render the disease inactive. However, there is a potential for reactivation years later.

Symptoms of TB include fever, night sweats, malaise, and weight loss. Productive cough and pleuritic pain are the pulmonary symptoms.[3] Up to 80% of patients without HIV infection show only pulmonary involvement, but the majority of patients with HIV infection show extrapulmonary symptoms involving the genitourinary tract, bones, joints, meninges, and peritoneum.

Treatment of active TB has two goals: to cure the infection and to prevent spread to others. Patients with active TB are kept in ventilated isolation rooms in which high-efficiency particulate air (HEPA) filtration and UV germicidal irradiation are provided.[38] Health care workers entering the room of an infected patient must wear personal respirators with HEPA-filtered masks that must be tested for proper fit annually to ensure close facial contact with the mask. Isolation may be discontinued when three consecutive sputum samples (taken on different days) are negative for the bacilli and the patient is improving clinically. This may take up to 3 weeks or longer if the patient is infected with a resistant strain.

The initial phase of treatment consists of at least three different medications, possibly four if the organism is suspected to be resistant, and includes isoniazid, rifampicin, pyrazinamide, and ethambutol.[1] This phase lasts a minimum of 2 months. The second, continuation phase lasts at least 4 months and consists of isoniazid and rifampin. If there is TB located in the bone or brain or if there is evidence of resistance, this phase is longer.

Isoniazid

Isoniazid is the most critical drug for the treatment of TB. This drug inhibits the synthesis of mycolic acid, an important lipid constituent of the mycobacterium cell wall. It is absorbed well orally and even achieves concentrations in the cerebrospinal fluid to treat tuberculous meningitis. Common side effects include hepatitis and peripheral neuropathy, but hematological changes, arthritic symptoms, and vasculitis have also been reported. For active disease this drug is *always* used in combination with rifampin plus at least one other antimycobacterial drug. Treatment is given two to three times per week for at least 6 months but may be as long as 12 months if the patient is also infected with HIV. Persons with a positive tuberculin skin test result but no evidence of TB on a chest x-ray film may be treated with isoniazid alone.[39] The protocol for this is isoniazid treatment two to three times a day for 6 to 9 months.

Rifampin

Rifampin is used along with isoniazid as a first-line agent against *M. tuberculosis.*[1] However, it is also used to treat other infections, such as *M. leprae* (causes Hansen's disease), legionellae, *N. meningitidis, H. influenzae,* and staphylococci. Rifampin binds to the DNA-dependent RNA polymerase to inhibit RNA synthesis. Rifampin induces hepatic P450 enzymes, and therefore metabolism of other drugs is increased. Other effects of these drugs include thrombocytopenia, nephritis, and orange discoloration of most secretions, including tears (which results in staining of contact lenses).

Pyrazinamide

Pyrazinamide is also a first-line agent against TB and is given along with rifampin and isoniazid.[1] It is a prodrug converted to pyrazinoic acid, which is toxic to an enzyme present only in the bacilli. Its main side effect is hepatotoxicity.

Ethambutol

The fourth drug commonly included in this regimen is ethambutol. It is thought to inhibit the bacteria's production of RNA, but the exact mechanism is not known. It has some rather bizarre side effects, mainly on vision. It produces retrobulbar neuritis, which begins as red-green color blindness and progresses to a generalized loss of visual acuity.

Other Antimycobacterial Drugs

Other antimicrobial drugs are effective against TB, especially when given in combination.[40] Capreomycin, an aminoglycoside, can be injected in the event that a patient has difficulty with any of the standard drugs. Adverse effects include renal failure and injury to the eighth cranial nerve producing deafness and ataxia. Cycloserine is a broad-spectrum agent that is bacteriostatic against the mycobacterium. Its primary mechanism of action is to inhibit cell wall synthesis. This drug primarily produces neurological symptoms including headache, depression, convulsions, and psychotic episodes.

Multidrug-Resistant Tuberculosis

Multidrug resistant TB is a growing problem and a dangerous public health issue. It is defined as strains resistant to at least isoniazid and rifampin. Primary

multidrug-resistant TB develops when a person acquires a strain of TB that is already resistant, whereas secondary multidrug-resistant TB develops in an individual who was noncompliant with treatment or who received inadequate treatment.[38] It is related both to noncompliance with treatment and HIV status. The noncompliance issue encompasses not only premature drug withdrawal but also treatment devoid of some of the key drugs used for TB.[38] In several parts of the world, the complete four-drug protocol is not available. Patients may receive only one of the four drugs, giving the mycobacterium an opportunity to develop resistance. Even in New York City, this has become a problem and is related to socioeconomic conditions. Poverty is a risk factor for TB, and from 1979 to 1993, the poverty rate in the city rose almost 10%, corresponding to a 33% increase in the incidence of TB. In the United States in the 1950s, drug resistance accounted for 1% to 2%, but by 1991, this had increased to 23%.

Several strategies have been developed to stem the growth of resistant TB.[41] An individual drug protocol is designed based on the drugs "thought to be most sensitive." Medications are added one at a time until five effective drugs are found. More than five may be used if sensitivity of the bacterium is unclear. Another strategy includes "directly observed therapy." This method refers to requiring patients to attend a local health clinic where they can be directly observed taking their medication. If appointments are missed, the patient may then be incarcerated. In some cases, health care professionals visit the patient at home to ensure compliance with treatment. Other strategies include providing vouchers for transportation to the health clinic, food coupons, housing assistance, support groups, and educational activities.

SOME SPECIFIC BACTERIAL INFECTIONS AND THEIR TREATMENT

Microorganisms invade the body tissue, somehow evading normal host defenses. They multiply and create an infective process that usually consists of fever, chills, sweats, redness, pain, pus, and swelling. In addition, the white blood cell count increases as the host begins to fight back. In most cases, the host's defense systems along with standard antibiotic treatment are enough to eradicate the infection.

However, because of the ever-changing nature of bacteria, treatment of infection does not always follow a standard protocol. Some infections the physical therapist may see in the clinic and their current treatment regimens are discussed in the following sections.

Clostridium difficile

C. difficile is a gram-positive, spore-forming anaerobic bacillus that produces colitis, voluminous infectious watery diarrhea, abdominal cramping, and sometimes fever.[42] Dehydration, electrolyte depletion, and other complications including hemorrhage, reactive arthritis, sepsis, and death may occur. C. difficile infection often occurs after administration of a broad-spectrum antibiotic but can also follow chemotherapy or immunosuppressive treatments. Antimicrobial agents are often to blame because they eradicate the normal GI flora needed to keep the C. difficile level to a minimum.[43] Elderly patients commonly have this illness after antibiotic treatment of a diabetic or vascular wound. Some individuals may be asymptomatic or only show mild symptoms but carry high levels of C. difficile. Patient-to-patient transmission occurs, and the organisms can be cultured from hands, clothing, and stethoscopes of health care workers who have been in the rooms of infected patients. These bacteria can survive up to 5 months in the environment. Colonization occurs by the fecal-oral route. Ingested spores survive the acid environment of the stomach and grow in the colon. The drug of choice for C. difficile is intravenous metronidazole, with vancomycin coming in second.[44] Successful treatment of this infection has also been documented with intracolonic vancomycin.[21] This mode of administration eliminates the neurotoxicity and nephrotoxicity associated with the drug.

Methicillin-Resistant Staphylococcus aureus

Staphylococcus aureus is present on the skin of many people but generally does not cause a problem for those who are healthy. However, it is a significant threat to the sick and elderly population, particularly in the resistant form, MRSA. MRSA poses a significant health risk because it is immune to the effects of the standard first-line antibiotics used for Staphylococcus infections. MRSA spreads through direct contact, often from contamination of hands from hospital staff members to patients. It can also be spread through contact with contaminated surfaces in the environment. It can survive for long periods (up to 79 days) in dry environmental conditions, existing on paper, foil, cotton, Formica, and other surfaces.[45] In an effort to control these bacteria, patients with MRSA infections are usually isolated in single rooms. They remain in isolation until they are free from infection (three consecutive cultures taken on different days). Drug choices for the treatment of MRSA are becoming increasingly limited. For several years, vancomycin was one of the most effective remedies for this infection, but now there are several reports of vancomycin-resistant Staphylococcus aureus. At the time of this writing, only two other drugs have Food and Drug Administration approval for the treatment of MRSA, linezolid and quinupristin/dalfopristin. Of the two, linezolid is preferred because of its favorable pharmacokinetic properties. It is one of the few drugs with bioavailability nearing 100% for the oral form (making the transition from intravenous to oral administration easy), and it is metabolized without any P450 enzymes. In addition, the dosing interval is every 12 hours, and no dose adjustment is required for patients with renal problems. Fluoroquinolones, tetracyclines, and TMP-SMZ may occasionally be effective.[44] Linezolid, as well as other drugs used to treat resistant infections, must be used sparingly. Appropriate laboratory testing must be performed to ensure that the correct drugs are used to fight infection and to prevent indiscriminate use. Their use must be preserved for only difficult infections.

Pneumonia

Community-acquired bacterial pneumonia is often caused by Streptococcus pneumoniae (pneumococci).[46] In the United States, more than 15% of these bacteria are resistant to penicillin, and they are becoming increasingly resistant to cephalosporins, macrolides, and the fluoroquinolones. For Streptococcus pneumoniae, a fluoroquinolone (levofloxacin, gatifloxacin, or moxifloxacin) is the choice of therapy. Doxycycline (a macrolide) is also recommended. Atypical pathogens including Mycoplasma pneumoniae, Chlamydia pneumoniae, and Legionella pneumophila cause up to 40% of cases of this community-acquired disease. For these atypical infections, a macrolide (e.g., erythromycin, azithromycin, or clarithromycin) is given.

Urinary Tract Infections

Uncomplicated cystitis is treated with a 3-day course of oral TMP-SMZ or a single dose of three double-strength tablets. In areas where there is TMP-SMZ–resistant *E. coli*, a fluoroquinolone is substituted. When urinary tract infections have been acquired in a hospital or nursing home, the infectious agent is presumed to be resistant gram-negative bacilli, *Staphylococcus aureus*, or enterococci. A fluoroquinolone, third-generation cephalosporin, or amoxicillin/clavulanic acid may be used.

ANTIMICROBIAL PROPHYLAXIS IN SURGERY

Antimicrobial prophylaxis can decrease the incidence of infection, particularly wound infection, after certain surgeries, but this benefit must be weighed against risks, such as allergic reactions or the development of resistant bacteria. It is recommended for procedures associated with high infection rates such as those involving implantation of prosthetic material, those involving the GI tract, and those involving trauma in which the wound is already dirty.[47] Host factors such as immunosuppression or the presence of valvular and other cardiac diseases also warrant prophylaxis. Long preoperative hospitalizations are associated with increased risk of infection with a resistant organism, and therefore prophylaxis may be required. Antimicrobial prophylaxis to prevent bacterial endocarditis in patients with prosthetic heart valves, rheumatic heart disease, or other cardiac abnormalities is also recommended before dental procedures.

In most cases, a single intravenous or intramuscular dose of an antimicrobial administered between 30 minutes and 1 hour before the initial incision provides adequate tissue concentrations throughout the surgery. If the surgery is prolonged (more than 4 hours) or if major blood loss occurs, another dose is given. For "dirty surgery" such as that for a perforated abdominal cavity, a compound fracture, or a laceration caused by an animal or human bite, the use of antimicrobial drugs is considered therapy rather than prophylaxis and should be continued for several days. Cefazolin is recommended for many procedures because of its long half-life; however, in hospitals where MSRA is present, vancomycin may be used. For colorectal surgery and appendectomies, cefotetan is the drug of choice because it is more active against bowel anaerobes. Endocarditis prophylaxis commonly includes amoxicillin, cephalexin, azithromycin, or cefazolin. Many different protocols are used, depending on the type of surgery.

PREVENTING ANTIBIOTIC RESISTANCE AND THE SPREAD OF INFECTION

Antibiotic resistance was at one time confined to hospitals, but today it is quite prevalent in the community at large. One of the main reasons for this prevalence, as discussed previously, is related to the unnecessary use of antibiotics. In fact, it is thought that between 20% and 50% of all antibiotic prescriptions are unnecessary.[13] To meet this challenge, several groups of physicians and scientists have come together to develop strategies for preventing the spread of infection and antibiotic resistance. One group in particular that has been very active in providing information for physicians, particularly those in the community, is the Alliance for the Prudent Use of Antibiotics.[48] Some of the recommendations made by this group include "appropriate prescribing." This requires that physicians make use of diagnostic methods to identify the causative bacteria and then prescribe only the selected targeted-spectrum antibiotic. Care should be taken not to prescribe antimicrobials for viral infections. In addition, patients should receive appropriate medications to reduce symptoms such as decongestants, cough medicine, and antipyretics; and explanations should be provided regarding why an antibiotic might not be prescribed. The Centers for Disease Control and Prevention has developed special prescription pads for patients with cold or flu explaining why antibiotics may not be prescribed.[13]

Strategies to prevent the spread of infection include detailed attention to hygiene before and after seeing a patient with an infection.[45] This includes disinfecting any equipment that comes in contact with the patient, especially if it will be used on another patient. Items left in the hospital room after a patient is discharged, such as the phone and bedside table also need attention. Other strategies are use of only disposable items and storing items away from other patients until the organisms are nonviable. It is important to understand that nosocomial pathogens can be transmitted not only from wet surfaces but also from dry ones.

ADVERSE EFFECTS OF ANTIBIOTICS AND THERAPEUTIC CONCERNS

The most common side effect of antimicrobial treatment is GI upset. Patients commonly experience nausea, vomiting, diarrhea, and abdominal discomfort. These symptoms are often minimized when the drug is taken with food, but some antibiotics will have reduced absorption if taken at mealtime. Other side effects include ototoxicity and nephrotoxicity if the drug is administered for long periods. In addition, tetracyclines, sulfonamides,

and the fluoroquinolones all increase the patient's sensitivity to UV light. Nearly all the antibiotics can cause *C. difficile* enteritis.

Physical therapists must take extreme precautions when treating patients who are receiving metronidazole, vancomycin, linezolid, or quinupristin/dalfopristin. Administration of these drugs usually means that the patient has a resistant type of infection. Mask, gown, and glove protection is often necessary but depends on the type of organism and whether the infection is spread by respiratory droplets or contact with infected bodily secretions.[23] Strict adherence to infection control measures, especially hand washing, is imperative, and equipment that has contact with the patient, such as walkers and weights, must be disinfected. Therapists should also be aware of the psychological stress induced by isolation and refer the patient to the appropriate health care provider.[49]

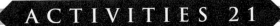

ACTIVITIES 21

■ 1. Briefly discuss one topical agent used for the treatment or prevention of wound infection commonly seen in physical therapy practice. Please discuss the type of organism against which the drug is active, how the drug is administered, and any side effects that may occur. Also, if possible, report on any personal experience you have had with the drug and your thoughts on its effectiveness.

■ 2. Discuss how physical therapists can help stop the spread of infection. What infection control strategies have been used in clinics with

which you have been affiliated and do you think physical therapists do enough to protect themselves and their patients?

■ 3. Search the literature for information regarding what clinical signs a patient should demonstrate before receiving a prescription for an antibiotic.

■ 4. Visit the website of the Alliance for the Prudent Use of Antibiotics, http://www.apua.org. Review and discuss strategies for preventing infection after surgical procedures.

References

1. Rang HP, Dale MM, Ritter JM, Moore JL. *Pharmacology.* 5th ed. New York: Churchill Livingstone; 2003.
2. Livermore DM. The threat from the pink corner. *Ann Med.* 2003;35(4):226-234.
3. Infectious diseases. In: Braunwald E, Fauci AS, Kasper DL, Hauser SL, Longo DL, Jameson JL, eds. *Harrison's Manual of Medicine.* 15th ed. New York: McGraw-Hill; 2002:325-334.

4. Poole K. Multidrug resistance in gram-negative bacteria. *Curr Opin Microbiol.* 2001;4:500-508.
5. Thielman NM, Neu HC. Principles of antimicrobial use. In: Brody MJ, Larner J, Minneman KP, eds. *Human Pharmacology: Molecular to Clinical.* 3rd ed. Philadelphia: Mosby; 1998:641-654.
6. Pankey GA, Sabath LD. Clinical relevance of bacteriostatic versus bactericidal mechanisms of action in the treatment of gram-positive bacterial infections. *Clin Infect Dis.* 2004;38(6):864-870.

7. Shafran SD. Drugs and bacteria. In: Page C, Curtis MJ, Sutter MC, Walker MJ, Hoffman BB, eds. *Integrated Pharmacology.* 2nd ed. Philadelphia: Mosby; 2002:111-136.

8. Tan YT, Tillett DJ, McKay IA. Molecular strategies for overcoming antibiotic resistance in bacteria. *Mol Med Today.* 2000;6:309-314.

9. Amyes SG. Resistance to beta-lactams—the permutations. *J Chemother.* 2003;15(6):525-535.

10. Markham PN, Neyfakh AA. Efflux-mediated drug resistance in gram-positive bacteria. *Curr Opin Microbiol.* 2001;4:509-514.

11. Levy SB. Antimicrobial resistance: bacteria on the defence. *BMJ.* 1998;317:612-613.

12. Huovinen P, Cars O. Control of antimicrobial resistance: time for action. *BMJ.* 1998;317:613-614.

13. Hooton TM, Levy SB. Antimicrobial resistance: a plan of action for community practice. *Am Fam Physician.* 2001;63(6):1087-1096.

14. Thielman NM, Neu HC. Bacterial cell wall inhibitors. In: Brody MJ, Larner J, Minneman KP, eds. *Human Pharmacology: Molecular to Clinical.* Philadelphia: Mosby; 1998:655-682.

15. Klein JO. Amoxicillin/clavulanate for infections in infants and children: past, present and future. *Pediatr Infect Dis J.* 2003;22(suppl 8):S139-S148.

16. Augmentin XR. *Med Lett Drugs Ther.* 2003;45(1148):5-6.

17. White AR, Kaye C, Poupard J, Pypstra R, Woodnutt G, Wynne B. Augmentin (amoxicillin/clavulanate) in the treatment of community-acquired respiratory tract infection: a review of the continuing development of an innovative antimicrobial agent. *J Antimicrob Chemother.* 2004;53(suppl 1):13-20.

18. Cefditoren (Spectracef)—a new oral cephalosporin. *Med Lett Drugs Ther.* 2002;44(1122):5-6.

19. Leviton I. Separating fact from fiction: the data behind allergies and side effects caused by penicillins, cephalosporins, and carbapenem antibiotics. *Curr Pharm Des.* 2003;9(12):983-988.

20. Ertapenem (Invanz)—a new parenteral carbapenem. *Med Lett Drugs Ther.* 2002;44(1126):25-26.

21. Apisarnthanarak A, Razavi B, Mundy LM. Adjunctive intracolonic vancomycin for severe *Clostridium difficile* colitis: case series and review of the literature. *Clin Infect Dis.* 2002;35:690-696.

22. Kikuchi K. Genetic basis of neonatal methicillin-resistant *Staphylococcus aureus* in Japan. *Pediatr Int.* 2003;45(2): 223-229.

23. Slaughter S, Hayden MK, Nathan C, et al. A comparison of the effect of universal use of gloves and gowns with that of glove use alone on acquisition of vancomycin-resistant enterococci in a medical intensive care unit. *Ann Intern Med.* 1996;125(6):448-456.

24. Dunbar LM. Current issues in the management of bacterial respiratory tract disease: the challenge of antibacterial resistance. *Am J Med Sci.* 2003;326(6):360-368.

25. Brown J, Freeman BB. Combining quinupristin/dalfopristin with other agents for resistant infections. *Ann Pharmacother.* 2004;38(4):677-685.

26. Diekema DJ, Jones RN. Oxazolidinone antibiotics. *Lancet.* 2001;358:1975-1982.

27. Linezolid (Zyvox). *Med Lett Drugs Ther.* 2000;42(1079): 45-46.

28. Ament PW, Jamshed N, Horne JP. Linezolid: its role in the treatment of gram-positive, drug-resistant bacterial infections. *Am Fam Physician.* 2002;65(4):663-670.

29. Alberts B, Bray D, Lewis J, Raff M, Roberts K, Watson JD. *Molecular Biology of The Cell.* New York: Garland Publishing, Inc.; 1989.

30. Post-exposure anthrax prophylaxis. *Med Lett Drugs Ther.* 2001;43(1116-1117):91-92.

31. Gatifloxacin and moxifloxacin: two new fluoroquinolones. *Med Lett Drugs Ther.* 2000;42(1072):15-17.

32. Edwards R, Harding KG. Bacteria and wound healing. *Curr Opin Infect Dis.* 2004;17(2):91-96.

33. Dye C, Scheele S, Dolin P, Patharia V, Raviglione MC. Consensus statement. Global burden of tuberculosis: estimated incidence, prevalence, and mortality by country. *JAMA.* 1999;282:677-686.

34. de Jong BC, Israelski DM, Corbett EL, Small PM. Clinical management of tuberculosis in the context of HIV infection. *Annu Rev Med.* 2004;55:283-301.

35. Stewart GR, Robertson BD, Young DB. Tuberculosis: a problem with persistence. *Nat Rev Microbiol.* 2003;1:97-105.

36. Cosma CL, Sherman DR, Ramakrishnan L. The secret lives of the pathogenic mycobacteria. *Annu Rev Microbiol.* 2003;57:641-676.

37. Chan J, Flynn J. The immunological aspects of latency in tuberculosis. *Clin Immunol.* 2004;110:2-12.

38. Paolo W, Nosanchuk JD. Tuberculosis in New York City: recent lessons and a look ahead. *Lancet.* 2004;4:287-293.

39. Enarson DA. Use of the tuberculin skin test in children. *Paediatr Respir Rev.* 2004;5(suppl A):S135-S137.

40. Cohn DL. Treatment of latent tuberculosis infection. *Semin Respir Infect.* 2003;18(4):249-262.

41. Mukherjee JS, Rich ML, Socci AR, et al. Programmes and principles in treatment of multidrug-resistant tuberculosis. *Lancet.* 2004;363:474-481.

42. Mylonakis E, Ryan E, Calderwood SB. *Clostridium difficile*–associated diarrhea. *Arch Intern Med.* 2001; 161:525-533.

43. Safdar N, Maki D. The commonality of risk factors for nosocomial colonization and infection with antimicrobial-resistant *Staphylococcus aureus, Enterococcus,* gram-negative bacilli, *Clostridium difficile* and *Candida. Ann Intern Med.* 2002;136:834-844.

44. The choice of antibacterial drugs. *Med Lett Drugs Ther.* 2001;43(1111-1112):69-78.

45. Dietze B, Rath A, Wendt C, Martiny H. Survival of MRSA on sterile goods packaging. *J Hosp Infect.* 2001;49:255-261.

46. Thibodeau KP, Viera AJ. Atypical pathogens and challenges in community-acquired pneumonia. *Am Fam Physician.* 2004;69:1699-1706.

47. Antimicrobial prophylaxis for surgery. *Treat Guidel Med Lett.* 2004;2(20):27-32.

48. Alliance for the Prudent Use of Antibiotics. Available at: http://www.apua.org. Accessed March 30, 2005.

49. Tarzi S, Kennedy P, Stone S, Evans M. Methicillin-resistant *Staphylococcus aureus*: psychological impact of hospitalization and isolation in an older adult population. *J Hosp Infect.* 2001;49:250-254.

CHAPTER 22

ANTIVIRAL AGENTS AND SELECTED DRUGS FOR FUNGAL INFECTIONS

TREATMENT OF VIRAL INFECTIONS

Viruses represent one of the smallest classes of microorganisms. Unlike bacteria, they can only replicate in the cells of their hosts. They can enter the body through the respiratory tract, gastrointestinal (GI) tract, or the skin or mucous membranes; and they can cross the placenta. Viruses may be transferred through the skin as a result of sharing syringes, sexual contact, blood transfusions, or animal bites.

Virus Structure and Function

Viruses are extremely small parasites that consist of nucleic acids (RNA or DNA) contained in a protein shell or capsid.[1] The protein shell plus the nucleic acid is called the *nucleocapsid*. In some viruses, the nucleocapsid is encased in a lipoprotein envelope. This entire structure is then called a *virion* (Figure 22-1). Some viruses also contain enzymes necessary to initiate replication in the host cell; however, for the most part, they use the host enzyme systems.

Viral Entry and Uncoating

When a virion reaches a possible host cell, it attaches itself to the surface and prepares to deliver its capsid and enzymes in a form that favors replication.[2] The virion is extremely skilled at entering the host cell with minimal detection. The receptors on the host can be cytokines, neurotransmitters, hormones, ion channels, or membrane glycoproteins. Some host cell structures that are used as receptors include the CD4 glycoprotein on helper T lymphocytes for the HIV virus, the acetylcholine receptor at the neuromuscular junction for the rabies virus, and major histocompatibility complexes for adenoviruses that produce a sore throat. The virion is aided by certain attachment factors and viral surface glycoproteins, which help to determine the cell types and tissues a virus can invade.

Many viruses depend on endocytosis to enter the host cell, including the adenovirus and the influenza virus.[2] One of the advantages to this method of entry is that the endocytic vesicles are able to traverse barriers imposed by the cytoskeleton and cytoplasm of the host cell. Another advantage is that the virus is exposed to an acidic environment in the endosome, which provides a trigger for uncoating of the protein shell. In addition, if the virus enters an endosomal compartment, it leaves no viral glycoproteins exposed on the cell surface for the immune system to detect.

Other viruses, especially those with a lipoprotein envelope, enter the cell by fusion and penetration.[2] Fusion proteins exist in the viral envelope and are triggered by receptor binding or low pH. They produce irreversible conformational changes, exposing hydrophobic protein sequences that insert into the target membrane and deliver viral capsids into the cytosol. Essentially, the viral envelope acts as the

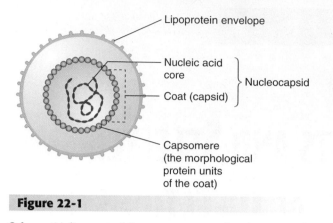

Lipoprotein envelope

Nucleic acid core

Coat (capsid)

Nucleocapsid

Capsomere (the morphological protein units of the coat)

Figure 22-1

Schematic diagram of the components of a virus particle or virion. (From Rang HP, Dale MM, Ritter JM, Moore JL. *Pharmacology*. 5th ed. New York: Churchill Livingstone; 2003.)

transport vesicle. Nonenveloped viruses penetrate the cell either by lysing part of the host membrane or by creating a channel or pore-like structure.

After the virus penetrates the host cell, the nucleic acids must be transported to either the nucleus (for DNA viruses) or to specific cytosolic membranes.[2] At this point, endocytic vesicles can ferry the virus to the appropriate target, or the capsid itself can take advantage of certain motors within the cytoplasm, such as actin filaments. Actin has been found to drive virus-containing vesicles through the cytoplasm. Entering the nucleus represents the next challenge for the capsid, which must traverse through the nuclear pore complexes to reach the host's supply of DNA and RNA polymerases, as well as splice and modify the enzymes necessary for viral reproduction. The small viruses and capsid can enter the nuclear pore complexes without difficulty, but larger viruses must undergo deformation or be disassembled to allow the genome to pass into the nucleus.

Infection can also be transmitted directly from cell to cell with or without virus infection. Viruses, such as measles that can fuse at a neutral pH, can often induce fusion of infected cells with uninfected cells and pass the viral genes directly from cell to cell.

This simplified discussion highlights the mechanisms involved in viral entry into a cell. This is a complex multistep process involving many host and viral proteins that presumably can act as targets for antiviral agents. In the past, drug therapy was focused primarily on blocking viral replication. However, new drugs that target the entry and uncoating processes have been developed, specifically, an inhibitor against the influenza virus and an inhibitor against the fusion protein used by HIV-1.

Viral Replication

DNA viruses enter the host cell nucleus and provide the directions for creation of a new virus. Transcription of the viral DNA into messenger RNA (mRNA) is carried out by the host cell RNA polymerase.[3] Translation of the mRNA into virus-specific proteins is next. Some of these proteins are then used to make the protein shell and envelope, and others are used to synthesize more viral DNA. The amount of information that the virus brings to the host cell varies greatly, but even the smallest DNA virus codes for proteins that initiate the synthesis of their own DNA.

RNA viruses do not need to enter the host cell nucleus (with the exception of the influenza virus) but must undergo some specialized procedures to replicate. They must copy RNA molecules first by encoding their own RNA-dependent polymerase enzymes. The virus's RNA can then serve as its own mRNA, or the enzymes in the virion can synthesize its mRNA.

Retroviruses were first known as RNA tumor viruses because infection leads to a permanent genetic change, making the cell cancerous.[3] These viruses became known as retroviruses because they reverse the normal process in which DNA is transcribed into RNA. They contain a reverse-transcriptase enzyme (virus RNA–dependent DNA polymerase), which makes a DNA copy of the single-stranded viral RNA. This forms a DNA-RNA hybrid, which is then transcribed by the same enzyme into a double helix with two DNA strands. This DNA copy then integrates into a host cell chromosome. Large numbers of new viral RNA molecules are then constructed by the host cell RNA polymerase.

After synthesis of either viral DNA or viral RNA and the structural proteins, assembly of the coat proteins around the viral genome occurs, and the virion is ready to be released.[1] The mechanism of release may be budding or host cell lyses. The new viral particles are then free to infect other host cells. Examples of retroviruses include HIV and T-cell leukemia virus.

Host Warfare Against Viruses and Viral Defenses

The host cell launches a rather sophisticated campaign against an invading virus. There are a variety of innate and adaptive immune responses to viruses.[4] Innate immunity acts as the body's first line of defense and includes the skin and its mucosal barriers and a nonspecific inflammatory response. The nonspecific response involves the phagocytes (leukocytes), cytokines (interferons and tumor necrosis factor-α), and natural killer (NK) cells. The interferons are especially important, acting as messengers both within the immune system and between the immune system and other parts of the body, signaling invasion. In addition, interferons have an important defense role against viruses. They are produced by virus-infected cells and act to interrupt the viral life cycle at many steps. They also coat surrounding cells to make them more virus-resistant and up-regulate major histocompatibility complex expression to target infected cells. The specific interferons involved include interferon (IFN)-α and IFN-β, which become potent inducers of NK cell–mediated cytotoxicity.[5] The NK cells, which are specialized lymphocytes, recognize virally infected cells and launch a direct attack, killing the organism by releasing lytic proteins on the infected cell, triggering the apoptotic pathway, and releasing cytokines.

In the adaptive immune response, the key cells are the lymphocytes: B cells, which produce antibodies; T cells, which are essential for the induction phase of the cell-mediated immune reaction; and cytotoxic T cells (derived from CD8 cells) (Figure 22-2). During the induction phase the antigen is presented to the T lymphocytes on the surface of antigen presenting cells. At this point, the T cell becomes activated, meaning that it can now recognize the antigen. The T cell develops interleukin 2 receptors and also generates this interleukin. The T cells also give rise to two different subsets of helper cells, Th1 and Th2 cells. Each type of helper cell produces its own interleukins. The Th2 cells produce cytokines, which stimulate B cells to proliferate and mature into plasma cells that produce antibodies. The effector phase is the antibody-mediated phase in which the antibody recognizes the specific antigen and then activates several of the host's defense systems. Antiviral antibodies are observed late in most infections and

are thought to be responsible for prevention of cell-to-cell spread. The additional host resources are reinforcement of the cell-mediated reactions and include CD8 cytotoxic T cells, which kill virus-infected cells; cytokine-releasing CD4 T cells, which stimulate macrophage killing; and memory cells, which are produced so that cells are ready to react more rapidly the next time the antigen invades.

Viruses use a variety of methods to overcome the host's reactions.[6] Viruses can limit the action of some cytokines by expressing a receptor on their cell surfaces to match the cytokine. These act as pseudoreceptors that bind cytokines, preventing them from reaching their real receptors. Another ploy is to express a major histocompatibility complex that the NK cells are unable to recognize. Still another method is the production of viral proteins that interfere with apoptosis.[7] For the virus to keep functioning, it requires a live host cell.

Antiviral Agents

Viruses, for the most part, are difficult to eradicate for several reasons.[8] First, replication of the virus generally reaches its peak (host contains a large viral load) before any clinical symptoms appear. Second, the available antiviral drugs are virustatic as opposed to virucidal and depend on a normal host immune system for cure. A diseased host immune system will lead to impaired recovery and a prolonged and more severe illness. In addition, in vitro susceptibility testing for viruses is less predictive than testing sensitivity to antimicrobials. Resistant viruses are also a problem similar to resistant bacteria.

Several sites that act as targets for drug action within the viral reproductive cycle are currently available (Figure 22-3).[8] Some drugs inhibit uncoating of the virus, which is necessary to unleash the genome into the host cell. Other drugs block RNA and DNA replication, as well as production of the viral proteins by inhibiting transcription and translation. Some fairly new compounds on the market prevent release and budding of the new virions.

Antiviral Agents That Inhibit Uncoating

Amantadine, approved for the prevention of influenza A, and rimantadine inhibit uncoating of the virus by blocking the H$^+$ channel, which would normally acidify the inside of the virion.[8]

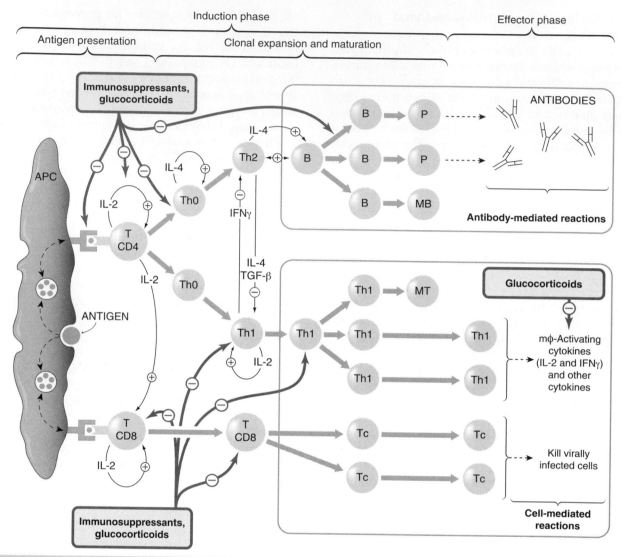

Figure 22-2

Simplified diagram of the induction and effector phases of lymphocyte activation with the sites of action of immunosuppressants. Antigen-presenting cells *(APC)* ingest and process antigen (●) and present fragments of it (•) to naive, uncommitted CD4 T cells in conjunction with major histocompatibility complex (MHC) class II molecules and to naive CD8 T cells in conjunction with MHC class I molecules (-[), arming them. The armed CD4 T cells synthesize and express interleukin (IL)-2 receptors and release IL-2, which stimulates the cells by autocrine action, causing generation and proliferation of T helper zero (Th0) cells. Autocrine cytokines (e.g., IL-4) cause proliferation of some Th0 cells to produce Th2 cells, which are responsible for the development of antibody-mediated immune responses. These Th2 cells cooperate with and activate B cells to proliferate and give rise eventually to memory B cells *(MB)* and plasma cells *(P)*, which secrete antibodies. Autocrine cytokines (e.g., IL-2) cause proliferation of some Th0 cells to produce Th1 cells, which secrete cytokines that activate macrophages (responsible for some cell-mediated immune reactions). The armed CD8 T cells also synthesize and express IL-2 receptors and release IL-2, which stimulates the cells by autocrine action to proliferate and give rise to cytotoxic T cells. These can kill virally infected cells. IL-2 secreted by CD4+ cells also plays a part in stimulating CD8+ cells to proliferate. Note that the "effector phase" depicted here relates to the "protective" deployment of the immune response. When the response is inappropriately deployed—as in chronic inflammatory conditions such as rheumatoid arthritis—the Th1 wing of the immune response is dominant, and the activated microphages (mφ) release IL-1 and tumor necrosis factor α *(TNF-α)*, which in turn triggers the release of the various chemokines and inflammatory cytokines that have a major role in the pathogenesis of the disease. (From Rang HP, Dale MM, Ritter JM, Moore JL. *Pharmacology.* 5th ed. New York: Churchill Livingstone; 2003.)

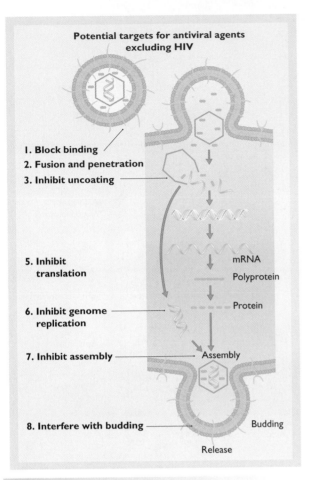

Figure 22-3

Currently available antiviral drugs and their sites of action in the non-HIV replicative cycle. (From Page C, Curtis MJ, Sutter MC, Walker MJ, Hoffman BB, eds. *Integrated Pharmacology.* 2nd ed. Philadelphia: Mosby; 2002.)

Acidification of the virion is necessary for uncoating. Both drugs are used to treat the influenza A virus but have no effect on influenza B and C viruses. Treatment must be initiated within 2 days of the start of illness to be 10% to 27% effective, but it may take at least 4 to 5 more days for the host to shed the virus. In the healthy individual, these drugs decrease flu duration by 1 day, and in the high-risk elderly patient, by 2.5 days.[9] Although a reduction in duration of 1 to 2.5 days does not seem very impressive, for the high-risk unvaccinated patient, these drugs could make a difference in overall morbidity and could significantly shorten a hospital stay. The two drugs are equally effective in the treatment of flu and exhibit a 70% prophylactic efficacy

in unvaccinated patients.[10] However, they are less effective in immunocompromised patients and may even produce resistant viral strains.

Side effects of amantadine and rimantadine are dose related.[11] Amantadine produces some mild reversible central nervous system (CNS) effects such as dizziness, insomnia, orthostatic hypotension, and slurred speech but can also produce livedo reticularis in elderly patients. This drug has high oral bioavailability, which is somewhat of a problem for older patients who have some renal impairment, so dosing must be reduced in this population. This drug also enhances release of dopamine so it has a dopaminergic effect on the CNS and cardiovascular system. Rimantadine is better tolerated, producing only some GI complaints.

Inhibitors of Viral Transcription

Interferons are the antiviral drugs that prevent transcription.[8] There are three classes of interferons—α, β, and γ—but only IFN-α and IFN-β are primary antiviral agents. Their mechanism of action is rather complex, but essentially they bind to cell surface receptors that activate Janus-activated kinases, further activating signal transducers and transcription to produce proteins that enhance cellular resistance. Interferons inhibit virus entry into cells, uncoating, and especially transcription of different viruses by inducing ribosomal enzymes that inhibit viral mRNA.

IFN-α-2a is useful against chronic hepatitis B virus (HBV), hepatitis C virus (HCV), Kaposi's sarcoma caused by human herpes virus 8, and skin conditions associated with human papilloma virus.[11] IFN-α-2b is also effective for human papilloma virus, HBV, and HCV. Commercial preparations of IFN-α are produced by recombinant DNA techniques. They are not orally bioavailable and must be administered either by intramuscular or subcutaneous injection or intravenously. For chronic HBV and HCV, subcutaneous injections three times weekly for 24 to 48 weeks are recommended.

Adverse effects of interferons include a flu-like syndrome, probably caused by the synthesis of interleukin 1.[8] Symptoms will lessen in severity after several weeks of treatment. Myelosuppression (neutropenia and thrombocytopenia), as well as some neurotoxic effects (headache, anxiety, and dizziness), may occur. However, fatigue is quite common and may be profound enough to interfere with physical therapy interventions. Autoimmune responses, primarily the development of auto-antibodies against the thyroid gland and anti-double-stranded DNA, have also been reported with this therapy.[12] Clinical manifestations may include systemic lupus erythematosus and thyroid disease. Depression is also a significant side effect of the interferons.

Ribavirin is a guanosine analog that interferes with viral transcription by preventing elongation of mRNA.[13] Its mechanism of action is similar to that of acyclovir (see discussion of drugs that inhibit viral RNA or DNA replication in that it acts as a chain terminator. It is predominantly used as an aerosol to decrease morbidity in children with respiratory syncytial virus, bronchiolitis, and pneumonia. Oral ribavirin has been used as part of a combination treatment along with IFN-α for hepatitis C (hepatitis C virus). It does not reduce viral load but does reduce fatigue and hepatic inflammation. Intravenous (IV) ribavirin decreases mortality among patients with Lassa fever and hemorrhagic fever associated with the hantavirus. In addition, it is also active against West Nile virus.[14] Because ribavirin accumulates in erythrocytes and produces hemolysis, one of the side effects is anemia. The drug is also carcinogenic and teratogenic in animals.

Drugs that Inhibit Viral RNA or DNA Replication (Chain Terminators)

The prototypic drug that inhibits viral RNA or DNA replication is acyclovir. This drug undergoes intracellular phosphorylation to the active form, acyclovir triphosphate, by using a virus-specific thymidine kinase and then subsequent host enzymes (Figure 22-4). Next, the active drug competes with deoxyguanosine triphosphate for the viral DNA polymerase. The drug becomes incorporated into the growing viral DNA chain, but because it is not a true nucleic acid (lacks a phosphodiester linkage for the next nucleic acid), chain termination occurs (Figure 22-5). Acyclovir and the other drugs in this category (valacyclovir, penciclovir, ganciclovir, and cidofovir) are used to inhibit replication of herpes simplex virus (HSV-1 and HSV-2), varicella zoster virus, cytomegalovirus, and the Epstein-Barr virus.[11] They are somewhat effective for a clinical infection but offer no immunity for a latent infection. They all have slightly different sensitivities for the different viruses; ganciclovir is more effective than acyclovir against cytomegalovirus, and valacyclovir is more effective than acyclovir for the treatment of herpes.

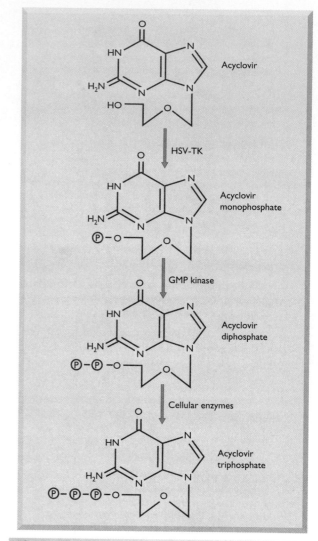

Figure 22-4

Enzymatic conversion of acyclovir to its monophosphate, diphosphate, and triphosphate forms. Herpes simplex virus thymidine kinase *(HSV-TK)* avidly catalyzes the formation of acyclovir monophosphate. Cellular kinases convert the monophosphate to the diphosphate and triphosphate forms. Acyclovir triphosphate is the active antiviral moiety. (From Page C, Curtis MJ, Sutter MC, Walker MJ, Hoffman BB, eds. *Integrated Pharmacology.* 2nd ed. Philadelphia: Mosby; 2002. Adapted from Elion GB. Mechanism of action and selectivity of acyclovir. *Am J Med.* 1982; 20;73[1A]:7-13; Acyclovir Symposium: 7-13, with permission from Excerpta Medica, Inc.)

Valacyclovir is a prodrug of acyclovir with greater bioavailability, which allows a more convenient dosing schedule. For a genital herpes infection, this drug may be given two times a day for 5 days, instead of the more frequent dosing schedule

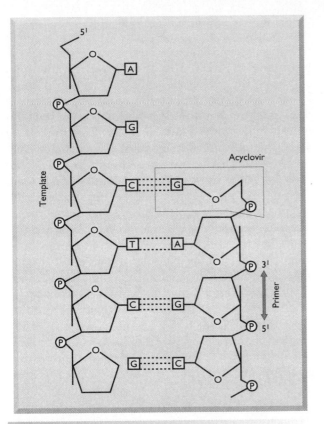

Figure 22-5

Representation of acyclovir triphosphate termination of DNA chain elongation. Absence of the 3'-C molecule on the acyclic ribose molecule precludes formation of the 3'-5'-phosphodiester linkage needed to allow DNA chain elongation. (From Page C, Curtis MJ, Sutter MC, Walker MJ, Hoffman BB, eds. *Integrated Pharmacology.* 2nd ed. Philadelphia: Mosby; 2002. Adapted from Elion GB. Mechanism of action and selectivity of acyclovir. *Am J Med.* 1982; 20;73[1A]:7-13; Acyclovir Symposium: 7-13, with permission from Excerpta Medica, Inc.)

required for acyclovir. It is also approved for once-a-day dosing to suppress frequently recurring herpes infections.

Side effects of acyclovir include neurotoxicity (lethargy, confusion, tremor, and seizures), but this drug is generally well tolerated. Discontinuation of the drug reverses the adverse effects.

Foscarnet is another drug in this category, but it inhibits viral DNA polymerase and HIV reverse transcriptase directly without undergoing any transformations.[8] It binds to and blocks the binding site for viral polymerase. It is a nonnucleoside herpes virus inhibitor because it does not resemble any of the purines or pyrimidines. Foscarnet is

approved for the treatment of cytomegalovirus retinitis in AIDS and acyclovir-resistant HSV infections. Adverse effects include reversible serious organ toxicity, affecting the urinary tract, CNS, and hematological system.

Drugs That Inhibit Viral Release

Zanamivir and oseltamivir inhibit influenza neuraminidase, which is necessary for cleaving the budding virion from its parent cell.[15] They are equally effective for the treatment of influenza A and B viruses, reducing the severity of illness by about 25% to 35% when treatment is initiated within 2 days of the onset of symptoms. They also reduce symptom duration by an average of 0.8 days in otherwise healthy adults and by 1 day in children.[16] In patients older than 65 years or in those who have chronic medical conditions, zanamivir reduced the duration of symptoms by 2.0 days, but oseltamivir only reduced duration by 0.4 day. Postexposure prophylaxis for both drugs is between 70% and 90%. Side effects are nausea and vomiting, but there have also been a few reports of bronchospasm.

Drug Treatment for HIV

HIV is a retrovirus that selectively targets the immune system, particularly the CD4+ T lymphocytes, severely compromising the individual's ability to prevent infection or certain types of cancer. There is currently no cure for this infection, but some drugs can reduce the viral load, giving the immune system a chance to recover function. Without treatment, most patients will die within 2 years after the onset of symptoms.[1] HIV infection is a global health problem, with at least 30 million people worldwide positive for HIV and with epidemic proportions, particularly in sub-Saharan Africa.[17] As of 2001, more than 20 million people had died from this disease, and although drugs are available, they do not reach everyone who needs them. Hence, the infection continues to spread.

Pathophysiology

Two distinct viruses, HIV-1 and HIV-2, actually produce AIDS. HIV-1 is responsible for most of the infections worldwide, but in West Africa, HIV-2 is predominant. The routes of transmission of the two viruses are the same: exchange of bodily fluids through sexual contact, sharing of syringes, exposure to infected blood, and vertical transmission from mother to fetus in utero and from mother to neonate during delivery and through breast milk.

Once infected, a patient may remain free of symptoms for a long time. Initially, the cytotoxic T lymphocytes are recruited to prevent the spread of HIV, mainly by killing the HIV-infected cells. However, a depletion of noninfected T cells occurs as well.[18] Sources of T-cell production also fail, but the exact cause is not known. The virus continues to multiply, producing 10^{10} new particles each day, and many of these particles mutate to a slightly different form. The immune system tries to keep up with the viral load, but eventually the mutated virus escapes detection, the CD4 cell count decreases, and the immune system fails.

Disease Progression and Clinical Signs and Symptoms

There is much variation in the progression and clinical manifestations of AIDS. After exposure to the virus, an initial acute flu-like illness develops, resulting from the increase in HIV particles in the blood and the formation of antibodies.[19] This phase is known as primary HIV infection (Figure 22-6). Symptoms may include fever, diarrhea, arthralgias, headaches, maculopapular rash, and occasionally,

neurological symptoms such as meningitis, neuropathy, or encephalopathy. This syndrome is not specific and thus is rarely recognized as the beginning of AIDS. This is followed by the quiet stage as the cytotoxic cells reduce viral load. However, virus replication continues, silently damaging the lymph nodes and depleting the CD4 lymphocytes and dendritic cells. This period of asymptomatic infection may last as long as 10 years, but eventually, the immune system fails and the signs of AIDS appear. As the disease progresses, the infected patient may demonstrate generalized lymphadenopathy, constitutional symptoms (fever, diarrhea, weight loss), hematological abnormalities (anemia, thrombocytopenia, lymphopenia, and neutropenia), and dermatological problems (dermatitis, candidiasis, and oral hairy leukoplakia).

AIDS is defined by the CD4 cell count and whether the patient has an AIDS-defining condition (opportunistic infection). Manifestations of AIDS are not common with CD4 cell counts above 500 cells/mm³.[20] However, as this count drops, opportunistic infections develop. These infections include but are not limited to tuberculosis, toxoplasmosis, Kaposi's sarcoma, cytomegalovirus, *Pneumocystis carinii* pneumonia, leishmaniasis, and

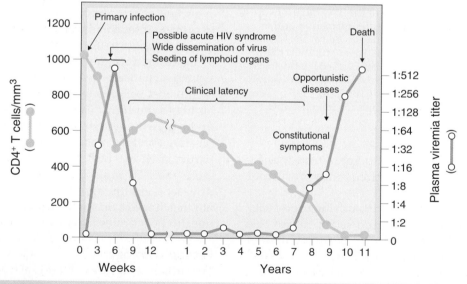

Figure 22-6

Schematic outline of the course of HIV infection. (CD4⁺ T cell titer is often given as cells/mm³, which is equivalent to cells × 10⁶ cells/L. (From Rang HP, Dale MM, Ritter JM, Moore JL. *Pharmacology*. 5th ed. New York: Churchill Livingstone; 2003. Adapted from Pantaleo G, Graziosi C, Fauci AS. New concepts in the immunopathogenesis of human immunodeficiency virus infection. *N Engl J Med*. 1993;328:327-335.)

cryptococcosis. They are more likely to develop when the CD4 cell count drops below 200 cells/mm^3.

Life Cycle of HIV

Several potential targets for anti-HIV drugs have been identified in the viral replication cycle (Figure 22-7).[1] Step 1 in this cycle involves the binding of the virus to the host cell surface receptor. The HIV recognizes the CD4 receptor on helper T lymphocytes and the CCR5 receptor on macrophages and dendritic cells. The surface glycoprotein, gp120, on the HIV envelope binds to these receptors and also to a chemokine co-receptor (CXCR4) on the T cell. After binding, the virion penetrates the cell and uncoats, exposing its RNA. At step 4, the viral RNA is converted to viral DNA by the reverse transcriptase enzyme. The virus draws from the infected cell's supply of deoxynucleosides (thymidine, guanosine, adenosine, and cytidine) to make a double-stranded DNA copy of the viral RNA. The viral DNA can then remain in the cytoplasm or be transported to the nucleus, where the viral DNA is integrated into the host DNA via the integrase enzyme. At step 6, transcription of the host cell's DNA and the viral DNA occurs and is followed by translation and production of viral proteins. The protease enzyme then hydrolyzes the newly formed proteins into smaller units and assembles them with the viral RNA to produce new virions. The last step is budding and release of the new HIV particles.

Antiretroviral Drugs

There are currently three main classes of anti-HIV drugs: nucleoside reverse transcriptase inhibitors, nonnucleoside reverse transcriptase inhibitors, and protease inhibitors (PIs). Effective treatment requires the administration of a combination of these drugs known as highly active antiretroviral therapy (HAART).[21] It is important for patients to understand that these medications do not cure HIV infection, and they should be reminded that while they are taking these drugs, they can still transmit the virus to others. In addition, patients must continue to take these drugs to keep viral load down and to raise CD4 cell counts. Viral rebound in the plasma and seminal fluids occurs after therapy interruption and results in a greater viral load compared with pretreatment viremia after early discontinuation of antiviral therapy (8 to 9 days after the initiation of therapy).[22,23] In one small study, reintroduction of therapy resulted in a reduction

in HIV-RNA, and in 1 to 2 months, approximately 50% of patients had undetectable HIV-RNA levels in plasma.

Nucleotide Reverse Transcriptase Inhibitors

Nucleoside reverse transcriptase inhibitors (NRTIs) were the first group of drugs used to fight HIV infection.[21] The prototypic drug in this category is zidovudine (also known as azidothymidine or AZT). It is a dideoxynucleoside analog that lacks a hydroxyl group that is needed to add bases to the growing DNA strand. The reverse transcriptase enzyme incorporates zidovudine into the growing chain, thus eliminating further elongation. This drug also has an inhibitory effect on the enzyme itself.

Serious side effects are associated with most of the drugs in this category, with the exception of lamivudine, the best-tolerated anti-HIV drug. All of the drugs in this group have the potential to produce a fatal lactic acidosis and have been associated with fat redistribution and hyperlipidemia. Zidovudine causes anemia, neutropenia, myopathy, headaches, and nausea and vomiting. Myelosuppression is a major problem. Didanosine produces pancreatitis, diarrhea, and peripheral neuropathy. Stavudine and zalcitabine are also associated with a high incidence of peripheral neuropathy. However, because HIV produces neuronal injury, including an AIDS dementia, it is often difficult to determine whether this manifestation is disease related or an adverse effect of the drugs.[24,25]

Tenofovir disoproxil fumarate is a fairly new drug that has a slightly different structure than the NRTIs; however, it has similar actions.[21] It is a nucleotide that is a phosphorylated nucleoside. This drug is generally well tolerated, although it produces nausea, vomiting, and diarrhea. The significance of this drug is that it is active against some resistant strains of HIV and is also active against HBV.

Nonnucleoside Reverse Transcriptase Inhibitors

Nonnucleoside reverse transcriptase inhibitors (NNRTIs) inhibit HIV replication by binding to a portion of the reverse transcriptase, which changes the shape of the enzyme, thus directly inactivating it.[21] The drugs that fall within this category include nevirapine, delavirdine, and efavirenz. Combinations of NNRTIs with NRTIs or PIs are at least additive in reducing HIV replication. HIV strains that are resistant to the NRTIs may be sensitive to the NNRTIs. Adverse effects include maculopapular

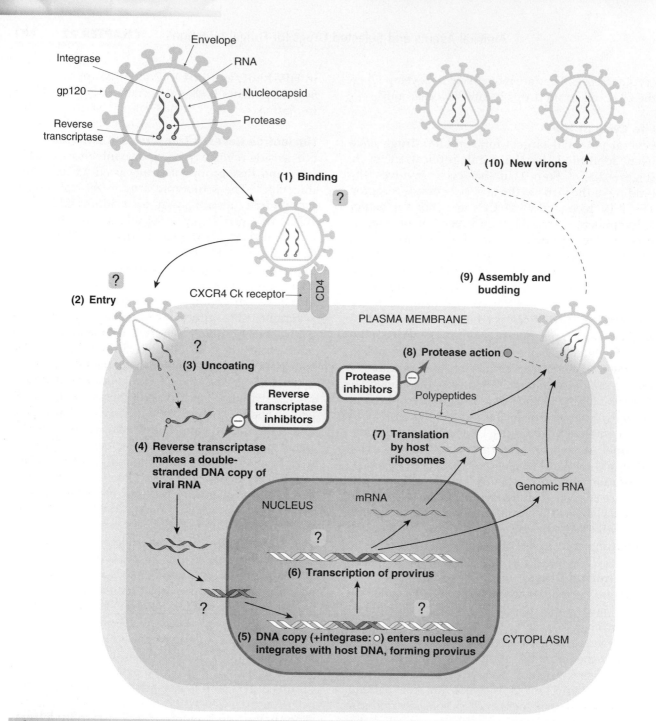

Figure 22-7

Schematic diagram of infection of CD4+ T cell by an HIV virion with the sites of action of the two main classes of drug and sites for possible new drugs. The 10 steps, from attachment to the cell to release of new virions, are shown. The virus uses the CD4 co-receptor and the chemokine (Ck) receptor CXCR4 as binding sites. Step 6, transcription, occurs when the T cell itself is activated; when this happens, transcription factor NF-κB initiates transcription of both host cell DNA and the provirus. Step 8, the action of the viral protease, involves the cleaving of the polypeptides into structural proteins and enzymes (integrase, reverse transcriptase, protease) for the new virion (the protease and thus the protease inhibitors actually act on the immature virions after budding). Sites of action of potential new drugs, each indicated by a question mark, include binding of the virion (by modification of the gp120-CD4 or gp120-CXCR4 interaction), entry of virion, uncoating of virion, translocation of viral complementary DNA into nucleus, integration of viral cDNA into host cell DNA, inhibition of the gene coding for the HIV core protein, inhibition of budding. (From Rang HP, Dale MM, Ritter JM, Moore JL. *Pharmacology.* 5th ed. New York: Churchill Livingstone; 2003.)

rashes that require discontinuation of treatment in about 10% to 20% of patients. In addition, hepatitis and neuropsychiatric symptoms (vivid dreams, nightmares, and hallucinations) have been reported. The CNS effects tend to occur between 1 and 3 hours after each dose but may subside within a few weeks. These drugs are metabolized by the cytochrome P450 enzyme system and therefore have many drug interactions, including a potential for interaction with PIs.

Protease Inhibitors

PIs bind to the protease enzyme of HIV-1 and HIV-2, preventing the breakdown of viral polyprotein into the components needed for viral assembly and budding.[21] The use of a PI in combination with other drugs has led to a marked improvement and prolonged survival, even in patients with advanced HIV infection. In addition, resistance to the PIs requires more mutations for loss of effectiveness than resistance to some other drugs. The drugs in this category include saquinavir, ritonavir, indinavir, nelfinavir, amprenavir, and lopinavir-ritonavir. The principal side effects are GI symptoms and a syndrome of lipodystrophy.[26] This syndrome includes peripheral fat wasting, central obesity, high serum triglyceride and cholesterol levels, and insulin resistance. Because of these side effects, some physicians treating patients with AIDS discuss heart disease and myocardial infarctions as new complications of HIV disease. Studies are ongoing to determine whether antidiabetic drugs could reduce lipodystrophy, but so far, they have not been useful.[27] However, some studies have demonstrated improvement in insulin levels when an NNRTI was substituted for a PI.[28]

Fusion Inhibition

Enfuvirtide is the first in a new class of HIV drugs that bind to the surface glycoprotein on the viral envelope, preventing fusion of the virus to the host cell. This drug, when given to patients already receiving a standard HIV protocol, resulted in a lowered viral load and higher CD4 cell counts compared with the protocol alone.[29] Almost all patients receiving this drug have local injection-site reactions consisting of mild to moderate pain, erythema, induration, and cysts. Other effects include eosinophilia and an increase in bacterial pneumonia.

Use of Antiretrovirals in Pregnancy

In European nations and the United States, the use of HAART in pregnant women has lowered the rate of mother-to-child transmission of HIV-1 from 25% to 1% to 2%.[30] However, in poorer countries where HAART is not available and breast-feeding and vaginal deliveries are standard practice (both of which facilitate transmission), mother-to-child transmission is a major component of the AIDS epidemic.[31]

Zidovudine is typically used during pregnancy to reduce transmission of HIV to the infant. When started at 14 to 32 weeks' gestation and continued in the neonate for 6 weeks after delivery, transmission is reduced from 26% to 8% globally.[21] This 8% is higher than what was reported in the previous paragraph because of the breast-feeding practices and lack of medications in developing nations, which lead to an overall risk of transmission at 18 to 24 months as high as 15% to 25%. For added protection, many clinicians are now offering zidovudine plus another NRTI and a PI. Single-dose nevirapine or single-dose lamivudine along with a short course of zidovudine (from weeks 32 to 36 of pregnancy) have shown the highest efficacy among women with CD4 cell counts of $200/mm^3$ or less and viral loads of at least 2500 HIV-1 RNA copies/mL.[32] If infection is not detected until delivery, nevirapine can be administered to the mother during labor, and then zidovudine and nevirapine can be subsequently given to the infant for effective reduction in transmission.[33]

Combination Therapy for HIV

Potent combination drug regimens have proved to be the most efficacious approach to the treatment of HIV. Standard therapy for HIV infection requires at least a three-drug regimen. The goal of using multiple drugs is to stop the replication of the virus at a number of different steps in its reproductive cycle. It has also been found that administering just one or two drugs increases the chance of developing drug resistance. In fact, most resistance to treatment is due to partial suppression of the virus rather than acquisition of a resistant form.[34] In the United States, 50% of patients are resistant to at least one drug.[35] Combination therapy has also been found to be much more effective for reducing viral load than sequential administration of the same drugs.

The most common regimens are as follows:
1. Two NRTIs + one PI
2. Two NRTIs + one NNRTI
3. Two NRTIs + ritonavir + another PI (Ritonavir has been added to this protocol because it has been found to act as a PI enhancer.)[36]

Of these protocols, the one that appears to be most effective at this time is two NRTIs with one NNRTI, specifically use of zidovudine, lamivudine, and efavirenz.[37] Addition of a fourth drug has the potential to increase potency of the regimen but may also be associated with increased toxic effects. The addition of a fourth drug may also reduce adherence to the drug routine and limit future treatment options if resistance develops, because many of the drugs are cross-resistant within the same category. A four-drug regimen compared with the three-drug regimen of zidovudine, lamivudine, and efavirenz was not significantly different in terms of the length of time to failure, defined as an increase in viral load or viral rebound.[38] However, it is clear that much more work is necessary to determine the optimal protocol for controlling viral load.

The optimal time to begin therapy with the available anti-HIV drugs has not yet been determined.[20,39] At one time, some clinicians were waiting until the CD4 cell count dropped below 200 cells/mm^3, and others began therapy when the count was at 500 cells/mm^3. Fear of developing resistance was the main factor in waiting until the CD4 cell count was at a critical level, which is 200 cells/mm^3. It was believed that if a patient developed resistance to the drugs early in the disease, there would be no medications left to try when the illness became critical. Treatment is now begun earlier, when the CD4 cell count drops to 350 cells/mm^3 or when opportunistic infections develop. Other factors that determine when to initiate therapy include willingness of the patient to start and adhere to therapy, drug toxicity, pill burden, dosing schedule, sensitivity of the particular strain of HIV to treatment, and drug-drug interactions.

Once the patient begins the treatment regimen, viral load and CD4 cell counts should be tested. It is recommended that viral load testing be performed 2 to 8 weeks after therapy is started and then every 4 to 6 months throughout treatment.[40] CD4 cell counts should be done every 3 to 6 months throughout therapy. This count should increase, or at least not decrease, while the patient is taking medication.

If the level decreases, it may mean that the drugs are not working and there is "regimen failure."

There are three types of regimen failure: virologic failure in which the virus is still detected in the blood 48 weeks after the start of treatment or virus that was originally undetected becomes apparent; immunological failure, which reflects decreases in CD4 cell count; and clinical failure, indicating that physical health is deteriorating or the patient has acquired an HIV-related infection.[40] Virologic failure is most common, and patients who maintain their present drug regimen despite this development usually experience immunological failure within 3 years.

Therapeutic Concerns

Therapy protocols for HIV are very difficult to follow. Some of the drugs must be taken with food, some must be taken either 1 hour before meals or 2 hours after, and some must be taken with large amounts of water.[21] In addition, some of the protocols require taking a large number of pills at one time. The full dose of amprenavir requires swallowing 16 capsules daily, and the dose of saquinavir may require as many as 18 pills per day. Many of the capsules are large and difficult to swallow, particularly if the patient has mucosal ulcers or oral candidiasis. The drugs may also need to be mixed or crushed. Didanosine must be chewed or crushed and mixed with water. It is a full-time job to keep track of when and how these drugs must be administered. When you add this to the adverse effects—particularly the severe nausea, vomiting, and diarrhea—it is not surprising that patients have trouble being compliant with the program. In clinical studies, these drugs are effective in reducing viral load and raising CD4 cell counts. However, when patients continue to take the drugs without the benefit of close supervision afforded by a clinical trial, many become noncompliant, and viral loads begin to climb. In one study, only about half of the patients took all antiretroviral medication as directed in terms of timing and dietary instructions during a preceding week.[41] Patients who reported compliance issues were less likely to have HIV-1 RNA levels below 500 copies/mL, approximately four times higher than those of compliant patients. It is suggested that initially patients practice following their drug regimen with jelly beans or mints to determine ahead of time if the regimen chosen for them is doable.[40] Other suggestions to improve compliance include sorting the drugs into a pill box, using a timer or alarm clock to signal when it is time to take medications, and keeping a medication diary in which the patient can write the names of the drugs and then later check off each dose as it is administered.

A physical therapist may see patients with HIV because of some virus-related events, as well as drug-related events, especially peripheral neuropathies. The therapist needs to be sensitive to the patient's drug regimen when arranging therapy so that it does not interfere with his or her medication schedule.

Hepatitis B

Hepatitis B is a major viral infection. There are more than 350 million chronic carriers of HBV worldwide, and HBV causes 1 million deaths yearly.[42] If untreated or unresponsive to therapy, chronic HBV infection leads to cirrhosis of the liver and hepatocellular carcinoma. An HBV vaccine has been developed, but this prophylactic treatment is unavailable to many.

Hepatitis B Virus

HBV is transmitted through blood and other bodily secretions and is 100 times more infectious than HIV.[43] HBV can remain alive outside the body in dried blood for more than 1 week. In the United States, transmission of the virus primarily occurs though sexual contact or IV drug use; but in Southeast Asia, China, and in sub-Saharan Africa, hepatitis is primarily transmitted from mother to child in the perinatal period. Progression to chronic HBV occurs in 25% to 30% of children and in 3% to 5% of adults.

HBV consists of double-stranded circular DNA enclosed in a nucleocapsid (core antigen), which is surrounded by an envelope (surface antigen).[43] The entire virus is also known as the Dane particle. HBV infects hepatocytes, and when it enters the nucleus, the genome encodes a DNA polymerase that also acts as a reverse transcriptase enzyme. The DNA provides a template for mRNA, which then undergoes transcription to produce other viral proteins including a "pre-genomic" RNA. The HBV genome also produces a circulating protein called *the e antigen* that correlates with high viral replication and provides a useful laboratory marker for active disease.

Signs and Symptoms

Infection with HBV produces nausea, fatigue, low-grade fever, elevated liver transaminase levels, and right upper quadrant pain or epigastric pain. Jaundice may also be present. Extrahepatic signs include myalgias, arthralgias, and urticaria. Symptoms do not occur immediately after exposure but have an incubation period of 1 to 4 months. In most cases the host immune system can control the infection, and the illness resolves. However, some patients have chronic HBV infection. In addition, about 1% of acute infections develop quickly into fulminant hepatic failure.

Chronic disease is defined as seropositivity for HBV surface antigen for more than 6 months, HBV DNA levels >100,000 copies/mL, persistent elevation in liver enzyme levels, and detection of necrosis on a liver biopsy specimen. Asymptomatic carriers are seropositive for HBV surface antigen and seronegative for hepatitis B e antigen (HBeAg) and have lower levels of HBV DNA (<100,000 copies/mL). Patients who demonstrate resolution of the illness are seropositive for antibody B and seronegative for HBsAg.

Drug Treatment for Chronic Hepatitis B

Drugs for HBV fall mainly into two categories: immune modulators (IFN-α-2a and IFN-α-2b) and those that inhibit HBV replication (lamivudine and adefovir dipivoxil). The goals of therapy include lowering viral load and preventing end-stage liver disease. Rarely is drug treatment curative.

IFN-α-2b was approved as therapy for chronic HBV in 1992.[43] It appears to have the most success in patients who have low HBV DNA levels, elevated liver enzyme levels without fibrosis of the liver, and no HIV co-infection. Overall, approximately 46% of subjects who are treated with IFN-α-2b seroconvert from HBeAg to the antibody within the first year after treatment. However, a small percentage of these patients will lose their HBeAg seronegativity over time and have further liver damage. An additional meta-analysis of 16 randomized, controlled trials showed that seroconversion occurred in 33% of IFN-treated patients compared with 12% in the control group.[44] Long-term follow-up of IFN-treated patients demonstrated a 5-year survival rate of 95% in those who seroconverted but less than 50% in those patients who were still seropositive for HBeAg.[45] So even though interferons are quite helpful for a certain subset of patients with hepatitis B, many individuals do not benefit from this treatment. There are also patients who must stop taking the drug because its side effects: the flu-like symptoms, mood alterations, thyroid abnormalities, bone marrow suppression, and excessive fatigue. In addition, the rigorous dosing schedule of 5 million units injected subcutaneously daily or 10 million units injected three times per week for 16 weeks is difficult to tolerate. In some cases, dosing lasts a full year. Regular follow-up is still needed after seroconversion to monitor liver enzyme levels and viral load.

Lamivudine is another first-line treatment for chronic hepatitis B. It was briefly discussed earlier as a drug for HIV but was also approved for treatment of hepatitis B in 1999. The drug inhibits the reverse transcriptase action of the DNA polymerase. Advantages over interferons include a more rapid response, oral administration, and a good tolerability profile with few adverse effects. The disadvantages of this drug include uncertainty about the durability of HBeAg seroconversion and the development of lamivudine-resistant strains. The 3-year relapse rate has varied between 38% and 77%.[46]

Adefovir dipivoxil is the third drug approved for the treatment of chronic HBV.[47] It has action similar to that of lamivudine in that it inhibits the DNA reverse transcriptase action. It was approved for use in 2002, so there are few long-term data on efficacy or safety. However, in the short run, this drug may rival IFN in its efficacy and surpasses IFN in its safety. Adverse reactions have been described as being no different from those that occur with placebo.[48] In addition, this drug shows efficacy in lamivudine-resistant infections. The drug is administered orally for 48 weeks and demonstrates improved liver histologic findings in approximately 28% of patients who are HBeAg-seropositive compared with placebo. Even though drug therapy for patients with chronic hepatitis is available, the percentage of patients for whom drug therapy has long-term efficacy is not ideal.

Hepatitis C

There are more than 170 million chronic carriers of hepatitis C worldwide.[49] Because this virus is extremely robust, with more than 85% of those infected developing chronic infection, it has become a major health concern. Transmission occurs mostly through the blood-borne route (blood transfusions,

organ transplants, and IV drug use). Like HBV, chronic infection with HCV is associated with liver cirrhosis and hepatocellular carcinoma. HCV is also associated with some autoimmune diseases including arthritis and glomerulonephritis, and it has been linked to diabetes mellitus, neuropathy, lymphoma, Sjögren's syndrome, and mixed cryoglobulinemia.

Hepatitis C Virus

HCV is an RNA virus that targets hepatocytes and possibly B lymphocytes.[49] It is a rapidly replicating virus producing 10^{10} to 10^{12} copies per day. Replication occurs by an RNA-dependent RNA polymerase that lacks the ability to detect and repair mutations, so that at any one time, an individual may have several forms of HCV. More than 90 genotypes have been identified and distributed into six main types numbered from 1 to 6.[50] Subtypes are further identified by lowercase letters, starting with a, b, c, and so on. In fact, variability within a region of gene that codes for nonstructural proteins has significance, particularly in Japan where many individuals have this isolate called *subtype 1b*.[51] Unfortunately, this subtype confers resistance to IFN-α-2b.

The HCV encodes a single chain of 3011 amino acids, which then becomes 10 structural and regulatory proteins. The structural components include the core and two envelope proteins. The envelope has a specialized region for binding to the CD81 marker expressed on hepatocytes and B lymphocytes. HCV also encodes a virus-specific helicase, protease, and polymerase for replication. All of these structures represent potential targets for drug therapy, but successful treatment has been difficult to achieve.

Signs and Symptoms

Like HBV, diagnosis of HCV in the acute phase of infection is not common.[52] Symptoms usually occur within 7 to 8 weeks after infection, but many patients have either no symptoms or only mild complaints. When there are symptoms, they are usually nausea, jaundice, and general malaise. Acute infection will lead to chronic disease in 74% to 86% of patients. Chronic infection leads to hepatic fibrosis and some nonspecific symptoms such as fatigue. Once the infection becomes chronic, a reduction in viral load is unlikely. It may take 30 or more years to develop fulminant liver disease, but at least one third of patients become seriously ill in less than 20 years after infection. Progression of the disease depends on alcohol intake, co-infection with HIV, male sex, and an older age at the time of infection.

Drug Treatment of HCV

Even though drug treatment has yielded disappointing results, the National Institutes of Health recommends that all patients with chronic HCV be considered candidates for drug treatment. Factors that need to be taken into consideration are comorbid illness that would make drug treatment more dangerous, patient motivation, and HCV genotype. Treatment of HCV genotype 1 has a success rate of only 40% to 50%, but patients with HCV type 2 or 3 have a 70% to 80% treatment success rate, meaning that they are asymptomatic and have minimal hepatic damage.

In 1989, the first cases of HCV successfully treated with IFN-α were reported with great enthusiasm.[52] However, it quickly became apparent that there was a high rate of relapse. Later, it was shown that a combination of IFN-α-2b with ribavirin for 24 or 48 weeks resulted in normalization of liver enzyme levels and a loss of HCV RNA in 30% to 50% of previously untreated patients.[53] The treatment response depended on the viral genotype, with genotype 1 being more resistant to treatment. Genotype 1 was found to require 1 year of treatment instead of 6 months. About half of the patients who experienced relapse after monotherapy with IFN had success with the combination of IFN-α-2b and ribivarin.[54]

The success rate of drug therapy for HCV has recently been improved by the attachment of polyethylene glycol to IFN-α (called *peginterferon alfa*).[55-57] It has been found that this alteration in drug structure extends its duration of action. Peginterferon alfa is given only once a week at a dose that is calculated based on the patient's weight. Studies evaluating the combination of peginterferon with ribavirin are ongoing. Side effects of combination therapy are similar to those of IFN-α and include a flu-like syndrome, depression, alopecia, bone marrow depression, erythema at injection sites, cough, and ribavirin-induced anemia.

A combination of factors leads to the failure of IFN-ribavirin treatment to eradicate HCV and includes the genotype of the virus, the presence of marked liver disease, alcohol intake, co-infection, and the remarkable ability of the virus to withstand rigorous treatment.[58] It is likely that the problem in finding successful treatment for hepatitis has to do with our own lack of understanding about how this virus infects host cells and what strategies it uses to resist drug treatment. Much additional research is needed in this area.

Therapeutic Concerns with Antiviral Agents

Most individuals taking antiviral medication may be coping with a serious chronic illness. Constitutional symptoms, particularly of fatigue and general malaise, will affect a patient's performance in physical therapy. These symptoms may be exacerbated by drug therapy, particularly with the interferons because they produce flu-like symptoms. However, these symptoms do respond to acetaminophen and symptom-modified activity, and they do disappear with continued drug treatment.

Myelosuppression causing anemia may be caused by antiviral agents or by the illnesses themselves. In either case, it affects exercise performance. Hemoglobin levels tend to be reduced in patients with HIV, which in turn reduces maximal oxygen uptake and induces an earlier lactic acidosis threshold.[59] This higher lactate level is observed at lower exercise intensities, leading to hyperventilation and the sensation of dyspnea. Similar expectations are present for chronic hepatitis.

In terms of the effect of exercise on viral load, there is evidence that prolonged intense training may impair some immune functions, such as neutrophil function, immunoglobulin levels, and NK cell cytotoxic activity.[60] Therefore the viral load would be expected to increase during periods of intense workouts. These parameters have not been seen to increase with moderate exercise. Regardless, patients with chronic infections need regular monitoring of their viral load and immune function. It is also recommended that persons with chronic hepatitis keep a record of their liver transaminase levels along with their activity levels and be prepared to reduce exercise intensity if these become elevated.[61] Participation in either contact or semicontact sports will also need to be limited if the patient has any palpable hepatomegaly or splenomegaly, and those patients who have rather severe cirrhotic disease with ascites, jaundice, edema, bleeding varices, hypersplenism, or coagulopathy will only be able to participate in a very low level of activity.

Because many of the viral infections are transmitted through blood and secretions, therapists need to take appropriate measures to prevent transmission of pathogens during physical therapy intervention. Caring properly for exposed skin lesions and making sure equipment is disinfected after use is important. Following "standard precautions" guidelines is mandatory.

DRUGS AND FUNGAL INFECTIONS

Most fungi that cause human infection produce relatively minor or superficial infections. A fungal infection, particularly in the cool and temperate climatic zones, is usually athlete's foot or an oral or vaginal yeast infection.[1] These are somewhat bothersome infections but hardly life-threatening. However, in the last 20 years, there has been an upsurge of some serious systemic fungal infections so that a discussion of antifungal agents is necessary. The spread of fungal diseases has increased in large part because of pervasive use of broad-spectrum antimicrobials, which eliminate bacteria (nonpathogenic) that compete with fungi. Another reason for the growth of fungal infections is the impaired immunity seen in AIDS or produced by immunosuppressive and chemotherapeutic agents. Fungal infections are also more common in the elderly, patients with diabetes, pregnant women, and those who have sustained a burn injury.[62,63]

Fungal infections are known as mycoses and can be divided into superficial infections affecting the skin, nails, or mucous membranes and systemic infections affecting major organ systems.[1] Superficial fungal infections include dermatomycoses and candidiasis. Dermatomycoses are most commonly caused by *Trichophyton, Microsporum,* and *Epidermophyton* and produce various types of ringworm (tinea) (Table 22-1). Tinea cruris affects the groin, tinea pedis affects the feet, and tinea capitis affects the scalp. Superficial candidiasis is caused by a yeast-like organism that infects the mucous membranes, leading to oral thrush (mouth), vaginal candidiasis, or infection of the skin (diaper rash).

Serious systemic fungal diseases include cryptococcal meningitis, endocarditis pulmonary aspergillosis, blastomycosis, histoplasmosis, and coccidiomycosis. The last three are considered to be primary infections, meaning that they are not a result of immunosuppression.

Characteristics of Fungi

Approximately 50 species of fungi can cause human infection. Fungi are considered to be plantlike parasitic microorganisms. These plants lack chlorophyll and therefore cannot make their own food. They also lack leaves, true stems, and roots. Fungi reproduce by means of spores, but the reproductive process is not completely understood.

The first encounter that the fungi have with the human host is at the plant's cell wall. The cell wall of most fungi consists of glycoproteins embedded within a polysaccharide scaffolding.[64] Carbohydrate groups on the exterior cell wall are presumed to be the first structures to make contact with the host cell. It is hoped that further study of the carbohydrate groups will help in the development of a drug to prevent attachment of the fungi to the host cell. At present, the antifungal agents attempt to disrupt the internal milieu of the fungal cell by punching a hole through the cell wall.

Antifungal Agents

Only a few antifungal agents are currently available. The main reason for this is that high concentrations of the drugs are needed to kill the fungi, yet these concentrations usually cannot be tolerated by the patient. The three main classes of antifungal drugs are polyene macrolides, antifungal azoles, and allylamines. A few other miscellaneous agents are also used to treat fungal infections.

Polyene Macrolide Antibiotics

Amphotericin B is one of the original antifungal agents, developed in the 1950s. It binds to ergosterol and then produces a channel in the fungal cell membrane (Figure 22-8). This opening allows potassium and magnesium ions to flow out of the cell, leading to cell death. Ergosterol is a substance similar to cholesterol in humans and is a major constituent in the fungi cell wall. Amphotericin B has high affinity for the cell wall of fungi and some protozoa but not for mammalian cells or bacteria because cholesterol is the main sterol in the membrane of human cells.

Amphotericin B is considered a broad-spectrum agent and the drug of choice for treatment of severe systemic fungal infections.[65] It is available in parenteral, topical, and oral forms. Topical forms are used for oral or cutaneous candidiasis. Oral

Table 22-1

Mycotic Infections

Mycosis	Fungus	Endemic Location	Reservoir	Transmission	Primary Tissue Affected
SYSTEMIC INFECTION					
Aspergillosis	*Aspergillus* spp.	Universal	Soil	Inhalation	Lungs
Blastomycosis	*Blastomyces dermatitidis*	North America	Soil, animal droppings	Inhalation	Lungs
Coccidioidomycosis	*Coccidioides immitis*	Southwestern United States	Soil, dust	Inhalation	Lungs
Cryptococcosis	*Cryptococcus neoformans*	Universal	Soil, pigeon droppings	Inhalation	Lungs/meninges of brain
Histoplasmosis	*Histoplasma capsulatum*	Universal	Soil, bird and chicken droppings	Inhalation	Lungs
CUTANEOUS INFECTION					
Candidiasis	*Candida abicans*	Universal	Humans	Direct contact, nonsusceptible antibiotic overgrowth	Mucous membrane/skub disseminated (may be systemic)
Dermatophytes, tinea	*Epidermophyton* spp., *Microsporum* spp., *Trichophyton* spp.	Universal	Humans	Direct and indirect contact with infected persons	Scalp, skin
SUPERFICIAL INFECTION					
Tinea versicolor	*Malassezia furfur*	Universal	Humans	Unknown*	Skin

From Lilley LL, Harrington S, Snyder JS. *Pharmacology and the Nursing Process*. 4th ed. St Louis: Mosby; 2005.
Malassezia spp. are a usual part of the normal human flora and appear to cause infection in only select individuals.

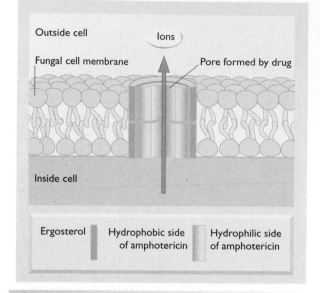

Outside cell

Ions

Fungal cell membrane

Pore formed by drug

Inside cell

| Ergosterol | Hydrophobic side of amphotericin | Hydrophilic side of amphotericin |

Figure 22-8

Mechanism of action of polyene antifungal agents. Binding to ergosterol damages the membrane with leakage of ions and irreversible fungal cell damage. (From Page C, Curtis MJ, Sutter MC, Walker MJ, Hoffman BB, eds. *Integrated Pharmacology.* 2nd ed. Philadelphia: Mosby; 2002. Adapted with permission from Brody T, Larner J, Minneman KP. *Human Pharmacology: Molecular to Clinical.* St Louis,: Mosby; 1994.)

formulations tend to be used for infections in the GI tract because this form of the drug is poorly absorbed and thus mostly stays in the GI tract near the site of infection. IV amphotericin is used for systemic fungal infections such as candidiasis, cryptococcosis, aspergillosis, and blastomycosis. The IV formulation is complexed with sodium deoxycholate, which causes significant side effects. There is an ongoing search for an improved formulation or a different delivery system.[66]

Side effects of amphotericin B include renal toxicity; impaired hepatic function; thrombocytopenia; and infusion-related effects such as tachycardia, chills, fever, tinnitus, and headache.[67] In addition, about one in five patients experience vomiting. For some infections, daily IV treatment is needed, sometimes lasting for a period of 6 to 12 weeks. The drug is also very irritating to the endothelium of veins, sometimes resulting in thrombophlebitis after injection. Pretreatment with acetaminophen, antihistamines, and antiemetics may be provided to decrease these infusion-related side effects and make the duration of treatment

more tolerable. The newer formulations, lipid-complexed agents, produce fewer complications. In addition to some of the annoying adverse effects of this drug, the renal toxicity is the most common and also the most significant. Nearly 80% of patients treated with this drug experience renal impairment. Even after the drug is discontinued, impairment of glomerular filtration may remain.

Nystatin is another polyene macrolide antibiotic, similar in structure to amphotericin, and it has the same mechanism of action.[65] Because it is poorly absorbed, its use is limited to *Candida* infections of the skin and GI tract. Oral administration may cause nausea, vomiting, diarrhea, and cramps, and topical application can lead to rash and urticaria. It is available as a lozenge for treatment of oral candidiasis

Antifungal Azoles

The azoles inhibit ergosterol synthesis and interfere with the action of membrane-associated enzymes. They are a group of synthetic fungistatic agents with broad-spectrum activity. Ketoconazole, fluconazole, itraconazole, miconazole—and the newest azole— voriconazole are mainly administered orally, although fluconazole and voriconazole are also available in IV forms. Miconazole and clotrimazole are available in topical forms for use in the treatment of vaginal yeast infections.

Ketoconazole is a prototypic agent in this category, and it is used for serious chronic resistant mucocutaneous candidiasis, dermatophyte infections, and systemic infections, with the exception of fungal meningitis. Adverse effects include nausea, vomiting, photophobia, cardiac dysrhythmias, rashes, hepatotoxicity, gynecomastia, and menstrual irregularities. The azoles also inhibit the P450 enzymes and, in particular, increase plasma concentrations of phenytoin, oral hypoglycemics, anticoagulants, and cyclosporine.

Allylamines

Terbinafine also inhibits ergosterol synthesis by a different mechanism than the azoles. It is available as a topical cream, a gel, and a spray for the treatment of tinea pedis, tinea cruris, and tinea corporis. An oral formulation is available and is a popular mode for treating onychomycosis of the fingernails or toenails. It is quite lipophilic and therefore becomes concentrated in the dermis, epidermis, hair follicles, and adipose tissue within a few hours after oral administration. It enters the nail beds and distal nails, but this takes a few weeks. Treatment for 6 weeks is required for fingernail infections, and 12 weeks is needed for the toenails. After the drug is withdrawn, antifungicidal concentrations remain for several more weeks, reducing the chance for relapse. In a large clinical trial on onychomycosis and in a meta-analysis of randomized clinical trials, terbinafine demonstrated superior effectiveness compared with some other antifungal agents, including itraconazole.[68-70] Terbinafine also shows high efficacy in patients with high-risk conditions such as diabetes and those awaiting organ transplantation. In the treatment of tinea capitis, terbinafine was as effective in 4 weeks as griseofulvin (see discussion of other antifungal agents) was in 8 weeks.[71] The drug also works well when given in pulsed doses for this condition. (Pulsed dosing is administration of the drug for 1 week, followed by 3 weeks without administration.) The cycle is repeated until infection clears.[72] Side effects of terbinafine are mild but may include nausea, abdominal pain, and less commonly, elevated liver enzyme levels. This drug is well tolerated, which is especially important, given the very long duration of treatment.

Other Antifungal Agents

Griseofulvin is an oral, narrow-spectrum agent that acts by interfering with mitosis. It has been used to treat dermatophyte infections of the skin and nails and is the preferred agent for tinea capitis in children.[73] However, this drug is far from ideal. Tinea capitis requires treatment for 6 to 12 weeks, and some nail infections (tinea unguium, a dermatophyte infection of the nail) may require treatment for 12 to 24 months. In addition, relapse rates are high because the drug clears rapidly from the skin once it is discontinued.

Flucytosine is another antifungal agent that is effective mostly against those infections caused by yeast.[67] Resistance is common with monotherapy, so it is often combined with amphotericin, particularly for cryptococcal meningitis. In fungal cells, flucytosine is converted to fluorouracil, which inhibits DNA synthesis. It is available in either an oral or IV form. Infrequent adverse effects include GI disturbances, bone marrow depression, and alopecia.

Caspofungin is a new drug in a new category of antifungal agents called *echinocandins*.[74,75] Caspofungin acts by inhibiting the synthesis of 1,3 β-glucan, a glucose polymer that is an important constituent in the fungal cell wall. It is effective against candidiasis and some resistant forms of aspergillosis. It is administered intravenously once per day. Adverse effects are generally mild and reversible and include fatigue, vomiting, flushing, hypokalemia, eosinophilia, and proteinuria.

Amorolfine is another new antifungal agent formulated as a nail lacquer for dermatophytes. It interferes with fungal sterol synthesis. Although application is easy, monotherapy with amorolfine is not nearly as effective as treatment with the azoles. However, when amorolfine was combined with itraconazole, a greater mycological cure (but not statistically significant) was attained compared with itraconazole alone.[76]

Therapeutic Concerns

The main therapeutic concerns with antifungal agents are elevated serum transaminase levels and renal damage. These concerns are especially important if patients are taking amphotericin B. An easy way to watch for renal impairment is to have patients weigh themselves weekly and document a gain of more than 2 lb. Rapid weight gain may indicate retention of fluid cause by renal impairment.

Another general concern is the length of time required for treatment. Many patients take antifungal agents from 6 months to a year or longer, depending on the type of infection they have and their immune status. Continued motivation and diligence are often necessary for patients to complete the therapeutic protocol. Individuals who require IV medications spend a considerable amount of time with an infusion pump. The therapist must be sensitive to the psychosocial issues that may develop as a result of prolonged treatment and the impact it has on lifestyle.

ACTIVITIES 22

■ 1. You are treating a patient with HIV for complaints of lower-extremity weakness associated with muscle wasting. The patient has a CD4 cell count of 250 cells/mm³ and is currently taking a three-drug regimen consisting of zidovudine, lamivudine, and efavirenz.

Questions

a. What are the side effects of these drugs?
b. Outline the patient's drug schedule.
c. When is the best time of day to schedule physical therapy services?
d. What red flags should you look for that warrant a call to the physician.
e. Are there any physical therapy interventions that should be avoided when treating this patient?

■ 2. The following are case vignettes of patients with HCV infection. Discuss therapeutic options for each patient.

Questions

a. Mr. England is a 40-year-old man who contracted HCV infection more than 20 years ago, probably during a period of drug use. He has received treatment for his addictions and has been clean and sober for the last 15 years. He reports feeling fatigue but has no other specific complaints. A biopsy specimen of his liver shows moderate inflammation and fibrosis (3 on a 4-point scale, with 0 being no fibrosis and 4 being cirrhosis).

b. Mr. Jones is a 45-year-old construction worker who just found out he is infected with HCV. He consumes large quantities of alcohol daily and has been in an alcohol detoxification unit at least two times in the past year. He refuses to go to AA meetings. He also admits to having multiple sex partners, many of whom were prostitutes during drinking binges. A liver biopsy specimen shows moderate inflammation, level 3 fibrosis.

c. Ms. Snowden is a 35-year-old single mother of two young children. She contracted HCV (genotype 2) years ago in her teens from a blood transfusion. After years of being asymptomatic, she now complains of extreme fatigue and nausea. Her medical history is significant for chronic depression that is currently being treated with a selective serotonin reuptake inhibitor. Her liver biopsy specimen shows only minimal inflammation. She also works in the housekeeping department of a local hospital and has no family close by.

References

1. Rang HP, Dale MM, Ritter JM, Moore JL. *Pharmacology.* 5th ed. New York: Churchill Livingstone; 2003.
2. Smith AE, Helenius A. How viruses enter animal cells. *Science.* 2004;304(5668):237-242.
3. Alberts B, Bray D, Lewis J, Raff M, Roberts K, Watson JD. *Molecular Biology of the Cell.* New York: Garland Publishing, Inc.; 1989.
4. Guidotti LG, Chisari FV. Noncytolytic control of viral infections by the innate and adaptive immune response. *Annu Rev Immunol.* 2001;19:65-91.
5. Biron CA, Nguyen KB, Pien GC, Cousens LP, Salazar-Mather TP. Natural killer cells in antiviral defense: function and regulation by innate cytokines. *Annu Rev Immunol.* 1999;17:189-220.
6. Tortorella D, Gewurz BE, Furman MH, Schust DJ, Ploegh HL. Viral subversion of the immune system. *Annu Rev Immunol.* 2000;18:861-926.
7. Polster BM, Pevsner J, Hardwick JM. Viral Bcl-2 homologs and their role in virus replication and associated diseases. *Biochim Biophys Acta.* 2004;1644(2-3):211-227.
8. Aoki FY, Rosser S. Drugs and viruses. In: Page C, Curtis MJ, Sutter MC, Walker MJ, Hoffman BB, eds. *Integrated Pharmacology.* 2nd ed. Philadelphia: Mosby; 2002.
9. Rothberg MB, Bellantonia S, Rose DN. Management of influenza in adults older than 65 years of age: cost-effectiveness of rapid testing and antiviral therapy. *Ann Intern Med.* 2003;139(5):321-329.
10. Couch RB. Prevention and treatment of influenza. *N Engl J Med.* 2000;343(24):1778-1787.
11. Balfour HH. Antiviral drugs. *N Engl J Med.* 1999; 340(16):1255-1268.
12. Krause I, Valesini G, Scrivo R, Shoenfeld Y. Autoimmune aspects of cytokine and anticytokine therapies. *Am J Med.* 2003;115(5):390-397.
13. Drugs for non-HIV viral infections. *Med Letter Drugs Ther.* 2002;44(1126):28.

14. Jordan I, Briese T, Fischer N, Johnson YL, Lipkin WI. Ribavirin inhibits West Nile virus replication and cytopathic effect in neural cells. *J Infect Dis*. 2000; 182:1214-1218.

15. Garman E, Laver G. Controlling influenza by inhibiting the virus's neuraminidase. *Curr Drug Targets*. 2004; 5(2):119-136.

16. Cooper NJ, Sutton AJ, Abrams KR, Wailoo A, Turner D, Nicholson KG. Effectiveness of neuraminidase inhibitors in treatment and prevention of influenza A and B: systematic review and meta-analyses of randomised controlled trials. *BMJ*. 2003;326(7401):1235.

17. Grant AD, De Cock K. HIV infection and AIDS in the developing world. *BMJ*. 2001;322:1475-1478.

18. McCune JM. The dynamics of CD4+ T-cell depletion in HIV disease. *Nature*. 2001;410:974-979.

19. Mindel A, Tenant-Flowers M. Natural history and management of early HIV infection. *BMJ*. 2001;322: 1290-1293.

20. Weller IVD, Williams IG. Antiretroviral drugs. *BMJ*. 2001; 322:1410-1412.

21. Drugs for HIV infection. *Treat Guidel Med Lett*. 2004; 2(17):1-8

22. de Jong MD, de Boer RJ, de Wolf F, et al. Overshoot of HIV-1 viraemia after early discontinuation of antiretroviral treatment. *AIDS*. 1997;11(11):F79-F84.

23. Liuzzi G, D'Offizi G, Topino S, et al. Dynamics of viral load rebound in plasma and semen after stopping effective antiretroviral therapy. *AIDS*. 2003;17(7):1089-1092.

24. Lipton SA. Neuronal injury associated with HIV-1: approaches to treatment. *Annu Rev Pharmacol Toxicol*. 1998;38:159-177.

25. Kaul M, Garden GA, Lipton SA. Pathways to neuronal injury and apoptosis in HIV-associated dementia. *Nature*. 2001;410:988-994.

26. Carr A, Emery S, Law M, et al. An objective case definition of lipodystrophy in HIV-infected adults: a case-control study. *Lancet*. 2003;361:726-735.

27. Carr A, Workman C, Careyk D, et al. No effect of rosiglitazone for treatment of HIV-1 lipoatrophy: randomised, double-blind, placebo-controlled trial. *Lancet*. 2004;363:429-438.

28. Koutkia P, Grinspoon S. HIV-associated lipodystrophy: pathogenesis, prognosis, treatment, and controversies. *Annu Rev Med*. 2004;55:303-317.

29. Lalezari JP, Henry K, O'Hearn M, et al. Enfuvirtide, an HIV-1 fusion inhibitor, for drug-resistant HIV infection in North and South America. *N Engl J Med*. 2003; 348(22):2175-2185.

30. Coovadia H. Antiretroviral agents: how best to protect infants from HIV and save their mothers from AIDS. *N Engl J Med*. 2004;351(3):289-292.

31. World Health Organization. *Anti-retroviral regimens for the prevention of mother-to-child HIV-1 transmission: the programmatic implications*. World Health Organization; 2000. Available at: http://www.who.int/reproductive-health/rtis/MTCT/. Accessed March 31, 2005.

32. Lallemant M, Jourdain G, Le Coeur S, et al. Single-dose perinatal nevirapine plus standard zidovudine to prevent mother-to-child transmission of HIV-1 in Thailand. *N Engl J Med*. 2004;351(3):217-228.

33. Taha TE, Kumwenda NI, Hoover DR, et al. Nevirapine and zidovudine at birth to reduce perinatal transmission of HIV in an African setting. *JAMA*. 2004;292(2):202-209.

34. Deeks SG. Treatment of antiretroviral-drug-resistant HIV-1 infection. *Lancet*. 2002;362:2002-2011.

35. Clavel F, Hance AJ. HIV drug resistance. *N Engl J Med*. 2004;350(10):1023-1035.

36. Walmsley S, Bernstein B, King M, et al. Lopinavir-ritonavir versus nelfinavir for the initial treatment of HIV infection. *N Engl J Med*. 2002;346(26):2039-2046.

37. Robbins GK, De Gruttola V, Shafer RW, et al. Comparison of sequential three-drug regimens as initial therapy for HIV-1 infection. *N Engl J Med*. 2003;349(24):2293-2303.

38. Shafer RW, Smeaton LM, Robbins GK, et al. Comparison of four-drug regimens and pairs of sequential three-drug regimens as initial therapy for HIV-1 infection. *N Engl J Med*. 2003;349(24):2304-2315.

39. Skolnik PR. HIV therapy—what do we know, and when do we know it? *N Engl J Med*. 2003;349(24):2351-2352.

40. AIDSinfo: A Service of the U.S. Department of Health and Human Services. Available at: http://www.aidsinfo.nih.gov/guidelines/. Accessed June 28, 2004.

41. Nieuwkerk PT, Sprangers M, Burger DM, et al. Limited patient adherence to highly active antiretroviral therapy for HIV-1 infection in an observational cohort study. *Arch Intern Med*. 2001;161:1962-1968.

42. World Health Organization. *Hepatitis B. Fact Sheets*. Available at: http://www.who.int/inf-fs/en/fact204.html. Accessed June 26, 2004.

43. Lin KW, Kirchner JT. Hepatitis B. *Am Fam Physician*. 2004;69:75-82.

44. Malik AH, Lee WM. Chronic hepatitis B virus infection: treatment strategies for the next millennium. *Ann Intern Med*. 2000;132(9):723-731.

45. Niederau C, Heintges T, Lange S, et al. Long-term follow-up of HBeAg-positive patients treated with interferon alfa for chronic hepatitis B. *N Engl J Med*. 1996; 334(22):1422-1427.

46. Lok ASF, McMahon BJ. Chronic hepatitis B: update of recommendations. *Hepatology*. 2004;39(3):857-861.

47. Qaqish RB, Mattes KA, Ritchie DJ. Adefovir dipivoxil: a new antiviral agent for the treatment of hepatitis B virus infection. *Clin Ther*. 2003;25(12):3084-3099.

48. Rivkin A. Adefovir dipivoxil in the treatment of chronic hepatitis B. *Ann Pharmacother*. 2004;38:625-633.

49. Eisen-Vandervelde A, Yao ZQ, Hahn YS. The molecular basis of HCV-mediated immune dysregulation. *Clin Immunol*. 2004;111:16-21.

50. Penin F, Dubuisson J, Rey FA, Moradpour D, Pawlotsky JM. Structural biology of hepatitis C virus. *Hepatology*. 2004; 39(1):5-19.

51. Omata M, Yoshida H. Prevention and treatment of hepatocellular carcinoma. *Liver Transpl*. 2004;10(S2):S111-S114.

52. Lauer GM, Walker BD. Hepatitis C virus infection. *N Engl J Med*. 2001;345(1):41-52.

53. McHutchison JG, Gordon SC, Schiff ER, et al. Interferon alfa-2b alone or in combination with ribavirin as initial treatment for chronic hepatitis C. Hepatitis Interventional Therapy Group. *N Engl J Med*. 1998; 338(21):1485-1492.

54. Davis GL, Esteban-Mur R, Rustgi VK, et al. Interferon alfa-2b alone or in combination with ribavirin for the treatment of relapse of chronic hepatitis C. *N Engl J Med*. 1998;339(21):1493-1499.

55. Ward RP, Kugelmas M, Libsch KD. Management of hepatitis C: evaluating suitability for drug therapy. *Am Fam Physician*. 2004;69(6):1429-1436.

56. Hadziyannis SJ, Sette H, Morgan TR, et al. Peginterferon-alpha2a and ribavirin combination therapy in chronic hepatitis C: a randomized study of treatment duration and ribavirin dose. *Ann Intern Med.* 2004;140(5):346-355.

57. Camma C, Di Bona D, Schepis F, et al. Effect of peginterferon alfa-2a on liver histology in chronic hepatitis C: a meta-analysis of individual patient data. *Hepatology.* 2004;39(2):333-342.

58. Pawlotsky JM. The nature of interferon-[alpha] resistance in hepatitis C virus infection. *Curr Opin Infect Dis.* 2003; 16(6):587-592.

59. Stringer WW. Mechanisms of exercise limitation in HIV+ individuals. *Med Sci Sports Exerc.* 2000;32(7):S412-S214.

60. Mackinnon LT. Chronic exercise training effects on immune function. *Med Sci Sports Exerc.* 2000;32(7):S369-S376.

61. Harrington D. Viral hepatitis and exercise. *Med Sci Sports Exerc.* 2000;32(7):S422-S430.

62. Kauffman CA. Fungal infections in older adults. *Clin Infect Dis.* 2001;33:550-555.

63. Lionakis MS, Kontoyiannis DP. Glucocorticoids and invasive fungal infections. *Lancet.* 2003;362:1828-1838.

64. Masuoka J. Surface glycans of *Candida albicans* and other pathogenic fungi: physiological roles, clinical uses, and experimental challenges. *Clin Microbiol Rev.* 2004; 17(2):281-310.

65. Lilley LL, Harrington S, Snyder JS. Antifungal agents. In: *Pharmacology and the Nursing Process.* 4th ed. St Louis: Mosby; 2005:689-699.

66. Linden PK. Amphotericin B lipid complex for the treatment of invasive fungal infections. *Exp Opin Pharmacother.* 2003;4(11):2099-2110.

67. Eggimann P, Garbino J, Pittet D. Management of *Candida* species infections in critically ill patients. *Lancet Infect Dis.* 2003;3:772-785.

68. Sigurgeirsson B, Billstein S, Rantanen T, et al. L.I.O.N. Study: efficacy and tolerability of continuous terbinafine (Lamisil) compared to intermittent itraconazole in the treatment of toenail onychomycosis. Lamisil vs. Itraconazole in Onychomycosis. *Br J Dermatol.* 1999; 141(suppl 56):5-14.

69. Evans EG, Sigurgeirsson B. Double blind, randomised study of continuous terbinafine compared with intermittent itraconazole in treatment of toenail onychomycosis. The LION Study Group. *BMJ.* 1999;318(7190): 1031-1035.

70. Haugh M, Helou S, Boissel JP, Cribier BJ. Terbinafine in fungal infections of the nails: a meta-analysis of randomized clinical trials. *Br J Dermatol.* 2002;147:118-121.

71. Chan YC, Friedlander SF. New treatments for tinea capitis. *Curr Opin Infect Dis.* 2004;17(2):97-103.

72. Gupta AK, Adam P. Terbinafine pulse therapy is effective in tinea capitis. *Pediatr Dermatol.* 1998;15:56-58.

73. Hainer BL. Dermatophyte infections. *Am Fam Physician.* 2003;67:101-108.

74. Wong-Beringer A, Kriengkauykiat J. Systemic antifungal therapy: new options, new challenges. *Pharmacotherapy.* 2003;23(11):1441-1462.

75. Klastersky J. Empirical antifungal therapy. *Int J Antimicrob Agents.* 2004;23:105-112.

76. Rigopoulos D, Katoulis AC, Ioannides D, et al. A randomized trial of amorolfine 5% solution nail lacquer in association with itraconazole pulse therapy compared with itraconazole alone in the treatment of candida fingernail onychomycosis. *Br J Dermatol.* 2003;149(1): 151-156.

9

Chemotherapeutic Drugs and Agents Acting on the Immune System

CHEMOTHERAPY AND IMMUNE MODULATION

ETIOLOGY AND PATHOPHYSIOLOGY OF CANCER

Cancer encompasses more than 300 diseases that are characterized by cellular transformation and uncontrolled cellular growth, with the potential to invade surrounding tissue and metastasize to sites distant from the site of origin.[1] Some other terms (*neoplasm, malignancy,* and *tumor*) have been used interchangeably with the term *cancer,* but technically, they have different meanings.[2] Neoplasms and tumors both refer to masses of new cells that show unrestrained growth. A neoplasm can be either benign or malignant. Benign tumors tend to be solid or encapsulated and slow growing, and they show no tendency to metastasize but may still cause death by growing into or pressing against vital tissue. A malignant tumor, however, is different in that it invades surrounding tissues, has an unpredictable rate of growth, and spreads by either direct extension into surrounding tissues or through the lymphatic system or circulating blood. The growth of cancer is called *carcinogenesis* or *tumorigenesis* and is considered to be a complex multistep process arising from a single normal cell that undergoes a transformation (Figure 23-1).

Tissue categories for tumors include sarcomas, carcinomas, leukemias, and tissue of neural origin[2] (Table 23-1). Identifying the source of the tumor is extremely important because it often determines the type of chemotherapy that will be effective. Carcinomas originate from epithelial tissue, which is the tissue that lines body surfaces. Examples include the skin, the mucosal lining of the gastrointestinal (GI) tract, and the bronchial lining in the lungs. Sarcomas arise from connective tissue, which is composed of bone, cartilage, muscle, and vascular structures. Nerve tumors consist of constituents of the nervous tissue and exist in the cells of the central nervous system (CNS) or peripheral nervous systems. Lymphomas come from lymphatic tissue; and the last tissue category, leukemia, arises from leukocytes. These two types of neoplasms are also known as circulating cancers or hematological malignancies because they are diffuse and do not form a distinct solid tumor.

In addition to the signs and symptoms produced by the loss of a particular tissue from the invasion of cancerous cells, neoplastic tissue may cause symptoms far from the tumor or its site of metastasis.[2] These symptoms are referred to as *the paraneoplastic syndrome* and may include hypercalcemia and syndrome of inappropriate antidiuretic diuretic hormone secretion with lung cancer; disseminated intravascular coagulation with leukemia; Cushing's syndrome with adrenal, lung, or thyroid cancer; and addisonian syndrome with cancer of the adrenal gland. These syndromes may be caused by biologically active substances, such as hormones, secreted by the primary tumor. Patients who

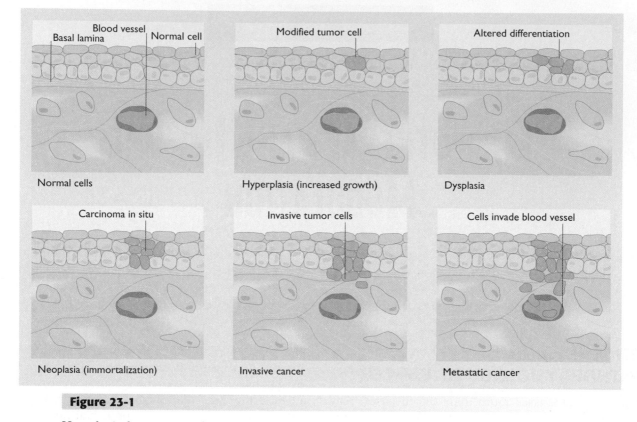

Figure 23-1

Hypothetical progression from normal to malignant cells. (From Page C, Curtis MJ, Sutter MC, Walker MJ, Hoffman BB, eds. *Integrated Pharmacology*. 2nd ed. Philadelphia: Mosby; 2002.)

experience these symptoms will need additional drug treatment above and beyond the standard anticancer agents.

Principles of Cancer Cell Growth

Neoplastic growths are initiated by a variety of factors. Extrinsic factors, such as exposure to chemical carcinogens, play a significant role in many cancers, as do intrinsic factors such as genetic predisposition. Oncogenes, DNA sequences that code for proteins involved in tumorigenesis, are also at fault.[3] Oncogenes may be overexpressed and promote proliferation of a neoplasm once cell growth has been initiated. In addition, proliferation can proceed without difficulty as a result of mutations or loss of tumor suppressor genes such as the *p53* gene, mutated DNA repair genes, or overexposure of anti-apoptotic proteins such as Bcl-2.[4,5] The *p53* gene is responsible for halting DNA replication and initiates apoptosis. A loss of this gene allows the damaged DNA to replicate. High levels of Bcl-2

immortalize cancer cells because there is a re-expression of certain enzymes that are usually lost in normal cells with each growth cycle. A great deal of research on gene therapy is being conducted to find methods to enhance the suppressor genes and inhibit Bcl-2.[6]

Cell Growth Cycle

Cancer cells spread by directly invading surrounding tissue or by traveling through the lymphatic or vascular circulation. Cancer cells express collagenases and other activators that help the cells move through tissues. Angiogenesis, the production of blood vessels supplying a tumor, is stimulated by vascular endothelial growth factor; and fibroblast growth factor helps to create a scaffold to aid in the attachment of cells at metastatic sites. In addition, at any one time, neoplastic cells are actively dividing (progressing through a cell cycle period), differentiating, or at rest.

Cellular reproduction has four distinct phases[2] (Figure 23-2). The G1 phase is the pre-DNA period

Table 23-1

Tumor Classification Based on Specific Tissue of Origin	
Tissue of Origin	**Malignant Tissue**
EPITHELIAL = CARCINOMAS	
Glands or ducts	Adenocarcinomas
Respiratory tract	Small- and large-cell carcinomas
Kidney	Renal cell carcinomas
Skin	Squamous cell, epidermoid, and basal cell carcinoma; melanoma
CONNECTIVE = SARCOMAS	
Fibrous	Fibrosarcoma
Cartilage	Chondrosarcoma
Bone	Osteogenic sarcoma (Ewing's tumor)
Blood vessels	Kaposi's sarcoma
Synovia	Synoviosarcoma
Mesothelium	Mesothelioma
LYMPHATIC = LYMPHOMAS	
Lymph tissue	Lymphomas (Hodgkin's disease and multiple myeloma)
NERVE	
Glial	Glioma
Adrenal medulla nerves	Pheochromocytoma
BLOOD	
White blood cells	Leukemia

From Lilley LL, Harrington D, Snyder JS. Pharmacology and the Nursing Process. 4th ed. St Louis: Mosby; 2005.

in which the enzymes necessary for DNA production are synthesized. During the S phase, DNA synthesis occurs. During this time, the enzymes involved in DNA synthesis—DNA polymerase, RNA polymerase II, and topoisomerases I and II—become active. In addition, the enzymes involved in the folate pathway for purine and pyrimidine synthesis, such as dihydrofolate reductase, also become quite active. The next phase is G2 or the pre-mitosis phase during which synthesis of the cellular and structural components needed for mitosis occurs. By the end of this phase, the usual numbers of chromosomes have doubled. The M phase (mitosis) is next and begins cell division. G0 is the resting stage in which there is a temporary or permanent halt to proliferation. Currently, some drugs act on one particular phase in this cycle (cell cycle–specific [CCS] agents), and some act throughout the entire cycle (cell cycle–nonspecific [CCNS] agents)

Each type of neoplastic cell runs through the cycle at a variable but rapid pace. Each phase takes only hours to complete (12 to 18 hours for some cells but as little as 1 to 2 hours for other cells). The entire cycle may take 48 to 72 hours. However, tumor growth is not linear. It has been described as "Gompertzian kinetics," which means that there is slow growth at the smallest and largest tumor sizes and greater growth in between.[7]

CYTOTOXIC STRATEGY IN CHEMOTHERAPY AND ITS CONSEQUENCES

Chemotherapy is indicated for neoplasms that are known to or likely to have spread and for those that cannot be cured by surgery.[1] It is also used as an adjunct to surgery and radiation to make sure as many cells as possible are eradicated. The drugs mount an attack against rapidly proliferating cells, interrupting processes necessary for cell replication. Many drugs block synthesis of precursors for DNA and RNA or set out to destroy the DNA or RNA once it is made. Other drugs block transcription and translation. Chemotherapy agents tend to be most successful against cells that are cycling as opposed to those in the G0 stage at rest. Surgically debulking the tumor is a technique used to increase cell kill because this procedure usually causes the remaining cells to begin cycling again.

Chemotherapy agents kill a constant fraction of tumor cells with each treatment cycle.[1] This means that there will always be some cells that survive therapy. However, the idea is that each drug cycle will lower the tumor burden further, so that eventually, the patient's immune system can control the cancer. If the immune system cannot keep the cancer at bay, then the cells will continue to grow, although undetectably at first. This corresponds to the remission phase of cancer. By the time clinical

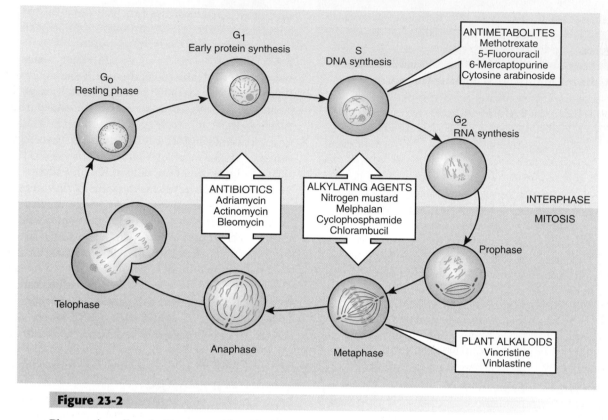

Figure 23-2

Phases of a cell cycle. Drugs are identified by where they exert their effect. (From Beare PG, Meyers JL. *Adult Health Nursing.* 3rd ed. St Louis: Mosby; 1998.)

symptoms reoccur, or the tumor is detected, the tumor may have as many as 10^9 cells (about the size of a pea). If chemotherapy resumes and is effective in killing 99.9% of cells, unfortunately there will still be plenty of cells left alive to multiply again. Hence, complete eradication of cancer cells is difficult.

Consequences of the Cytotoxic Strategy

Chemotherapy targets cells that undergo extremely rapid cell division. However, because cancer cells are not the only actively proliferating cells in the human body, the drugs are not selectively toxic. They affect the bone marrow, GI tract and buccal mucosa, reproductive organs, and hair follicles.[7] Hence, the side effects of most agents used for cancer include myelosuppression, more commonly known as bone marrow suppression (resulting in thrombocytopenia, leukopenia, and anemia); nausea and vomiting; diarrhea; stomatitis; amenorrhea with possible ovarian failure; lowered sperm count; and

hair loss. These signs are generally dose limiting, occur early in treatment, and, for the most part, are reversible when treatment is discontinued. The gonadal dysfunction may or may not be reversible but tends to be less severe when therapy is given to prepubertal children. However, males at puberty are more susceptible than any other patient group. Chemotherapy agents may also produce secondary cancers later on. Specifically, a group of drugs called *alkylating agents* may produce hematopoietic malignancies. This is because these drugs cause permanent genetic mutations.

Contraindications for all cancer drugs include a very low white blood cell count, infection, and poor nutritional or hydration status. The time at which the white blood cells reach their lowest levels is called *the nadir* and may occur from 10 to 28 days after chemotherapy. The anticancer agents are withheld at this time, and the patient may be given prophylactic antibiotics and also special growth factors (see discussion of hematopoietic agents and stem cell replacement).

RESISTANCE TO CHEMOTHERAPY

Resistance to chemotherapy may occur for several reasons. Cancer cells may produce abnormal transport mechanisms, resulting in decreased uptake of the drug.[8] Another transport problem that may occur is the development of an efflux pump.[9] This is a transport mechanism that pumps the drug out of the cell and is responsible for much of the multidrug-resistant cancers. If the drug makes it into a cell, enzymes may inactivate it by metabolism to inactive forms. Enhanced DNA repair inside the cancer cell is another means by which carcinoma may develop resistance to chemotherapy. In addition, some cancers are innately difficult to treat because of their location. Brain cancers are more difficult to treat with chemotherapy because the drug must penetrate the blood-brain barrier. The testes represent another difficult area to treat because this tissue tends to be acidic, causing the drugs to become ionized, which decreases diffusion across the membranes. These areas are sometimes called *pharmacological sanctuaries.*

CHEMOTHERAPY (ANTINEOPLASTIC) DRUG CLASSES

The major chemotherapy drug classes include alkylating agents, mitotic spindle poisons, cytotoxic antibiotics, antimetabolites, hormones, and various miscellaneous agents.

Alkylating Agents

Alkylating drugs are CCNS antineoplastics that are effective at various stages in the growth cycle, although most effective against rapidly growing cancer and rapidly growing normal body cells. These agents covalently bind to DNA by nucleophilic substitution with an alkyl group (saturated carbon atom, e.g., $-CH_3$) (Figure 23-3). Normally, the two DNA strands are linked together by the nucleic bases (adenine [A], guanine [G], thymine [T], or cytosine [C]) through covalent hydrogen bonds forming the molecular bridge between strands. The presence of an alkyl group, however, creates an abnormal chemical bond between adjacent DNA strands. The three categories of alkylating agents are classic alkylators (nitrogen mustards), nitrosoureas, and a group of probable alkylators.

Classic Alkylators

Mechlorethamine is a derivative of nitrogen mustard, which was originally discovered during World War I when mustard gas was used for chemical warfare. It gives off two chloride ions and develops a reactive intermediate that binds to the ^7N nitrogen of a guanine residue in one or both strands of DNA. It is also capable of alkylating ^6O guanine and ^3N cytosine.[2] These interstrand cross-links produce DNA damage and prevent DNA replication and RNA transcription. Binding to a single strand of DNA produces strand breaks.

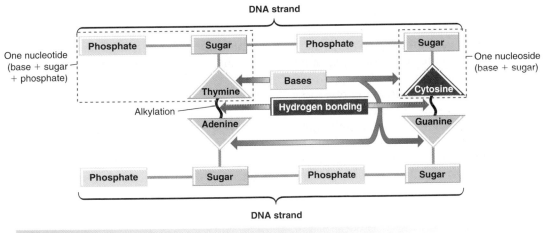

Figure 23-3

Organization of DNA and site of action of alkylating agents. (From Lilley LL, Harrington D, Snyder JS. *Pharmacology and the Nursing Process.* 4th ed. St Louis: Mosby; 2005.)

Mechlorethamine is part of the MOPP (mechlorethamine, Oncovin, prednisone, and procarbazine) protocol for the treatment of Hodgkin's disease. It is also used to treat non-Hodgkin's lymphomas, chronic leukemia, and certain solid tumors. It is administered intravenously or into a cavity such as the lungs or peritoneum. Adverse effects include severe vomiting, bone marrow depression, neurotoxicity, weakness, alopecia, hyperuricemia, and gonadal atrophy. Ototoxicity has also been reported. Lymphocytopenia begins within 24 hours of the first dose, and granulocytopenia begins 6 to 8 days later and lasts for 10 days to 3 weeks. Additionally, this drug produces severe blistering if it comes into contact with skin. If extravasation occurs, drug administration must stop immediately and the physician must be notified. Usually, attempts are made to aspirate any residual drug through the intravenous (IV) tubing, and an antidote is prepared. Mechlorethamine is prepared fresh, just before use, and requires the preparer to use a mask and rubber gloves to avoid inhalation of vapors or contact with the skin.

Cyclophosphamide is among the most commonly used alkylating agents in part because it can be given orally, as well as parenterally. It is used in the treatment of Hodgkin's and non-Hodgkin's lymphomas, multiple myeloma, breast cancer, and some sarcomas. Ifosfamide is a similar drug that has a longer half-life but is only available for parenteral administration.[10] In addition to bone marrow suppression, GI complaints, and alopecia, these agents produce hemorrhagic cystitis leading to bladder fibrosis.[11] A toxic metabolite (acrolein) of these drugs is eliminated in the urine but not before it causes damage to the bladder. Adequate hydration and IV injection of MESNA (sodium 2-mercaptoethane sulfonate) help to inactivate the toxic compound. MESNA binds to the irritant metabolites in the bladder to prevent cystitis. It is given either intravenously or orally 15 minutes before and again at 4 hours and 8 hours after the alkylating agent has been administered. Neurotoxicity has also been reported with ifosfamide, mostly in the form of sedation; but seizures, ataxia, hallucinations, and extrapyramidal symptoms have rarely been seen.[12]

Nitrosureas

Carmustine and lomustine are nitrosureas. They act like the classic alkylators by cross-linking strands of DNA to inhibit DNA and RNA replication. Their cytotoxicity is greater during cell division. Because of their great lipid solubility, these drugs are able to penetrate the CNS for treatment of brain tumors. Carmustine is also available in a wafer form for implantation into the resection cavity of patients undergoing surgery for glioblastomas.[13] Polymer release systems containing carmustine are currently under study for implantation in the brain. Survival is longer with the wafers and release systems, but the risk of intracranial infection is higher. The major problems with these drugs are myelosuppression and vomiting. Other adverse effects that may occur include pain at the injection site, pulmonary fibrosis, and nephrotoxicity.

Probable Alkylators

Cisplatin and carboplatin are two drugs that fall within the category of probable alkylators. Cisplatin is a chemotherapeutic drug that contains platinum in its chemical makeup.[14,15] It consists of a platinum atom surrounded by chloride atoms and ammonia molecules. Both drugs bind to purine bases in DNA, forming intrastrand links.[16] The result is an unwinding of the DNA helix and ultimate cell inactivation. These drugs have dramatically improved survival rates for patients with testicular cancer, including those with the metastatic form. They are also used to treat ovarian, bladder, breast, and lung cancers. The major adverse effect, other than GI symptoms, is renal toxicity, which may be reduced by hydration and diuresis. Myelosuppression is less of a problem with these drugs than with the other alkylating agents. The nadir for white blood cells and platelets occurs 18 to 23 days after a dose and returns to normal within 39 days. Peripheral neuropathy and ototoxicity are also quite common. At the first sign of numbness or tingling, cisplatin must be discontinued because peripheral neuropathy may be irreversible. Carboplatin is better tolerated than cisplatin because it is associated with less vomiting.

Mitotic Spindle Poisons (Tubulin-Binding Agents)

The drugs in this category originate largely from plants: the vinca alkaloids, vinblastine, vincristine, and vinorelbine, come from the periwinkle plant; the epipodophyllotoxin derivatives, etoposide and teniposide, are semisynthetic derivatives from extracts of the mandrake plant; and the taxanes, paclitaxel and docetaxel, are derived from the bark of the Western (Pacific) yew tree. In general, they are CCS agents working before and during mitosis to inhibit cell division.

Vinca Alkaloids

The vinca alkaloids bind to the protein tubulin during the metaphase of mitosis.[17] Tubulin is a major protein that helps to form the intracellular skeleton of the mitotic spindle. Binding to this protein prevents formation and assembly of the microtubules, and without mitotic spindles, cell division cannot proceed. Spindle disassembly is also promoted.

Vincristine is the O (trade name of Oncovin) in the MOPP regimen for the treatment of Hodgkin's disease and acute leukemias. It is also used in the treatment of acute lymphoblastic leukemia, Wilms' tumor, Ewing's sarcoma, and non-Hodgkin's lymphomas. Vinblastine may be given with bleomycin and cisplatin for treatment of metastatic testicular cancer.

Both drugs can cause phlebitis or cellulitis if extravasation occurs during injection. Nausea, vomiting, diarrhea, and alopecia occur with both drugs; however, surprisingly, vincristine is not very myelosuppressive. Both are extremely neurotoxic, producing paresthesias, painful peripheral neuropathy, loss of reflexes, foot drop, wrist drop, and ataxia. Specifically, these agents induce a nociceptor hyperresponsiveness to both heat and mechanical stimulation.[18] They may also induce the syndrome of inappropriate antidiuretic hormone secretion.

Epipodophyllotoxin Derivatives

The epipodophyllotoxin derivatives include etoposide and teniposide. These drugs are believed to kill cancer cells in the late S phase and the G2 phase of the cell cycle. They are used for the treatment of testicular and small-cell lung cancer. Side effects include the usual GI and myelosuppressive symptoms, as well as liver and kidney toxicity.

Taxanes

Paclitaxel was originally isolated from the Western yew tree in 1958. However, because of purification and formulation problems, it did not reach the pharmacy until 25 years later, although it is now made synthetically. It binds to tubulin, but instead of promoting disassembly of the mitotic spindle like the vinca alkaloids, it promotes stability.[17,19] However, the result is the same in that the mitotic spindle becomes nonfunctional.

Paclitaxel is approved for the treatment of ovarian cancer, metastatic breast cancer, squamous cell carcinoma of the head and neck, and bladder cancer. Docetaxel is used for breast cancer and non-small-cell lung cancer.

Both of these drugs produce the usual side effects that accompany chemotherapeutic agents. However, they may also produce neuropathic pain and peripheral neuropathy, as well as an occasional anaphylactic reaction. Because paclitaxel is insoluble in water, it must be emulsified in a substance called *Cremophor*, which in some individuals may result in an anaphylactic reaction (dyspnea, chest pain, bronchospasm, urticaria, and hypotension). Pretreatment with glucocorticosteroids and antihistamines can be used to prevent this reaction. In terms of the peripheral neuropathy, there are some case reports documenting recovery from paresthesia with venlafaxine.[20]

Anti-Tumor Antibiotics

Cytotoxic antibiotics are CCNS agents, although depending on the drug, one phase may be favored over another.[2] Most of these drugs act by intercalation, involving the insertion of the drug between the two strands of DNA. Specifically, a cytotoxic antibiotic binds to the base pairs, causing the DNA helix to assume an unstable structure. Doxorubicin and daunorubicin are examples of two antitumor antibiotics. They are effective in treating multiple cancers including breast, bone, and ovarian cancer; leukemias; lymphomas; and neuroblastomas. Stomatitis, nausea, and vomiting are common complications of this treatment. Myelosuppression is also expected. In addition, these drugs may produce darkening of the palms and soles of the feet and reddening of urine. Doxorubicin is also associated with a dose-related cardiotoxicity that is more common in patients older than 70 years and very young children.[21] Patients should be observed for pedal edema, dysrhythmias, and shortness of breath. Doxorubicin is now available in a liposomal drug delivery system, which reduces systemic effects and increases the duration of action.

Antimetabolites

Chemotherapeutic antimetabolites are CCS agents that mimic the action of substances necessary for the synthesis of DNA and RNA. They are used against solid tumors of the colon, breast, stomach, ovary, pancreas, and liver, as well as for acute leukemia and non-Hodgkin's lymphomas.

Methotrexate

Methotrexate blocks dihydrofolate reductase, an enzyme necessary for converting folic acid to its active form.[2] Folic acid is a necessary cofactor in purine and pyrimidine synthesis. Specifically, thymidine, adenine, and guanine levels will be depressed and thus lead to decreased synthesis of DNA and RNA (Figure 23-4). Methotrexate is most active in the S phase. This drug can also inhibit lymphocyte production, giving it immunosuppressive activity. Side effects of methotrexate include myelosuppression, nausea, vomiting, diarrhea, stomatitis, rash, urticaria, and alopecia. Long-term use may lead to hepatic toxicity with fibrosis, and renal damage occurs with administration of high-dose methotrexate. A reversible pulmonary toxicity may occur with symptoms of cough, dyspnea, fever, and cyanosis. Neurological toxic effects have occurred when the drug was given intrathecally. Some of these adverse effects can be avoided by means of "leucovorin rescue." Leucovorin is a drug that bypasses the blocked dihydrofolate reductase and replenishes folate stores. However, the dose of leucovorin must be kept low so as not to negate the action of methotrexate. It is administered 24 to 42 hours after the initiation of high-dose methotrexate therapy.

Fluorouracil

Fluorouracil is a pyrimidine analog (mimics uracil) that ultimately inhibits thymidylate synthase and the formation of thymidine (Figure 23-4).[22] This drug is considered a false nucleic acid that competes with deoxyuridine monophosphate for thymidylate synthetase. The enzyme does not recognize the difference between deoxyuridine monophosphate and the drug, but ultimately, no product is made when the drug is the substrate for the enzyme. Myelosuppression and GI problems are the major side effects, although dermatitis on the extremities can also occur. The usual dose is daily IV treatments for 4 days or continuous infusion. If no toxicity occurs during the next 3 days, the dose may be administered every 3 to 4 days for 2 weeks. A topical preparation for the treatment of precancerous skin lesions and basal cell carcinomas also exists. Ongoing studies are evaluating its use in chemoradiotherapy, a method of hastening the effects of radiotherapy with an anti–S-phase radiosensitizer. In this treatment, fluorouracil is administered for 24 to 48 hours after external beam radiation therapy.

Mercaptopurine

Mercaptopurine reduces purine levels in tumor cells by inhibiting the first step in purine synthesis (inhibition of glutamine 5-phosphoribosylpyrophosphate aminotransferase).[2] It is a synthetic analog of adenine and works by incorporating itself into the metabolic pathway instead of a nucleic base. It is primarily used to treat leukemias. Myelosuppression and GI problems are the primary side effects.

Topoisomerase-1 Inhibitors (Camptothecins)

Topoisomerase-1 inhibitors are a new class of chemotherapy agents presently consisting of two agents, topotecan and irinotecan.[23] Both are semisynthetic

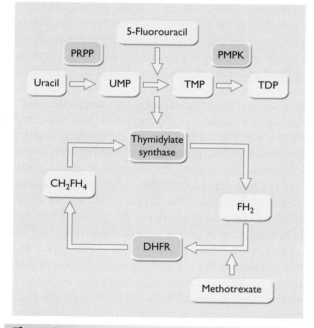

Figure 23-4

The thymidine pathway showing the inhibition of thymidylate synthase by 5-fluorouracil. Methotrexate and 5-fluorouracil both act to decrease the synthesis of thymidine. *DHFR,* Dihydrofolate reductase; *CH₂FH₄,* methylene tetrahydrofolate, the donor of a methyl group to uracil; *FH₂,* dihydrofolate; *PMPK,* pyrimidine monophosphate kinase; *TDP,* thymidine diphosphate; *TMP,* thymidine monophosphate; *UMP,* uracil monophosphate. (From Page C, Curtis MJ, Sutter MC, Walker MJ, Hoffman BB, eds. *Integrated Pharmacology.* 2nd ed. Philadelphia: Mosby; 2002.)

analogs of camptothecin, which was originally isolated from a Chinese shrub. These drugs are CCS agents and bind to the DNA–topoisomerase-1 complex during the S phase. Normally, this complex creates temporary strand cleavage and then reattachment, which is necessary for unwinding of DNA. Both drugs are used primarily to treat ovarian and colorectal cancer. Common side effects are similar to those of the other chemotherapeutic agents and include GI disturbance and bone marrow depression. Irinotecan, in particular, is associated with severe diarrhea, which may occur during drug infusion or may begin 2 to 10 days after infusion. The diarrhea can be quite severe and even life-threatening. Aggressive treatment with loperamide is necessary.

Hormone Therapy

Many tumors are hormone sensitive, meaning that they may regress when a hormone is administered or when a hormone's action is blocked. An example is estrogen-sensitive breast cancer. When a drug is given to block estrogen receptors, the tumor shrinks. In general, these drugs are more selective and less toxic than the other chemotherapeutic agents.

Prednisone

Steroids (glucocorticoids, not anabolic steroids) can induce remission in acute lymphocytic leukemia and Hodgkin's and non-Hodgkin's lymphomas.[2] In particular, prednisone slows lymphocytic growth, produces lymphocytopenia, and reduces lymphoid tissue. Other steroids, such as dexamethasone, are used in cancer treatment to prevent extravasation injury during IV infusion of chemotherapeutic agents, as well as to prevent hypersensitivity reactions to these drugs, and to retard emesis. Prednisone is also useful in reducing cerebral edema from a growing brain tumor or from edema induced by radiation.

Tamoxifen

Tamoxifen is a mixed estrogen antagonist and agonist.[24] Tamoxifen binds to estrogen receptors and blocks estrogen activation in the breast. The result is a decrease in growth factors involved in the proliferation of breast tissue and an increase in certain antiproliferative proteins. Tamoxifen offers palliation and tumor regression in advanced metastatic disease and may produce a cure when given along with other agents in the early stages of the disease. In addition, tamoxifen has been shown to significantly reduce the incidence of breast cancer in women who are at high risk for the disease.[25] This drug also produces estrogen-like effects in bone, so osteoporosis is not a problem with long-term treatment. Common side effects include menopausal symptoms, including hot flashes, nausea, irregular menstruation, and vaginal bleeding. In addition, because tamoxifen is an estrogen agonist in the uterus, there is a small increased risk of endometrial cancer with its use. Tamoxifen is also associated with a greater risk of venous thrombosis (see Chapter 14). Tamoxifen is not routinely given to premenopausal women because natural estrogen competes with tamoxifen for receptors and will limit its effectiveness.

Raloxifene is a compound similar to tamoxifen, except that it is also an estrogen antagonist in endometrial tissue.[26] It is currently used to prevent postmenopausal osteoporosis but is also under study for the treatment of breast cancer. Initial studies show a reduction in new breast cancers by 50%, but further studies are needed to compare it with tamoxifen.

Aromatase Inhibitors (Exemestane, Letrozole)

Postmenopausal women continue to have circulating estrogen levels despite ovarian shutdown.[2] This estrogen results from the conversion of adrenal androstenedione and testosterone to estrone in the adrenal glands and fatty tissue by the aromatase enzyme. In many patients with breast cancer, aromatase activity is increased, which in turn is responsible for higher estrogen levels.

The aromatase inhibitors are generally nonsteroidal competitive inhibitors of the aromatase enzyme.[27] Reduction in this enzyme leads to reduced estrogen levels. Ongoing studies show that these drugs may be equivalent to tamoxifen as first-line therapy.[28,29] Side effects are fairly mild and include hot flashes, skin rashes, nausea, fatigue, headache, and dizziness.

Luteinizing Hormone–Releasing Hormone Agonists and Gonadotropin-Releasing Hormone Agonists

Leuprolide and goserelin are analogs of luteinizing hormone–releasing hormone and gonadotropin-releasing hormone, respectively.[2] These hormones control the secretion of luteinizing hormone and follicle-stimulating hormone to stimulate sex hormone production in the testes and ovaries. Follicle-stimulating hormone and luteinizing hormone are initially released, but continued dosing produces a drop in their levels. The result is regression of hormone-dependent tumors of the prostate, breast, endometrium, and ovaries. Adverse drug reactions are equivalent to those of menopause or castration. Both sexes experience hot flashes, weight gain, GI disturbances, osteoporosis, and loss of libido and muscle mass. Men become impotent, and women show breast atrophy and vaginitis. A flare of prostate cancer symptoms may occur initially and cause urinary retention.

Antiandrogens (Flutamide)

Flutamide competitively inhibits binding of testosterone to androgen receptors in the testes and prostate gland. It is used in conjunction with leuprolide or goserelin in the treatment of prostate cancer. Adverse drug reactions include gynecomastia and GI discomfort.

Miscellaneous Chemotherapeutic Agents

A variety of chemotherapeutic agents do not fall within the structural or mechanistic categories outlined previously, but nevertheless, are strong contenders in the fight against cancer.

Imatinib

Imatinib is a fairly new drug, approved for use as a chemotherapeutic agent by the Food and Drug Administration in 2001.[30] It is primarily indicated for the treatment of chronic myelogenous leukemia (CML). CML results from a mutation in a pluripotent stem cell expressing a chromosome identified as the Philadelphia chromosome (a translocation of chromosomes 9 and 22, resulting in a shortened chromosome 22). This mutation produces progressive granulocytosis, marrow hypercellularity, and splenomegaly. CML is usually diagnosed in the chronic or stable phase, but within 4 to 6 years, an accelerated phase that leads to a fatal acute leukemia may occur. An accumulation of molecular abnormalities leads to the loss of terminal differentiation into a mature myeloid cell, and instead, immature or blast cells are released from the bone marrow. Until now, treatment has consisted of stem cell transplantation and administration of hydroxyurea (a chemotherapeutic agent that closely resembles

the antimetabolite antineoplastics) or interferon (IFN)-α; however, the cure rate is still less than 20%.[31]

The translocation of the chromosomes produces a tyrosine kinase fusion gene called BCR-ABL, which phosphorylates proteins that drive cellular proliferation.[30] Imatinib inhibits BCR-ABL–mediated transfer of phosphate to its substrates. This drug is one of the first in a series of agents developed to target specific proteins expressed by human cancers. Imatinib inhibits or kills proliferating myeloid cell lines containing the BCR-ABL gene with little harm to normal cells. In a group of 532 patients with CML in the chronic phase for whom interferon treatment had previously failed, 88% experienced clinically a complete clinical response, and 30% experienced a complete genetic response.[32-34] Sixty-three percent of patients given imatinib during the accelerated phase of CML also demonstrated response to the drug, with 28% achieving a complete hematological response and 14% achieving a complete genetic response. Patients in blast crisis did not fare as well, although 19% reverted to the chronic phase. Median duration of response in the chronic phase was 1 month; 6 months of treatment was necessary for patients in the accelerated phase. Side effects included nausea (55% to 68%), vomiting (28% to 54%), and diarrhea (33% to 49%). Edema—in the form of pleural effusion, ascites, or pulmonary edema—has also been reported, as well as neutropenia and thrombocytopenia, but these side effects were much less frequent than the GI disturbances.

Cyclooxygenase-2 Inhibitors

Epidemiological studies have shown a significant reduction in the incidence of colorectal cancer in individuals who take nonsteroidal antiinflammatory drugs (NSAIDs).[35-37] Specifically, there is evidence supporting a cyclooxygenase-2 (COX-2) contribution to tumorigenesis. Normally, COX-2 is not expressed unless induced by cytokines, growth factors, and oncogenes—all of which promote the synthesis of prostaglandins in malignant tissue and under inflammatory conditions. There is also a positive correlation between expression of this enzyme and inhibition of apoptosis. In addition, metabolic products in the COX-2 pathway may contribute to the vascularization necessary to support tumor growth. Overexpression of COX-2 in the intestinal epithelial cells has been seen in several different cancers, but especially in colorectal disease. Currently, several ongoing clinical trials are evaluating the effectiveness of COX-2 inhibitors in treatment of colon, lung, bladder, and esophageal tumors.

Combination Therapy

The majority of anticancer agents act primarily on the production or function of DNA, RNA, or protein. Chemotherapy often consists of two or more drugs that are used together to attack the cancer cells at several stages in the replication cycle.[2] In addition, because single agents are unable to produce cures or significant remissions, multiple agents are usually administered concurrently or sequentially. However, the drugs used in the combination protocols must not have overlapping toxic effects. A common protocol used for lymphoma is CHOP: cyclophosphamide, hydroxydaunomycin (doxorubicin), Oncovin (vincristine), and prednisone. Cyclophosphamide is an alkylating agent whose major toxic effects are myelosuppression and bladder irritation. Hydroxydaunomycin (doxorubicin) is an antibiotic whose major toxic effects are myelosuppression and cardiac toxicity. Oncovin (vincristine) is a vinca alkaloid with peripheral nerve toxicity but little myelosuppression (tubulin-binding drug). Prednisone shrinks lymphoid tissue; it has no myelosuppression but affects glucose metabolism and bone matrix formation.

Other nonmarrow-suppressive drugs, such as methotrexate with leucovorin rescue, may also be used with the CHOP protocol when blood cell counts are low.

Other common drug combinations include the following:

MOPP (mechlorethamine/vincristine/procarbazine/prednisone)

CMF (cyclophosphamide/methotrexate/fluorouracil)

CAF (cyclophosphamide/doxorubicin/fluorouracil)

The reader should be aware that more than 200 drug combinations have been developed by oncologists.

CHEMOTHERAPY SIDE EFFECTS, RECOMMENDATIONS FOR TREATMENT, AND PHYSICAL THERAPY IMPLICATIONS

Patients with cancer experience multiple problems, some related to the drugs and others related to the cancer, which may adversely affect their ability to continue taking the drugs.

Malnourishment

In general, patients with cancer are cachectic and anorexic, which obviously decreases their ability to tolerate chemotherapy. Nutritional supplementation may be necessary before drug therapy begins. This may include placement of a nasogastric feeding tube, use of central venous hyperalimentation (total parenteral nutrition), or simply instructing the family to find nutritious and appealing foods for the patient to eat.

Nausea

Nausea and vomiting are common complaints with chemotherapeutic agents, especially with the cisplatin-based protocols.[38] GI disturbances caused by chemotherapy usually begin 3 to 6 hours after treatment but may be delayed for 2 to 5 days. Nausea may result from irritation to the GI tract or from stimulation of the central vomiting center and chemoreceptor trigger zone that attempts to protect humans from toxic chemicals. See Table 23-2 for the emetic potential of several chemotherapeutic agents.

A number of drugs can help reduce vomiting.[39] Granisetron and ondansetron are selective antagonists at the 5-hydroxytryptamine 3 (5-HT3) receptor both in the CNS and at peripheral sites in the GI tract. The 5-HT3 receptors are in abundance on vagal afferent neurons in the vomiting center and in the GI tract. These drugs can be given intravenously in three doses (30 minutes before chemotherapy and then at 4 and 8 hours after therapy). They are available in the oral form for continued treatment. Dexamethasone is also used, but its exact

Table 23-2

Emetic Potential of Some Chemotherapy Agents		
Strong	Moderate	Low
Cisplatin	Daunorubicin	Vincristine
Cyclophosphamide	Cytarabine	Tamoxifen
Doxorubicin	Methotrexate	Bleomycin
Lomustine		Fluorouracil
Mechlorethamine		

mechanism for reducing emesis is unknown. The antipsychotic drug prochlorperazine reduces nausea and vomiting but is avoided because of its side effect, extrapyramidal reactions. Marijuana and tetrahydrocannabinol have also been used.

Diarrhea and Stomatitis

The epithelial lining of the GI tract is extremely sensitive to chemotherapy agents.[2] Stomatitis may develop within a few days of chemotherapy and persist for a few weeks after treatment. Oral inflammation causes pain with eating, speaking, and swallowing. Thus many functional activities are affected. Topical anesthetics and antifungal drugs may be helpful, and certain foods should be avoided such as those high in citric acid, those that are spicy, and those that have rough texture. It is also recommended that the patient remain hydrated. This is very important if the patient is losing fluid as a result of diarrhea or emesis. Ten to twelve glasses of fluid per day plus a diet high in fiber and binding foods, such as cheese and rice, are recommended.

Bone Marrow Suppression

Because many of the antitumor drugs cause bone marrow suppression and immunosuppression, patients may have infection and bleeding tendencies. See Table 23-3 for the myelosuppressive potential of the chemotherapy agents.

Low levels of platelets, less than $20,000/mm^3$, are associated with spontaneous and life-threatening bleeding in the GI tract and brain. This bleeding is recognized by the development of petechiae, purpura, ecchymoses, hematuria, or anemia and the presence of blood in the stool (GI bleeding). Patients may also experience nosebleeds and bleeding from the mouth and gums after tooth-brushing. Platelet transfusions are usually given if the count falls below $20,000/mm^3$. Activity levels must be modified to ensure that patients do not injure themselves during exercise (Table 23-4). In addition, agents that impair platelet function, such as aspirin and NSAIDs, should be avoided; and if the platelet count falls too low, oprelvekin can be added to the drug routine (see the discussion of hematopoietic agents and stem cell replacement).

Infection as a result of neutropenia is another major problem with chemotherapy.[2] The normal neutrophil count is between 2500 and $7000/mm^3$,

Table 23-3

Myelosuppressive Potential of Chemotherapy Drugs

Strong	Moderate	Mild
Vinblastine	Methotrexate	Bleomycin
Nitrosoureas	Fluorouracil	Vincristine
Cyclophosphamide	Etoposide	Tamoxifen
Doxorubicin		Hormone
Mercaptopurine		treatments
Ifosfamide		

Table 23-4

Activity Guidelines for Patients with Thrombocytopenia

Platelet Count	Acceptable Activities
50,000-150,000	Light resistance Swimming Bicycling (no grade)
30,000-50,000	Stationary bicycling Walking
20,000-30,000	Active range of motion
<20,000	Activities of daily living (If spontaneous bleeding occurs, notify physician immediately.)

Adapted from Goodman CC, Boissonnault WG, Fuller KS. Laboratory tests and values. In: Goodman CC, Boissonnault WG, eds. *Pathology: Implications for the Physical Therapist.* New York: WB Saunders; 1998.

and when the count falls below $1000/mm^3$, the risk of infection is increased. The risk is escalated when the count falls below $500/mm^3$.

The physical therapist should be alert for fever, sore throat, or chills because these may be the first signs of infection.[2] Temperatures should be taken every 4 hours during the neutrophil nadir periods. A temperature above $38°$ C requires prompt evaluation. Other symptoms may include myalgias, tachycardia, tachypnea, irritability, and lethargy. As the infection worsens, shock, adult respiratory distress syndrome, GI hemorrhage, and death may occur. Standard practice is to begin administration of a broad-spectrum antibiotic or an antifungal agent immediately when fever occurs.[40] Granulocyte colony-stimulating factor may be used after a bout of chemotherapy to build up the granulocyte count to prevent infection. A granulocyte-macrophage colony-stimulating factor is also available (see discussion of hematopoietic agents and stem cell replacement). They both stimulate differentiation and proliferation of myeloid progenitor cells into granulocytes. With most chemotherapeutic agents, the lowest peripheral granulocyte count (without growth factors) occurs at approximately 10 to 14 days after treatment, so this is the time when the patient is most susceptible to infectious agents. Recovery takes about 3 to 4 weeks. In general, the next scheduled chemotherapy session will be cancelled if the neutrophil count falls below $500/mm^3$, the platelet count is below $100,000/mm^3$, and/or the white blood cell count is below $4000/mm^3$.[2] From a physical therapy point of view, activity will need to be limited (Box 23-1).

Anemia is another problem associated with bone marrow suppression. Erythropoietin is a hormone produced in response to tissue hypoxia in the kidneys. Sensors in the tubular cells of the kidneys are responsive to tissue oxygen content, and when hypoxia is present, they release erythropoietin. In the bone marrow, erythropoietin binds to erythroid progenitor cells and activates tyrosine protein kinase signal pathways to stimulate cell proliferation into red blood cells. Recombinant erythropoietin is now available (see discussion of hematopoietic agents and stem cell replacement) and is used to treat anemia caused by chronic renal failure, anemia associated with HIV disease, and chemotherapy-induced anemia in patients with cancer. For patients with cancer and anemia, the usual regimen is subcutaneous injections, three times a week for 8 weeks.

Fatigue—whether it is due to bone marrow suppression, vomiting, drug treatment, or the cancer itself—can be overwhelming. It is described as being unusual, persistent, and not reduced by rest.[41] The cause is unknown, but it is speculated to result from muscle wasting caused by inflammatory cytokines or tumor necrosis factor. It tends to be more severe midway through the treatment cycle. Fatigue is also inversely proportional to activity level, and it has been found to be reduced on days when patients exercise. Recommendations for treatment include aerobic exercise programs at low intensity. Initially, patients may only be able to exert themselves for a few minutes, but if activity is continued, gains can be made. Patients are encouraged to keep a diary, documenting the exercise mode, duration, intensity, heart rate, time of day, and any symptoms. Drug treatment consisting of psycho-stimulants such as methylphenidate or dextro-amphetamine may be helpful.

Pain

Pain is another symptom that may result from the cancer or from chemotherapy. The majority of patients with cancer require some analgesic therapy while awaiting a response to chemotherapy. Regular administration of NSAIDs is the usual starting point for mild pain associated with cancer. However, the beneficial response of pain control needs to be balanced against the risks (GI problems, bleeding tendencies, and masking of fever that indicates infection). When these drugs are no longer effective, a weak opioid may be added to or substituted for the NSAID. Codeine and hydrocodone, combined with aspirin or acetaminophen, are recommended. When combinations of codeine-like drugs and NSAIDs are not sufficient and pain is severe, strong opioids are recommended. Morphine, hydro-morphone, transdermal fentanyl, and oxycodone are appropriate. These drugs can be administered in a variety of ways. Immediate-release preparations, which have a short latency and short duration, and controlled-release preparations such as MS Contin, which may be administered every 8 to 12 hours, are

---

Box 23-1	**Activity Guidelines for Patients with Bone Marrow Suppression**

- Leukopenia
  $<5000/mm^3$ with fever: no exercise
  $>5000/mm^3$: light exercise and progress as tolerated
- Decreased Hemoglobin
  <8 g/dL: no exercise
  8-10 g/dL: light exercise
  >10 g/dL: begin resistive exercise

Adapted from Goodman CC, Boissonnault WG, Fuller KS. Laboratory tests and values. In: Goodman CC, Boissonnault WG, eds. *Pathology: Implications for the Physical Therapist*. New York: WB Saunders; 1998.

available. Transdermal fentanyl provides a stable level of pain control. NSAIDs may also be given along with these drugs.

Most patients require a basal, long-acting analgesic, administered around the clock at regular intervals, and a short-acting analgesic given on an as-needed basis. Compliance and quality of analgesia are enhanced by regular administration. The supplemental drugs are used for breakthrough pain. Oral transmucosal fentanyl (in the form of a lollipop) can provide relief from breakthrough pain within 5 minutes. This strategy promotes consistent therapeutic plasma levels that will keep pain at a minimum. Opioids may also be given. The route of administration may be rectal, subcutaneous, IV, subdural, or intrathecal; or an implantable pump system may be used.

Bone is one of the most common sites of metastatic disease from breast, prostate, and lung cancers. Pain from bone lesions produces significant morbidity, and complete responses of bone lesions to chemotherapy are fairly rare. However, a partial response and disease stabilization can be achieved, particularly if surgery for stabilization of weight-bearing bones is possible. Bone pain has been described as "a unique pain state," involving neuro-chemical changes in afferent neurons. Mechanical allodynia often develops and becomes so severe that coughing, turning in bed, or gentle limb movements can produce pain.[42] Bone pain is correlated with the extent of osteolysis. From a chemical standpoint, bone disease is related to the expression of dynorphin, a prohyperalgesic peptide. Treatment includes external beam radiation and bisphosphonates. The bisphosphonates inhibit bone resorption and have been shown to reduce morbidity in terms of pain, fracture, and hypercalcemia, although the exact mechanism of action in bone cancer is not known.[43,44]

Alopecia

Alopecia, or hair loss, occurs most frequently with cyclophosphamide, vincristine, doxorubicin, and bleomycin.[2] It begins 7 to 10 days after treatment is initiated, with the peak effect seen at 2 months. Patients are encouraged to take a before-treatment photograph so that a wig that closely matches their pretreatment hair type and color can be made. They should also be reassured that the hair will usually grow back, even with continuing maintenance therapy, although color and texture may change.

Extravasation Injury

Extravasation of some of the chemotherapeutic drugs may lead to severe tissue damage and skin sloughing.[2] In some cases, skin grafting will be necessary. As mentioned earlier, the caregivers administering these agents must be very careful to monitor the infusion site every hour. If extravasation occurs, administration of the drug must be stopped immediately, and an antidote should be given. In some cases, the physical therapist will need to treat a patient for an upper extremity or hand injury.

Organ Toxicity

Specific organ toxicity is another problem associated with chemotherapy and usually involves the kidneys, liver, heart, lungs, CNS, gonads, and even the brain.[2] Renal tubular necrosis can result from the use of cisplatin. Hydration and diuretics are necessary to ensure sufficient flow of urine. Creatinine clearance from the kidneys, as well as serum creatinine values, must be monitored regularly. Liver toxicity may result from prolonged treatment with methotrexate or mercaptopurine. Cardiotoxicity is associated with the anticancer antibiotics, especially doxorubicin and daunorubicin. It may be sudden in onset, irreversible, and fatal; or there may be transient electrocardiographic changes with delayed cardiomyopathy with congestive heart failure. Those patients with preexisting cardiac disease must be monitored extra carefully. Frequent monitoring of left ventricular ejection fraction is warranted.

Peripheral neuropathy characterized by loss of deep tendon reflexes, paresthesias, motor weakness, and neuropathic pain is commonly associated with vincristine and the other mitotic spindle inhibitors.[18,45] Improvement is slow and may take more than a year after drug withdrawal, and in some cases, the neuropathy is permanent. Evaluation of hand sensibility for light touch, moving touch, two-point discrimination, and vibration is helpful in the assessment of chemotherapy-induced neuropathy and is also useful for tracking sensory return.[46,47]

In general, the red flags that may indicate organ toxicity include signs and symptoms of infection, yellowing of the skin, abdominal pain, decreased urine production, rapid respiration, poor skin turgor, skin lesions, and rashes. In addition, there is some evidence that chemotherapeutic agents can produce cognitive changes and even delirium.[48,49]

Future Cancers

Second malignancies resulting from genetic damage caused by chemotherapy have become a concern among long-term survivors. The incidence of these cancers (usually leukemias) is greater when chemotherapy was originally combined with radiation therapy. Peak incidence of the secondary leukemia is between 3 and 9 years after treatment and is greater among those patients who were older than 40 years at the time of the initial cancer.

Hypersensitivity Reactions

Hypersensitivity reactions are not uncommon, but when they occur with chemotherapeutic drugs, they can present a significant challenge. Some mild reactions can be treated with diphenhydramine, acetaminophen, and steroids. For life-threatening reactions, patients are treated with epinephrine, bronchodilators, and saline solution. If the reaction proves to be non–life-threatening, infusion may be restarted after symptoms subside.

Chemotherapy Performance Scale

Not every patient can tolerate the side effects of chemotherapy, either physically or emotionally. Some attempts have been made to develop a simple performance scale to predict whether a patient will respond to chemotherapy and be able to tolerate the side effects. The Eastern Cooperative Oncology Group, a multicenter cooperative group for cancer studies, uses a simple activities of daily living scale (Box 23-2).[50] If a patient has a performance status below 3, chemotherapy is not recommended unless a response is highly likely and the patient is motivated enough to tolerate treatment. Level 3 corresponds to being in bed more than 50% of the time. The word *motivated* is the key word because the discomfort and pain associated with these drugs are tremendous. Patients often become noncompliant

<table>
<tr><td>**Box 23-2**</td><td>**Eastern Cooperative Oncology Group (ECOG) Performance Status Scale**</td></tr>
</table>

- 0: Normal Activity
- 1: Symptoms but ambulatory
- 2: Bed rest <50% of the time
- 3: Bed rest >50% of the time
- 4: Total bed rest

Adapted from Bakermeier RF, Qazi R. Basic concepts of cancer chemotherapy and principles of medical oncology. In: Rubin P, ed. *Clinical Oncology*. 8th ed. New York: Saunders; 2001.

with the treatment because they cannot tolerate the side effects. At this point the patient must decide whether to stop treatment or to begin palliative treatment (symptom-controlling treatment).

TUMOR IMMUNOTHERAPY

As knowledge of the immune system has grown, efforts have been directed at using the patient's own immune system for cancer destruction. Active immunotherapy refers to the administration of agents that mimic or enhance a patient's immune response (by giving interferons and interleukins) to recognize tumor-specific antigens. Passive immunotherapy involves giving active immunological agents that can directly produce tumor regression. These agents include tumor vaccines, monoclonal antibodies (MABs), adoptive transfer of cytotoxic cells, and genetic manipulation. At this time the majority of these interventions are either at their earliest stage of development or are experimental; nevertheless, they represent a new classification of anticancer drugs called *biological response modifiers*.[2] The current subclasses of biological response modifiers include hematopoietic agents, interferons, MABs, and interleukins.

Normal Immune System

Although the immune system has been covered in various chapters in this text, a review at this point will be helpful and assist the reader in understanding the biological response modifiers. The immune system is vitally important in helping the body distinguish between self and an invading virus or

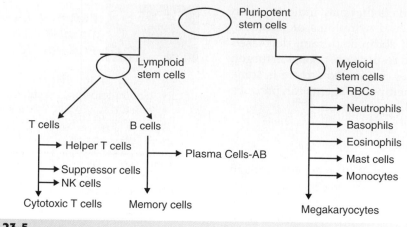

Figure 23-5

The origin of hematological cells. *NK*, Natural killer; *RBCs*, red blood cells.

bacterium.[2] However, even though tumors are not really foreign invaders, they may have undergone significant differentiation and may no longer resemble the cells from which they originated. Tumor cells also express markers on their surfaces that signal impending danger to the immune system. These chemical markers are called *tumor antigens*, and they label the cancer as *non-self*.

The major components of the immune system originate from the pluripotent stem cell and consist of humeral immunity, which is mediated by B cells producing antibodies, and cell-mediated immunity, which is mediated by T cells (Figure 23-5). Cytokines (interferons and interleukins) produced by T cells represent the specialized chemical communication system between the two components that fosters synchronization and coordination.

The humeral immune system has as its main component the B lymphocytes, also known as B cells, because they originate from the bone marrow. When antigen is detected, the B cells mature into plasma cells, which then produce antibodies that bind to the antigen, inactivating it (Figure 23-6). The B cells also produce memory cells that "study" the exact nature of the foreign invader, so that the next time exposure to the antigen occurs, the system can launch a faster and stronger immune response.

The cell-mediated immune system consists of T lymphocytes, also known as T cells, because they mature in the thymus. There are three main types of T cells: cytotoxic T cells, which kill their targets by causing cell lysis; T suppressor cells, which work opposite to the cytotoxic cells to limit the actions of the immune system; and the T helper cells, the

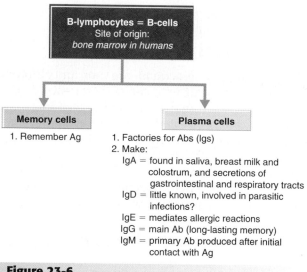

Figure 23-6

Cells of the humoral ("antibody-mediated") immune system. *Ab*, Antibody; *Ag*, antigen; *Ig*, immunoglobulin. (From Lilley LL, Harrington D, Snyder JS. *Pharmacology and the Nursing Process*. 4th ed. St Louis: Mosby; 2005.)

masters or directors of the entire system. The T helper cells initiate the actions of other components of the immune system, such as the lymphokines and cytotoxic T cells. Lymphokines are a subset of the cytokines produced by the T lymphocytes. Through the lymphokines, the T cells help the B cells to produce immunoglobulin G, activate monocytes, directly kill target cells, and mobilize the inflammatory response (Figure 23-7). The healthy individual has about two times as many T helper cells as T suppressor cells. There is speculation that an

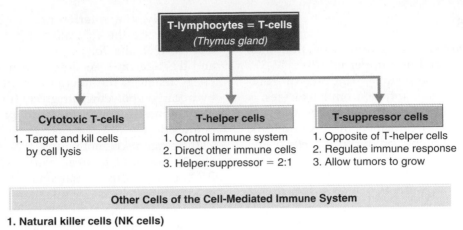

Figure 23-7

Cells of the cellular immune system. (From Lilley LL, Harrington D, Snyder JS. *Pharmacology and the Nursing Process.* 4th ed. St Louis: Mosby; 2005.)

Table 23-5

Effects of Selected Cytokines

Cytokine	Cell Source	Function
IL-1	Macrophage	T-cell and B-cell activation
IL-2	T cells	T-cell and B-cell activation
IL-3	T cells	Stem cell proliferation and differentiation
IL-4	T cells	B-cell differentiation into IgE; Th2
IL-5	T cells	Eosinophil activation
IL-6	T cells	B-cell differentiation
IL-7	Stromal cells	B-cell differentiation
IL-8	Macrophages	Neutrophil attraction
IL-10	T cells	Inhibition of Th1 cells
IL-12	Macrophages	Th1 differentiation
GM-CSF	T cells	Activation of eosinophils
IFN-γ	T cells, NK cells	Inhibition of Th2 cells, macrophage activation, MHC class I and II activation
IFN-α	Leukocytes	NK cell activation, MHC class I activation
TNF-α	Macrophages	Activation macrophages, granulocytes

IL, Interleukin; *IgE,* immunoglobulin E; *GM-CSF,* granulocyte-macrophage colony-stimulating factor; *NK,* natural killer; *MHC,* major histocompatibility complex; *IFN,* interferon; *TNF-α,* tumor necrosis factor α.

abundance of T suppressor cells permits tumor growth.

Additional cells of the immune system function as active cancer killers. These include macrophages, neutrophils (polymorphonuclear leukocytes), lymphokine-activated killer cells, and natural killer (NK) cells.[51] The NK cells contain perforin (a pore-forming protein), serine proteases, and other enzymes capable of lysing tumor cells. Lymphokine-activated killer cells are capable of lysing some tumors resistant to the NK cells. Macrophages possess some toxic properties, are capable of producing cytokines, and are also the cells that "present antigen to lymphocytes." Activation of many of these cells comes from interleukins and interferons—the cytokines (Table 23-5).

Interferons

Interferons are proteins that have antiviral, antitumor, and immunomodulating properties (Box 23-3).[2] There are three types, alpha (α), beta (β), and gamma (γ). The alpha subtype, from leukocytes, is used in the treatment of viral infections; the beta subtype is used in the treatment of multiple sclerosis; and the gamma subtype, produced by cells of the immune system, is proinflammatory. In terms of designating interferons, the word *alfa* is synonymous with the Greek letter alpha, but the word *alfa* seems to be used more in clinical contexts.

The exact mechanism of action of the interferons in cancer is not known. Possibilities include oncogene modulation and activation of immune host defenses, resulting in an increase in cytotoxic T cells, helper T cells, NK cells, and antigen-presenting cells. IFN-α also has anti-angiogenic effects on tumor endothelial cells by inhibiting fibroblast growth factors.

The interferons can be produced from genetically modified *Escherichia coli* bacteria by using recombinant DNA technology. There are currently six IFN alfas, two IFN betas, and one IFN gamma.

Specifically, the interferons involved in cancer treatment are the IFN alfas: IFN alfa-2a, pegIFN alfa-2a, IFN alfa-2b, pegIFN alfa-2b, IFN alfa-n3, and IFN alfacon-1. As described in Chapter 22, the "peg" refers to the interferon's attachment to the hydrocarbon polyethylene glycol (PEG). This attachment reduces its antigenicity and prolongs its therapeutic effect.

In terms of chemotherapy, IFN alfa-2a and IFN alfa-2b are used to treat hairy-cell leukemia and AIDS-related Kaposi's sarcoma. IFN alfa-2a is also used to treat chronic myelogenous leukemia, and IFN alfa-2b is used in the treatment of malignant melanoma and certain lymphomas. Side effects of these drugs include fever, chills, myalgias, headache, fatigue, neutropenia, GI disturbances, and elevated liver enzyme levels. Other adverse effects include cardiovascular (tachycardia, orthostatic hypotension, electrocardiographic changes) and CNS disturbances (confusion, poor concentration, seizures, paranoid psychoses).

Interleukins

Interleukins are soluble proteins released from activated lymphocytes, especially NK cells. There are many different interleukins (IL-2-8, IL-10, and IL-12), and more are being recognized as knowledge of the immune system grows. There are currently four interleukins commercially available, three that are IL-2, and used in cancer treatment, and a fourth, anakinra, actually an IL-1 receptor blocker, which is used in the treatment of rheumatoid arthritis.

The most widely used interleukin is aldesleukin. This is an IL-2 analog that binds to T-cell receptors to induce a differentiation into lymphokine-activated killer cells in the blood and tumor-infiltrating lymphocytes in specific tumors. It is given intravenously for metastatic renal cell carcinoma every 8 hours for 14 doses. After 9 days of rest, the regimen is repeated for a total of 28 doses. It is currently under investigation for use in breast, ovarian, colon, brain, head and neck, and lung cancer.

Aldesleukin is associated with a syndrome known as capillary leak syndrome. This is a condition in which capillaries allow the passage of colloids, albumin, and other proteins out of the vasculature. The result of this movement creates fluid overload in the surrounding tissues. Massive fluid retention can lead to respiratory distress, heart failure, and

---

Box 23-3	**Interferon: Current FDA-Approved Indications**

Antiviral uses (type of interferon)
Condylomata acuminata (genital warts: HPV)
Hepatitis (alfa-2a*, alfa-2b*, alfacon-1)

Antineoplastic uses (type of interferon)
Chronic myelogenous leukemia (alfa-2a)
Follicular lymphoma (alfa-2b)
Hairy-cell leukemia (alfa-2a, alfa-2b)
Kaposi's sarcoma (alfa-2a, alfa-2b)
Malignant melanoma (alfa-2b)

Other immunomodulatory uses (type of interferon)
Chronic granulomatous disease (gamma-1b)
Multiple sclerosis (beta-1a, beta-1b)
Osteopetrosis (gamma-1b)

From Lilley LL, Harrington D, Snyder JS. *Pharmacology and the Nursing Process.* 4th ed. St Louis: Mosby; 2005. *FDA*, U.S. Food and Drug Administration; *HPV*, human papilloma virus.
*Including pegylated dosage forms (pegIFNs).

myocardial infarction. These effects are reversible if the drug is promptly discontinued. Close patient monitoring is necessary, and visible edema or rapid weight gain needs to be reported to the physician. Milder effects include GI disturbances, fever, chills, rash, myalgias, hepatotoxicity, and eosinophilia.

Monoclonal Antibodies

MABs are genetically engineered murine (mouse) or human antibodies that are directed against certain specific antigens expressed on cancer cells. Because specificity is high, destruction of other cells is limited, and therefore many side effects produced by the traditional chemotherapeutic agents are avoided. MABs were originally made by immunizing a mouse with antigen and then removing the spleen several weeks later.[52] From the spleen, a mixture of lymphocytes and plasma cells were obtained and then fused in vitro with myeloma cells (cancerous B cells that produce large numbers of antibodies). The result was significant amounts of homogenous antibodies tailor-made to act against a specific antigen. Nowadays, they are manufactured with recombinant DNA techniques.

An MAB is made up of two regions: the Fab fragment containing the antigen-binding site and the Fc region containing the binding site for monocytes, macrophages, NK cells, and other similar effector cells. Using these regions, the antibody blocks tumor growth by several different mechanisms.[53] The traditional mechanism involves binding of the antibody to the antigen and the activation of the complement components, opsonization by phagocytic cells, and then direct lysis. The second mechanism occurs when the MAB binds to the Fc receptors on macrophages or NK cells, resulting in release of cytokines. A sort of cross-linkage forms between the effector cells, the MAB, and the tumor. Another method used by the MAB is to bind directly to growth factor receptors on the cancer cell. The drugs rituximab for B-cell lymphomas and trastuzumab for breast cancer both work in this manner.

Rituximab was the first MAB to be approved for use in humans. It binds to the CD20 antigen on the surface of normal and cancerous B lymphocytes.[54] It is primarily used against B-cell non-Hodgkin's lymphoma, but its use has expanded to include other lymphomas as well. The CD20 antigen is a transmembrane protein that exists on almost all B cells, from the stage at which they become committed to becoming B cells up to the stage in which they become plasma cells. This marker does not exist on multiple myeloma cells, which arise from the more mature B cells. The drawback to use of rituximab is that it also kills normal B cells. Yet surprisingly, the absence of normal B cells for 6 months has not been associated with pronounced infectious disease. Because normal B cells recover in about 6 months after treatment, a schedule of 4 weeks of the drug every half year has been used.

Once the rituximab binds to the CD20 marker, it is not exactly clear how cell death occurs. Complement activation occurs, but NK cells and cytokine secretion are also involved.[54] Unfortunately, because not all the patients reach remission and relapses are common, resistance mechanisms are hard at work. The response rate is 48%, with duration of response lasting about a year.[55] Response was significantly improved when the MAB was added to chemotherapy, resulting in complete response in 58% of patients and partial responses in 42%. In addition to flu-like symptoms during infusion, this drug can produce severe bronchospasm, angioedema, and hypotension.

Trastuzumab is another MAB with a different mechanism of action. It has been approved for use in the United States since 1998 as a treatment for metastatic breast cancer. It is a genetically engineered anti–human epidermal growth factor receptor 2 (HER2) MAB that binds to the HER2 expressed on human breast cancer cells. Approximately 25% to 30% of patients with breast disease have amplification of the *HER2* gene, resulting in overexpression of the HER2 protein. Abundance of this growth factor leads to rapid growth of the tumor and a particularly virulent and resistant form of the disease. Therefore blocking this receptor on the cancer cell appears to be a reasonable approach to treatment.

The initial studies on trastuzumab, when used as monotherapy in the first-line treatment of metastatic disease, demonstrated that the drug was not only effective but also produced improvements in quality-of-life measures.[56] This outcome measure has been chosen by many chemotherapeutic studies, because in the majority of metastatic diseases, there is a prolongation of survival but no overall decrease in mortality rate. Any increase in survival should be matched by an improvement in function or the drug would not be considered very effective. When trastuzumab was added to a regimen of chemotherapy, the overall response rate was 45%, compared with 29% for chemotherapy alone.[55,57] Specifically, the chemotherapy agents doxorubicin, paclitaxel, and vinorelbine all potentiate the effectiveness of trastuzumab.[58] Time to progression of the disease was also significantly increased with combination therapy. However, when the drug is withdrawn, tumor growth resumes.

Side effects of trastuzumab are mild to moderate in severity and are usually infusion related.[59] Symptoms include fever, chills, nausea, and headache; but these usually dissipate during the infusion. In addition, symptoms are worse with the initial dose. However, cardiac dysfunction has been reported when trastuzumab is used in combination with chemotherapy, particularly anthracycline or doxorubicin.

Gemtuzumab ozogamicin is another MAB with a unique makeup.[2] The antibody is attached to the antineoplastic antibiotic ozogamicin. This complex binds to leukemic blast cells for the treatment of acute myelocytic leukemia. Attachment of the antibody portion of the drug leads to internalization of the compound. Once in the cell, the ozogamicin component is released into the lysosomes and leads to DNA damage.

Ibritumomab tiuxetan, like gemtuzumab ozogamicin, is also an interesting compound.[2] It is administered along with a radioactive isotope. The MAB binds to the CD20 antigen on the surfaces of normal and cancerous B lymphocytes. Once this binding occurs, the tiuxetan binds the radioisotope, which in turn damages the cell containing the drug. It is used to treat non-Hodgkin's lymphoma. Other MABs include cetuximab for the treatment of metastatic colorectal cancer and alemtuzumab for B-cell chronic lymphocytic leukemia.[60,61]

Hematopoietic Agents and Stem Cell Replacement

The hematopoietic agents are not directly involved in the killing of cancer cells but rather enhance the effects of the chemotherapeutic agents by allowing higher and more frequent chemotherapy dosing with quicker recovery between antineoplastic cycles. They are also known as *colony-stimulating factors*, promoting the growth and differentiation of the progenitor cells.

The colony-stimulating factors are produced by recombinant DNA technology and therefore are identical to the natural endogenously produced chemicals. They bind to receptors in the bone marrow to increase the production of specific cell lines. Epoetin alfa is the synthetic version of erythropoietin that stimulates red blood cell production.[62] Darbepoetin alfa is a newer agent that is longer acting.[63] Filgrastim and lenograstim stimulate the production of granulocytes and are also called *granulocyte colony-stimulating factors.*[64] Sargramostim stimulates the production of both granulocytes and macrophages and hence is known as *granulocyte-macrophage colony-stimulating factor.* Oprelvekin works a bit differently from the other colony-stimulating factors in that it is an IL-11 analog that stimulates megakaryocytes to produce platelets.

The benefits of these colony-stimulating agents include a reduction in chemotherapy-induced neutropenia, thrombocytopenia, and anemia. Clinically, this results in reduced fever, mouth sores, infections, antibiotic use, and hospital stay among patients with cancer treated with chemotherapy.[65] However, studies have not shown tremendous benefit unless the patient has a grade 4 neutropenia (defined as an absolute neutrophil count of <500 cells/mm^3) or a fever.[66] An example of how these drugs may be used is the administration of docetaxel in the treatment of metastatic disease.[67] The recommended dose and cycling of this drug is $100 \, mg/m^2$ every 21 days. Neutropenia limits greater concentrations and a shorter dosing interval. However, in one small study, the addition of lenograstim reduced the dosing interval to once every 2 weeks. In general, filgrastim is given until the absolute neutrophil count is about $10,000/mm^3$ after the neutrophil nadir.[2] Hematological recovery (neutropenic status) may take as little as 7 days, whereas the return of hematological status after straight chemotherapy may take 3 weeks or more.[68] This shortened time cuts down on mortality from infection and bleeding and also allows the next cycle of chemotherapy to begin earlier, if indicated.

In general, these stimulating factors are well tolerated, but there are a few things to watch out for. For example, erythropoietin may force the hematocrit and hemoglobin values to rise too high and too quickly, producing hypertension and seizures. There is also some concern that the platelet-inducing agents might cause deep vein thrombosis and pulmonary embolism.[69]

The benefits of colony-stimulating treatments may be more evident in patients undergoing hematopoietic stem cell mobilization or transplantation. Hematopoietic stem cell mobilization refers to the expansion of circulating stem cells in preparation for autologous and allogeneic peripheral blood stem cell replacements.[68] Administration of granulocyte colony-stimulating factor and granulocyte-macrophage colony-stimulating factor is used to cause the progenitor cells to leak out into the circulation so they can be collected. Chemotherapy agents may also be combined with the growth factors because it has been observed that when the two therapies are combined, a synergistic effect occurs, resulting in substantially larger numbers of peripheral blood progenitor cells. In the early 1970s, it was observed that the use of chemotherapy agents with myelosuppressive, as opposed to myeloablative, characteristics produced a mobilization of hematopoietic stem cells from the marrow about 2 weeks after recovery from the nadir. Cyclophosphamide and paclitaxel have been commonly used for this purpose.

In the autologous transplant, the growth factors are administered first, followed by collection of the progenitor cells with leukapheresis. The cells range the gamut of stem cells and include megakaryocytic, erythroid, and myeloid types, as well as mature neutrophils. The patient then undergoes high-dose chemotherapy to eradicate malignant cells and to make space in the bone marrow for new cells. This is followed by reinfusion of the patient's own progenitor cells, approximately 48 to 72 hours after the last chemotherapy dose. The neutropenia that occurs with the stem cell transplantation may last from 9 to 21 days.[70] If the neutropenia continues, it usually means the graft has failed. Mature T lymphocytes and lymphocyte subtypes may take a minimum of 6 months or as long as 2 years to recover, and B lymphocytes may also take up to 2 years to recover. Advantages of using the growth factors include the avoidance of marrow harvesting from the iliac crest, enhanced engraftment, and the avoidance of graft-versus-host disease (GVHD).

IMMUNOSUPPRESSION

Drugs that are used to prevent organ or tissue rejection are known as immunosuppressant agents. Commonly used agents include cyclosporine, muromonab-CD3, tacrolimus, sirolimus, and basiliximab.[2,71] Steroids are often combined with these drugs for added immunosuppression. Each agent differs in the exact mechanism of action, but the result is always inhibition of T-cell activation. See Figure 23-8 for the sites of action of these agents. Patients who take these drugs become immunocompromised like patients with AIDS or patients with bone marrow depression resulting from high-dose chemotherapy. Therefore many of the concerns expressed earlier can be applied to the patient who has undergone transplantation surgery.

Immunosuppressant Agents

Cyclosporine is the primary agent used to prevent the rejection of a transplanted kidney, heart, or liver or bone marrow. It is also beneficial in the treatment of some autoimmune disorders. This is a potent drug that has a narrow therapeutic index. Acute nephrotoxicity is a common side effect that generally occurs within the first month of use. Reduction of the dose may reverse the toxicity. Hepatotoxicity can also occur. Some other effects include hypertension (50% of patients), neurotoxicity including tremors (20% of patients), hyperkalemia, hirsutism, glucose intolerance, and gingival hyperplasia.

Tacrolimus is similar to cyclosporine but more potent. It is used primarily to prevent liver rejection. It produces a lower incidence of rejection, and lower doses of glucocorticoids are needed, reducing the incidence of infections. Because this agent is more potent, it also produces a greater incidence of nephrotoxicity and neurotoxicity than cyclosporine. Other toxic effects are similar to those caused by cyclosporine, with the exceptions of hirsutism and gingival hyperplasia. Sirolimus is very similar to tacrolimus in chemical structure and in mechanism of action. It is used to prevent organ rejection but also has been used as a coating on stents during angioplasty to prevent restenosis.

Basiliximab and daclizumab are both IL-2 receptor antagonists. They are MABs that bind to the IL receptor present on the cell surface of activated lymphocytes. Both drugs are used to prevent kidney rejection in a regimen that includes cyclosporine and a steroid. They are better tolerated than cyclosporine.

Muromonab-CD3 is another MAB directed against the CD3 antigen of the human T cell. It is unique for a variety of reasons. It is very similar to the antibodies naturally produced by the human body, but it is derived from mice. In addition, it is the only immunosuppressant agent indicated for

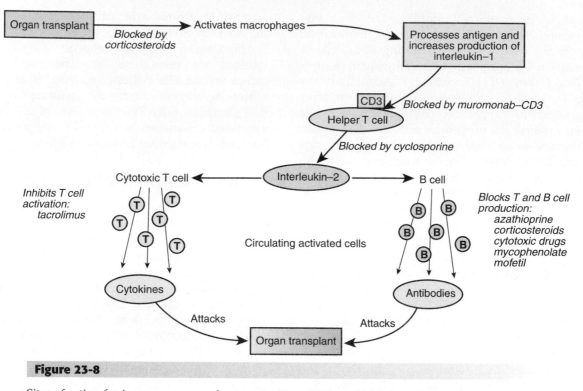

Figure 23-8

Sites of action for immunosuppressive agents. (From McKenry LM, Salerno E. *Mosby's Pharmacology in Nursing.* 21st ed. St Louis: Mosby; 2003.)

the treatment of organ rejection once it has started. However, because initial use is associated with cytokine release, it is necessary to premedicate the patient with methylprednisolone, diphenhydramine, and acetaminophen. This cytokine release syndrome leads to flu-like illness. A high fever may occur, as well as seizures, encephalopathy, and cerebral edema.

Implications for the physical therapist are similar to those outlined for some of the chemotherapy agents. Therapists must watch for signs of infection and bone marrow depression. Therapists must also watch for signs of GVHD, which can be devastating.

Graft-versus-Host Disease

Acute GVHD occurs very quickly after transplantation or bone marrow infusion. It is caused by alloantigen-activated donor T cells that travel into target organs and cause tissue destruction.[72] It is a primary cause of morbidity and mortality among transplant recipients. In terms of hematopoietic cell transplantation, it causes death in 15% to 40% of

patients. Symptoms include hepatitis, dermatitis, and GI problems. The rashes are maculopapular and often begin on the palms and soles. This syndrome results from inflammatory cytokines and has been called *cytokine storm* as a result of the continued release of cytokines.

Chronic GVHD develops in 15% to 50% of patients who survive 3 months after transplantation.[72] It involves multiple organ toxicity. The skin becomes fragile, and rashes are also present. Nails also become fragile and cracked with vertical ridging. Even hair becomes thin and delicate. Dryness, photophobia, and burning are symptoms occurring in the eyes. The mouth becomes similarly dry, and symptoms include sensitivity to spicy food. GI problems such as reflux, dysphagia, diarrhea, and malabsorption occur, as well as cholestasis. Liver disease also becomes a problem. Chronic GVHD even displays some musculoskeletal signs, including muscle cramps and fascitis (diminished slide of the skin over muscles).[73] Physical therapy may be required to monitor range of motion. Respiratory involvement includes bronchiolitis, and lastly, the immune system displays severe immunodeficiency.

Therapeutic Concerns

As with patients receiving chemotherapy, physical therapists must be on alert for any signs of infection in patients with GVHD. The physician must be contacted immediately if fever, rash, sore throat, or unusual fatigue develops. Patients must be monitored for signs of bone marrow depression, such as increased bleeding or bruising. Frequent laboratory monitoring is necessary, and the drugs may be withheld if the leukocyte count drops below $30,000/\text{mm}^3$.

Patients who have undergone transplant surgery must continue to receive immunosuppressants on a long-term basis. Side effects are not pleasant and often lead to noncompliance with treatment.[74] In addition to the hypertension or hypercholesterolemia, transplant recipients also experience changes in their physical appearance and emotional baseline. Weight gain, sleep deprivation, tremors, hirsutism, sexual dysfunction, and psychiatric symptoms (depression and anxiety) may develop and affect the patient's quality of life. Physical therapy can help with some of these side effects by providing gentle stretching modalities, a conditioning program, and biofeedback to help with the drug-induced myalgias, weight gain, or even some of the musculoskeletal symptoms of chronic GVHD. Patients should be scheduled for therapy at times when the gym is least crowded and should be kept away from any person with a cold, infection, or other contagious illness.

ACTIVITIES 23

■ 1. Multiple organ toxicity is a sign of GVHD. What are some of the early signs that indicate multiple organs are involved and what dysfunction do they represent?

■ 2. How would you monitor for the complications of multiple toxicity?

■ 3. Provide some strategies that the physical therapist can implement to help protect the immunocompromised patient.

■ 4. Chemotherapy agents are potentially hazardous not just to the patient but also to the caregiver who administers the drug. Therefore all drugs, vials, needles, syringes, and other equipment must be discarded with extreme caution. Discuss some of the methods for drug disposal, as well as for disposal of body fluids that may contain the chemotherapy agent.

References

1. McKenry LM, Salerno E. Principles of antineoplastic chemotherapy. In: *Mosby's Pharmacology in Nursing.* 21st ed. St Louis: Mosby; 2003:928-939.
2. Lilley LL, Harrington D, Snyder JS. Antineoplastic agents. In: *Pharmacology and the Nursing Process.* 4th ed. St Louis: Mosby; 2005:773-811.
3. Norman KL, Farassati F, Lee PWK. Oncolytic viruses and cancer therapy. *Cytokine Growth Factor Rev.* 2001; 12:271-282.
4. Lane DP, Lain S. Therapeutic exploitation of the p53 pathway. *Trends Mol Med.* 2002;8(suppl 4):S38-S42.
5. Reed JC. Apoptosis-based therapies. *Nat Rev Drug Discov.* 2002;1:111-121.
6. Sikic BI. New approaches in cancer treatment. *Ann Oncol.* 1999;10(suppl 6):149-153.
7. Eder JP. Drugs and neoplasms. In: Page C, Curtis MJ, Sutter MC, Walker MJ, Hoffman BB, eds. *Integrated Pharmacology.* 2nd ed. Philadelphia: Mosby; 2002:163-187.
8. Damaraju VL, Damaraju S, Young JD, et al. Nucleoside anticancer drugs: the role of nucleoside transporters in resistance to cancer chemotherapy. *Oncogene.* 2003; 22:7524-7536.
9. Kruh GD, Belinsky MG. The MRP family of drug efflux pumps. *Oncogene.* 2003;22:7537-7552.
10. Furlanut M, Franceschi L. Pharmacology of ifosfamide. *Oncology.* 2003;65(suppl 2):2-6.
11. Klastersky J. Side effects of ifosfamide. *Oncology.* 2003; 65(suppl 2):7-10.
12. Nicolao P, Giometto B. Neurological toxicity of ifosfamide. *Oncology.* 2003;65(suppl 2):11-16.
13. Parney IF, Chang SM. Current chemotherapy for glioblastoma. *Cancer J.* 2003;9(3):149-156.

14. Hartmann JT, Lipp HP. Toxicity of platinum compounds. *Expert Opin Pharmacother.* 2003;4(6):889-901.

15. Boulikas T, Vougiouka M. Cisplatin and platinum drugs at the molecular level [review]. *Oncol Rep.* 2003; 10(6):1663-1682.

16. Siddik ZH. Cisplatin: mode of cytotoxic action and molecular basis of resistance. *Oncogene.* 2003;22:7265-7279.

17. Dumontet C, Sikic BI. Mechanisms of action of and resistance to antitubulin agents: microtubule dynamics, drug transport, and cell death. *J Clin Oncol.* 1999; 17(3):1061-1070.

18. Tanner KD, Reichling DB, Levine JD. Nociceptor hyper-responsiveness during vincristine-induced painful peripheral neuropathy in the rat. J Neurosci. 1998; 18(16):6480-6491.

19. Orr GA, Verdier-Pinard P, McDaid H, Horwitz SB. Mechanisms of taxol resistance related to microtubules. *Oncogene.* 2003;22:7280-7295.

20. Durand J, Goldwasser F. Dramatic recovery of paclitaxel-disabling neurosensory toxicity following treatment with venlafaxine. *Anticancer Drugs.* 2002;13(7):777-780.

21. Schimmel K, Richel D, van den Brink R, Guchelaar HJ. Cardiotoxicity of cytotoxic drugs. *Cancer Treat Rev.* 2004; 30:181-191.

22. Rich TA, Shepard RC, Mosley ST. Four decades of continuing innovation with fluorouracil: current and future approaches to fluorouracil chemoradiation therapy. *J Clin Oncol.* 2004;22(11):2214-2232.

23. Rasheed ZA, Rubin EH. Mechanisms of resistance to topoisomerase I-targeting drugs. *Oncogene.* 2003; 22(47):7296-7304.

24. Osborne K. Drug therapy: tamoxifen in the treatment of breast cancer. *N Engl J Med.* 1998;339(22):1609-1618.

25. Tamoxifen for prevention of breast cancer. *Med Lett Drugs Ther.* 1999;41(1043):1-2.

26. Cummings SR, Eckert S, Krueger KA, et al. The effect of raloxifene on risk of breast cancer in postmenopausal women. *JAMA.*1999;281(23):2189-2197.

27. Piccart-Gebhart MJ. New stars in the sky of treatment for early breast cancer. *N Engl J Med.* 2004;350(11):1140-1142.

28. Toremifene and letrozole for advanced breast cancer. *Med Lett Drugs Ther.* 1998;40(1024):43-45.

29. Coombes RC, Hall E, Gibson LJ, et al. A randomized trial of exemestane after two to three years of tamoxifen therapy in postmenopausal women with primary breast cancer. *N Engl J Med.* 2004;350(11):1081-1092.

30. Savage DG, Antman KH. Imatinib mesylate: a new oral targeted therapy. *N Engl J Med.* 2002;346(9):683-693.

31. Druker BJ. ST1571 (Gleevec) as a paradigm for cancer therapy. *Trends Mol Med.* 2002;8(4):S14-S18.

32. Druker BJ, Talpaz M, Resta DJ, et al. Efficacy and safety of a specific inhibitor of the BCR-ABL tyrosine kinase in chronic myeloid leukemia. *N Engl J Med.* 2001; 344(14):1031-1037.

33. Druker BJ, Sawyers CL, Kantarjian H, et al. Activity of a specific inhibitor of the BCR-ABL tyrosine kinase in the blast crisis of chronic myeloid leukemia and acute lymphoblastic leukemia with the Philadelphia chromosome. *N Engl J Med.* 2001;344(14):1038-1042.

34. Gleevec (STI-571) for chronic myeloid leukemia. *Med Lett Drugs Ther.* 2001;43(1106):49-50.

35. Dempke W, Rie C, Grothey A, Schmoll HJ. Cyclooxygenase-2: a novel target for cancer chemo-therapy? *J Cancer Res Clin Oncol.* 2001;127:411-417.

36. Xu XC. Cox-2 inhibitors in cancer treatment and prevention, a recent development. *Anticancer Drugs.* 2002;13(2):127-137.

37. Gupta RA, DuBois RN. Colorectal cancer prevention and treatment by inhibition of cyclooxygenase-2. *Nat Rev Cancer.* 2001;1:11-21.

38. Hornby PJ. Central neurocircuitry associated with emesis. *Am J Med.* 2001;111(suppl 8A):106S-112S.

39. Grunberg SM, Hesketh PJ. Drug therapy: control of chemotherapy-induced emesis. *N Engl J Med.* 1993; 329(24):1790-1796.

40. Rolston K. Management of infections in the neutropenic patient. *Annu Rev Med.* 2004;55:519-526.

41. Watson T, Mock V. Exercise and cancer-related fatigue: a review of current literature. *Rehabil Oncol.* 2003; 21(1):23-30.

42. Clohisy DR, Mantyh PW. Bone cancer pain. *Cancer.* 2003; 97(suppl 3):866-873.

43. Fine PG. Analgesia issues in palliative care: bone pain, controlled release opioids, managing opioid-induced constipation and nifedipine as an analgesic. *J Pain Palliat Care Pharmacother.* 2002;16(1):93-97.

44. Rogers MJ, Watts DJ, Graham R, Russell G. Overview of bisphosphonates. *Cancer.* 1997;80(8):1652-1660.

45. Tanner K, Levine J, Topp K. Microtubule disorientation and axonal swelling in unmyelinated sensory axons during vincristine-induced and painful neuropathy in rat. *J Comp Neurol.* 1998;395(4):481-492.

46. Ruppert M, Croarkin E. A review of four vibration sensation assessments used to examine chemotherapy induced neuropathy. *Rehabil Oncol.* 2003;21(3):11-18.

47. Perkins BA, Olaleye D, Zinman B, Bril V. Simple screening tests for peripheral neuropathy in the diabetes clinic. *Diabetes Care.* 2001;24(2):250-256.

48. Minisini A, Atalay G, Bottomley A, Puglisi F, Piccart M, Biganzoli L. What is the effect of systemic anticancer treatment on cognitive function? *Lancet Oncol.* 2004; 5:273-282.

49. Fann JR, Sullivan AK. Delirium in the course of cancer treatment. *Semin Clin Neuropsychiatry.* 2003;8(4):217-228.

50. Bakemeier RF, Quazi R. Basic concepts of cancer chemotherapy and principles of medical oncology. In: Rubin P, ed. *Clinical Oncology.* 8th ed. New York: Saunders; 2001:146-159.

51. Papamichail M, Perez SA, Gritzapis AD, Baxevanis CN. Natural killer lymphocytes: biology, development, and function. *Cancer Immunol Immunother.* 2003;53(3):176-186.

52. Kawabata TT. Immunopharmacology. In: Brody MJ, Larner J, Minneman KP, eds. *Human Pharmacology: Molecular to Clinical.* 3rd ed. St Louis: Mosby; 1998: 621-640.

53. Houghton AN, Scheinberg DA. Monoclonal antibody therapies: a 'constant' threat to cancer. *Nat Med.* 2000; 6(4):373-374.

54. Smith MR. Rituximab (monoclonal anti-CD20 antibody): mechanisms of action and resistance. *Oncogene.* 2003; 22:7359-7368.

55. White CA, Weaver RL, Grillo-Lopez AJ. Antibody-targeted immunotherapy for treatment of malignancy. *Annu Rev Med.* 2001;52:125-145.

56. Vogel CL, Cobleign MA, Tripathy D, et al. Efficacy and safety of trastuzumab as a single agent in first-line treatment of HER2-overexpressing metastatic breast cancer. *J Clin Oncol.* 2002;20(3):719-726.

57. Osoba D, Slamon DJ, Burchmore M, Murphy MB. Effects on quality of life of combined trastuzumab and chemotherapy in women with metastatic breast cancer. *J Clin Oncol.* 2002;20(14):3106-3113.
58. Mitchell MS. Combinations of anticancer drugs and immunotherapy. *Cancer Immunol Immunother.* 2003; 52:686-692.
59. Bell R. Duration of therapy in metastatic breast cancer: management using Herceptin. *Anticancer Drugs.* 2001; 12:561-568.
60. Reynolds NA, Wagstaff AJ. Cetuximab: in the treatment of metastatic colorectal cancer. *Drugs.* 2004;64(1):109-118.
61. Harris M. Monoclonal antibodies as therapeutic agents for cancer. *Lancet Oncol.* 2004;5:292-302.
62. Erythropoietin (Procrit; Epogen) revisited. *Med Lett Drugs Ther.* 2001;43(1104):40-41.
63. Darbepoetin (Aranesp): A long-acting erythropoietin. *Med Lett Drugs Ther.* 2001;43(1120):109-110.
64. Martin-Christin F. Granulocyte colony stimulating factors: how different are they? How to make a decision? *Anticancer Drugs.* 2001;12:185-191.
65. Dale DC. Where now for colony-stimulating factors? *Lancet.* 1995;346:135-136.
66. Hoelzer D. Hematopoietic growth factors: not whether, but when and where. *N Engl J Med.* 1997;336(25):1822-1824.
67. Culine S, Romieu G, Fabbro M, et al. Reducing the time interval between cycles using standard doses of docetaxel and lenogastrim support. *Cancer.* 2004;101:178-182.
68. Fu S, Liesveld J. Mobilization of hematopoietic stem cells. *Blood Rev.* 2000;14:205-218.
69. Fanucchi M, Glaspy J, Crawford J, et al. Effects of polyethylene glycol-conjugated recombinant human megakaryocyte growth and development factor on platelet counts after chemotherapy for lung cancer. *N Engl J Med.* 1997;336(6):404-409.
70. Trigg ME. Hematopoietic stem cells. *Pediatrics.* 2004; 114(4):1051-1057.
71. First MR, Fitzsimmons WE. New drugs to improve transplant outcomes. *Transplantation.* 2004;77(9):S88-S92.
72. Anasetti C. Advances in the prevention of graft-versus-host disease after hematopoietic cell transplantation. *Transplantation.* 2004;77(9):S79-S83.
73. Arai S, Vogelsang GB. Management of graft-versus-host disease. *Blood Rev.* 2000;14:190-204.
74. Galbraith CA, Hathaway D. Long-term effects of transplantation on quality of life. *Transplantation.* 2004; 77(9):S84-S87.

The Relationship Between Drug Therapy and Exercise

INTERACTION BETWEEN SELECTIVE CARDIOPULMONARY AND DIABETIC MEDICATIONS AND EXERCISE

The beneficial effects of exercise for those with cardiac, pulmonary, and metabolic diseases are well documented in the literature.[1-3] The American Heart Association Scientific Statement on Cardiac Rehab and Secondary Prevention of Coronary Heart Disease cites the cardioprotective mechanisms of exercise training for those with coronary artery disease (CAD).[1] Among them were the increased flow-mediated shear stress on artery walls during exercise, the decrease in C-reactive proteins, the reduction in rate pressure product, the improvement in coronary artery compliance and endothelium-dependent vasodilatation, and the increase in the luminal area of conduit vessels through arteriogenesis and myocardial capillary density by angiogenesis.

The most recent Official Statement of the American Thoracic Society on Pulmonary Rehabilitation states that "the efficacy and scientific foundation of pulmonary rehabilitation have been firmly established."[2] The American Thoracic Society has stated that pulmonary rehabilitation reduces symptoms, increases functional ability, and improves quality of life in individuals with chronic respiratory disease, even in the face of irreversible abnormalities of lung architecture. According to the report, exercise training is the foundation of pulmonary rehabilitation and has a positive effect on dyspnea.

The Clinical Practice Recommendations 2004: Position Statement of the American Diabetic Association cites the beneficial aspects of physical activity for both type 1 and type 2 diabetes.[3] The benefits include glycemic control, prevention of cardiovascular disease, a decrease in triglyceride-rich very low density lipoprotein, a decrease in blood pressure (BP), enhancement of weight loss, and prevention of type 2 diabetes.

The question therefore is not whether to exercise patients with cardiac, pulmonary, or metabolic diseases, but how can these patients be safely exercised and what are the effects of the medications on the exercise responses?

The basic principles of exercise training must be used when the prescription is formulated. The principles of overload, specificity, individuality, and reversibility must be applied to achieve the desired training outcomes.[4] *Overload* refers to the application of a load that enhances physiological function to bring about a training response, that is, the exercise prescription. Manipulation of frequency, intensity, and duration will achieve the appropriate training overload. *Specificity* refers to the adaptations in metabolic and physiological functions that depend on the overload imposed. Exercise outcomes are specific to the muscles and energy systems trained, as well as to the type of training mode. Specificity focuses on the "how to" of goal achievement. *Individuality* refers to the individual variation in the training response. This principle takes into account the person's level of fitness and other specific factors to gear the prescription to the person's needs and capacities. It focuses on the skilled interventions that are required to safely exercise these patients. *Reversibility* focuses on the detraining response, which occurs rapidly when the overload is removed. In a sense, it refers to "use it or lose it." This principle focuses on the need for exercise compliance. These basic principles must be followed when the physical therapist is preparing an effective and safe exercise prescription for a patient.

The normal responses to exercise for a healthy individual are well documented in exercise physiology textbooks, as well as in the guidelines for an exercise prescription[4] (Table 24-1). Also, a plethora of research has been done on the responses to exercise in healthy individuals receiving medication. What are not well documented are the responses to exercise for those receiving medications who have an actual disease. More specifically, the responses to long-term training versus a brief bout of exercise are sparse in the literature. Interpretation of the literature is also difficult because studies vary with respect to drug doses, drugs examined, time of day when the patients exercise, and exercise parameters used as outcome measures. The purpose of this chapter is to discuss the response to exercise by subjects with cardiac, pulmonary, or metabolic disease who are taking appropriate medications.

CARDIAC MEDICATIONS

The American College of Sports Medicine Guidelines for Exercise Testing and Prescription delineates the exercise responses during treatment with certain cardiac medications.[4] This section focuses on two of the most prescribed medications for those with cardiac disease: β-blockers and calcium channel blockers. These medications are used to treat hypertension and angina pectoris. Their mechanisms of action on cardiac parameters are discussed to help explain the exercise responses. The population considered consists of patients with CAD because these medications produce different responses depending on the disease. For example, patients with hypertension show a decrease in exercise capacity while taking a β-blocker, but patients with CAD demonstrate an increase in exercise capacity.

β-Blockers

β-Blockers are classified as selective and nonselective, depending on the receptors on which they act. *Selective* refers to those that act primarily on the heart, whereas nonselective agents will affect the heart, bronchi, peripheral vasculature, pancreas, and liver.[5] This will have implications during exercise, depending on which type of β-blocker is prescribed. Actions of the β–adrenoreceptors are controlled by their link to the sympathetic nervous system. They

Table 24-1

Normal Aerobic Exercise Responses in Healthy Sedentary Individuals		
Variable	Rest	Exercise
HR	60-90 beats/min	↑10-12 beats/min/MET level
SBP	<120 mm Hg	↑ 7 mm Hg/MET level
DBP	<80 mm Hg	↑↓ 10 mm Hg in entire session
SpO2	97-98	↔ or ↑
V_{O_2}	3.5 mL/kg/min^{-1}	↑
CO	5 L/min	↑ to 20-22 L/min
SV	71 mL/beat	↑ to 100 mL/beat but plateaus at 40% to 50% $V_{O_{2max}}$

↑, Increase; ↓, decrease; ↔, no effect; *HR*, heart rate; *MET*, metabolic equivalent; *SBP*, systolic blood pressure; *DBP*, diastolic blood pressure; *SpO₂*, saturation of oxygen with hemoglobin; *V$_{O_2}$*, oxygen consumption; *CO*, cardiac output; *SV*, stroke volume.

promote sympathetic control of the body's response to daily stresses of gravitational strain, muscular exercise, and emotional stimulation. β-Blockers are referred to as the treatment that mimics the effect of fitness on the heart rate (HR).

β-Blocking drugs, regardless of their selectivity, cause a reduction in HR, BP, and cardiac output (CO) during rest and exercise; a decrease in myocardial contractility; and a decrease in coronary and muscle blood flow, thus increasing myocardial efficiency as a result of a reduction in oxygen consumption.[6,7] Studies have shown a reduction in exercising HR by 20% to 30% and CO by 5% to 23%.[8,9] During exercise of moderate intensity (50% to 60% of maximum oxygen consumption [VO_{2max}]), the reduction in HR becomes more pronounced and produces compensatory adjustments in the cardiovascular system, such as an increase in stroke volume to maintain the CO and exercise level.[9,10] HR is a major determinant of myocardial oxygen consumption; this decrease in HR allows for an increase in diastolic filling time of coronary arteries, which allows for an increase in myocardial oxygen supply in comparison with the "unblocked" state.[6]

All β-blocking drugs (selective > nonselective β-blockers) produce an increase in exercise capacity in patients who have CAD but may decrease physical work capacity in those who only have hypertension.[11-25] The increase noted in physical work capacity with those who have CAD is documented by an increase in VO_{2max} with a decrease in HR and a lower rate pressure product at maximum levels, suggesting myocardial efficiency (Table 24-2). The oxygen economy of the myocardium may also be influenced by the interference of its cellular metabolism.[17] Propranolol, a nonselective β-blocker, has been found to decrease the myocardial use of free fatty acids with a consequent rise in myocardial carbohydrate utilization.[26] This could indicate an oxygen-saving shift in myocardial energy metabolism.[27] Despite the increase in work capacity with a lower rate pressure product, chest pain has been documented to occur, suggesting myocardial insufficiency.[14,20,21] This mechanism is not fully understood but may be explained by an increase in left ventricular volume and ejection time caused by the decrease in HR and contractility, which may increase myocardial oxygen demand.[16]

Another finding in the literature is that despite a further decrease in ejection fraction seen with β-blockade during exercise in patients whose

Table 24-2

Central (Cardiac) Responses during Exercise of Patients with Coronary Artery Disease while Taking a β-Blocker.	
Variable	**Response**
RHR	↓
MHR	↓ 20%-30%
SBP	↓
RPP	↓
CO	↓ 5%-23%
MVO_2	↑
CBF	↓
TET	↑
DFT	↑
Exercise capacity	↑
VO_{2max}	↑
SV	↑ Moderate exercise
DF	↑
Myocardial contractility	↓
ST depression	↓
Myocardial efficiency	↑
Ischemic threshold	↓

↑, Increase; ↓, decrease; *RHR*, resting heart rate; *MHR*, maximum heart rate; *SBP*, systolic blood pressure; *RPP*, rate pressure product; *CO*, cardiac output; *MVO_2*, myocardial oxygen consumption; *CBF*, coronary blood flow; *TET*, total exercise time; *DFT*, diastolic filling time; *VO_{2max}*, maximum oxygen consumption; *SV*, stroke volume; *DF*, diastolic function.

ejection fraction is less than 40% at rest, an increase in work capacity was still demonstrated.[13,14,28] This is in keeping with the fact that left diastolic function, and not left systolic function, predicts exercise tolerance.[29,30] β-Blockers have the potential to increase exercise tolerance by improving diastolic function.[31] They lengthen the diastolic period and improve subendocardial perfusion, in addition to decreasing left ventricular filling pressure and increasing left ventricular compliance.[13]

β-Blockers, particularly propranolol, may prevent the coronary steal phenomenon. Bortone et al.[32] found that despite coronary constriction at rest, coronary constriction of the stenosed segments during exercise was prevented with propranolol. Drug administration causes "reverse coronary steal" by the redistribution of the coronary blood flow from normal to ischemic regions, perhaps by way of collaterals. This decreases the ischemic threshold and allows the patient to exercise longer before chest pain occurs.

Selective and nonselective β-blockers have the same effect on cardiac parameters as described previously. However, differences lie in the pharmaco-kinetics; pulmonary influence; and metabolic, thermo-regulation, and vascular resistance effects.[6,7,24,33] Nonselective β-blockers have adverse effects on these parameters, so when medication is prescribed for active patients, the β_1 drugs tend to be preferred (Table 24-3). It is important to note that β-blockers with intrinsic sympathomimetic activity confer no advantage during exercise training.[6,7,24]

Some of the nonselective drugs are lipophilic and readily cross the blood-brain barrier to enter the central nervous system.[6,7] This may account for the central nervous system side effects (nightmares, fatigue, depression) seen with these agents.[34] It is presumed that these side effects can have implications for the individual's perception of the exercise bout and should be kept in mind because the physical therapist is attempting to promote a positive feeling regarding exercise.[6]

Thermoregulation is also affected by β-blockers as a result of an accelerated sweating response of approximately 10%.[24] This mechanism is not fully understood because nonselective agents cause peripheral constriction. Nevertheless, dehydration may occur if fluid replacement is not provided during exercise. Skin blood flow is also impaired as a result of a reduction in CO during exercise.[25] Even though the stroke volume does increase to compensate for the decrease in HR to maintain the CO, stroke volume plateaus at 40% of the person's VO_{2max} despite his or her disease.[35] Fluid replacement is important during exercise to prevent the decrease in BP that has been seen in patients participating in cardiac rehabilitation programs, especially those taking propranolol (anecdotal findings).

Metabolically, both the selective and nonselective β-blockers have effects on fat, glucose, and triglyceride utilization during exercise, but it appears that the nonselective blockers have a greater effect. The review by Head[7] goes into detail regarding this subject. This abnormality of metabolism can contribute to the premature fatigue experienced during exercise and also contributes to the unpleasantness sometimes associated with exercise during treatment with these drugs. The kinetics of drug release

Table 24-3

Nonselective β-Blockade Metabolic and Thermoregulatory Responses during Exercise

Variable	Responses
Fatigue	↑
Thermoregulation	Accelerated sweating response, dehydration
Fat utilization	Inhibition of intramuscular lipolysis, Reduction in adipose tissue lipolysis
Glucose utilization	Inhibitory effect on muscle glycogen breakdown
	Decrease in blood glucose levels:
	Impaired hepatic glycogenolysis
	Reduced hepatic gluconeogenesis
	Possible inhibitory effect on glucose uptake by exercising muscles

can also affect metabolic changes and exercise performance. Exercising at peak plasma concentrations can cause more fatigue and thus decrease exercise performance. Peak concentrations generally occur about 90 minutes after administration of the β-blockers.[36] Also, at higher doses, the selectivity appears to decrease, and the benefits of a selective β-blocker are lost.[37]

Exercise Prescription for Patients Taking β-Blockers

It is accepted that patients with CAD are able to attain a physiological training effect, regardless of the type of β-blocker they are taking.[7,24,38] The general principles of exercise training and prescription apply to this population as well.[4,35] The only exceptions are due to the pharmacokinetic properties of the β-blockers. The exercise prescription needs to be individualized according to the results of an exercise test while the person is taking the β-blocker.[6,24] Also, the exercise should take place at the same time each day to avoid differences in the plasma concentrations of the β-blocker and thus different exercise responses. If the patient experiences any of the adverse effects during exercise, appropriate action needs to be taken.[4] An exercise prescription should be based on the following information:

Type of exercise: aerobic for both upper and lower extremities and anaerobic for both upper and lower extremities if the patient meets the American Association of Cardiovascular and Pulmonary Rehabilitation criteria[39]

Mode: walking, stationary biking, upper extremity endurance training, rowing, dual-action devices

Frequency: 3 to 5 days per week

Duration: 20 to 60 minutes of continuous exercise

Intensity: 40% to 75% of Karvonen's formula ([(max HR − resting HR [RHR]) × %] + RHR) with HR max taken from the peak HR obtained during the stress test

Monitoring:

1. All patients should exercise based on the calculated intensity of their target heart rate (THR).
2. Rate of perceived exertion can only be used as an adjunct to HR monitoring.[6, 40-42]

Guidelines:

1. Exercise should occur at the same time each day.
2. Fluid replacement needs to be provided during the exercise session.
3. Pulse taking is required of the patient to monitor the THR during exercise.
4. The training HR must always be obtained by the patient's performance during the stress test conducted while he or she is taking medication.
5. If the patient does not take the medication, the exercise intensity is limited to an HR of 20 beats/min above resting value.[4]
6. If the medication is changed to another β-blocker or if the dose is adjusted, then the exercise HR is limited to 20 beats/min above resting value.[4]
7. The patient still requires a THR for skilled physical therapy.
8. The intensity of exercise should be limited to the THR so as not to violate the ischemic threshold during training.[43,44]
9. If nitroglycerin is prescribed, the patient should carry it at all times.

Calcium Channel Blockers

The introduction of calcium channel blockers for the treatment of cardiovascular disease has been considered the most significant advance in therapy since the introduction of β-blockers.[45,46] Calcium ion antagonists are used to decrease myocardial contractility, reduce peripheral vascular resistance, and dilate coronary arteries.[47] The resulting increase in coronary blood flow and reduced pressures is believed to decrease myocardial oxygen demand during exercise and thus prevent exertional angina pectoris.[48] Calcium channel blockers are not equal in their reactions and differ in their primary antianginal mechanisms because of their different chemical structures.[49-51] This will result in different exercise effects based on the type of calcium channel blocker administered.

The dihydropyridines (amlodipine, nicardipine, nifedipine) increase HR at rest and at maximal exercise levels but are more vascular selective with less effect on nodal tissue than the other calcium channel blockers.[47] This increase in HR can increase the myocardial oxygen consumption and possibly induce angina pectoris.[52] However, in general, this class of drugs will increase exercise time, increase the time before ST-segment depression, increase time to angina, and decrease the incidence of angina.[47,53,54]

The dihydropyridines are also known for decreasing BP—both the systolic and diastolic readings in normotensive as well as hypertensive individuals. In some individuals, when BP is lowered to a great extent, the heart compensates by producing a reflex tachycardia.[53,55, 56] The ensuing increase in myocardial oxygen consumption, caused by the increase in HR, creates additional angina. Amlodipine and nifedipine are the two drugs in this class that produce this side effect. Amlodipine is also known for producing lower extremity edema as a result of local effects on the microcirculation.[47,52,57] Another serious side effect with this group is coronary steal.[58,59] This phenomenon is explained by the fact that the blood is shunted away from the ischemic region to the nonischemic region, which worsens myocardial ischemia and thus increases episodes of angina.[60] This phenomenon will occur only in patients with good collateral blood flow.

The other commonly used calcium channel blockers, diltiazem and verapamil, influence cardiac muscle and nodal activity to a greater degree than do the dihydropyridines. This property makes them more effective for the treatment of exertional angina than the dihydropyridines.[54] They reduce HR at rest and during exercise because of their nonspecific inhibition of sympathetic drive, and they are effective for the treatment of supraventricular tachycardia and atrial fibrillation because they slow conduction through the atrioventricular node, thereby increasing the PR interval.[47,48,53,57] The reduction in HR reduces the myocardial oxygen consumption in these patients and the incidence of exertional angina, thus having a greater impact on effort-induced indices of myocardial ischemia. Diltiazem and verapamil therefore reduce myocardial oxygen demand better than the dihydropyridines.[53] They also dilate the coronary arteries and have negative chronotropic and mild inotropic effects, while also reducing peripheral vascular resistance to a lesser extent than the dihydropyridines.[47,53] They will decrease submaximal and maximal BP but not resting BP, thus preventing the reflex tachycardia seen with the dihydropyridines.[48] This class of drugs will also increase exercise time, increase the time before ST-segment depression, increase time to angina, and decrease the incidence of angina.[47,48,53]

Therefore, given the varying effects of the calcium channel blockers, it seems logical that an active patient with mild to moderate hypertension would probably perform better with a dihydropyridine, whereas a lower-functioning patient with exertional angina would do better with either verapamil or diltiazem. Because emerging evidence indicates that many patients with exertional angina have both CAD and increased vasomotor tone, these patients may perform better with diltiazem.[61,62] This "dynamic obstruction" is superimposed on a fixed obstruction, resulting in variability of the anginal threshold during exercise, and may be a contributing factor to the pathogenesis of myocardial ischemia.[63] Diltiazem has also been shown to increase resting coronary blood flow, increase resting and exercise levels of the left ventricular ejection fraction, and produce less depression of ventricular muscle.[57,64] Table 24-4 presents a summary of the hemodynamic responses produced by calcium channel blockers.

Exercise Prescription for Patients Taking Calcium Channel Blockers

The guidelines for patients taking calcium channel blockers are similar to those for patients taking a β-blocker. The general principles of exercise training apply as well to patients taking calcium ion antagonists. The most important consideration would be the class of calcium blockers the patient is taking. This would provide a general idea of what to expect during rest, as well as during the exercise session. If the patient experiences any of the

Table 24-4

Hemodynamic Responses of Calcium Channel Blockers		
Variable	Dihydropyridines	Benzothiazepines
RHR	↑	↓
MHR	↑	↓
MVO_2	↑	↓
TET	↑	↑
Time to ST depression	↑	↑
Time to angina	↑	↑
Anginal incidence	↓	↓
RSBP	↓	↔
RDBP	↓	↔
Reflex tachycardia	⊕	↔
Edema (LEs)	⊕	↔
Coronary steal	⊕	↔
Dilatation of coronary arteries	↔	⊕

↑, Increase; ↓ decrease; ↔, no effect; ⊕, has an effect; *RHR*, resting heart rate; *MHR*, maximum heart rate; *MVO_2*, myocardial oxygen consumption; *TET*, total exercise time; *RSBP*, resting systolic blood pressure; *RDBP*, resting diastolic blood pressure; *LEs*, lower extremity adverse effects to exercise, appropriate action must be taken.[1]

Type of exercise: aerobic for both upper and lower extremities and anaerobic for both upper and lower extremities if the patient meets the American Association of Cardiovascular and Pulmonary Rehabilitation criteria[39]

Mode: walking, stationary biking, upper extremity endurance training, rowing, dual-action devices

Frequency: 3 to 5 days per week

Duration: 20 to 60 minutes of continuous exercise

Intensity: 40% to 75% of Karvonen's formula ($[(max HR - RHR) \times \%] + RHR$) with HR max taken from the peak HR obtained during the stress test

Monitoring:

1. All patients should exercise based on the calculated intensity of their THR.
2. Rate of perceived exertion can only be used as an adjunct to HR monitoring.[6,40-42]

Guidelines:

1. Exercise should occur at the same time each day.
2. Pulse taking is required of the patient to monitor HR during exercise.
3. Side effects are more common with the dihydropyridines: reflex tachycardia, edema of the ankles, increase in RHR, and possible increase in angina during exercise.
4. If the patient does not take his or her medication, the exercise intensity should be limited to an HR of 20 beats/min above RHR.[4]
5. If the medication is changed to another calcium channel blocker or if the dose is adjusted, then the exercise HR is limited to 20 beats/min above resting HR.[4]
6. The patient still requires a THR for skilled physical therapy.
7. The intensity of exercise should be limited to the THR so as not to violate the ischemic threshold during training.[43,44]
8. If nitroglycerin is prescribed, the patient should carry it at all times.

β-Blockers or Calcium Channel Blockers for the Exercising Patient with Cardiac Disease

In a meta-analysis Heidenreich et al.[56] compared the relative efficacy and tolerability of treatment with β-blockers and calcium channel blockers in patients who have stable angina pectoris. A total of 143 articles were identified by MEDLINE and EMBASE searches, and a total of 90 fulfilled their inclusion criteria. Their results showed the following: (1) there was no significant difference in the cardiac death and myocardial infarction rates for patients taking β-blockers and those taking calcium channel blockers; (2) significantly fewer episodes of angina were observed per week in patients taking β-blockers than in those taking calcium channel blockers; (3) calcium channel blockers were discontinued significantly more often than β-blockers because of adverse events; and (4) no significant differences were found between the drugs in time to ischemia or in exercise time to ischemia. Heidenreich et al.[56] concluded "β-Blockers should be considered first-line agents because they are as effective as and better tolerated than calcium antagonists and have been shown to improve prognosis in other populations with coronary disease."

PULMONARY MEDICATIONS

Chronic obstructive pulmonary disease (COPD) is a major cause of morbidity and mortality in the United States. Currently, it is ranked as the fourth major cause of death, affecting an estimated 11.2 million people. It is estimated that 24 million more adults have some evidence of impaired lung function, indicating an underdiagnosis of the disease.[65] In 2004 the annual cost to the nation for COPD was $37.2 billion according to estimates made by the National Heart, Lung, and Blood Institute. Currently, there is no cure for COPD, although two treatments, smoking cessation and long-term oxygen therapy, will increase survival.[66,67] Bronchodilators will increase exercise capacity, but there is no evidence that this will increase the survival rate. However, an increase in exercise capacity will improve quality of life and the patient's ability to perform activities of daily living. The focus of this section is the bronchodilators and their effect on exercise capacity.

Bronchodilator Therapy

A main goal of bronchodilator therapy is to decrease airflow limitation in the airways, thus decreasing dyspnea and improving exercise tolerance.[68] Dyspnea can be caused by many factors including airway obstruction, impaired gas exchange, thoracic hyperinflation, impaired ventilatory mechanics and diaphragmatic function, loss of elastic lung recoil, respiratory and peripheral muscle weakness, and deconditioning.[67] Despite these differences in physiology, according to the literature, it is fairly clear that dyspnea is relieved by bronchodilators, regardless of the cause of impairment or class of bronchodilators administered. However, the reductions in dyspnea during exercise noted in response to these drugs appear to be closely related to the reduction in dynamic hyperinflation.[69]

Although bronchodilators seemingly improve exercise capacity, it is difficult to determine from the literature which type is best for which patient. Comparisons between studies are often difficult to make. Liesker et al.[68] present the following five reasons for this confusion: (1) lack of clarity regarding whether the patients were actually limited in exercise because of their ventilatory capacity or limited by nonventilatory reasons such as cardiovascular limitations, a decrease in muscle performance or motivation, or diminished diffusion capacity; (2) exclusion, in some studies, of patients with reversible airway disease such as asthma; (3) variability in dosing of the bronchodilator; (4) administration of tests that were sensitive to a learning effect; and (5) the small number of patients in the studies.[68] Oga et al.[70] added to this list by reporting on the variability of exercise tests used to measure the outcome of improved exercise capacity.[70] They discovered that a cycle endurance test was much more sensitive in detecting the effects of an anticholinergic drug on exercise capacity than the 6-minute walk test or a progressive cycle ergometry test. Other researchers criticize the use of forced expiratory volume in 1 second (FEV_1) as a measure of exercise capacity, stating that it is not a sensitive marker of bronchodilator responsiveness.[71] They use inspiratory capacity as a marker of responsiveness because dynamic hyperinflation is responsible for the dyspnea noted during exercise. Moreover, inspiratory capacity is predictive of an improvement in exercise tolerance and a reduction in dyspnea, and FEV_1 is not.[72]

In a systematic review of the effects of bronchodilators on exercise capacity by Liesker et al.,[68] 33 double-blind, randomized, placebo-controlled studies were selected and reviewed. Exercise capacity was measured by either a steady-state or an incremental exercise test, both of which measure cardiorespiratory endurance. Dyspnea was measured by using the Borg scale slope (ΔBorg score/ΔVO_{2max}). This parameter indicates the rise in dyspnea when patients increase their oxygen consumption during exercise. Only half of the studies reviewed demonstrated a significant positive effect of the bronchodilation on exercise capacity. Anticholinergics showed the most significant effects, with a trend toward high-dose rather than low-dose therapies being more effective. Short-acting β_2 sympathomimetics also produced significant positive effects on exercise capacity, but this was not the case for the longer-acting ones. Methylxanthines showed negative effects on exercise capacity. The review also indicated that with the addition of a second bronchodilator, there was no proven advantage for improving exercise capacity. Finally, the majority of the studies demonstrated a reduction in dyspnea, even in the absence of improvement in exercise capacity.

In a newer study by Oga et al.,[73] the effects of salbutamol (a short-acting β_2 sympathomimetic) on exercise endurance were compared with those of ipratropium (an anticholinergic bronchodilator). Improvement in exercise capacity, as measured by time on a cycle endurance test, was equal with both types of bronchodilators. Oga et al.[73] concluded that both types could be used as first-line drugs for the treatment of patients with COPD who want to exercise. They also found that the effects on exercise capacity varied within individuals, possibly because of a complex mechanism responsible for the different effects of the bronchodilators on exercise capacity versus airflow limitation.

Weiner et al.[74] investigated the cumulative effects of the long-acting bronchodilator (LABD) salmeterol, exercise, and inspiratory muscle training on the perception of dyspnea in patients with advanced COPD. The LABD had no effect on exercise capacity, FEV_1, or the perception of dyspnea. The nonsignificant results of the FEV_1 are in keeping with the conclusion of Newton et al.,[71] who found that this was not a sensitive measure for airway responsiveness. The significant results, however, indicated that inspiratory muscle training decreased the perception of dyspnea and the endurance exercise increased the 6-minute walk test time.

Brusasco et al.[75] examined health outcomes after treatments with tiotropium (anticholinergic) and salmeterol (LABD) in patients with COPD. The outcome measures consisted of exacerbations, health resource use, dyspnea, health-related quality of life, and spirometry. The results showed that the anticholinergics had more significant effects on all these measures. Exacerbations and health resource use were significantly less, and there were significant improvements in responses to the health-related quality-of-life survey, spirometric test results demonstrating an improved FEV_1, and the perception of dyspnea.

It appears that the anticholinergics and short-acting β_2 sympathomimetics improve exercise capacity and reduce dyspnea in patients with COPD. The anticholinergics also improve quality-of-life measures as compared with an LABD. The methylxanthines appear to have negative effects on exercise capacity in patients with COPD. Their side effects appear to be deleterious as well. They include tachycardia, hypertension, palpitations, chest pain, agitation, dizziness, and headache.[76] The side effects for the β_2 sympathomimetics include tremor, palpitation, headache, nervousness, dizziness, nausea, and hypertension; and the anticholinergics appear to have fewer side effects: delirium, hallucinations, and decreased gastrointestinal activity.[76]

The anticholinergics are used more frequently than the β-agonists for patients with COPD because of their more effective bronchodilator properties and fewer side effects.[77,78] β–Agonists are also known to cause side effects at rest after administration (i.e., a significant drop in PaO_2) after inhalation through the mechanism of a worsening ventilation/perfusion ratio.[79] Saito et al.[80] looked at the effects of an anticholinergic (oxitropium) and a β_2 sympathomimetic (fenoterol) on pulmonary hemodynamics at rest and during exercise in patients with COPD. The purpose of the study was to determine whether the resting effects of the β_2 sympathomimetic improved or worsened during exercise. Fenoterol caused a significant increase in HR, CO, mixed venous oxygen tension, and oxygen delivery and a significant decrease in pulmonary vascular resistance, PaO_2, and $PaCO_2$. Oxitropium caused a significant decrease during rest in HR and oxygen delivery. These differences between the drugs were not seen during exercise. Both classes of drugs significantly attenuated exercise-induced increases in pulmonary artery pressure, pulmonary capillary wedge pressure, and right arterial pressure. Thus both classes of drugs were equally effective in attenuating right heart afterloads during exercise in patients with COPD, with the main differences in pulmonary hemodynamics occurring at rest. This is an important

consideration because in most patients these values have a tendency to stay at resting levels.

In summary, the anticholinergics increase exercise capacity, decrease dyspnea, have fewer central effects at rest, improve quality of life, and attenuate right heart afterloads during exercise with fewer side effects than the other classes of bronchodilators when they are used for the treatment of COPD. See Table 25-5 for the summary of rest and exercise responses of the bronchodilators.

COPD is now considered a systemic disease, with cardiovascular and musculoskeletal impairments starting early in the disease process.[81] Exercise performance is limited because of physical deconditioning, even in patients with only mild degrees of airway obstruction.[82] It is vital that all patients with COPD start an exercise program that is safe with regard to their impairments and the effects of the medication on their exercise response.

Exercise Prescription for the Patient Taking Bronchodilators

It is well accepted that patients with COPD benefit from exercise training, even though exercise has not resulted in measurable effects on the respiratory system.[4,83] Its positive effects on dyspnea and the importance of physical deconditioning as a comorbid factor in advanced lung disease make exercise a very important factor in the treatment of patients with COPD. Some of the benefits of exercise training include increased exercise capacity, increased functional ability, decreased severity of dyspnea, and improved quality of life. The prescription follows the basics of exercise training and is individually based on the patient's severity of disease, exercise test results, and individual impairments.[4,83] If a patient experiences any of the adverse effects during exercise, appropriate action must be taken.[4]

Type of exercise: aerobic for both upper and lower extremities and anaerobic for both upper and lower extremities

Mode: walking, stationary biking, upper extremity endurance training, rowing, dual-action devices

Specific respiratory techniques: pursed lip breathing, respiratory muscle training, supplemental oxygen therapy, breathing exercises, ventilatory strategies, energy conservation techniques, posture re-education, airway clearance techniques if necessary

Frequency: 3 to 5 days per week

Table 24-5

Responses of Bronchodilators at Rest and during Exercise

Variable	β-Mimetics	Xanthines	Anticholinergics
Dyspnea	↓	↓	↓
Exercise capacity	↓ (LABD) ⇑ (SABD)	∅	↑
Exacerbations	↔	NS	↓
Health resource usage	↔	NS	↓
Quality of life	↔	NS	↑
Side effects	↑	↑↑	↓
RHR	↑	↑	↓
RPaO$_2$	↓	NS	↔
EPaO$_2$	↑	↑	↑
BP	↑	↑↓	↔

↑, Increase; ↓, decrease; ↔, no effect; ↑↓, increase or decrease; ∅, negative effects; *LABD*, long-acting bronchodilator; *SABD*, short-acting bronchodilator; *RHR*, resting heart rate; *RPaO$_2$*, resting partial pressure of oxygen; *EPaO$_2$*, exercising partial pressure of oxygen; *BP*, blood pressure.

Duration: 20 to 30 minutes of continuous exercise; initially, intermittent training may be necessary with rest periods of 3 to 5 minutes between bouts

Intensity: 60% of Karvonen's formula([(max HR − RHR) × %] + RHR) with HR max taken from the peak HR obtained during the stress test

Monitoring:
1. All patients should exercise based on the calculated intensity of their THR.
2. Symptoms must be monitored (e.g., shortness of breath, paradoxical breathing pattern, leg fatigue).
3. SpO$_2$ saturation of oxygen with hemoglobin.

Guidelines:
1. Paradoxical breathing is the first clinical sign of respiratory muscle fatigue.
2. RHR will be elevated in patients taking β-agonists and methylxanthines.
3. More serious side effects will occur with the methylxanthines.
4. Monitor for signs of right ventricular failure.
5. Exercise at the same drug plasma levels by exercising at the same time each day.
6. If a rescue inhaler is prescribed, the patient should carry it, especially during physical therapy.

DIABETIC MEDICATIONS

Diabetes mellitus (DM) is a metabolic disorder characterized by hyperglycemia resulting from defects in insulin secretion, insulin action, and glucose sensing by the pancreas.[84] Complications of DM include heart disease, stroke, hypertension, blindness, kidney disease, nervous system disease, amputations, dental disease, complications of pregnancy, and susceptibility to illness, and biochemical imbalances.[85] Disturbances in fat, protein, and carbohydrate metabolism also exist, causing additional complications during exercise. The most potentially lethal complication is hypoglycemia, which occurs more frequently in type 1 DM than in type 2 DM. The microvascular and macrovascular complications are directly related to the level of glycemic control, and patients with type 1 DM that is tightly controlled exhibit more frequent episodes of hypoglycemia. Patients with DM, regardless of the type, also demonstrate endothelial dysfunction, decrease in baroreflex sensitivity, autonomic dysfunction of the parasympathetic nervous system or both the parasympathetic and sympathetic nervous systems, impaired cardiac function, and altered energetic properties of both skeletal and cardiac muscle—all of which potentially alter exercise capacity. The focus of this section is on the interaction between exercise and drug therapy.

Antidiabetic Medications

The use of exercise as a treatment for diabetes is critical to the well-being of patients who have this metabolic disorder. Although there are not a lot of rules to follow, some very specific guidelines must be followed for patients taking antidiabetic medications

Sulfonylureas

The main class of oral antidiabetic medications that produce hypoglycemia is the sulfonylureas. These drugs increase insulin production with a subsequent lowering of plasma glucose concentrations.[86-88] Exercise is also known to cause a decrease in plasma glucose and insulin concentrations in both the postabsorptive and postprandial states.[89] The important question to answer is whether the combined effect of exercise and a sulfonylurea will cause an increase in the hypoglycemic response. Three recent studies have attempted to examine this response, but design flaws weaken their conclusions.[90-92] Riddle et al.[90] examined the effect of exercise combined with glipizide in 25 moderately obese subjects with type 2 DM. Subjects underwent an exercise test consisting of treadmill walking at 2.5 mph for 90 minutes before and after 9 weeks of either glipizide or placebo treatment. Outcome measures included plasma glucose, insulin, and C-peptide concentrations. No real conclusions could be made regarding the effect of the drug on exercise performance or plasma glucose concentration because testing was conducted at too low an intensity, and "exercise only" and "medication only" treatment groups were not included in the study. Massi et al.[91] demonstrated that a greater decrease in plasma glucose levels occurred when exercise was combined with either glibenclamide or glimepiride than when exercise was done alone; however, a "drug only" treatment group was not included in this study. A third study by Larsen et al.[92] did succeed in demonstrating an enhanced hypoglycemic response with the combination of exercise and glibenclamide. In this study the design flaws were minimized, the exercise intensity was individualized for each patient, and the appropriate guidelines were followed. Glibenclamide increased plasma insulin concentrations, thus lowering hepatic glucose production while glucose clearance was unchanged. Exercise, on the other hand, decreased plasma glucose concentrations by increasing glucose clearance.

This is in keeping with the fact that patients with type 2 DM have defective insulin-stimulated glucose uptake and insulin-stimulated GLUT 4 translocation but have normal contraction-stimulated glucose uptake and GLUT 4 translocation.[93-95] Patients with type 2 DM retain the capacity to translocate GLUT 4 to the sarcolemma in response to exercise. The actual risk of developing serious hypoglycemia will depend on the pharmacokinetics and pharmacodynamics of the particular sulfonylurea and the increase in the plasma insulin levels before the start of exercise.

Concerns regarding the safety of the sulfonylureas in the area of cardiac mortality, especially in combination with exercise, have been expressed.[96-99] In the University Groups Diabetes Program and the Bypass Angioplasty Revascularization Investigation, patients taking the sulfonylureas experienced a higher mortality rate as a result of cardiac dysfunction than those taking alternatives.[100,101] One explanation may be that the sulfonylureas cause the loss of *ischemic preconditioning. Ischemic preconditioning* refers to a protective mechanism in the heart that reduces ischemia and subsequent myocardial damage after temporary blockages of coronary blood flow or after a short-term increase in myocardial oxygen demand, as in exercise. Essentially, this is the heart's "warm-up." In terms of exercise, this phenomenon reduces ischemia during a closely followed second bout of exercise.[102] The adenosine triphosphate–sensitive potassium channel located in cardiomyocytes and in vascular smooth muscle is believed to mediate this ischemic preconditioning. The open channel has a role in regulation of coronary blood flow and also in protecting cardiac muscle from ischemia.[103] Therefore when this channel is blocked by the sulfonylureas, there is "no flow" after ischemia.[104-106] Övünç[107] studied this phenomenon in 18 patients with type 2 DM. Subjects underwent two consecutive treadmill tests with a 15-minute rest period between each test, with and without the sulfonylurea. It was found that glibenclamide eliminated the warm-up phenomenon and diminished the improvement in the ischemic threshold and exercise tolerance during the second bout of exercise. The author concluded that this drug should be used carefully in patients with CAD.

Glimepiride, a third-generation sulfonylurea, differs from the other sulfonylureas in that it is associated with a lower risk of hypoglycemia and less weight gain.[108] There is also evidence that myocardial preconditioning is preserved with this drug because glimepiride was shown to have less influence on the cardiovascular mitochondrial adenosine triphosphate–sensitive potassium (K_{ATP}) channels.[109] The other oral antidiabetic agents do not produce such serious side effects, especially when they are combined with exercise. Generally, if hypoglycemia results from other agents besides the sulfonylureas, it is due to the patient taking an increased dose to offset his or her "sugar" intake.

Metformin and Rosiglitazone

As discussed previously, patients with type 2 DM still have normal contracted-stimulated glucose uptake and GLUT 4 translocation.[12] A study by Musi et al.[110] demonstrated that an acute bout of exercise in patients with type 2 DM increases glucose uptake via an insulin-independent pathway mediated by activation of adenosine monophosphate–activated protein kinase (AMPK). AMPK is a protein consisting of one catalytic subunit and two regulatory subunits.[111,112] Two isoforms of the catalytic subunit have been identified—α_1 and α_2. AMPK α_1 is widely distributed; AMPK α_2 is predominantly localized in the skeletal muscle, heart, and liver.[113] Musi et al.[110] found that exercise significantly increased AMPK α_2 activity 2.7-fold over basal activity; this protein expression was also found in those without diabetes.

In another study, Musi et al.[114] demonstrated a significant increase in AMPK α_2 activity in the skeletal muscle after 10 weeks of treatment with metformin. The increase in AMPK activity results in the stimulation of glucose uptake in muscle, fatty acid oxidation in muscle and liver, and inhibition of hepatic glucose production. In a 26-week double-blind trial in which patients received rosiglitazone or metformin, metformin was shown to improve contraction-stimulated glucose uptake via the AMPK pathway but had no effect on the insulin-stimulated glucose uptake.[115] Rosiglitazone (a thiazolidinedione), however, improved insulin responsiveness in resting skeletal muscle and doubled the insulin-stimulated glucose uptake during physical exercise by improving insulin-stimulated glucose uptake.

Insulin

Much of the research surrounding the insulins examines their effect with regard to hypoglycemia and glycemic control with no exercise component. However, comparisons have been made between the short-acting insulin and regular insulin. Insulin lispro was formulated to act more like physiological insulin in terms of rapidity of action.[116] Research has indicated that the use of lispro results in a lower incidence of hypoglycemia; however, little is known about how this formulation performs with exercise.[117] Yamakita et al.[118] found that the decrease in plasma glucose level with exercise was greater after the administration of lispro than after the administration of regular insulin. But even though the level showed a significant difference in glucose concentration, hypoglycemia did not result in either case. The length of the exercise session was 30 minutes, and the timing of the session was at peak levels of action to ascertain a better understanding of their effects.

In contrast to patients with type 2 DM, patients with type 1 DM, who are also insulin resistant, appear to have a defect in both pathways for glucose uptake, insulin-stimulated and contraction-stimulated.[119] In a study by Peltoniemi et al.,[119] it was shown that patients with type 1 DM had a blunted effect with the two pathways; thus even exercise did not increase glucose uptake in these patients. They hypothesized that the increase in free fatty acids seen in this population could account for the diminished ability of exercise to stimulate glucose uptake. The higher free fatty acid concentrations might have caused a lower rate of glucose uptake, either through impaired insulin signaling or substrate competition.[120,121] Insulin resistance can be reversed in patients with type 1 DM if glycemic control is normalized.[122,123]

Exercise Guidelines for the Patient with Diabetes It is important to note that exercise will increase glucose utilization several-fold; thus hypoglycemia is a frequent problem for patients with insulin-treated diabetes and one of most common reasons that patients do not exercise. Insulin dosage may need to be adjusted, or carbohydrate ingestion before exercise may be needed. The physician needs to be consulted when hypoglycemia is limiting the patient's ability to exercise. Also, alcohol inhibits gluconeogenesis (in all people) and will contribute to hypoglycemia. Thus exercising and drinking alcohol is not a good combination.

Before starting an exercise program, the patient is required to be cleared by his or her physician for macrovascular or microvascular disease. An electrocardiographic stress test is recommended if the individual meets any of the following criteria[63]:

1. Age >40 years, with or without cardiovascular disease risk factors other than diabetes
2. Age >30 years and
   - Type 1 or type 2 diabetes of >10 years' duration
   - Hypertension
   - Cigarette smoking
   - Dyslipidemia
   - Proliferative or preproliferative retinopathy
   - Nephropathy, including microalbuminuria
3. Any of the following, regardless of age:
   - Known or suspected CAD, cerebrovascular disease, and/or peripheral vascular disease
   - Autonomic neuropathy
   - Advanced nephropathy with renal failure

Type of exercise: aerobic for both upper and lower extremities and anaerobic for both upper and lower extremities

Mode: walking, stationary biking, upper extremity endurance training, rowing, dual-action devices

Frequency: 3 to 5 days per week because of the duration of increased insulin sensitivity, which is not >72 hours, the time between the sessions should not be more than 72 hours

Duration: 20 to 60 minutes of continuous exercise
150 min/wk of moderate intensity aerobic exercise (40% to 60% of Karvonen)
90 min/wk of vigorous intensity aerobic exercise (–60% to 75% of Karvonen)

Intensity: 40% to 75% of Karvonen's formula ([(max HR – RHR) × %] + RHR) with HR max taken from the peak HR obtained during the stress test

Monitoring:
1. All patients should exercise based on the calculated intensity of their THR.
2. Rate of perceived exertion can only be used as an adjunct to HR monitoring.

Guidelines:
1. Proper footwear must be worn.
2. Identification must be carried at all times.
3. Fast-acting carbohydrate must be carried at all times.
4. No exercise should be done if fasting glucose levels are >280 mg/dL.

5. Patient should ingest a carbohydrate if glucose levels are <70 mg/dL before exercise.
6. Glucose needs to be monitored before, during, and after exercise for those with type 1 DM and before and after exercise for those with type 2 DM. DM.
7. Glucose needs to be monitored 4 to 8 hours after an exercise bout for those with type 1 DM.
8. Fluid ingestion should occur before, during, and after exercise.
9. No head-jarring activities should be done if the patient has retinopathy.
10. The patient should not exercise at peak insulin levels (see Table 24-6).
11. Insulin injection sites should be rotated away from active muscles.
12. Exercise should be avoided during illness; illness can increase glucose levels.
13. Alcohol should be avoided 3 hours before exercise and after exercise.
14. Vigorous exercise above 80% of Karvonen can cause hyperglycemia after exercise.

Table 24-6

Action of Insulin			
Type of Insulin	**Onset**	**Peak**	**Duration**
ULTRA SHORT-ACTING			
Lispro	5 min	1 hr	3 hr
Aspart	5 min	1 hr	3 hr
SHORT-ACTING			
Regular	30 min	2-4 hr	6-8 hr
Semilente	30 min	2-8 hr	12-16 hr
INTERMEDIATE-ACTING			
NPH	1-4 hr	6-12 hr	14-20 hr
Lente	1-4 hr	6-12 hr	14-20 hr
LONG-ACTING			
Ultralente	4-6 hr	6-18 hr	20-36 hr
Protamin	4-6 hr	14-20 hr	24-36 hr

REFERENCES

1. Leon AS (Chair), Franklin BA, Costa F, et al. Cardiac rehabilitation and secondary prevention of coronary heart disease. AHA Scientific Statement. *Circulation.* 2005;111;369-376.
2. American Thoracic Society. Pulmonary rehabilitation: 1999. *Am J Respir Crit Care Med.* 1999;159:1666-1682.
3. American Diabetes Association. Clinical practice recommendations 2004: Position Statement. Physical activity/exercise and diabetes. *Diabetes Care.* 2004;27(1): S58-S62.
4. Franklin B, Whaley M, Howley E, eds. *ACSM's Guidelines for Exercise Testing and Prescription.* 6th ed. New York: Lippincott Williams & Wilkins; 2000.
5. Lands AM, Arnold A, McAuliff JP, et al. Differentiation of receptor systems activated by sympathomimetic amines. *Nature.* 1967;214:597-598.
6. Eston R, Connolly D. The use of ratings of perceived exertion for exercise prescription in patients receiving β-blocker therapy. *Sports Med.* 1996;21(3):176-190.
7. Head A. Exercise metabolism and β-blocker therapy. *Sports Med.* 1999; 27(2):81-96.
8. Joyner MF, Freund BJ, Jilka SM, et al. Effects of beta adrenergic blockade on exercise capacity of trained and untrained men: haemodynamic comparison. *J Appl Physiol.* 1986;60:1429-1434.
9. Reybrouck T, Amery A, Fagard R, et al. Haemodynamic responses to graded exercise after chronic beta adrenergic blockade. *J Appl Physiol.* 1977;42:133-138.
10. Lund-Johansen P. Haemodynamic changes at rest and during exercise in long-term beta-blockade therapy of essential hypertension. *Acta Med Scand.* 1974;195: 117-121.
11. Todd IC, Ballantyne D. Antianginal efficacy of exercise training: a comparison with β-blockade. *Br Heart J.* 1990; 64(1):14-19.
12. Kaski JC, Rodriguez-Plaza L, Brown J, et al. Efficacy of carvedilol in exercise-induced myocardial ischemia. *J Cardiovasc Pharmacol.* 1987;10(suppl.11):S137-S140.
13. Poulsen SH, Jensen SE, Egstrup K. Improvement of exercise capacity and left ventricular diastolic function with metoprolol XL after acute myocardial infarction. *Am Heart J.* 2000; 140(1):6e-11e.
14. Steele P, Gold F. Favorable effects of acebutolol on exercise performance and angina in men with coronary artery disease. *Chest.* 1982;82(1):40-43.
15. Magder S, Sami M, Ripley R, et al. Comparison of the effects of pindolol and propranolol on exercise performance in patients with angina pectoris. *Am J Cardiol.* 1987;59:1289-1294.
16. Lee G, DeMaria A, Favrot L, et al. Efficacy of acebutolol in chronic stable angina using single-blinded and randomized double-blinded protocol. *J Clin Pharmacol.* 1982;22:371-378.
17. Uusitalo A, Keyriläinen O, Johnsson G. A dose-response study on metoprolol in angina pectoris. *Ann Clin Res.* 1981;13(suppl.30):54-57.
18. Thadani U, Davidson C, Chir B, et al. Comparison of the immediate effects of five β-adrenoreceptor-blocking drugs with different ancillary properties in angina pectoris. *N Engl J Med.* 1979;300(14):750-755.
19. Shapiro W, Park J, DiBianco R, et al. Comparison of nadolol, a new long-acting beta-receptor blocking agent, and placebo in the treatment of stable angina pectoris. *Chest.* 1981;80(4):425-430.
20. Thadani U, Parker JO. Propranolol in angina pectoris: duration of improved exercise tolerance and circulatory effects after acute oral administration. *Am J Cardiol.* 1979; 44:118-125.
21. Biron P, Tremblay G. Acebutolol: basis for the prediction of effect on exercise tolerance. *Clin Pharmacol Ther.* 1975;19(3):333-338.
22. Tzivoni D, Medina A, David D, et al. Effect of metoprolol in reducing myocardial ischemic threshold during exercise and during daily activity. *Am J Cardiol.* 1998;81(6):775-777.
23. Miller L, Crawford M, O'Rourke R. Nadolol compared to propranolol for treating chronic stable angina pectoris. *Chest.* 1984;86(2):189-193.
24. Gordon NF, Duncan JJ. Effect of beta-blockers on exercise physiology: implications for exercise training. *Med Sci Sports Exerc.* 1991;23(6):668-676.
25. Gordon NF, Van Rensburg JP, Van Den Heever DP, et al. Effect of dual β-blockade and calcium antagonism on endurance performance. *Med Sci Sports Exerc.* 1987; 19(1):1-6.
26. Marchetti G, Merlo L, Noseda V. Myocardial uptake of free fatty acids and carbohydrates after β-adrenergic blockade. *Am J Cardiol.* 1968;22:370-374.
27. McKenna DH, Curliss RJ, Sialer S, Zarnstorff WC, Crumpton CW, Rowe GG Effect of propranolol on systemic and coronary haemodynamics at rest and during stimulated exercise. *Circ Res.* 1966;19:520-527.
28. Steele PP, Maddoux G, Kirch DL, et al. Effects of propranolol and nitroglycerin on left ventricular performance in patients with coronary arterial disease. *Chest.* 1978;73:19-23.
29. Finkelhor RS, Sun J-P, Bahler RC. Left ventricular filling shortly after an uncomplicated myocardial infarction as a predictor of subsequent exercise capacity. *Am Heart J.* 1990;119:85-91.
30. Yuasa F, Sumimoto T, Hattori T, et al. Effects of left ventricular peak filling rate on exercise capacity 3 to 6 weeks after acute myocardial infarction. *Chest.* 1997;111:590-594.
31. Mueller HS. Propranolol in acute myocardial infarction in man: effects of hemodynamics and myocardial oxygenation. *Acta Med Scand.* 1976;(suppl)587:177-183.
32. Bortone AS, Hess OM, Gaglione A, et al. Effect of intravenous propranolol on coronary vasomotion at rest and during dynamic exercise in patients with coronary artery disease. *Circulation.* 1990;81:1225-1235.
33. Chick TW, Halperin AK, Gacek EM. The effect of antihypertensive medications on exercise performance: a review. *Med Sci Sports Exerc.* 1988;20(5):447-454.
34. Van Camp S. Pharmacologic factors in exercise and exercise testing. In: ACSM. *Resource Manual for Guidelines for Exercise Testing and Prescription.* Philadelphia: Lea and Febiger; 1988:135-152.
35. McArdle WD, Katch FI, Katch VL. *Exercise Physiology: Energy, Nutrition, and Human Performance.* 5th ed. New York: Lippincott Williams & Wilkins; 2001.

36. Brown HC, Carruthers SG, Johnstone GB, et al. Clinical pharmacologic observations on atenolol, a beta-adrenoceptor blocker. *Clin Pharmacol Ther.* 1976;20:524-534.

37. Silas JH, Freestone S, Leard MS, et al. Comparison of two slow release preparations of metoprolol with conventional metoprolol and atenolol. *Br J Clin Pharmacol.* 1985;20:387-391.

38. Blood SM, Ades PA. Effects of beta-adrenergic blockade on exercise conditioning in coronary patients: a review. *J Cardiopulm Rehab.* 1988;8:141-144.

39. Robertson L, Reel K, Crist R, et al, eds. *Guidelines for Cardiac Rehabilitation and Secondary Prevention Programs.* 3rd ed. Champaign, IL: Human Kinetics; 2000.

40. Dunbar C, Glickman-Weiss E, Bursztyn D, et al. A submaximal treadmill test for developing target ratings of perceived exertion for outpatient cardiac rehabilitation. *Percept Mot Skills.* 1998;87:755-759.

41. Eston RG, Thompson M. Use of ratings of perceived exertion for predicting maximal work rate and prescribing exercise intensity in patients taking atenolol. *Br J Sports Med* 1996;31:114-119.

42. Joo KC, Brubaker PH, MacDougall A, et al. Exercise prescription using heart rate plus 20 or perceived exertion in cardiac rehabilitation. *J Cardiopulm Rehabil.* 2004;24(3):178-184.

43. Mittleman MA, Maclure M, Tofler GH, et al. Triggering of acute myocardial infarction by heavy physical exertion: protection against triggering by regular exertion. *N Engl J Med.* 1993;329:1677-1683.

44. Hassock K, Hartwig R. Cardiac arrest associated with supervised cardiac rehabilitation. *J Cardiopulm Rehabil.* 1982;2:402-408.

45. Schamroth L. The philosophy of calcium ion antagonists. In: Zanchetti A, Krikler DM, eds. *Calcium Antagonism in Cardiovascular Therapy. Exercise with Verapamil.* Amsterdam: Excerpta Medica; 1981:5-9.

46. Zelis R, Flaim SF. Calcium blocking drugs for angina pectoris. *Annu Rev Med.* 1982;33:465-478.

47. Khurmi NS, Raftery EB. A comparison of nine calcium ion antagonists and propranolol: exercise tolerance, heart rate, and ST-segment changes in patients with chronic stable angina pectoris. *Eur J Clin Pharmacol.* 1987;32:539-548.

48. Hossack KF, Bruce RA. Improved exercise performance in persons with stable angina pectoris receiving diltiazem. *Am J Cardiol.* 1981; 47:95-101.

49. Henry PD. Comparative pharmacology of calcium antagonists: nifedipine, verapamil and diltiazem. *Am J Cardiol.* 1980;46:1047-1058.

50. Millard RW, Lathrop DA, Grupp G, et al. Differential cardiovascular effects on calcium channel blocking agents: potential mechanisms. *Am J Cardiol.* 1982;49:499-506.

51. Fleckenstein A. Specific pharmacology of calcium in myocardium, cardiac pacemakers and vascular smooth muscle. *Annu Rev Pharmacol Toxicol.* 1977;17:149-166.

52. Davies RF, Habibi H, Klinke WP, et al. Effect of amlodipine, atenolol and their combination on myocardial ischemia during treadmill exercise and ambulatory monitoring. *J Am Coll Cardiol.* 1995;25:619-625.

53. Chugh SK, Digpal K, Hutchinson T, et al. A randomized, double-blind comparison of the efficacy and tolerability of once-daily modified-release diltiazem capsules with once-daily amlodipine tablets in patients with stable angina. *J Cardiovasc Pharmacol.* 2001;38(3):356-364.

54. Van Der Vring JA, Daniëls MC, Holwerda NJ, et al. Combination of calcium channel blockers and beta-adrenoceptor blockers for patients with exercise-induced angina pectoris: a double-blind parallel-group comparison of different classes of calcium channel blockers. *Br J Clin Pharmacol.* 1999;47(5):493-498.

55. Hung J, Lamb IH, Connoly ST, et al. The effect of diltiazem and propranolol, alone and in combination, on exercise performance and left ventricular performance in patients with stable effort angina: a double-blind, randomized, and placebo-controlled study. *Ther Prev- Coron Artery Dis.* 1983;;68(3):560-566.

56. Heidenreich PA, McDonald KM, Hastie T, et al. Meta-analysis of trials comparing beta-blockers, calcium antagonists, and nitrates for stable angina. *JAMA.* 1999;281(20):1927-1936.

57. Opie LH. Pharmacological differences between calcium antagonists. *Eur Heart J.* 1997;18(suppl A):A71-A79.

58. Egstrup K, Andersen PJ. Transient myocardial ischemia during nifedipine therapy in stable angina pectoris, and its relation to coronary collateral flow and comparison with metoprolol. *Am J Cardiol.* 1993;71:177-183.

59. Schultz W, Jost S, Kober G, et al. Relation of antianginal efficacy of nifedipine to degree of coronary arterial narrowing and to presence of coronary collateral vessels. *Am J Cardiol.* 1985;55:26-32.

60. Kaufmann PA, Mandinov L, Seiler C, et al. Impact of exercise-induced coronary vasomotion on anti-ischemic therapy. *Coron Artery Dis.* 2000;11(4):363-369.

61. Maseri A, Chierchia S. A new rationale for the clinical approach to the patient with angina pectoris. *Am J Med.* 1981;71:639-644.

62. Maseri A, L'Abbate A, De Nes M, et al. "Variant" angina: one aspect of a continuous spectrum of vasospastic myocardial ischemia. *Am J Cardiol.* 1978;42:1019-1035.

63. Boden WE, Bough EW, Reichman MJ, et al. Beneficial effects of high-dose diltiazem in patients with persistent effort angina on β-blockers and nitrates: a randomized, double-blind, placebo-controlled cross-over study. *Circulation.* 1985;71(6):1197-1205.

64. Millard RW, Lathrop DA, Grupp G, et al. Differential cardiovascular effects of calcium channel blocking agents: potential mechanisms. *Am J Cardiol.* 1982;49:499-506.

65. National Center for Health Statistics. National Health Interview Survey, 1997-2002. Information cited in: American Lung Association, Epidemiology and Statistics Unit. *Trends in chronic bronchitis and emphysema: Morbidity and Mortality, April 2004,* retrieved from the American Lung Association's website: http://www.lungusa.org/site/pp.asp?c=dvLUK9O0E&b=35019. Accessed May 3, 2005.

66. BTS guidelines for the management of chronic obstructive pulmonary disease. The COPD Guidelines Group of the Standards of Care Committee of the BTS. *Thorax.* 1997;52(suppl 5):S1-S28.

67. Roche N. Recent advances: pulmonary medicine. *BMJ.* 1999;318;171-176.

68. Liesker JJW, Wijkstra PJ, Ten Hacken NHT, et al. A systematic review of the effects of bronchodilators on exercise capacity in patients with COPD. *Chest.* 2002; 121(2):597-608.

69. Belman MJ, Botnick WC, Shin JW, et al. Inhaled bronchodilators reduce dynamic hyperinflation during exercise in patients with chronic obstructive pulmonary disease. *Am J Respir Crit Care Med.* 1996;153:967-975.

70. Oga T, Nishimura K, Tsukino M, et al. The effects of oxitropium bromide on exercise performance in patients with stable chronic obstructive pulmonary disease: a comparison of three different exercise tests. *Am J Respir Crit Care Med.* 2000;161:1897-1901.

71. Newton MF, O'Donnell DE, Forkert L. Response of lung volumes to inhaled salbutamol in large population of patients with severe hyperinflation. *Chest.* 2002;121(4): 1042-1050.

72. O'Donnell DE, Lam M, Webb KA. Measurement of symptoms, lung hyperinflation and endurance during exercise in chronic obstructive pulmonary disease. *Am J Respir Crit Care Med.* 1998;158:1557-1565.

73. Oga T, Nishimura K, Tsukino M, et al. A comparison of the effects of salbutamol and ipratropium bromide on exercise endurance in patients with COPD. *Chest.* 2003;123(6):1810-1816.

74. Weiner P, Magadle R, Berar-Yanay N, et al. The cumulative effects of long-acting bronchodilators, exercise, and inspiratory muscle training on the perception of dyspnea in patients with advanced COPD. *Chest.* 2000;118(3):672-678.

75. Brusasco V, Hodder R, Miravittles M, et al. Health outcomes following treatment for six months with once daily tiotropium compared with twice daily salmeterol in patients with COPD. *Thorax.* 2003;58(5): 399-404.

76. Cahalin LP, Sadowsky HS. Pulmonary medications. *Phys Ther.* 1995;75(5):397-414.

77. Chapman KR. The role of anticholinergic bronchodilators in adult asthma and chronic obstructive pulmonary disease. *Lung.* 1990;168(suppl):295-303.

78. Chapman KR. Anticholinergic bronchodilators for adult obstructive airway disease. *Am J Med.* 1991; 91(suppl):13S-16S.

79. Wagner PD, Dantzker DR, Iacovoni VE, et al. Ventilation-perfusion inequality in asymptomatic asthma. *Am Rev Respir Dis.* 1978;118:511-524.

80. Saito S, Miyamoto K, Nishimura M, et al. Effects of inhaled bronchodilators on pulmonary hemodynamics at rest and during exercise in patients with COPD. *Chest.* 1999;115(2):376-382.

81. Petty TL. COPD in perspective. *Chest.* 2002;121(5 suppl): 116S-120S.

82. Carter R, Nicrota B, Blevins W, et al. Altered exercise gas exchange and cardiac function in patients with mild chronic obstructive pulmonary disease. *Chest.* 1993; 103:745-750.

83. Lareau SC, ZuWallack R, Carlin B, et al. Pulmonary rehabilitation: 1999. Official Statement of The American Thoracic Society. *Am J Respir Crit Care Med.* 1999; 159:1666-1682.

84. The Expert Committee on the Diagnosis and Classification of Diabetes Mellitus. Report of the Expert Committee on the Diagnosis and Classification of Diabetes Mellitus. *Diabetes Care.* 1997;20:1183-1197.

85. Centers for Disease Control and Prevention. *National Diabetes Fact Sheet 2002.* Atlanta, GA: U.S. Department of Health and Human Services, Centers for Disease Control and Prevention; 2003.

86. Jennings AM, Wilson RM, Ward JD. Symptomatic hypoglycemia in NIDDM patients treated with oral hypoglycemic agents. *Diabetes Care.* 1989;12:203-208.

87. Seltzer HS. Drug-induced hypoglycemia: a review of 1,418 cases. *Endocrinol Metab Clin North Am.* 1989; 18:163-183.

88. Ferner RE, Neil HA. Sulphonylureas and hypoglycemia. *BMJ Clin Res Ed.* 1998;296:949-950.

89. Martin IK, Katz A, Wahren J. Splanchnic and muscle metabolism during exercise in NIDDM patients. *Am J Physiol.* 1995;269:E583-E590.

90. Riddle MC, McDaniel PA, Tive LA. Glipizide-GITS does not increase the hypoglycemic effect of mild exercise during fasting in NIDDM. *Diabetes Care.* 1997; 20(6): 992-994.

91. Massi B, Herz M, Pfeiffer C. The effects of acute exercise on metabolic control in type II diabetic patients treated with glimepiride or glibenclamide. *Horm Metab Res.* 1996;28:451-455.

92. Larsen JJ, Dela F, Madsbad S, et al. Interaction of sulfonylureas and exercise on glucose homeostasis in type 2 diabetic patients. *Diabetes Care.* 1999; 22(10): 1647-1654.

93. Zierath JR, He L, Guma A, et al. Insulin action on glucose transport and plasma membrane GLUT4 content in skeletal muscle from patients with NIDDM. *Diabetologia.* 1996;39:1180-1189.

94. Garvey WT, Maianu L, Zhu JH, et al. Evidence for the defects in the trafficking and translocation of GLUT4 glucose transporters in skeletal muscle as a cause of human insulin resistance. *J Clin Invest.* 1998;101: 2377-2386.

95. Kennedy JW, Hirshman MF, Gervino EV, et al. Acute exercise induces GLUT4 translocation in skeletal muscle of normal human subjects with type 2 diabetes. *Diabetes.* 1999; 48:1192-1197.

96. Willett LL, Albright ES. Achieving glycemic control in type 2 diabetes: a practical guide for clinicians on oral hypoglycemics. *South Med J.* 2004; 97(11):1088-1092.

97. Panunti B, Kunhiraman B, Fonseca V. The impact of antidiabetic therapies on cardiovascular disease. *Curr Atheroscler Rep.* 2005;7:50-7.

98. Jadhav S, Petrie J, Ferrell W, et al. Insulin resistance as a contributor to myocardial ischemia independent of obstructive coronary atheroma: a role for insulin sensitization? *Heart.* 2004; 90:1379-1383.

99. Jia EZ, Yang ZJ, Chen SW, et al. Significant association of insulin and proinsulin with clustering of cardiovascular risk factors. *World J Gastroenterol.* 2005;7: 149-153.

100. Klimt CR, Knatterud GL, Meinert CL, et al. A study of the effects of hypoglycemic agents on vascular complications in patients with adult onset diabetes. *Diabetes.* 1970;19:744-830.

101. The BARI (Bypass Angioplasty Revascularization Investigation) Investigators: Influence of diabetes on 5 year mortality and morbidity in a randomized trial comparing CABG and PTCA in patients with multivessel disease. The Bypass Angioplasty Revascularization Investigation (BARI). *Circulation*. 1997;96:1761-1769.

102. Noma A. ATP-regulated K channels in cardiac muscle. *Nature*. 1983;305:147-148.

103. Farouque HM, Worthley SG, Meredith IT. Effect of ATP-sensitive potassium channel inhibition on coronary metabolic vasodilation in humans. *Arterioscler Thromb Vasc Biol*. 2004:5:905-910.

104. Miura T, Miki T. ATP-sensitive K+ channel openers: old drugs with new clinical benefits for the heart. *Curr Vasc Pharmacol*. 2003;1(3):251-258.

105. Huizar JF, Gonzalez LA, Alderman J, Smith HS. Sulfonylureas attenuate electrocardiographic ST-segment elevation during an acute myocardial infarction in diabetics. *J Am Coll Cardiol*. 2003;42(6):1017-1021.

106. Leibowitz G, Cerasi E. Sulphonylurea treatment of NIDDM patients with cardiovascular disease: a mixed blessing? *Diabetologia*. 1996;5:503-514.

107. Övünç K. Effects of Glibenclamde, a KATP channel blocker on warm up phenomenon in type II diabetic patients with chronic stable angina pectoris. *Clin Cardiol*. 2000; 23:535-539.

108. Massi-Benedetti M. Glimepiride in type 2 diabetes mellitus: a review of the worldwide therapeutic experience. *Clin Ther*. 2002;25(3):799-816.

109. Smits P, Bijlstra PJ, Russel FG, et al. Cardiovascular effects of sulphonylurea derivatives. *Diabetes Res Clin Pract*. 1996;31(suppl):S55-S59.

110. Musi N, Fujii N, Hirshman MF, et al. AMP-activated protein kinase (AMPK) is activated in muscle of subjects with type 2 diabetes during exercise. *Diabetes*. 2001; 50(5):921-927.

111. Hardie DG, Carling D, Carlson M. The AMP-activated/SNF1 protein kinase subfamily: metabolic sensors of the eukaryotic cell? *Annu Rev Biochem*. 1998;67:821-855.

112. Kemp BE, Mitchelhill KI, Stapleton D, et al. Dealing with energy demand: the AMP-activated protein kinase. *Trends Biochem Sci*. 1999;24:22-25.

113. Stapleton D, Mitchelhill KI, Gao G, et al. Mammalian AMP-activated protein kinase subfamily. *J Biol Chem*. 1996;271:611-614.

114. Musi N, Hirshman MF, Nygren J, et al. Metformin increases AMP-activated protein kinase activity in skeletal muscle of subjects with type 2 diabetes. *Diabetes*. 2002; 51(7):2074-2081.

115. Hällsten K, Virtanen KA, Lönnqvist F, et al. Rosiglitazone but not metformin enhances insulin- and exercise-stimulated skeletal muscle glucose uptake in patients with newly diagnosed type 2 diabetes. *Diabetes*. 2002; 51(12):3479-3485.

116. Holleman F, Hoekstra JB. Insulin lispro. *New Engl J Med*. 1997;337:176-183.

117. Multicenter Insulin Lispro Study Group, Anderson JH, Brunelle RL, Koivisto VA, et al. Reduction of postprandial hyperglycemia and frequency of hypoglycemia in IDDM patients on insulin-analog treatment. *Diabetes*. 1997;46:265-270.

118. Yamakita T, Ishii T, Yamagami K, et al. Glycemic response during exercise after administration of insulin lispro compared with that after administration of regular human insulin. *Diabetes Res Clin Pract*. 2002;57:17-22.

119. Peltoniemi P, Yki-Järvinen H, Oikonen V, et al. Resistance to exercise-induced increase in glucose uptake during hyperinsulinemia in insulin-resistant skeletal muscle of patients with type 1 diabetes. *Diabetes*. 2001;50:1371-1377.

120. Griffin ME, Marcucci MJ, Cline GW, et al. Free fatty acid-induced insulin resistance is associated with activation of protein kinase C theta and alterations in the insulin signaling cascade. *Diabetes*. 1999;48:1270-1274.

121. Nuutila P, Koivisto VA, Knuuti J, et al. Glucose-free fatty acid cycle operates in human heart and skeletal muscle in vivo. *J Clin Invest*. 1992;89:1767-1774.

122. Yki-Järvinen H, Koivisto VA. Continuous subcutaneous insulin infusion therapy decreases insulin resistance in type 1 diabetes. *J Clin Endocrinol Metab*. 1984;58:659-666.

123. Revers RR, Kolterman OG, Scarlett JA, et al. Lack of in vivo insulin resistance in controlled insulin-dependent, type 1 diabetic patients. *J Clin Endocrinol Metab*. 1984; 58:353-358.

This text serves as a primer or introduction to the field of pharmacology with the goal of instructing the physical therapist on the "generalizations" of drug treatment. However, for a review of specific medications, the student is encouraged to become familiar with the *Physicians' Desk Reference* (*PDR*). The *PDR* provides information on all Food and Drug Administration (FDA)–approved pharmaceuticals, including prescribing information, side effects, and drug-drug interactions. In addition, results of early randomized placebo-controlled studies are often presented to prove the efficacy of the drugs.

The *PDR* is industry supported and thus represents only FDA-approved written communication provided by the drug manufacturers. Labeling and package inserts that are enclosed with drugs when purchased are similar to what can be found in the *PDR*. It is published yearly by Medical Economics in Montvale, New Jersey, which offers online and PDA versions as well. Medical Economics now publishes a *PDR* for nonprescription drugs and dietary supplements and an additional text for ophthalmic medicines.

At first glance, the *PDR* can be quite intimidating. It contains several color-coded sections that list medications in a variety of ways. The following is a brief guide that will help the student navigate this rather large book.

SECTION 1: THE MANUFACTURERS' INDEX

The Manufacturers' Index lists all the companies that contribute to the PDR. They are listed in alphabetical order, beginning with Abbot Laboratories. Under the company names, you will find the addresses and phone numbers of the manufacturers' headquarters, as well as numbers to dial for product information and medical emergencies. The medical departments at each of the pharmaceutical companies are accessible to provide information on dosage, side effects, and results of clinical trials if requested.

SECTION 2: THE BRAND AND GENERIC NAME INDEX

The Brand and Generic Name Index, also known as the **Pink Pages**, lists all the drugs supplied by the participating pharmaceutical companies in alphabetical order by both trade and generic names. The trade names are followed by the manufacturer's name and page numbers in boldface type, which indicate where full prescribing information can be found. Generic names are underlined. In some cases, a boldface diamond symbol can be found to the left of a drug name. This indicates that there is a picture of the drug in the Product Identification Guide. The pink pages offer the ideal place to start your research if you know the drug name.

SECTION 3: PRODUCT CATEGORY INDEX

The Product Category Index, also known as the **Blue Pages**, lists the drugs according to their mechanism of action or therapeutic uses. For example, if you wanted to know what drugs are available for low back pain, you would first look under the heading **ANALGESICS**. For the purpose of narrowing your search, each of these categories is further subdivided. For example, under the heading Analgesics, you can find drugs containing acetaminophen, narcotic agents, nonsteroidal antiinflammatory drugs, and of course, aspirin and other salicylates.

SECTION 3: PRODUCT IDENTIFICATION GUIDE

The Product Identification Guide provides glossy, actual-size pictures of pills, tablets, and capsules. The products are listed alphabetically under the name of the manufacturer.

This is a handy section for your patients to become familiar with because they can compare the medication that they just picked up from the pharmacy with the one pictured in the *PDR*. This confirms the drug's identity, helping to ensure that the correct medication has been purchased. However, the usefulness of this section has greatly diminished because most drugs are now dispensed as generics.

SECTION 5: PRODUCT INFORMATION

The Product Information section provides detailed information about all the drugs. It is the "meat and potatoes" of the *PDR* and takes up the majority of pages in the text. Each drug is again listed in alphabetical order under the manufacturer. This is the section to which you are referred by those boldface page numbers mentioned earlier.

Other useful information is also provided in the *PDR*, including a list of nationwide poison control centers, a key to pregnancy ratings, and a key to controlled substance categories.

The study of pharmacology is extremely fluid in that change in how drugs are prescribed, how patients are monitored, indications for use, and adverse events occur on an almost daily basis.[1] Although there are some excellent pharmacology texts to use for reference, by the time they reach publication, some of the information is outdated. Therefore it is important for the astute physical therapist to be able to search online sources for the most current and up-to-date medications.

A wide variety of health care information is available on the Web. Much of it is credible, but some is not. Health care organizations, health care agencies, and pharmaceutical companies usually provide accurate drug information. An example of an excellent industry site is http://www.merck.com, sponsored by the pharmaceutical giant Merck & Company.[2] Merck's home page provides links to "Product News," containing the latest information on the company's Food and Drug Administration (FDA)–approved medicines and vaccines; "Research and Development News," announcing drug approvals and partnerships for research, as well as new therapeutics under study; and links to sources of educational information such as *The Merck Manual.* There is also is a link to "Condition Guide," which is a site designed to provide easy-to-understand information on diseases for patients and caregivers. Abstracts of articles can be viewed by performing a MedlinePlus search, and you can even search for health centers and clinics on this site. Special features include Virtual Body Tours and the *Adam Encyclopedia.* Registered clients can have access to the *Harvard Health E-newsletter.*

Biomedical journals also provide current information on drugs and treatments for diseases. Many journals have their own websites and offer abstracts for free and full-text versions for a fee. An example is http://www.elsevier.com sponsored by Elsevier Publishing.[3] This company publishes many scientific journals and provides a link to the company sponsored "Sciencedirect," enabling full-text printing for registered members.[4]

Medical topics and drug-related information can be accessed on some of the health-related databases, especially PubMED, published by the National Library of Medicine at http://www.ncbi.nlm.nih.gov/entrez/query.fcgi. This site offers access to MEDLINE citations and in some cases direct links to the full-text article. Of course, any information about the safety of a drug can be retrieved from the FDA directly.[5] The FDA website contains a link to MEDwatch, the adverse drug event reporting service, as well as links to enormous volumes of information including the history of food and drug law in this nation, consumer advice, information on clinical trials, and even a kid's section discussing illicit drugs and prescription drugs commonly used by children and teens.

The Medical Letter, Inc., publishes a weekly newsletter reviewing new drugs and older drugs as information on them is updated.[6] This is a nonprofit publication authored by physicians and doctors of pharmacy (Pharm Ds). It is available on the Web for a fee at http://www.medicalletter.org. It is viewed as an extremely reliable publication, always providing evidence from the literature. The Medical Letter also publishes a quarterly issue that discusses treatment guidelines for a variety of conditions. Each issue illustrates just one disease, presenting its current pharmacological treatment. Topics that have been covered include drugs for psychiatric conditions, HIV, hypertension, and rheumatoid arthritis.

Drug information may also be obtained by typing the name of the drug into an Internet search engine. This method is especially useful if you are not sure which pharmaceutical company produces the drug of interest. For example, if you search for "Fosamax," you can link up to an industry-sponsored site that explains how the drug should be prescribed, lists side effects, and provides information on osteoporosis.[7]

In terms of websites directed toward the patient, MedlinePlus is an excellent and accurate source of health care information.[8] Like PubMED, this site is sponsored by the National Library of Medicine and the National Institutes of Health. Another patient-related site is MedicineNet.[9] This site is produced by a network of physicians and allied health care professionals and is assumed to be a reliable source of information because it displays the Health on the Net Foundation (HON) symbol on its homepage. The Health on the Net (HON) Foundation is an organization that evaluates the reliability and accuracy of health information on the Web.[1] In order to display the HON symbol, the website administrators must apply for site approval and demonstrate that they are following the code of conduct developed by the foundation. When seeking out websites for patients, you should keep in mind that many are either sponsored by or linked to online pharmacies that may be just as interested in selling something as they are in providing health information.

References

1. Slaughter RL. The future of drug information and the internet. In: Slaughter RL, Edwards DJ, eds. *Evaluating Drug Literature: A Statistical Approach.* New York: McGraw-Hill; 2001.
2. Merck & Company, Inc. Available at: http://www.merck.com. Accessed August 11, 2004.
3. Elsevier. Available at http://www.elsevier.com. Accessed August 11, 2004.
4. ScienceDirect. Available at: http://www.sciencedirect.com. Accessed August 11, 2004.
5. U.S. Food and Drug Administration. Available at: http://www.fda.gov. Accessed August 11, 2004.
6. The Medical Letter. Available at: http://www.medicalletter.org. Accessed August 11, 2004.
7. Fosamax. Available at: http://www.fosamax.com/fosamax/cns/home.html. Accessed August 11, 2004.
8. MedlinePlus. Available at http://www.medlineplus.org. Accessed August 11, 2004.
9. MedicineNet. Available at: http://www.medicinenet.com. Accessed August 11, 2004.

Drugs Affecting the Parasympathetic System

Trade Name	Generic Name	Comments
Urecholine	bethanechol	Direct acting
Pilocarpine	pilocarpine	Direct acting
Prostigmin	neostigmine bromide	Indirect acting
Antilirium	physostigmine	Indirect acting
Atropine	atropine	Anticholinergic
Transderm-Scöp	scopolamine	Anticholinergic
Robinul	glycopyrrolate	Antispasmodic

Diuretics

Trade Name	Generic Name	Comments
Bumex	bumetanide	Loop diuretic
Lasix	furosemide	Loop diuretic
Demadex	torsemide	Loop diuretic
HydroDIURIL, Esidrix	hydrochlorothiazide	Thiazide diuretic
Naturetin	bendroflumethiazide	Thiazide diuretic
Exna	benzthiazide	Thiazide diuretic
Aldactone	spironolactone	Potassium sparing
Dyrenium	triamterene	Potassium sparing

Cardiovascular Drugs

Trade Name	Generic Name	Comments
Adenocard	adenosine	Antiarrhythmic
Cordarone	amiodarone	Antiarrhythmic
Tikosyn	dofetilide	Antiarrhythmic
Procanbid/Pronestyl	procainamide	Antiarrhythmic
Betapace	sotalol	Antiarrhythmic
Tonocard	tocainide	Antiarrhythmic
Adrenalin	epinephrine	Inotropic
Primacor	milrinone	Inotropic
Dobutrex	dobutamine	Inotropic
Lanoxin	digoxin	Inotropic
Isordil	isosorbide dinitrate	Nitrate

Continued

Cardiovascular Drugs—cont'd

Trade Name	Generic Name	Comments
Imdur	isosorbide mononitrate	Nitrate
Nitrolingual, Nitrostat, Nitro-Bid, etc.	nitroglycerin	Nitrate
Cardura	doxazosin	α_1-Adrenergic blocker
Minipress	prazosin	α_1-Adrenergic blocker
Hytrin	terazosin	α_1-Adrenergic blocker
Catapres	clonidine	α_2-Agonist
Aldomet	methyldopa	α_2-Agonist
Nitropress	nitroprusside	Vasodilator
Apresoline	hydralazine	Vasodilator
Inderal	propranolol	β-Adrenergic blocker
Toprol-XL	metoprolol	β-Adrenergic blocker
Coreg	carvedilol	β-Adrenergic blocker
Tenormin	atenolol	β-Adrenergic blocker
Visken	pindolol	β-Adrenergic blocker
Capoten	captopril	Angiotensin-converting enzyme (ACE) inhibitor
Vasotec	enalapril	ACE inhibitor
Avapro	irbesartan	ACE receptor blocker
Diovan	valsartan	ACE receptor blocker
Atacand	candesartan	ACE receptor blocker
Procardia	nifedipine	Calcium blocker
Calan, Isoptin	verapamil	Calcium blocker
Cardizem	diltiazem	Calcium blocker
Norvasc	amlodipine	Calcium blocker

Hematological Drugs

Trade Name	Generic Name	Comments
Heparin	heparin	Anticoagulant
Coumadin	warfarin	Anticoagulant
Fragmin	dalteparin	Anticoagulant
Lovenox	enoxaparin	Anticoagulant
Integrilin	eptifibatide	Platelet inhibitor
Ticlid	ticlopidine	Platelet inhibitor
Aggrastat	tirofiban	Platelet inhibitor
Plavix	clopidogrel	Platelet inhibitor
ReoPro	abciximab	Platelet inhibitor
Activase	alteplase	Thrombolytic
Streptase	streptokinase	Thrombolytic
Retavase	reteplase	Thrombolytic
Abbokinase	urokinase	Thrombolytic

Hypolipidemic Drugs

Trade Name	Generic Name	Comments
Questran	cholestyramine resin	Bile acid–binding resin
WelChol	colesevelam	Bile acid–binding resin
Lopid	gemfibrozil	Fibric acid derivative
TriCor	fenofibrate	Bile acid–binding resin
Lipitor	atorvastatin	3-Hydroxy-3-methylglutaryl coenzyme A (HMG CoA) reductase inhibitor
Mevacor	lovastatin	HMG CoA reductase inhibitor
Zocor	simvastatin	HMG CoA reductase inhibitor

Pulmonary Drugs

Trade Name	Generic Name	Comments
Proventil, Ventolin	albuterol	Bronchodilator
Serevent	salmeterol	Bronchodilator
Foradil	formoterol	Bronchodilator
Brethaire	terbutaline	Bronchodilator
Theo-Dur	theophylline	Asthma controller
Tilade	nedocromil	Asthma controller
Gastrocrom	cromolyn	Asthma controller
Singulair	montelukast	Asthma controller
Zyflo	zileuton	Asthma controller
Atrovent	ipratropium	Anticholinergic for chronic obstructive pulmonary disease (COPD)
Zyrtec	cetirizine	Antihistamine
Clarinex	desloratadine	Antihistamine
Benadryl	diphenhydramine	Antihistamine
Tavist	fumarate	Antihistamine
Claritin	loratadine	Antihistamine
Beclovent	beclomethasone dipropionate	Corticosteroid
Pulmicort	budesonide	Corticosteroid
AeroBid	flunisolide	Corticosteroid
Flovent	fluticasone propionate	Corticosteroid
Azmacort	triamcinolone acetonide	Corticosteroid
Advair	salmeterol and fluticasone	Combination product
Combivent	albuterol and ipratropium	Combination product

Drugs for Gastrointestinal Disturbances

Trade Name	Generic Name	Comments
Tagamet	cimetidine	H_2 blocker
Pepcid	famotidine	H_2 blocker
Axid	nizatidine	H_2 blocker
Zantac	ranitidine	H_2 blocker
Nexium	esomeprazole	Proton pump inhibitor
Prevacid	lansoprazole	Proton pump inhibitor
Prilosec	omeprazole	Proton pump inhibitor
Protonix	pantoprazole	Proton pump inhibitor
Aciphex	rabeprazole	Proton pump inhibitor

Opioids

Trade Name	Generic Name
Alfenta	alfentanil
Stadol	butorphanol
Actiq, Sublimaze	fentanyl
Vicodin	hydrocodone and acetaminophen
Dilaudid	hydromorphone
Demerol	meperidine
MS-Contin	morphine
OxyContin	oxycodone
Percocet	oxycodone and acetaminophen
Percodan	oxycodone and aspirin
Sufenta	sufentanil
Ultram	tramadol
Darvon	propoxyphene
Dolophine	methadone

Nonsteroidal Antiinflammatory Drugs (NSAIDs)

Trade Name	Generic Name	Comments
Voltaren	diclofenac	Nonselective
Advil, Motrin	ibuprofen	Nonselective
Indocin	indomethacin	Nonselective
Toradol	ketorolac	Nonselective
Aleve, Naprosyn	naproxen	Nonselective
Clinoril	sulindac	Nonselective
Celebrex	celecoxib	Cyclooxygenase 2 (COX-2) inhibitor
Vioxx	rofecoxib	COX-2 inhibitor
Bextra	valdecoxib	COX-2 inhibitor

Drugs for Rheumatoid Arthritis

Trade Name	Generic Name	Comments
Ridaura	auranofin	Gold compound
Solganal	aurothioglucose	Gold compound
Imuran	azathioprine	Immunosuppressant agent
Enbrel	etanercept	Tumor necrosis factor α, TNF-α inhibitor
Plaquenil	hydroxychloroquine	Antimalarial
Remicade	infliximab	TNF-α inhibitor
Arava	leflunomide	Immunosuppressant agent
Rheumatrex	methotrexate	Antimetabolite
Cuprimine	penicillamine	T-cell inhibitor
Azulfidine	sulfasalazine	T-cell inhibitor

Systemic Glucocorticoids

Trade Name	Generic Name	Comments
Cortef, Hydrocortone	hydrocortisone	Short duration
Medrol	methylprednisolone	Intermediate
Orasone, Meticorten	prednisone	Intermediate
Aristocort	triamcinolone	Intermediate
Decadron, Hexadrol	dexamethasone	Long duration

Drugs for Diabetes

Trade Name	Generic Name	Comments
Diabinese	chlorpropamide	Sulfonylurea (1st generation)
Orinase	tolbutamide	Sulfonylurea (1st generation)
Glucotrol	glipizide	Sulfonylurea (2nd generation)
Glynase, DiaBeta	glyburide	Sulfonylurea (2nd generation)
Prandin	repaglinide	Sulfonylurea (2nd generation)
Starlix	nateglinide	Meglitinide
Actos	pioglitazone	thiazolidinedione
Avandia	rosiglitazone	thiazolidinedione
Precose	acarbose	α-Glucosidase inhibitor
Glyset	miglitol	α-Glucosidase inhibitor
Glucophage	metformin	Bioguanide
Humalog	lispro	Onset 0.25 hr
Novolog	aspart	Onset 0.25 hr
Humulin-R, Novolin-R	regular insulin	Onset 0.5 hr
Humulin N, Novolin N	NPH	Onset 1-1.5 hr
Lantus	glargine	Onset 6-14 hr
Humulin U	ultralente	Onset 6-14 hr

Drugs for Osteoporosis

Trade Name	Generic Name	Comments
Fosamax	alendronate	Bisphosphonate
Aredia	pamidronate	Bisphosphonate
Actonel	risedronate	Bisphosphonate
Didronel	etidronate	Bisphosphonate

Drugs for Anxiety

Trade Name	Generic Name	Comments
Xanax	alprazolam	Short-acting anxiolytic
Ativan	lorazepam	Short-acting anxiolytic
Librium	chlordiazepoxide	Longer-acting anxiolytic
Valium	diazepam	Longer-acting anxiolytic
Versed	midazolam	Short-acting hypnotic
Halcion	triazolam	Short-acting hypnotic
Ambien	zolpidem	Short-acting hypnotic
Restoril	temazepam	Short-acting hypnotic
Dalmane	flurazepam	Long-acting hypnotic

Drugs for Depression

Trade Name	Generic Name	Comments
Prozac	fluoxetine	Selective serotonin reuptake inhibitor (SSRI)
Paxil	paroxetine	SSRI
Zoloft	sertraline	SSRI
Elavil	amitriptyline	Tricyclic
Norpramin	desipramine	Tricyclic
Tofranil	imipramine	Tricyclic
Remeron	mirtazapine	Noradrenergic and specific serotonergic antidepressant
Effexor	venlafaxine	Serotonin and norepinephrine reuptake inhibitor
Wellbutrin	bupropion	Atypical antidepressant
Desyrel	trazodone	Atypical antidepressant

Drugs for Psychosis

Trade Name	Generic Name	Comments
Mellaril	thioridazine	Typical antipsychotic agent
Thorazine	chlorpromazine	Typical antipsychotic agent
Prolixin	fluphenazine	Typical antipsychotic agent
Haldol	haloperidol	Typical antipsychotic
Navane	thiothixene	Typical antipsychotic
Clozaril	clozapine	Atypical antipsychotic
Zyprexa	olanzapine	Atypical antipsychotic
Seroquel	quetiapine	Atypical antipsychotic
Risperdal	risperidone	Atypical antipsychotic
Lithane, Lithobid, Eskalith	lithium	Mood stabilizer

Drugs for Neurological Disorders (Anticonvulsants)

Trade Name	Generic Name	Comments
Tegretol	carbamazepine	Miscellaneous anticonvulsant
Klonopin	clonazepam	Misc. anticonvulsant
Zonegran	zonisamide	Misc. anticonvulsant
Neurontin	gabapentin	Misc. anticonvulsant
Lamictal	lamotrigine	Misc. anticonvulsant
Topamax	topiramate	Misc. anticonvulsant
Depakene	valproic acid	Misc. anticonvulsant
Barbita, Luminal	phenobarbital	Barbiturate
Dilantin	phenytoin	Hydantoin
Zarontin	ethosuximide	Succinimide

Drugs for Neurological Disorders (Alzheimer's Disease)

Trade Name	Generic Name	Comments
Aricept	donepezil	Cholinergic agent
Reminyl	galantamine	Cholinergic agent
Exelon	rivastigmine	Cholinergic agent

Drugs for Neurological Disorders (Parkinson's Disease)

Trade Name	Generic Name	Comments
Parlodel	bromocriptine	Dopamine agonist
Permax	pergolide	Dopamine agonist
Mirapex	pramipexole	Dopamine agonist
Requip	ropinirole	Dopamine agonist
Eldepryl	selegiline	Monoamine oxidase B inhibitor
Sinemet	carbidopa and levodopa	L-dopa
Cogentin	benztropine	Anticholinergic
Artane	trihexyphenidyl	Anticholinergic
Symmetrel	Amantadine	Antiviral agent
Tasmar	Tolcapone	Catechol-O-methyltransferase inhibitor

Drugs for Neurological Disorders (Multiple Sclerosis)

Trade Name	Generic Name
Avonex	Interferon-β-1a
Betaseron	Interferon-β-1b
Copaxone	Glatiramer
Novantrone	Mitoxantrone

Drugs for Musculoskeletal Relaxation

Trade Name	Generic Name
Lioresal	baclofen
Valium	diazepam
Zanaflex	tizanidine
Soma	carisoprodol
Flexeril	cyclobenzaprine
Robaxin	methocarbamol
Dantrium	dantrolene

Antimicrobial Agents

Trade Name	Generic Name	Comments
Primaxin	imipenem	Carbapenem
Duricef	cefadroxil	Cephalosporin (1st generation)
Ancef	cefazolin	Cephalosporin (1st generation)
Ceclor	cefaclor	Cephalosporin (2nd generation)
Cefotan	cefotetan	Cephalosporin (2nd generation)
Rocephin	ceftriaxone	Cephalosporin (3rd generation)
Azactam	aztreonam	Monobactam
Procaine	penicillin G	Penicillin
Pen Vee K	penicillin V	Penicillin
Tegopen	cloxacillin	Antistaphylococcal
Unipen	nafcillin	Antistaphylococcal
Bactocill	oxacillin	Antistaphylococcal
Ampicillin	ampicillin	Aminopenicillin
Amoxil	amoxicillin	Aminopenicillin
Pipracil	piperacillin	Antipseudomonal
Ticar	ticarcillin	Antipseudomonal
Augmentin	amoxicillin and clavulanate	Penicillin and β-lactam I
Unasyn	ampicillin and sulbactam	Penicillin and β-lactam I

Continued

Antimicrobial Agents—cont'd

Trade Name	Generic Name	Comments
Vancocin	vancomycin	Glycopeptide
Zithromax	azithromycin	Macrolide
Biaxin	clarithromycin	Macrolide
E-Mycin	erythromycin	Macrolide
Cipro	ciprofloxacin	Fluoroquinolone
Levaquin	levofloxacin	Fluoroquinolone
Vibramycin	doxycycline	Tetracycline
Tetracap	tetracycline	Tetracycline
Proloprim	trimethoprim	Sulfonamide
Synercid	quinupristin and dalfopristin	Streptogramin
Flagyl	metronidazole	Nitroimidazole
Garamycin	gentamicin	Aminoglycoside
Zyvox	linezolid	Oxazolidinone
Lamprene	clofazimine	Antimycobacterial
Myambutol	ethambutol	Antimycobacterial
INH, Laniazid	isoniazid	Antimycobacterial
Pyrazinamide	pyrazinamide	Antimycobacterial
Mycobutin	rifabutin	Antimycobacterial
Rimactane	rifampin	Antimycobacterial

Antifungal Agents

Trade Name	Generic Name	Comments
Diflucan	fluconazole	Systemic agent
Sporanox	itraconazole	Systemic agent
Nizoral	ketoconazole	Systemic agent
Lamisil	terbinafine	Systemic agent
Mycostatin	nystatin	Topical
Gyne-Lotrimin	clotrimazole	Topical

Antiviral Agents

Trade Name	Generic Name	Comments
Zovirax	acyclovir	Chain terminator
Valtrex	valacyclovir	Chain terminator
Vistide	cidofovir	Chain terminator
Famvir	famciclovir	Chain terminator
Denavir	penciclovir	Chain terminator
Foscavir	foscarnet	Chain terminator
Cytovene	ganciclovir	Chain terminator
Valcyte	valganciclovir	Chain terminator
Relenza	zanamivir	Neuraminidase inhibitor
Tamiflu	oseltamivir	Neuraminidase inhibitor
Flumadine	rimantadine	Viral uncoating inhibitor
Symmetrel	amantadine	Viral uncoating inhibitor

Drugs for HIV Disease

Trade Name	Generic Name	Comments
Ziagen	abacavir	Nucleotide reverse transcriptase inhibitor (NRTI)
Videx	didanosine	NRTI
Epivir	lamivudine	NRTI
Zerit	stavudine	NRTI
Hivid	zalcitabine	NRTI
Retrovir	zidovudine	NRTI
Combivir	zidovudine and lamivudine	NRTI
Trizivir	zidovudine, lamivudine, and abacavir	NRTI
Rescriptor	delavirdine	Nonnucleoside reverse transcriptase inhibitor (NNRTI)
Sustiva	efavirenz	NNRTI
Viramune	nevirapine	NNRTI
Agenerase	amprenavir	Protease inhibitor (PI)
Crixivan	indinavir	PI
Kaletra	lopinavir and ritonavir	PI
Viracept	nelfinavir mesylate	PI
Norvir	ritonavir	PI
Fortovase	saquinavir	PI
Invirase	saquinavir mesylate	PI

Chemotherapy Agents

Trade Name	Generic Name	Comments
Hexalen	altretamine	Alkylating agent
Busulfex	busulfan	Alkylating agent
Leukeran	chlorambucil	Alkylating agent
Platinol	cisplatin	Alkylating agent
Cytoxan	cyclophosphamide	Alkylating agent
Ifex	ifosfamide	Alkylating agent
Gliadel	carmustine	Alkylating agent
Cytosar-U	cytarabine	Antimetabolite
Gemzar	gemcitabine	Antimetabolite
Mexate	methotrexate	Antimetabolite
Purinethol	mercaptopurine	Purine analog
Proleukin	aldesleukin (interleukin 2)	Cytokine
Pegasys	peginterferon-alfa-2a	Cytokine
Intron A	interferon alfa-2b	Cytokine
Cerubidine	daunorubicin	DNA intercalating drug
Adriamycin	doxorubicin	DNA intercalating drug
Cosmegen	dactinomycin	DNA intercalating drug
Eulexin	flutamide	Antiandrogen
Nilandron	nilutamide	Antiandrogen
Cytadren	aminoglutethimide	Aromatase inhibitor
Arimidex	anastrozole	Aromatase inhibitor
Femara	letrozole	Aromatase inhibitor
Aromasin	exemestane	Aromatase inhibitor
Zoladex	goserelin acetate	Gonadotropin-releasing hormone
Lupron	leuprolide acetate	Gonadotropin-releasing hormone

Continued

Chemotherapy Agents—cont'd

Trade Name	Generic Name	Comments
Nolvadex	tamoxifen	Antiestrogen
Taxotere	docetaxel	Mitotic inhibitor
VePesid	etoposide	Mitotic inhibitor
Taxol	paclitaxel	Mitotic inhibitor
Velban	vinblastine	Mitotic inhibitor
Oncovin	vincristine	Mitotic inhibitor
Rituxan	rituximab	Monoclonal antibody
Herceptin	trastuzumab	Monoclonal antibody

Immunosuppressants

Trade Name	Generic Name
Imuran	azathioprine
Sandimmune	cyclosporine
Orthoclone OKT3	muromonab-CD3
Prograf	tacrolimus
Rapamune	sirolimus
Simulect	basiliximab

Index ❧

Note to reader: In the page references the use of t indicates tables, f indicates figures, and b indicates boxes.